Peri-operative Anesthetic Management in Liver Transplantation

Vijay Vohra • Nikunj Gupta
Annu Sarin Jolly • Seema Bhalotra
Editors

Peri-operative Anesthetic Management in Liver Transplantation

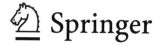

Springer

Editors
Vijay Vohra
Liver Transplant, GI Anesthesia
& Intensive Care
Medanta The Medicity
Gurgaon, India

Nikunj Gupta
Liver Transplant, GI Anesthesia
& Critical Care
Medanta The Medicity
Gurgaon, Haryana, India

Annu Sarin Jolly
Liver Transplant & General Anaesthesia
Narayana Superspeciality Hospital
Gurgaon, India

Seema Bhalotra
Liver Transplant, GI Anesthesia
& Critical Care
Formerly at Medanta The Medicity
Gurgaon, India

ISBN 978-981-19-6047-5   ISBN 978-981-19-6045-1   (eBook)
https://doi.org/10.1007/978-981-19-6045-1

This Springer imprint is published by the registered company Springer Nature Singapore Pte Ltd.
The registered company address is: 152 Beach Road, #21-01/04 Gateway East, Singapore
189721, Singapore

Preface

Liver transplantation is relatively a new specialty with first successful transplant being performed in the year 1967 by Thomas Starzl, and in India it was performed in 1998. The journey of transplantation in India has been very lucidly described in the chapter on history of liver transplantation in this book by Prof Samiran Nundy. Over the last 15–20 years, liver transplantation has gained momentum in the Asian subcontinent. If there were ten established centers in India doing liver transplantation in the year 2000, now there are over 135 centers doing liver transplantation and more centers are coming up. There are many textbooks available on the subject, but very few resources are available dealing with the perioperative care of patients with end-stage liver disease needing liver transplant. The surgical aspects are widely covered in these books with scant reference to the anesthetic and perioperative care of these patients. It was felt that there was a need to have a book which provided information on this aspect of patient care in patients with end-stage liver disease. There is another motivational reason to take on this assignment to get this book published. Our group under the leadership of Dr AS Soin were among the firsts to start liver transplants in India, initially at Sir Ganga Ram Hospital and then at Medanta Hospital, Gurgaon. On starting the training program of Fellowship in Liver Transplant Anaesthesia at Medanta from the year 2012, we felt at a loss to provide the fellows enough reading material or a textbook on the subject. Although in this era of Internet there is information available at the touch of a button, it is all scattered. Our fellows were provided with a collection of good articles to make a beginning. There was always something missing—a book to refer to, which had most of the basic information for perioperative care of liver transplant patients. Therefore our team of editors got together and decided to embark on this journey of getting this book together. The authors were identified who had good experience in this growing specialty. Of course everything was not straightforward and many authors had to be substituted for various reasons.

So the aim was to have a collection—book, which covers the perioperative care of liver transplant patients which would be useful for trainees as well as for practicing anesthesiologists, intensivists, and those responsible for the perioperative care of transplant patients. There is slightly more attention given towards living donation liver transplantation in the book as this is the dominant part of liver transplant program in India as of now.

In India, most of the transplantation activity is confined to living donor liver transplantation, whereas the deceased donor transplant is still not practiced very frequently due to lack of availability of organs. Looking at the figures for the year 2020, there were around 16.3% deceased donors (GODT— Global Observatory on Donation and Transplantation), the rest being living donor transplant. This is one area that needs to be looked at critically— improving deceased organ donation. I must express my sincere gratitude to Prof Samiran Nundy who has been motivating us in this venture and has been in constant touch regarding the progress of the book. He is the one who was also instrumental in bringing the Human Organ Transplant Act (1994) in India, initiating and giving impetus to the liver transplant activity.

Gurgaon, India   Vijay Vohra
Gurgaon, India   Nikunj Gupta
Gurgaon, India   Annu Sarin Jolly
Gurgaon, India   Seema Bhalotra

Contents

About the Editors

Vijay Vohra is Chairman, liver transplant, GI anesthesia, and intensive care at Medanta The Medicity, Gurgaon, India. He has 37 years' experience in anesthesiology after qualification. He headed the team that established liver transplant anesthesia and critical care at two major centers in India (SGRH and Medanta). He has 5 years' experience as Vice-Chairperson in policy making and running a large department of 40 anesthetists. Dr Vohra has imparted training in transplant anesthesia to visiting/fellow anesthetists and intensivists from 26 centers within India and abroad in the last 10 years. He has an experience of nearly 3000 liver transplants—among the highest anywhere. Dr Vohra is first in India to develop and introduce hemodynamic and coagulation monitoring protocol for bloodless liver transplant. He headed the anesthesia team that participated in almost all the firsts in liver transplantation in India. He has been a DNB teacher for 17 years. Dr Vohra has special expertise in anesthesia in liver transplant, kidney transplant, GI surgery, and vascular surgery. He is regularly invited as faculty to national and international conferences.

Nikunj Gupta is a Diplomate in National Board (DNB) qualified anesthesiologist and has an experience of over 20 years in the specialty. He has been involved in the care of liver transplant patients for nearly 18 years. For the last 12 years, he been practicing perioperative care of liver transplant patients at Medanta The Medicity, Gurgaon, India. He has been involved in the training of fellows admitted for liver transplant anesthesia at Medanta The Medicity.

Annu Sarin Jolly has over 20 years of experience as a consultant anesthesiologist in leading multispecialty hospitals of Delhi, India. Her area of interest is liver transplantation. She trained at the best centers of Delhi like Apollo, Sir Ganga Ram Hospital, and Medanta and had the privilege of working with pioneers in the field like Dr Soin and Dr Vijay Vohra, who have been her mentors. Currently, she is the clinical lead anesthesia at Narayana Health and conducts liver transplant anesthesia across its pan-India branches. She is also involved with pediatric transplants in NH SRCC Children's Hospital, Mumbai.Dr Annu has authored several national and international papers and contributed to a textbook on laparoscopic anesthesia before this. She has been actively involved in organizing seminars and teaching liver transplant fellows. She is also a DNB teacher and has several presentations to her credit.

Seema Bhalotra is a senior consultant, anesthesia and critical care medicine. Have practiced anesthesia in leading multispecialty hospitals like Ganga Ram hospital, New Delhi, and Medanta, The Medicity, Gurugram. Have a keen interest in liver transplant and gastrointestinal surgeries. Practiced liver transplant anesthesia for 8 years in a leading liver transplant center of India. Have been associated with teaching and training of DNB anesthesia and fellowship in liver transplant students. Have multiple national and international poster presentations and have contributed to chapters in anesthesia-related books.

The History of Liver Transplantation in India

1

Samiran Nundy

1.1 Introduction

In 1988 starting a liver transplantation programme in India seemed to be a distant dream for many of us because there were so many hurdles to overcome—it was an exorbitantly costly procedure, there was no local expertise available at that time, the trade in human organs especially kidneys was widespread and the law only recognised cardiorespiratory death and not brain death so that transplants from beating heart donors could not be done. However with a consistent and combined effort we were able to overcome most of these problems gradually and, although some still remain, we have reached a stage where there are now 135 centres in this country which have been registered to carry out liver transplants and, till May 2019, 16,806 procedures had been performed with the results in some centres matching the world's best. And India does the fourth largest number of liver transplants internationally following the USA, China and Korea.

In this chapter I will chronicle our journey from how it all started to where it has reached and although it is, of necessity, a rather personal account, I wish to pay tribute to many of the generally unnamed doctors, journalists, bureaucrats and politicians who helped bring about this momentous change.

1.2 Background

In 1988 there were an estimated 120 centres elsewhere in the world performing 4500 liver transplants annually with an 80% success and 70% five-year survival rates. In stark contrast, there was no liver transplant facility in India and there were an estimated 300,000 deaths from liver failure annually. A small group of us made an initial attempt to sensitise the public to this problem through popular television programmes like 'The World this Week' as well as articles in newspapers and medical journals. But probably the main impetus was provided by the then Prime Minister, Shri Rajiv Gandhi who, after one of his trips abroad, asked the Health Minister why heart and liver transplants were not being done in this country. The Health Secretary then constituted a small group of four people to report on this and we defined the problems that had to be overcome, i.e. the cost, the lack of local expertise, the organ trade and the absence of a law which recognised brain death. To move forward we identified the first move should be to educate the public on the benefits of starting a liver transplant programme in India.

S. Nundy (✉)
Department of Surgical Gastroenterology and Liver Transplantation, Sir Ganga Ram Hospital, New Delhi, India

1.3   Step I: Public Education

This was done through a series of newspaper articles and television appearances. Although there were major opponents to starting such a programme—it would cost 20 lakhs, there would be an enormous wastage of blood and blood products (the blood requirement for a single procedure was usually about 20 units at that time; now it is about 4–6 units); it would become the focus of hospital attention and distract from many other activities which benefited many more people. It was likened to having a 'CT scanner on a malarious swamp'!

The counterarguments were that the procedure would save many young productive lives, it would be available locally, the cost would be much lower than it was in western countries, the quality of doctors and hospitals would be upgraded and there would be national pride that such high-end medical care was available in our own country. No longer would our very rich compatriots need to go abroad for transplants where they were placed at the bottom of the waiting lists and often received 'marginal' livers that had been rejected for use in the indigenous population. We held conferences and workshops in Calcutta, Bombay, Madras and Delhi to which we invited prominent social workers, journalists and religious leaders to discuss whether the concepts of brain death and liver transplantation were acceptable and necessary. There was a generally positive response. The next step would be to try and change the existing law defining death and to allow beating heart organ transplantation.

1.4   Step 2: Changing the Law

After the conference in Delhi in 1991 the government appointed a small committee chaired by Dr. L.M. Singhvi, the eminent lawyer, to examine and report on the concept and definition of brain death, its desirability and implications, to suggest safeguards against misuse and how it might facilitate the availability of organs such as the heart and liver for transplantation.

The Singhvi Committee presented its report to the Cabinet and the Bill was placed in 1992 before the Rajya Sabha where it received overwhelming support. However when it went to the Lok Sabha there were serious objections raised to some of its clauses like including only first-degree relatives as living donors and it was referred to a Select Committee for further debate. Two years passed without any progress and we felt that the law would never be passed but in 1994 the Bill was placed before the Lok Sabha again and after a brief debate in a sparsely attended house it was accepted. The Transplantation of Human Organs Act became a law in 1995.

Its rules stated that only registered hospitals would be allowed to perform transplantation and listed the criteria for organ retrieval. Brain death would be determined by clinical tests alone, i.e. the cause of coma should be known, there would be an absence of cranial reflexes and there should be a positive apnoea test. All these would be verified twice by four specially designated doctors 6 h apart.

An 'Appropriate Authority' was also created which would be responsible for the registration of hospitals, maintenance of standards, would investigate breaches of the law and audit the indications and results of the transplant procedures. For living transplants only first-degree relatives would be allowed to donate organs but if the recipient did not have a suitable donor then someone 'emotionally' related would be permitted to donate. The 'emotional' attachment would by verified by a designated 'Authorisation Committee'.

Trading in human organs was made illegal and a non-cognisable offence.

1.5   Step 3: The Initial Procedures

The first procedure after the Bill was passed was a heart transplant done in the All India Institute of Medical Sciences (AIIMS), New Delhi, by Dr. P. Venugopal and was a success. It was announced by the then Prime Minister, Shri Atal Behari

Bajpayi, in Parliament to loud cheers. However liver transplantation took a long time to gain any sort of momentum. There were a few performed, mostly unsuccessfully, in 1995 in the Apollo Hospital, Chennai, and then at AIIMS Delhi. The first successful deceased donor liver transplant was done on a 43-year-old man in the Apollo Hospital, Delhi, on November 6, 1998, by Dr. AS Soin and Dr. MR Rajasekar. This patient lived for 12 years after the transplant. He had recidivism and died of recurrent alcoholic cirrhosis of his transplanted liver. The second successful transplant in India was a live donor (left lateral sector) liver transplant on November 15, 1998, on an 18-month-old male child with biliary atresia. This patient is alive and well.

1.6   Step 4: Sustainable Programmes

1.6.1   Numbers

In spite of the law being passed there were very few deceased donor transplants and the main activity, albeit small in number, was centred around living donors (Fig. 1.1).

There were very few done up to 2008 after which there was a spurt in activity after the year 2009 with a gradually increasing number of deceased donors especially in Tamil Nadu. The main impetus for this increase was the farseeing Tamil Nadu Government orders of 2008 which made brain death declaration mandatory and doc-

tors who were in charge of such patients were required to ask their relatives for organ donation. It also decreed that a State level waiting list be maintained, laid down norms on how the procured deceased organs should be distributed, required that Transplant Coordinators should be appointed in all registered hospitals, provided government subsidies of up to 30 lakhs towards the cost of the procedure, established 'green corridors' so that the harvested donor organs could be moved quickly in spite of heavy traffic to the recipient hospital and supported nongovernmental organisation such as the MOHAN Foundation which has done such sterling work in promoting deceased organ donation throughout the country.

In 2011 there were amendments to the existing law passed by Parliament which mandated a video recording of Authorisation Committee meetings, delinked transplantation registered institutions from those which could diagnose brain death, allowed intensivists and one other doctor to confirm the diagnosis (rather than the four designated doctors, including neurosurgeons, previously), included grandparents and uncles as near relatives and allowed 'swap' donations across family members according to blood group matching. It also established the NOTTO, ROTTO and SOTTO (National, Regional and State Organ and Tissue Transplant Organisations) in addition to the already existing ORBO (Organ Retrieval and Banking Organisation).

Thus Fig. 1.2 shows the rapid increase in liver transplant numbers since 2009 when there were

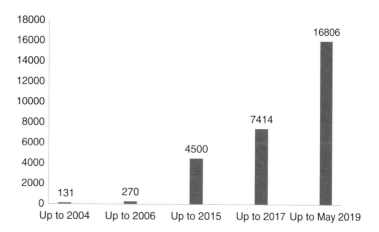

Fig. 1.1 Liver transplantation activity in India up to May 2019

Fig. 1.2 The total transplants performed annually in India between 2009 and 2018 with the numbers and proportions of deceased and living donor procedures

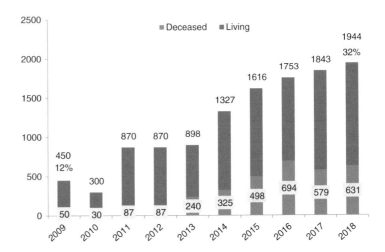

Fig. 1.3 Total liver transplants up to May 2019, Individual Centre Data (>500)

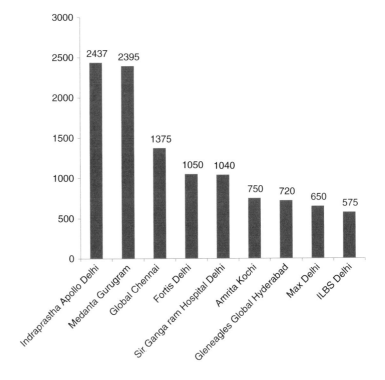

450 done with 12% from deceased donors to 2018 when 1944 were done and 32% were from deceased donors.

However in 2019 after we asked all members of the Liver Transplant Society of India to share their total numbers out of 135 registered centres 40 responded and the individual centre data are provided in Figs. 1.3, 1.4, 1.5, and 1.6.

The activity of hospitals in a single year (2018) is provided in Figs. 1.7, 1.8, and 1.9.

Thus only 4 institutions performed more than 200 in a single year (2018), 11 did 50–100, 30 did 1–50 and 90 others who were registered to perform the operation did not do any liver transplants or did not answer the questionnaire (Fig. 1.10).

When we repeated the same exercise recently in 2020 we only had one reply; perhaps because of the increasing competition or fall in numbers centres are now unwilling to disclose these figures.

Fig. 1.4 Total liver transplants up to May 2019, Individual Centre Data (100–500)

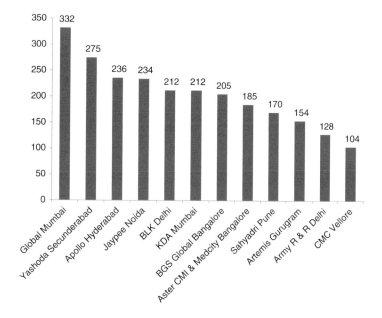

Fig. 1.5 Total liver transplants up to May 2019, Individual Centre Data (<100–30)

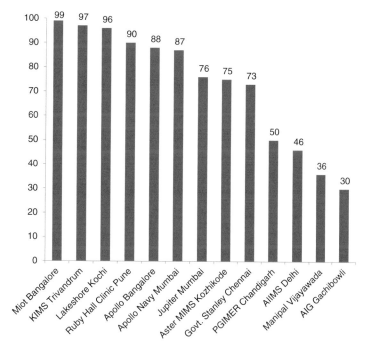

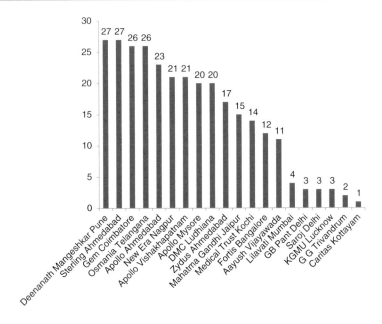

Fig. 1.6 Total liver transplants up to May 2019, Individual Centre Data (<30)

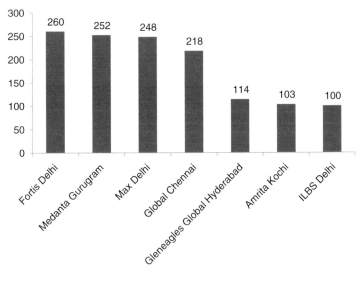

Fig. 1.7 Liver transplants in India in year 2018, Individual Centre Data (>100)

1.6.2 Statewise Distribution

Figure 1.11 shows the distribution of liver transplant centres in India with most in the South, West and North but very few in the Central and Eastern states.

The largest numbers of transplants done in 2018 were in Delhi (1161), which in 2020 has apparently 16 centres, but these were almost all from living donors (Fig. 1.12).

But if the numbers of deceased organ donations are depicted (Fig. 1.13), we will see that most of the activity has been in the Southern and

Fig. 1.8 Liver transplants in India in year 2018, Individual Centre Data (<100–50)

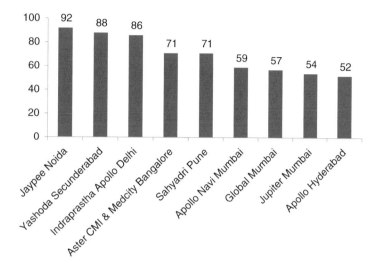

Fig. 1.9 Liver transplants in India in year 2018, Individual Centre Data (>50)

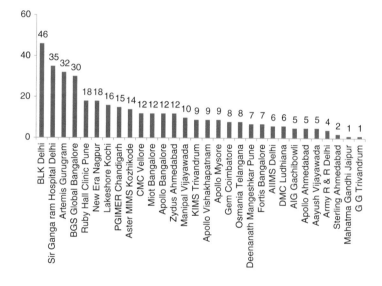

Western states with Tamil Nadu leading the way (Figs. 1.13 and 1.14).

In fact that state has been in the forefront of all deceased organ transplants including the lung, heart, liver and kidney (Fig. 1.15).

1.6.3   The Situation in 2020

The total number of centres registered to perform liver transplants in India is now 135 (compared to a total of 149 in the USA), and this is increasing rapidly as the procedure has become a marker for not only the prestige of a hospital but that of a state. However, it is rumoured that many of the centres although registered have not performed a single transplant or that they have had such bad results that there is little or no continuing activity. Thus the 'star' performing surgeons and their teams are sought after by most large hospital chains by being guaranteed astronomical salaries. Consequently the public sector is now performing only 3% of the transplants not only because it is losing its surgeons to private hospitals but it does not have the committed and dedicated large teams required to collaborate and perform such complex procedures. The cost of a living donor transplant is now anywhere between 16 and 30 lakh rupees.

Fig. 1.10 Overview of
liver transplants in India
in 2018

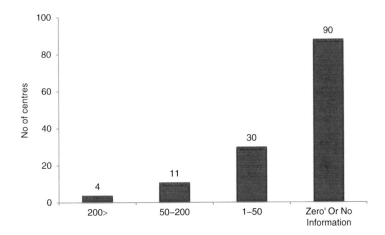

Fig. 1.11 Liver
transplant centres

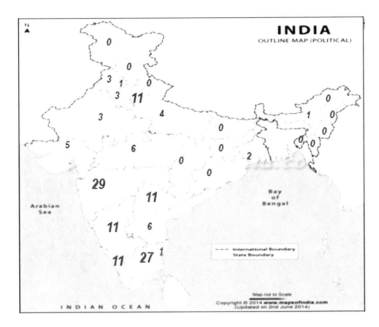

Fig. 1.12 Liver transplant numbers statewise

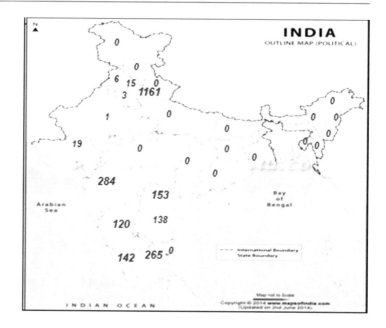

Fig. 1.13 States— deceased donations 2018

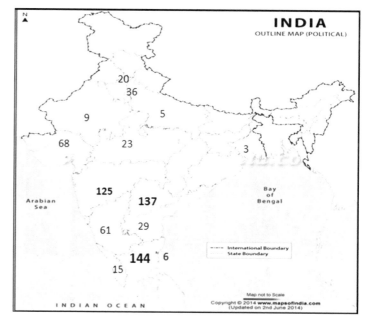

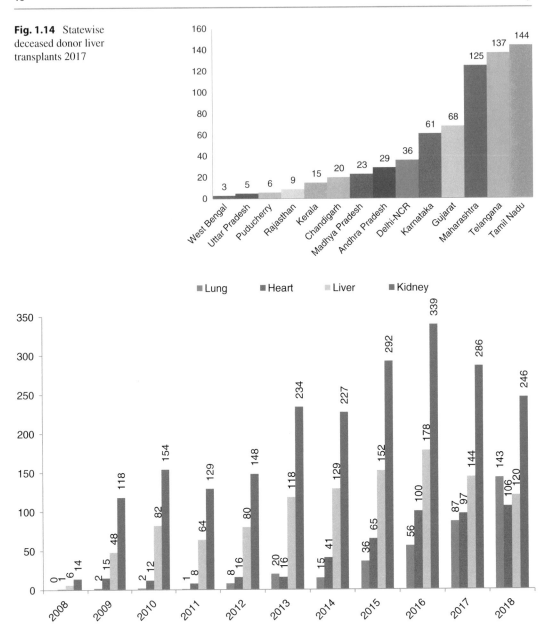

Fig. 1.14 Statewise deceased donor liver transplants 2017

Fig. 1.15 Tamil Nadu deceased organ transplants

1.7   India Vs the World

In 2018 there were a total of 1944 liver transplants performed in India which followed only the USA (8241), China (5149) and Korea (2854). However for the proportions of living donor liver transplants the figures vary considerably from Japan where 87% of transplants were from living donors to 4% and 2% in the USA and UK. In India and South Korea the majority of organs were taken from living donors (68% and 65%). In China although deceased donors are the largest source of organs for transplants most of these are alleged to have been obtained from condemned prisoners. This practice has been decried by the international transplant

Fig. 1.16 Liver transplants in India vs World (2009 and 2018)

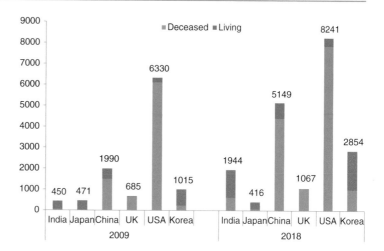

community and is now banned by the Chinese government. Figure 1.16 shows the changes in the numbers of transplants in some selected countries comparing 2009 and 2018.

All have shown increasing numbers except for Japan and what is noteworthy in that is India has probably shown the largest proportional increase of 4.3 times in total with an encouraging rise in the number of deceased donor transplants.

1.8   Concerns

But there are concerns. All the transplant programmes rely mainly on living donors and although deceased donation is increasing in the South and West in the central states, it remains poor in the North and East. This is because of a lack of awareness of the concept of brain death and the benefits of organ transplantation but also perhaps due to an absence of altruism in these areas. Public hospitals have not managed to mount regular programmes and the private sector where profit generation is the main concern this has resulted in large kickbacks to referring physicians, there is immense pressure to increase numbers and many 'marginal' livers which would not be used abroad are transplanted. The system continues to be opaque in that the living donor complications and deaths remain unknown and the results of transplantation are enormously variable ranging from

90-day recipient mortality rates of between 5% and 100%. There is a major gender gap with organ donors being predominantly female and the recipients male. In Tamil Nadu the proportion of females receiving kidney grafts is 23% and livers is 7%. The organ trade continues but it is small and clandestine.

1.9   Recommendations

The first priority should be to improve cadaver donation by strictly enforcing the law especially the 2011 amendments which delinked transplant hospitals from those from which organs could be harvested, enforce mandatory brain death declaration and required request, ensure a transparent and fair organ distribution system and even consider incentives to donor families like free lifetime railway passes. There should be many more centres in the public sector which would lower the cost of the procedure and perhaps improve the gender imbalance.

The dormant Appropriate Authority should collect data on the indications and results of transplantation, help raise public awareness, and encourage the exchange of problems, results and expertise between the private and public sectors. It should also punish unethical practices.

In spite of these problems the results have been gratifying as illustrated in Fig. 1.17.

Fig. 1.17 A three-and-
a-half-year-old Nigerian
girl with a large liver
tumour before and after
liver transplantation
(now well 5 years later)

Gratifying Results

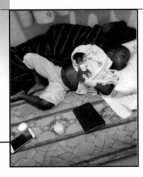
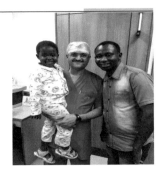

Pre-op   Post-op

1.10 Conclusions

Liver transplantation has had a major impact on
Indian health care. It has saved thousands of lives
of middle-class Indians who could not afford to
have the procedure done abroad, it has improved
the quality of surgery, anaesthesia, haematology,
nephrology, blood transfusion and pathology, the
results of the best centres match the world's best
and although there are attendant problems these
can be solved.

In fact liver transplantation has revolutionised
Indian medicine.

> **Key Points**
> 1. The Transplantation of Human Organs
>   Act of India in 1994 recognised brain
>   death and made the trade in human
>   organs illegal.
> 2. This allowed liver transplants to be per-
>   formed in this country.
> 3. After the first decade when few proce-
>   dures were done the main impetus came
>   in 2008 when the Tamil Nadu govern-
>   ment orders made the declaration of
>   brain death in hospitals mandatory and
>   required doctors to ask relatives for
>   organ donation.

> 4. There are now 135 centres registered to
>   perform liver transplants in 2020.
> 5. Most transplants are done in the private
>   sector and are from living related
>   donors.
> 6. Deceased organ donation occurs in the
>   Southern and Western states but in
>   Delhi, where 54% of the total liver
>   transplants in India are done, the major-
>   ity are from living donors.
> 7. India's total liver transplant numbers
>   rank only after the USA, China and
>   Korea.
> 8. Unfortunately the results regarding
>   indications and operative mortality are
>   opaque and there needs to be closer reg-
>   ulation of the activity throughout the
>   country.
> 9. Liver transplantation has enhanced the
>   quality and reputation of Indian health
>   care.

Acknowledgements I would like to thank Mr. Parmanand
Tiwari for his help in preparing this manuscript.

Part I

Basics Anatomy and Pathophysiology of Liver Disease

Physiological Role of Liver and Interpreting Liver Function Tests

2

Kamal Kajal, Venkata Ganesh, and Sameer Sethi

The purpose of this chapter is to review the anatomy and physiology of the liver as well as provide a brief interpretation of liver function tests. The anaesthetic management of the patient with chronic liver disease requires an in-depth understanding of the altered physiology of the cirrhosis along with pharmacokinetic and pharmacodynamic aspects of therapy. All types of liver surgery can induce transient or permanent injury to the liver, an understanding of which has improved the morbidity and mortality of hepatic transplant recipients and donors over the years.

The importance of the regenerative capacity of the liver cannot be overstressed as this is unique to the liver enabling partial transplants from live donors. This regenerative capacity is well illustrated in the myth of Prometheus [1]. Although potential liver replacement therapies such as Molecular Adsorbent Recirculating System (MARS) are available, these can never take over the extensive functions of this multi-tasking organ. These functions range across metabolic (including detoxification), synthetic, immunologic and homeostatic domains (Table 2.1).

K. Kajal (✉) · V. Ganesh · S. Sethi
Department of Anaesthesia and Intensive care,
Postgraduate Institute of Medical Education and
Research, Chandigarh, India

Table 2.1 Functions of the liver

Metabolic	Synthetic	Immunologic	Homeostatic
Glucose metabolism	Coagulation factor synthesis	Innate immunity	Intravascular homeostasis by acting as a blood reservoir, through renin-angiotensin-aldosterone axis and oncotic pressure regulation via albumin metabolism
Nitrogen metabolism	Procoagulants	Adaptive immunity	Glucose homeostasis
Lipid metabolism	Anticoagulants	Systemic antigen and allograft tolerance	Hepatic and portal blood flow regulation through hepatic arterial buffer response
Heme degradation	Fibrinolytics		
Drug metabolism and detoxification	Antifibrinolytics		
	Plasma protein synthesis		
	Albumin		
	Heme synthesis		
	Endocrine:		
	Steroid hormone synthesis		
	Cholesterol		
	Thrombopoietin		
	Angiotensinogen		
	IGF-1		

2.1   Gross Anatomy of the Liver

The liver derives from the ventral foregut endoderm during the fourth week of gestation [2–4]. Anatomy relevant to anaesthetic and surgical management includes the blood supply and the intrahepatic microscopic architecture.

The afferent blood to the liver is accounted for by both arterial and portal blood. The mean value of O_2-uptake in the liver, related to a blood flow of 110 mL/min/100 g, amounts to 6.08 ± 0.2 mL O_2/min [5]. This comprises 20–25% of the cardiac output. Although in terms of blood flow the portal vein supplies nearly 75% of the hepatic blood and the systemic artery supplies 25%, the oxygen supplied to the liver is equally shared between the two circulations [6]. The biliary tree is however supplied principally by the hepatic artery. The portal blood from the splenic vein brings in the hormones and cytokines from the pancreas whereas the superior mesenteric vein brings in the endotoxins and nutrients from the gut above the lower half of the rectum. In situations of increased portal vein pressure, portosystemic connections open up in areas such as the lower end of oesophagus, rectum, umbilicus, retroper-itoneal regions and bare area of the liver. This manifests as dilated veins/varices, bleeding and the shunting of unfiltered blood can manifest as sepsis and encephalopathy.

The venous outflow of the liver is through the three hepatic veins draining directly into the inferior vena cava (IVC) close to the diaphragm and any change in the intrathoracic and right heart pressures or beyond the hepatic vein (such as thrombosis in Budd-Chiari syndrome) can promote congestive injury to the hepatocytes.

Externally the liver can be seen to have the right and the left lobe divided by the IVC and the gall bladder fossa. However surgically, based on the vascular planar anatomy, the liver can be divided into eight segments [7]. Each segment has an afferent pedicle comprised of branches from the portal vein, hepatic artery and bile duct, and each segment drains into an individual tributary of the hepatic vein. The right lobe of the liver has segments V to VIII while the left lobe has slightly complicated segmental division with the true external left lobe comprising segments II and III and the medial portion of this or quadrate lobe is segment IV. The caudate lobe is named as segment I and independently drains into the central hepatic vein.

2.1.1 Hepatic Blood Flow Regulation

Blood flow to the liver is regulated by several intrinsic and extrinsic factors. These pathways work independently of each other.

Intrinsic Mechanisms

1. HABR (Hepatic arterial buffer response): The periportal tissues produce adenosine, the washout rate of which when decreased, as occurs during decreased portal blood flow, dilates the hepatic artery to preserve hepatic blood flow [8, 9]. The reverse also occurs when portal blood flow increases, increasing the washout of adenosine and constricting the hepatic artery. Endotoxemia and splanchnic vasoconstriction can abolish this response [6].
2. Metabolic control: Decrease in the oxygen content or pH of the portal venous blood can increase the hepatic arterial blood flow; post-prandial hyperosmolarity can also increase hepatic artery and portal venous flow.
3. Myogenic autoregulation: Vascular smooth muscle stretch during hypertensive episodes promotes vasoconstriction and decreased hepatic arterial flow protecting the liver from the hypertensive episode. The reverse also occurs with vasodilation of the hepatic artery during systemic hypotension. Inhaled volatile anaesthetic agents cause a dose responsive inhibition of this response.

Extrinsic Regulation

1. Neural control: Parasympathetic and sympathetic nerves that course along with the hepatic blood vessels help in regulating the vascular tone. During sympathoadrenal stimulation the blood volume within the hepatic and splanchnic circulation is squeezed into the systemic circulation. The hepatic artery has alpha 1,2 and beta 2 receptors while the portal vein has only alpha receptors [6].
2. Humoral control: Glucagon causes hepatic artery vasodilation whereas angiotensin II causes vasoconstriction of hepatic and portal venous circulation. Interestingly vasopressin raises splanchnic arterial resistance but

reduces the portal venous pressures and hence may be preferred in those with portal hypertension.

2.2 Cellular Anatomy of the Liver

The liver is composed of two groups of cells. The majority are parenchymal cells or hepatocytes which are responsible for the metabolic and most of the synthetic functions of the liver. The non-parenchymal cells are chiefly responsible in the liver acting as the immunological gateway especially for the enteric organisms. These include the Kupffer cells, Natural Killer (NK) cells, dendritic cells, T lymphocytes and B lymphocytes as well as the cholangiocytes, the sinusoidal endothelial cells and perisinusoidal pluripotent stellate or Ito cells. Table 2.2 summarizes the functions of these cells.

Table 2.2 Types of cells and their functions in the liver [10, 11]

	Function	Percentage of liver cells
Hepatocytes	• Hepatic regeneration	60–80
	• Detoxification	
	• Protein synthesis and metabolism	
	• Lipid oxidation	
	• Glucose metabolism	
	• Glycogen storage	
Perisinusoidal Ito cells	• Vitamin A and fat storage	5–15
	• Collagen secretion and contractile nature implicates these cells in liver cirrhosis and portal hypertension respectively	
	• Antigen-presenting cells	
Endothelial cells	• Exchange of substrates through fenestrations	15–20
	• Nitric oxide-mediated vascular tone regulation	
	• Antigen-presenting cells	

(continued)

Table 2.2 (continued)

	Function	Percentage of liver cells
Kupffer cells	• Antigen-presenting cells (macrophages) • Downregulate T cell activation in immune tolerance states • Produce nitric oxide, TNF alpha and other cytokines responsible for ischaemia reperfusion injury	15
Dendritic cells	• Antigen-presenting cells	<1
Lymphocytes NK cells	• Non-specific targeting of tumour cells and viruses	5–10
T cells	• Cell mediated adaptive immunity and immune memory	
B cells	• Antibody/humoral mediated adaptive immunity and immune memory	
Cholangiocytes	• Comprise the bile ducts	<1

2.2.1　Models of Liver Microanatomy

There are two prevalent models of liver microanatomy. In the lobular model, the terminal hepatic vein (central vein) is at the centre of a hexagonal "lobule" of hepatocytes while the subunits of the portal triad are at the periphery. These units are of individual metabolic capacity representing the fundamental unit of the liver.

In the acinar model, the hepatocytes are grouped in an approximately oval mass with the ends of the long diameter being the central veins of adjacent lobules and the short diameter being defined between two portal triad. This represents the functional microvascular unit of the liver and is based on the blood flow pattern to the hepatocyte. Each acinus is divided into three ill-defined zones, zone 1 being the richly oxygenated periportal, zone 2 intermediate and zone 3 closer to the central veins (Fig. 2.1).

Zone 1 being oxygen rich takes care of the aerobic glucose metabolism and is most resistant to ischaemic stressors. It is also responsible for fatty acid metabolism and urea cycle for ammo-

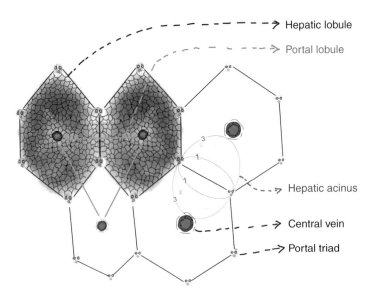

Fig. 2.1 Schematic representation of the microanatomy of the liver showing the hepatic lobule with the portal triads forming the borders of this hexagonal unit with the central vein at the centre of the mass of hepatocytes. The portal lobule is a triangular unit formed by joining three central veins with a portal triad at the centre. The hepatic acinus is a perfusion-based model with the hepatocytes distributed in three oval zones around the short axis of the oval being formed by joining two portal triads and the long axis being bounded by two central veins

nia metabolism. Zone 3 is perivenous and is most susceptible to hypoxia and ischaemia being involved in ketogenesis and drug detoxification. The functions of zone 2 overlap with the other two zones [12–14].

2.3 Liver, the Immunological Gateway

2.3.1 Innate and Adaptive Immunity

The non-parenchymal cells of the liver take part in the immune regulatory function, and both forms of immunity are closely linked within the liver. The hepatic circulation, unlike the systemic circulation, has more of the non-specific innate immune cells, as the major immune function of the liver is to regulate the massive antigen load from the enteric circulation before it reaches the systemic circulation. Hence it acts like an immunological gatekeeper for the body.

The non-specific innate immunity is mediated by the antigen-presenting cells (APC) as well as the NK cells. The APC form a bridge to the T and B lymphocytes that mediate adaptive immunity. These APC include Kupffer cells, dendritic cells, sinusoidal endothelial cells and Ito cells. The NK cells non-specifically target all foreign cells that do not contain self-major histocompatibility surface complex I (MHC-I) such as tumour cells and viruses [15]. These cells directly destroy their targets by secreting perforins that make the target's membrane more permeable and granzymes that lyse the cells internally. Decreased NK cell function has been associated with increased tumour burden [16].

The adaptive immune system is classically comprised of the cell-mediated and antibody-mediated acquired form of immunity which helps in mounting antigen-specific immune response with immunological memory. This memory response serves in quick processing of the antigens that enter the liver from the splanchnic and portal circulation. CD8 T cells can recognize tumour antigens and can help fight against hepatocellular carcinoma as well [17].

2.3.2 Immune Tolerance

Although early cases of transplantation were done exclusively in twins and in closely related individuals, it is a well-known fact that pigs, mice and rats accept unrelated liver transplants without immunosuppressants and even some human recipients are capable of weaning off immunosuppressive therapy [18]. There is also no immune response to the massive load of commensal bacteria in the gastrointestinal tract. This is because the liver manages to balance between acting as an immunological gateway and tolerating the commensal organisms whose antigens have been presented to the liver constitutionally over a prolonged period of time. This function of the liver is termed systemic or oral tolerance and a similar adaptation of the immune system is probably what is responsible for allograft tolerance and transplant success rates [19].

This "tolerogenicity" is thought to be mediated by the constitutive expression of antigens (for example the lipopolysaccharide or LPS of enteric organisms) on the antigen-presenting cells such as the Kupffer cells which tends to downregulate the activity of other antigen-presenting cells over time via TNF alpha and interleukin 10 [20]. This in turn decreases T cell activation [10]. Similar mechanisms underly allograft survival.

2.4 Hepatic Drug Metabolism

Most higher organisms are exposed to a lot of foreign chemical compounds in the environment. Evolution has provided pathways to transmute such xenobiotics to ensure their elimination, onset of action (prodrugs) or termination of effect by altering their susceptibility to excretion.

2.4.1 First Pass Effect

The first pass effect can be defined as the rapid uptake and metabolism of an agent into inactive compounds before it reaches systemic circulation. This phase of drug metabolism greatly reduces the bioavailability of enteral drugs. First pass effect occurs majorly in the liver but also to a certain extent in the GIT including the gastric secretions as well as intestinal mucosal enzymes. Parenterally administered drugs bypass the liver, have no first pass metabolism, reach their effect sites faster and hence are clinically more effective at lower doses with faster onset times.

2.4.2 Phases of Drug Metabolism

Phase I reactions involve oxidation, reduction or hydrolysis or a combination of these to make the drugs more polar by inserting or unmasking a hydroxyl, sulf-hydroxyl or amide groups in the chemical structure of a drug. These metabolites are then either excreted or undergo further phases of metabolism.

Phase II metabolism is where the by-products of phase I are attached to a glucuronate, glutathione, acetate or sulphate group to make them more water soluble and are then excreted via the bile and blood.

Absence or dysfunction of phase I or II enzymes results in encephalopathy, hyperbilirubinemia and drug toxicity. These phase I and II enzymes are chiefly located in zone III of the hepatic acinus and their dysfunction is hence most prone to occur in the state of ischaemic and oxidative stress. They chiefly belong to the cytochrome P-450 (CYP450) family. Gene mutations can affect metabolism and results in specific syndromes such as Crigler-Najjar and the milder Gilbert syndromes which result from mutations leading to a defective or decreased levels of bilirubin-UGT, presenting as unconjugated hyperbilirubinemia or kernicterus. Depletion of substrates of conjugation such as glutathione can lead to liver injury as is the case with paracetamol toxicity where NAPQI (*N*-acetyl-para-benzoquinone-imine) accumulates in zone II causing centrilobular necrosis. Being a precursor to glutathione *N*-Acetyl Cysteine (NAC) can be useful in treating acetaminophen toxicity. Its use as an organ protective agent is at best controversial [21].

Phase 0 and Phase III metabolism are misnomers and are merely carrier-mediated transport modes involved in the uptake and elimination via SLC transporters and ATP binding cassette (ABC) carriers in the basolateral and canalicular membranes respectively [22, 23].

These CYP450 enzyme systems are inducible as well as susceptible to inhibition by various substrates. Inducing these enzymes speeds up the metabolism of drugs decreasing their bioavailability rendering them clinically ineffective. For example barbiturates can induce the metabolism of phenytoin, steroids and warfarin. Conversely enzyme inhibitors such as azoles, amiodarone, SSRIs and omeprazole can dangerously elevate levels of warfarin and increase the risk of bleeding.

2.4.3 Drug Extraction Ratio

Since the quantity of hepatic enzymes as well as the hepatic blood flow can vary in various conditions, logically the rate of drug elimination should also fluctuate depending on these parameters. The drug extraction ratio is that between the intrinsic hepatic clearance of a drug and the hepatic blood flow. This ratio attempts to measure the efficiency of the liver in eliminating a given drug. Table 2.3 provides a summary of this concept [24].

Table 2.3 Hepatic extraction ratio with examples

Extraction ratio (ER)	Type of hepatic elimination	Saturable metabolism	Examples
High ER	Flow dependent	Non-saturable enzymes	Lignocaine, Mepivacaine, Morphine, Pethidine, Verapamil, Labetalol, Metoprolol, Propranolol
Low ER	Capacity dependant	Saturable (dose-dependent, non-linear, zero-order elimination)	Paracetamol, Aspirin, Diazepam, Digoxin, Ethanol, Phenobarbital, Phenytoin, Valproic acid, Warfarin

2.5 Energy Metabolism

2.5.1 Glucose Homeostasis

The liver is the seat of glucose metabolism and determines the fate of glucose whether it becomes glycogen for storage or it enters the Kreb's cycle and electron transport chain for ATP synthesis. The liver is also capable of producing glucose from glycogen (glycogenolysis) as well as from other sources such as amino acids, glycerol, pyruvate and lactate which is gluconeogenesis. Fasting induces these processes mediated by the hormones such as glucagon and epinephrine. This chiefly occurs in zone I of the acinus.

Glycogenesis is stimulated by insulin and takes place in non-fasted state especially in zone III of the hepatic acinus. As we can see, since precise regulation of glucose homeostasis occurs chiefly in the liver, the most apparent manifestation in acute terminal liver failure tends to be hypoglycaemia. Glycogen storage disorders such as Gaucher's manifest with recurrent hypoglycaemia, ketosis and hepatomegaly apart from musculoskeletal symptoms [25, 26].

2.5.2 Nitrogen Metabolism

In the presence of amino acid excess the liver engages in the urea cycle to produce ammonia and alpha-keto acids especially so in the zone I of the hepatic acinus. Glutamine synthetase then transforms ammonia and glutamate to glutamine. Hyperammonaemia resulting from liver dysfunction and portosystemic shunting produces encephalopathy as the neurotoxic ammonia and excessive glutamate, which is an excitatory neurotransmitter, elevate the intracranial pressure by increasing the osmotic intracellular gradient [27]. An alternate theory suggests that glutamine acts as a "Trojan horse" carrying the ammonia into the mitochondria of astrocytes causing free radical damage and cellular oedema [28]. Hence the predominant type of cerebral oedema that occurs in hepatic failure is cytotoxic as the blood brain barrier is mostly intact, rendering vasogenic oedema less likely preserving the response to osmotherapy with mannitol and hypertonic saline [29, 30].

The liver is also the site of major protein synthesis excepting gamma-globulin, especially albumin which is majorly responsible for the intravascular oncotic pressure as well as drug-protein binding. Catabolic states tend to reduce albumin and thus can lead to oedematous states which is characteristic of liver failure as well as in critical illness.

2.5.3 Fatty Acid Metabolism

The liver is responsible for both degradation and the de novo synthesis of fatty acids. Bile salt emulsified dietary fat is absorbed as micelles into the liver and the fatty acids undergo beta oxidation to yield ATP or these are converted to ketone bodies in insulin-deficient states and starvation. When there is defective insulin-mediated inhibition of lipolysis, as in obesity, the liver tends to store fat and this leads to steatosis and non-alcoholic fatty liver disease (NAFLD) [31, 32]. This may then progress to non-alcoholic steatohepatitis (NASH) and finally to cirrhosis and hepatic failure [33].

2.6 Role of the Liver in Coagulation

The liver is the major site for the synthesis of procoagulants, anticoagulants, fibrinolytics and antifibrinolytics as well as the stimulation of megakaryocyte production via the release of thrombopoietin [34]. The balance between procoagulants and anticoagulants in hepatic dysfunction determines bleeding or thrombosis. Routine markers of coagulation such as prothrombin time (PT) and partial thromboplastin time (PTT) are not accurate as they do not measure the anticoagulant profile of the patient. Hence functional tests of coagulation such as Thromboelastography and Sonoclot may be used to determine the risk of bleeding or thrombosis.

The liver synthesizes factors I, II, V, VII to XIII and the anticoagulants anti-thrombin III,

protein C and S; fibrinolytics such as plasminogen and antifibrinolytics alpha 2-antiplasmin
and TAFI (thrombin activable fibrinolysis
inhibitor) [35].

Extrahepatic factors that can worsen bleeding
include thrombocytopenia, portal hypertension,
sepsis and disseminated intravascular coagulation [36, 37].

2.7 Hepatic Endocrine Function

The liver is responsible for the production of 75%
of the total IGF-1 apart from thrombopoietin,
angiotensinogen and cholesterol which is
involved in steroid hormone synthesis. Growth
hormone stimulates the release of IGF-1 which
promotes tissue growth in times of puberty and
exercise. Thrombopoietin stimulates megakaryocyte and platelet production which explains why
platelet counts improve after orthotopic liver
transplantation [38]. Angiotensinogen, which
gets converted to angiotensin, that further partici-
pates in the renin-angiotensin-aldosterone pathway is also produced by the liver and is the
primary target of ACE inhibitors and angiotensin
receptor blockers (ARBs). The diuretic spironolactone is used to manage ascites in liver disease
by antagonizing the pathway's endpoint
aldosterone.

2.8 Chronic Liver Disease

Chronic liver disease is characterized by persistent injury to the liver for more than 6 months
after initial insult. Various causes are infections,
vascular, toxic, genetic and inflammatory aetiologies. The persistent episodes of injuries induce a
healing process that subsequently results in
hepatic fibrosis. Cirrhosis is a last stage fibrosis
of liver characterized by distorted liver architecture that results in increased intrahepatic resistance and subsequent development of portal
hypertension. Chronic liver diseases can induce

cellular death via apoptosis, necrosis or more
often a combination of the two, termed necrapoptosis or necroptosis [39, 40]. In chronic liver disease, the liver is subjected to repetitive tissue
damage resulting in alterations in regenerative
capacity, inflammatory response and eventually
fibrosis [41].

2.9 Interpreting Liver Function Tests

The term "Liver Function Tests" is commonly
used but it is potentially confusing since many
of the tests are not reflective of its function and
also, they may be abnormal even in patients
without liver disease. Nonetheless, these tests
are only initial tools for screening as well as
stratification of liver disease. Liver is an organ
that carries out numerous functions and measuring its function by a single or battery of tests
may not provide its entire assessment in different clinical scenarios. So, it becomes imperative
to classify these laboratory tests into broad categories. These categories include tests that (1)
*detect injury to hepatocytes or bile ducts, (2)
measure the liver's capacity to transport organic
anions and clear endogenous or exogenous substances from circulation, (3) measure the liver's
capacity to metabolize drugs, (4) measure
hepatic synthetic function and (5) contribute to
an accurate diagnosis of liver disease but do not
necessarily assess liver function.* Our aim is to
provide precise information about the utility of
these tests in routine clinical anaesthesia and
critical care.

2.10 Tests Detecting Hepatocyte Injury

2.10.1 Serum Aminotransferases

One of the sensitive indicators of hepatocyte
injury is a group of intracellular enzymes called

serum aminotransferases. These are alanine aminotransferase (ALT, serum glutamic-pyruvic transaminase [SGPT]) and aspartate aminotransferase (AST, serum glutamic-oxaloacetic transaminase [SGOT]). Their function is to catalyse the transfer of the alpha-amino groups of alanine and aspartate, respectively, to the alpha-keto group of ketoglutarate that results in the formation of pyruvate and oxaloacetate. ALT is situated entirely in cytosol, whereas AST is found in 80:20 ratio in mitochondria and cytosol of hepatocyte respectively. AST is not limited to liver only and has presence in other tissues like heart, skeletal muscles, kidney, brain, pancreas, lungs, leucocytes and erythrocytes. Therefore, AST levels are also elevated in cardiac and skeletal muscle diseases. Normal levels of AST and ALT are less than 30 IU/L for men and 20 IU/L for women, respectively. Levels decline in frail older patients and consumption of coffee [42]. Causes of elevated serum AST and ALT levels are shown in Table 2.4. Magnitude of serum aminotransferases elevation does not correlate with liver cell necrosis; in addition, the absolute elevation in serum aminotransferases is of little prognostic value since the liver can recover from majority of acute insults. Recovery of liver disease is often accompanied by faster decline in serum AST and ALT levels, but it may reflect poor prognosis due to massive loss of viable cells in acute liver failure. Rapid decline from initial elevation along

Table 2.4 Causes of elevated AST And ALT

	Causes
Mild elevations (less than 3 times the upper normal limit) or (100–249 IU/L)	Alcoholic steatohepatitis, NASH, drug hepatotoxicity, and chronic hepatitis C
Moderate elevations (3- to 20-fold of the upper normal limit) or (250–999 IU/L)	Drug hepatotoxicity, autoimmune hepatitis (AIH), acute and chronic viral hepatitis
Large elevations (more than 20-fold of the upper normal limit) or (>2000 IU/L).	Paracetamol poisoning, ischaemic hepatitis, acute viral hepatitis, massive hepatic necrosis

NASH non-alcoholic steatohepatitis

with rise in the plasma bilirubin concentration and prolongation of the prothrombin time indicates a poor prognosis in patients with acute liver failure.

2.10.2 AST to ALT Ratio

AST to ALT ratio is also useful in the diagnosis of certain hepatic diseases. For example, an AST-to-ALT ratio more than 4 is characteristic of Wilson disease, ratios between 2 and 4 are suggestive of alcoholic liver disease, and a ratio below 1 is suggestive of non-alcoholic steatohepatitis (NASH) [43]. In a study of 271 patients with biopsy-proven liver disease, almost 90% of the patients with AST to ALT ratio greater than or equal to 2 had alcoholic liver disease [44].

2.10.3 Lactate Dehydrogenase

There are other enzymes that can be measured but none is more specific and useful as aminotransferases for detecting hepatic disease. These are lactate dehydrogenase (LDH), glutamate dehydrogenase and isocitrate dehydrogenase. LDH is a cytoplasmic enzyme present in almost all tissues. It has five isoenzymes identified on electrophoresis. It has poor sensitivity and specificity compared with aminotransferases. In one study, profound elevation of LDH discriminates ischaemic hepatitis (ALT-to-LDH ratio less than 1.5) from viral hepatitis (ALT-to-LDH ratio greater than or equal to 1.5) with a sensitivity and specificity of 94% and 84%, respectively [45].

Glutathione-S-Transferase Glutathione-S-transferase (GST) is a sensitive and specific test for drug-induced liver injury. It has a short plasma half-life (90 min) and is released expeditiously in circulation following hepatocellular injury. GST is located in centrilobular region of acinus and is highly susceptible to hypoxia or reactive drug metabolites [46]. Therefore, serial measurements of GST may be a sensitive marker of centrilobular necrosis in its incipient stages.

Clinical significance The extent of liver cell necrosis correlates poorly with the magnitude of serum aminotransferase elevation; in addition, the absolute elevation in serum aminotransferases is of little prognostic value since the liver can recover from most forms of acute injury. There is, however, one pattern that is important to recognize: a rapid decrease in plasma AST and ALT levels, together with a rise in the plasma bilirubin concentration and prolongation of the prothrombin time, is indicative of a poor prognosis in patients with acute liver failure. Although a rapid decrease in serum aminotransferases is usually a sign of recovery from disease, it may also reflect the massive destruction of viable hepatocytes in patients with acute liver failure, signalling a poor prognosis.

2.11 Tests Detecting Injury to Bile Ducts

2.11.1 Alkaline Phosphatase

Alkaline phosphatase (ALK) is predominantly located in liver and bones. They are also found in other sites like intestine and placenta. Enhanced levels are usually due to hepatic and diseases related to bones. Cholestatic disorders induce the break in the lipid linkage that binds ALK to the canalicular surface lining the inner membrane of hepatocytes. In early stages of cholestatic pathologies, levels of ALK may be near normal and increase gradually as disease progresses. Elevation in serum alkaline phosphatase in hepatobiliary disease results from increased synthesis in the liver followed by release into the circulation The precise manner how it reaches circulation remains unclear. Causes of elevated alkaline phosphatase are shown in Table 2.5.

Table 2.5 Causes of elevated alkaline phosphatase

Marked elevation (≥4 times the upper limit of normal)	*Extrahepatic causes*	*Hepatic causes*
	Choledocholithiasis (most common)	Primary sclerosing cholangitis
	Malignant obstruction like pancreas, gallbladder, bile duct	Intrahepatic cholestasis of pregnancy
	Biliary strictures following invasive procedures and anastomotic stricture following liver transplantation	Primary biliary cholangitis
		Liver allograft rejection
Moderate elevation (<4 times upper limit normal)	*Liver-specific causes*	*Other causes*
	Hepatitis: viral, chronic, alcoholic	Pregnancy
	Cirrhosis	Physiologic (children)
	Hypoperfusion states: sepsis, heart failure	Disorders of bone
		Paget disease of bone
		Osteomalacia
		Hyperparathyroidism
		Hyperthyroidism

2.12 5′-Nucleotidase

5′-Nucleotidase is located in multiple sites like liver, heart, brain, blood vessels and pancreas. Its physiological function is not clear and is thought to catalyse hydrolysis of nucleotides such as adenosine 5′ phosphate and inosine 5′-phosphate. Along with serum alkaline phosphatase, its major valuable role is in establishing the diagnosis of obstructive biliary disease [47].

2.13 Gamma-Glutamyl Transferase

Gamma-glutamyl transferase (GGT) helps in catalysing the transfer of groups like gamma glutamyl peptides such as glutathione to L amino acids. It is located in canaliculi region and is released when cholestasis ensues. Higher levels of GGT along with alkaline phosphatase and 5′-nucleotidase corroborate the diagnosis of hepatobiliary disease. Drugs that induce the production of microsomal enzymes like ethanol, phenytoin and verapamil also promote the production of GGT [48]. Isolated elevations in GGT are due to extrahepatic causes.

2.14 Tests Assessing Biliary Organic Anion Transport

2.14.1 Serum Bilirubin

Bilirubin is produced from the catabolism of heme. It gives bile its characteristic colour and yellowish discoloration in patients with jaundice. Majority of bilirubin is produced from the destruction of old red blood cells in the reticuloendothelial system. Bilirubin is transferred into hepatocytes and conjugated with glucuronic acid to water-soluble bilirubin monoglucuronides and diglucuronides. Conjugation is catalysed by the enzyme uridine diphosphate glycosyltransferase (UGT). Unconjugated bilirubin is found in normal serum only. On the other hand, increased levels of conjugated bilirubin point towards liver injury. Albumin binds covalently with conjugated

Table 2.6 Causes of elevated bilirubin levels

Unconjugated hyperbilirubinemia	Conjugated hyperbilirubinemia
Gilbert syndrome	Bile duct obstruction
Haemolysis	Hepatitis
Blood transfusion	Cirrhosis
Crigler-Najjar syndrome	Primary biliary cholangitis
Ineffective erythropoiesis	Primary sclerosing cholangitis
Medications	Others
	Sepsis
	Total parenteral nutrition
	Postoperative jaundice
	Dubin-Johnson syndrome
	Rotor syndrome

bilirubin and thereby prolongs its half-life. Laboratory tests measure the direct reacting bilirubin and the total bilirubin. Difference between the two gives value of indirect bilirubin. Normal levels of total bilirubin are below 1 mg/dL. Up to 10% of adults have higher levels of unconjugated bilirubin due to Gilbert syndrome. Jaundice is found on physical examination when serum bilirubin levels are above 4 mg/dL. It is important to describe hyperbilirubinemias on the basis of direct or indirect bilirubin levels. Causes of hyperbilirubinemia are shown in Table 2.6. *Sepsis is often not accounted as a cause for jaundice, but its reported prevalence in 30% of ICU patients in one series with mortality as high as 51%* [49].

2.15 Tests Measure Hepatic Synthetic Capacity

2.15.1 Serum Proteins

Majority of serum proteins are produced by the liver (exception being immunoglobulins). Albumin is most widely used to determine the synthetic capacity of liver and is included in Child-Pugh scoring system for cirrhosis. Low albumin levels are usually a result of hepatic disease besides other factors. Albumin levels are an important predictor of prognosis in critically ill hospitalized patients [50]. The underlying processes include increased catabolism of albumin, increased capillary permeability to proteins and decreased albumin synthesis.

2.16 Prothrombin Time and International Normalized Ratio

Prothrombin time reflects the levels and function of clotting factors I, II, V, VII, X. All these factors are produced by the liver, and their reduced levels signify liver dysfunction. International normalized ration (INR) is reported along with prothrombin time. INR was introduced to standardize laboratory results for patients on warfarin. Patients with liver disease showed greater differences in their results, and now further attempts have been made to develop an INR specific to the liver [51]. Other potential cause of deranged prothrombin time and INR is vitamin K deficiency that can be either due to malabsorption or cholestatic disease.

2.17 Tests Measuring Blood Flow and Metabolic Capacity of Liver

They are also included as quantitative liver function tests. These tests are used as in the research tools as they are expensive and need a lot of time and efforts. Also, there is no convincing evidence of their superiority over standard liver function tests. Techniques for estimating hepatocellular mass include agents that are cleared avidly by the liver like bromsulphalein and indocyanine green (ICG). Mostly, they are crude computations as clearance of substance often influenced by many known and unknown factors. There are three methods to estimate blood flow to the liver: Clearance methods, indicator dilution method and direct measurements. Clearance methods are based on indirect Fick principle using agents with high hepatic and total body clearance. These include ICG dye, propranolol and lidocaine. ICG dye is the most consistent and reliable among them. The basic technique is that after injecting a

particular substance, the area under curve is obtained and computed for measuring liver blood flow assuming normal reticuloendothelial system. Direct measurements are obtained using electromagnetic probes through hepatic artery and portal vein.

On the other hand liver capacity to metabolize drugs can be measured by several methods, such as caffeine clearance, galactose elimination capacity, aminopyrine breath test and monoethyl-glycinexylidide (MEGX) [52]. Non-invasive methods are available for measuring caffeine clearance for which an oral dose of caffeine (150–300 mg) is administered to patients and subsequently its metabolites are measured in saliva for up to 24 h. One of the invasive methods currently gaining popularity for measuring liver blood flow is MEGX test especially in patients with critical illness. Patient is administered lidocaine (1 mg/kg) intravenously, and blood sample is retrieved after 15 min for MEGX, a metabolite of lidocaine.

2.18 Pattern of Liver Test Abnormalities

Evaluation of a patient presented with abnormal liver function tests starts with thorough history and physical examination to introspect for clues to the aetiology. Abnormalities in liver function tests provide information regarding the underlying cause of patient liver disease. Injury to hepatocytes presents with elevated aminotransferases and injury or obstruction to bile ducts represents cholestasis. In addition, the magnitude of derangement in liver function may help us in finding the causative factors. Apart from above, the ratio of the aspartate aminotransferase (AST) to alanine aminotransferase (ALT) may make few diagnoses more or less likely. The specificity of ALT as a marker of hepatic injury is more than AST.

Abnormalities in liver function tests can be grouped into one of these patterns: hepatocellular, cholestatic or isolated hyperbilirubinemia (Table 2.7). These abnormalities may manifest as acute (within weeks), subacute (6 weeks to 6 months) and chronic (more than 6 months).

Table 2.7 Pattern of liver test abnormalities

	Hepatocellular pattern	Cholestatic pattern
Serum transaminases		
AST and ALT	↑↑↑	↑
ALP	↑	↑↑↑
Serum bilirubin	↑ or ↔	Elevated
Synthetic function	May be abnormal	May be abnormal
Causes	Viral, toxic hepatitis, cirrhosis	

Most often, the aetiologies may present as mixed patterns in which there is escalation of both serum aminotransferases and alkaline phosphatases. Abnormalities of mixed origins can be characterized by the predominant abnormality; however it may not be possible to find this division. The magnitude of elevations of aminotransferases on few occasions differentiates between hepatocellular and cholestatic processes. Higher values of these enzymes usually indicate hepatocellular origin of disease. Synthetic function tests namely serum albumin and prothrombin time may be abnormal in both hepatocellular and cholestatic diseases. Normal albumin levels disfavour chronic aetiologies and signify acute processes like viral hepatitis or bile duct disease. Prolongation in prothrombin time indicates vitamin K deficiency due to malabsorption or significant hepatocellular dysfunction. No improvement in prothrombin time with parenteral vitamin K administration suggests severe hepatocellular injury.

Acute hepatitis is a serious insult to the liver that occurs in a short span of time. Majority of affected patients have complete recovery with only few patients progress to the extent that acute liver failure develops. Minority of patients may progress to chronic hepatic disease depending upon the cause. Most frequent causes of acute hepatitis include drug-induced liver injury (DILI), ischaemic hepatitis and alcoholic hepatitis, reliably diagnosed by elevated levels of aminotransferases.

Ischaemic liver injury occurs in patients with profound shock of any aetiology [53]. It is usually accompanied with striking elevations in

AST, ALT and INR. These enzymatic alterations often develop abruptly and rapidly return to normal on restoration of adequate perfusion. DILI is often difficult to diagnose and mostly it is the diagnosis of exclusion based on history of drugs intake. It is associated with elevations of AST, ALT and ALK and manifests after starting a medication. Majority of cases are an idiosyncratic reaction to drugs. Numerous drugs are associated with DILI but antibiotics are the common culprits.

Other major but rare cause of acute liver failure is acetaminophen toxicity. Patients usually presented with marked elevations of serum aminotransferases and INR but mild elevations in bilirubin. Levels of acetaminophen are needed to determine its exposure either accidental or intentional.

Acute viral hepatitis serologies are usually indicated for patients with acute hepatitis. Test panel includes: hepatitis B surface antigen (HBsAg), IgM anti-hepatitis B core antigen (anti-HBc), antibody to HBsAg, IgM anti-hepatitis A virus, anti-hepatitis C virus antibody (HCV), hepatitis C viral RNA and IgM anti-hepatitis E virus; in few cases, other non-specific viral illness based on patient history and risk factors like CMV antigen, anti-CMV antibodies, CMV antigen, and, for Epstein-Barr virus, heterophile antibody.

Ruling out autoimmune causes by evaluating for autoimmune markers (antinuclear antibodies, anti-smooth muscle antibodies, anti-liver/kidney microsomal antibodies type 1, IgG) is mandatory for unexplained jaundice. USG abdomen with doppler is also done routinely to look for any clue of a vascular occlusion (e.g. Budd-Chiari syndrome).

Supplementary tests like serum ceruloplasmin level and urinary copper quantitation should be done in patients suspected of Wilson disease. If the above testing is negative, sometimes a liver biopsy is needed if there is no decline in serum aminotransferases or if the patient progresses to acute liver failure.

Acute bile duct obstruction may manifest with clinical picture mimicking acute hepatitis. AST and ALT are often raised with near normal or slightly increased ALT in initial 1–2 days. Subsequently as disease progresses, typical gradual elevations in ALK occurs along with decline in AST and ALT. Imaging studies further substantiate the diagnosis and also help in discerning the cause of obstruction. Chronic cholestasis on the other hand if not associated with jaundice is benign to liver function. It is often recognized by the persistent elevations in ALT and GGT. Common causes of suspected chronic cholestasis are primary biliary cirrhosis and primary sclerosing cholangitis.

Chronic hepatitis does not pose major concern in anaesthesia during early stages. Mild impairment in metabolism of drugs may be the only concern [54]. There is usually mild increases in ALT with near normal AST. The majority of cases are due to HBV or HCV, or to non-alcoholic fatty liver disease. In late stages, major concern is progression to cirrhosis. It is estimated that up to 50% of patients infected with chronic HCV develop cirrhosis after 20–30 years [55].

2.19   Monitoring Liver Transplant

Orthotopic liver transplantation is the treatment of choice for patients with end-stage liver disease. There is typically a rapid improvement in liver function tests with normalization of bilirubin, INR, AST and ALT levels. Subsequently, about half of the patients may develop acute cellular rejection, often within the first several weeks after the procedure. The earliest manifestations of rejection are rising liver-associated enzymes, particularly GGT and ALK [56]. The escalation of ALK reflects likely injury to the bile ducts, that is a histologic feature of acute rejection. Increases in bilirubin, AST and ALT often occur late, but their rise correlates highly with the severity of rejection. Multiple factors contribute to the graft damage in the perioperative period. These are starting from graft procurement (cold and warm ischaemia), vascular injuries and most commonly bile duct injuries [57]. Because of multiple factors contributing to liver rejection, relying on laboratory tests is questionable. Liver biopsy is therefore sometimes required for recipients with unexplained abnormalities in liver-related tests.

References

1. Ankoma-Sey V. Hepatic regeneration—revisiting the myth of prometheus. Physiology. 1999;14(4):149–55.
2. Lemaigre FP. Mechanisms of liver development: concepts for understanding liver disorders and design of novel therapies. Gastroenterology. 2009;137(1):62–79.
3. Kaestner KH. The making of the liver: competence in the foregut endoderm and induction of liver-specific genes. Cell Cycle. 2005;4(9):1146–8.
4. Collardeau-Frachon S, Scoazec J-Y. Vascular development and differentiation during human liver organogenesis. Anat Rec. 2008;291(6):614–27.
5. Lutz J, Henrich H, Bauereisen E. Oxygen supply and uptake in the liver and the intestine. Pflugers Arch. 1975;360(1):7–15.
6. Mushlin PS, Gelman S. Miller's anesthesia. In: Miller RD, editor. Miller's anaesthesia. Hepatic physiology and pathophysiology. 8th ed. Philadelphia, PA: Elsevier Saunders; 2015. p. 525–6.
7. Bismuth H. Surgical anatomy and anatomical surgery of the liver. World J Surg. 1982;6(1):3–9.
8. Eipel C, Abshagen K, Vollmar B. Regulation of hepatic blood flow: the hepatic arterial buffer response revisited. World J Gastroenterol. 2010;16(48):6046–57.
9. Lautt WW. The 1995 Ciba-Geigy award lecture. Intrinsic regulation of hepatic blood flow. Can J Physiol Pharmacol. 1996;74(3):223–33.
10. Racanelli V, Rehermann B. The liver as an immunological organ. Hepatology. 2006;43(S1):S54–62.
11. Reynaert H, Thompson MG, Thomas T, Geerts A. Hepatic stellate cells: role in microcirculation and pathophysiology of portal hypertension. Gut. 2002;50(4):571–81.
12. Tortora GJ, Derrickson BH. Principles of anatomy and physiology. New York, NY: John Wiley & Sons; 2008, 946 p. Accessed 8 Jun 2019.
13. Gebhardt R. Metabolic zonation of the liver: regulation and implications for liver function. Pharmacol Ther. 1992;53(3):275–354.
14. Katz NR. Metabolic heterogeneity of hepatocytes across the liver acinus. J Nutr. 1992;122(Suppl 3):843–9.
15. Hepatic zonation of carbohydrate metabolism. Nutr Rev. 1989;47(7):219–21.
16. Gao B, Jeong W-I, Tian Z. Liver: an organ with predominant innate immunity. Hepatology. 2008;47(2):729–36.
17. Yoon JC, Yang CM, Song Y, Lee JM. Natural killer cells in hepatitis C: current progress. World J Gastroenterol. 2016;22(4):1449–60.
18. Shuai Z, Leung MW, He X, Zhang W, Yang G, Leung PS, et al. Adaptive immunity in the liver. Cell Mol Immunol. 2016;13(3):354–68.

19. Lau AH, Thomson AW. Dendritic cells and immune regulation in the liver. Gut. 2003;52(2):307–14.
20. Crispe IN. The liver as a lymphoid organ. Annu Rev Immunol. 2009;27:147–63.
21. Crispe IN, Giannandrea M, Klein I, John B, Sampson B, Wuensch S. Cellular and molecular mechanisms of liver tolerance. Immunol Rev. 2006;213:101–18.
22. Hilmi IA, Peng Z, Planinsic RM, Damian D, Dai F, Tyurina YY, et al. N-acetylcysteine does not prevent hepatorenal ischaemia-reperfusion injury in patients undergoing orthotopic liver transplantation. Nephrol Dial Transplant. 2010;25(7):2328–33.
23. Hediger MA, Clémençon B, Burrier RE, Bruford EA. The ABCs of membrane transporters in health and disease (SLC series): introduction. Mol Asp Med. 2013;34(2–3):95–107.
24. Ishikawa T. The ATP-dependent glutathione S-conjugate export pump. Trends Biochem Sci. 1992;17(11):463–8.
25. Mushlin PS, Gelman S. Miller's anesthesia. In: Miller RD, editor. Miller's anaesthesia. Hepatic physiology and pathophysiology. 8th ed. Philadelphia, PA: Elsevier Saunders; 2015. p. 531.
26. Bhattacharya K. Investigation and management of the hepatic glycogen storage diseases. Transl Pediatr. 2015;4(3):240–8.
27. Roscher A, Patel J, Hewson S, Nagy L, Feigenbaum A, Kronick J, et al. The natural history of glycogen storage disease types VI and IX: long-term outcome from the largest metabolic center in Canada. Mol Genet Metab. 2014;113(3):171–6.
28. Scott TR, Kronsten VT, Hughes RD, Shawcross DL. Pathophysiology of cerebral oedema in acute liver failure. World J Gastroenterol. 2013;19(48): 9240–55.
29. Albrecht J, Norenberg MD. Glutamine: a Trojan horse in ammonia neurotoxicity. Hepatology. 2006;44(4):788–94.
30. Detry O, De Roover A, Honore P, Meurisse M. Brain edema and intracranial hypertension in fulminant hepatic failure: pathophysiology and management. World J Gastroenterol. 2006;12(46):7405–12.
31. Ranjan P, Mishra AM, Kale R, Saraswat VA, Gupta RK. Cytotoxic edema is responsible for raised intracranial pressure in fulminant hepatic failure: in vivo demonstration using diffusion-weighted MRI in human subjects. Metab Brain Dis. 2005;20(3):181–92.
32. Tessari P, Coracina A, Cosma A, Tiengo A. Hepatic lipid metabolism and non-alcoholic fatty liver disease. Nutr Metab Cardiovasc Dis. 2009;19(4):291–302.
33. Alberti KGMM, Zimmet P, Shaw J, IDF Epidemiology Task Force Consensus Group. The metabolic syndrome--a new worldwide definition. Lancet. 2005;366(9491):1059–62.
34. Sheth SG, Gordon FD, Chopra S. Nonalcoholic steatohepatitis. Ann Intern Med. 1997;126(2):137–45.
35. Amitrano L, Guardascione MA, Brancaccio V, Balzano A. Coagulation disorders in liver disease. Semin Liver Dis. 2002;22(1):83–96.
36. Tripodi A. The coagulopathy of chronic liver disease: is there a causal relationship with bleeding? No. Eur J Intern Med. 2010;21(2):65–9.
37. Basili S, Raparelli V, Violi F. The coagulopathy of chronic liver disease: is there a causal relationship with bleeding? Yes. Eur J Intern Med. 2010;21(2):62–4.
38. Peck-Radosavljevic M, Wichlas M, Zacherl J, Stiegler G, Stohlawetz P, Fuchsjäger M, et al. Thrombopoietin induces rapid resolution of thrombocytopenia after orthotopic liver transplantation through increased platelet production. Blood. 2000;95(3):795–801.
39. Malhi H, Gores GJ. Mechanisms of liver injury. In: Schiff ER, Maddrey WC, Sorrell MF, editors. Schiff's diseases of the liver. 11th ed. Chichester: John Wiley and Sons; 2012. p. 216–31.
40. Lemasters JJ. V. Necrapoptosis and the mitochondrial permeability transition: shared pathways to necrosis and apoptosis. Am J Phys. 1999;276(1 Pt 1):G1–6.
41. Trautwein C, et al. Hepatic fibrosis: concept to treatment. J Hepatol. 2015;62(1Suppl):S15–24.
42. Ruhl CE, Everhart JE. Coffee and caffeine consumption reduce the risk of elevated serum alanine aminotransferase activity in the United States. Gastroenterology. 2005;128(1):24–32.
43. Davern TJ, Scharschmidt BF. Biochemical liver tests. In: Feldman M, Friedman LS, Sleisenger MH, editors. Sleisenger & Fordtran's gastrointestinal and liver disease pathophysiology, diagnosis, management. 7th ed. St. Louis, MO: Saunders; 2002. p. 1227.
44. Cohen JA, Kaplan MM. The SGOT/SGPT ratio--an indicator of alcoholic liver disease. Dig Dis Sci. 1979;24(11):835–8.
45. Cassidy WM, Reynolds TB. Serum lactic dehydrogenase in the differential diagnosis of acute hepatocellular injury. J Clin Gastroenterol. 1994;19(2):118–21.
46. Redick JA, Jakoby WB, Baron J. Immunohistochemical localization of glutathione S-transferases in livers of untreated rats. J Biol Chem. 1982;257:15200.
47. Pratt DS, Kaplan MM. Evaluation of abnormal liver-enzyme results in asymptomatic patients. N Engl J Med. 2000;342(17):1266–71.
48. Whitehead M, Hainsworth I, Kingham J. The causes of obvious jaundice in South West Wales: perceptions versus reality. Gut. 2001;48:409–13.
49. Vincent J, Dubois M, Navickis R, Wilkes M. Hypoalbuminemia in acute illness: is there a rationale for intervention? A meta-analysis of cohort studies and controlled trials. Ann Surg. 2003;237: 319–34.
50. Tripodi A, Chantarangkul V, Primignani M, Fabris F, Dell'era A, Sei C, et al. The international normalized ratio calibrated for cirrhosis (INR (liver)) normalizes prothrombin time results for model for end-stage liver disease calculation. Hepatology. 2007;46:520–7.
51. Jover R, Carnicer F, Sanchez-Paya J, et al. Salivary caffeine clearance predicts survival in patients with liver cirrhosis. Am J Gastroenterol. 1997;92:1905.
52. Schnegg M, Lauterburg BH. Quantitative liver function in the elderly assessed by galactose elimination

capacity, aminopyrine demethylation and caffeine clearance. J Hepatol. 1986;3:164.

53. Birrer R, Takuda Y, Takara T. Hypoxic hepatopathy: pathophysiology and prognosis. Intern Med. 2007;46:1063–70.

54. Everson G, Shiffman M, Morgan T, Hoefs J, Sterling R, Wagner D, et al. The spectrum of hepatic functional impairment in compensated chronic hepatitis C: results from the Hepatitis C Anti-viral Long-term Treatment against Cirrhosis Trial. Aliment Pharmacol Ther. 2008;27:798–809.

55. Davis G, Alter M, El-Serag H, Poynard T, Jennings L. Aging of hepatitis C virus (HCV)-infected persons in the United States: a multiple cohort model of HCV prevalence and disease progression. Gastroenterology. 2010;138:513–21.

56. Hickman P, Potter J, Pesce A. Clinical chemistry and post-liver-transplant monitoring. Clin Chem. 1997;43:1546–54.

57. Demetris A, Ruppert K, Dvorchik I, Jain A, Minervini M, Nalesnik M, et al. Real-time monitoring of acute liver-allograft rejection using the Banff schema. Transplantation. 2002;74:1290–6.

Surgical Anatomy of the Liver

3

Arvinder Singh Soin and Sanjay Kumar Yadav

A good knowledge of the anatomy of the liver is a prerequisite for modern surgery of the liver. (H. Bismuth).

3.1 Introduction

The liver, the largest internal organ in the body, accounts for approximately 2–3% of the total body weight of an adult. The precise knowledge of the architecture of the liver, biliary tract, and the related blood vessels and lymphatic drainage is essential for the successful performance of hepatobiliary surgery including liver transplantation.

3.2 Ligaments of the Liver (Fig. 3.1)

The liver itself is completely covered by a Glisson capsule (a peritoneal layer) except on the posterior surface and envelops all the three structures such as hepatic artery, portal vein, and bile duct at the hepatic hilum. The ligaments are actually

the fold of peritoneum which support the liver [1]. They are as follows:

- Round ligaments (Ligamentum Teres)
- Falciform ligament
- Coronary ligament
- Right and left triangular ligament
- Ligamentum venosum (Arantius Ligament)

The liver is suspended by the fibrous attachments (ligaments) and hepatic veins except at the bare area where it is connected to the diaphragm [2]. The two layer of the parietal peritoneum continues to the falciform ligament and surrounds the liver except for the bare area, where the two layers separate to form the coronary ligament and the left triangular ligament. The left layer of the falciform ligament becomes the superior layer of the left coronary ligament. The right layer becomes the upper layer of the coronary ligament, which meets the lower layer to form the right triangular ligament. The lower layer of the coronary ligament continues on the posterior surface of the liver and can reflect on the upper part of the right kidney to form the hepatorenal ligament. Then it passes in front of the groove for the inferior vena cava (IVC), and, after a semicircular course in front of the caudate lobe, it meets the right leaf of the lesser omentum. The leaf of the lesser omentum continues in the posterior leaf of the left triangular ligament [3].

A. S. Soin (✉)
Institute of Liver Transplantation & Regenerative Medicine, Medanta the Medicity, Gurgaon, India

S. K. Yadav
Medanta the Medicity, Gurgaon, India

© The Author(s), under exclusive license to Springer Nature Singapore Pte Ltd. 2023
V. Vohra et al. (eds.), *Peri-operative Anesthetic Management in Liver Transplantation*,
https://doi.org/10.1007/978-981-19-6045-1_3

Fig. 3.1 Ligaments of the liver

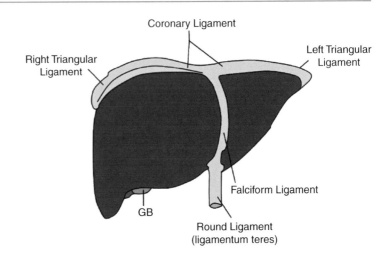

Fig. 3.2 (**a**) Arantius ligament. (**b**) Arantius ligament - diagramatic. (**c**) LHV-MHV looped after division of arantius ligament

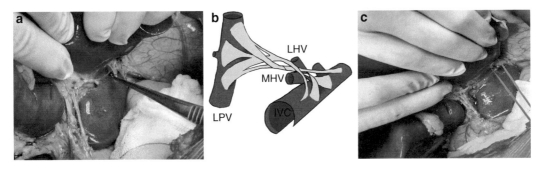

3.2.1 Ligamentum Venosum (Arantius Ligament)

This is the remnant of Arantius' canal (ductus venosus) that takes the oxygenated blood from the left umbilical vein through the left portal vein to the right atrium in fetal life. After birth the duct obliterates and persists as the ligamentum venosum or Arantius' ligament [4] (Fig. 3.2a).

The Arantius ligament usually inserts either into LHV or into the groove between the middle and the left hepatic vein [5] (Fig. 3.2b). The ligament can then be isolated, pulled upwards and to the left, and used to separate the veins when the left hepatic vein has to be controlled [6]. This maneuver is useful to pass a vessel loop around LHV for harvesting LLS graft in LDLT or in situ left lateral segment splitting. With further dissection, the maneuver can be used to encircle the common trunk of the left and middle hepatic

veins to prepare for harvesting of the left liver in living donor or split liver transplantation or for selective hepatic vein occlusion during liver resections (Fig. 3.2c). On the portal side, cutting the origin of the ligament close to the portal vein (i.e., when the vein is freed from the umbilical and the transverse plate) is a key maneuver to gain length in the left portal vein (in left donor hepatectomy, or during right hepatectomy along with portal vein bifurcation resection in perihilar cholangiocarcinoma), or exposure in the umbilical plate (in Kasai's operation).

3.3 Lobar and Segmental Anatomy of the Liver

Based on external appearance, the liver has been traditionally divided into four lobes, i.e., right, left, quadrate, and caudate lobe. The right and left lobes are separated by the falciform ligaments on the anterosuperior surface of the liver. The ligamentum teres and fissure for the ligamentum venosum separate both the lobes on the visceral surface of the liver (Fig. 3.3). However, hidden beneath this external gross appearance is the surgically and physiologically relevant detailed internal anatomy of the liver, also referred to as the functional anatomy of the liver.

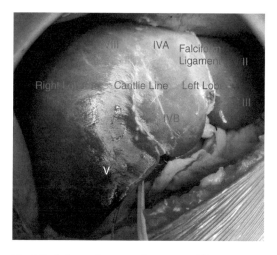

Fig. 3.3 Lobar and segmental anatomy of liver

3.3.1 Functional Surgical Anatomy of the Liver

The plane of division between the right and left lobes of the liver is not through the obvious falciform ligament but rather a plane passing through the bed of the gallbladder and the notch of the IVC, without other surface indications. This observation was first reported by Rex in 1888 and subsequently confirmed by Cantlie [7] in 1897 and Bradley [8] in 1909. However, it required another half century for wide acceptance of this concept [9]. This imaginary plane which divide the liver in right and left functional half is popularly known as Cantlie's line (or the principal plane, median fissure, Rex's line) (Fig. 3.3 *Cantlie Line*).

Based on arterial and portal venous blood supply, hepatic venous drainage, and biliary drainage, the liver is divided into functional lobes, sectors (sections), and segments (Fig. 3.4). Although various nomenclature exists, the Couinaud (1954) concept of hepatic segmentation is best known and widely accepted [10]. The internal architecture of the liver is composed of a series of segments that combine to form sectors

Fig. 3.4 Functional anatomy of liver. (Reprinted with permission from Blumgart's Surgery of the Liver, Biliary Tract and Pancreas, Sixth Edition, 2017)

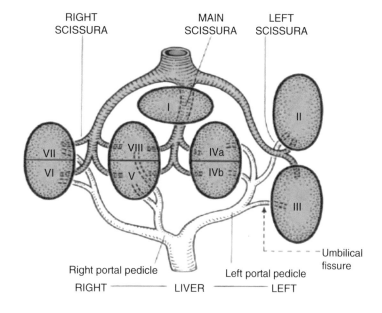

separated by scissurae that contain the hepatic veins (Fig. 3.5a, b). Essentially, the three main hepatic veins (right, middle, and left) within the scissurae divide the liver into four sectors, each of which receives a portal pedicle. The main portal scissura contains the middle hepatic vein and progresses from the middle of the gallbladder bed anteriorly to the left of the vena cava posteriorly. The right and left parts of the liver, demarcated by the main portal scissura, are independent in terms of portal and arterial vascularization and biliary drainage.

The right portal scissura separates the right liver into two sectors: anteromedial (anterior) and

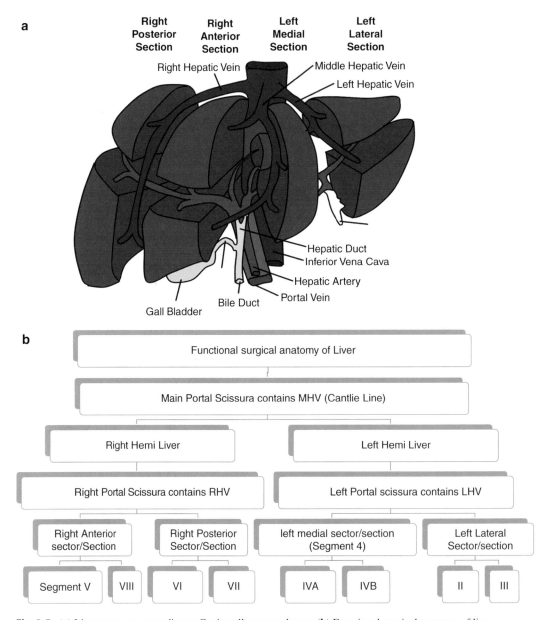

Fig. 3.5 (**a**) Liver segments according to Couinaud's nomenclature. (**b**) Functional surgical anatomy of liver

Table 3.1 Brisbane terminology of liver anatomy and resections (reprinted with permission from Blumgart's Surgery of the Liver, Biliary Tract and Pancreas, Sixth Edition, 2017)

Anatomic term	Couinaud segments	Surgical resections
Right hemiliver/right lobe	5–8	Right hepatectomy
Left hemiliver/left lobe	2–4	Left hepatectomy
Right anterior section	5, 8	Right anterior sectionectomy
Right posterior section	6, 7	Right posterior sectionectomy
Left medial section	4 (IVA/IVB)	Left median sectionectomy/resection of segment 4
Left lateral section	2, 3	Left lateral sectionectomy/bisectionectomy 2, 3
	4, 5, 6, 7, 8	Right trisectionectomy/extended right hepatectomy
	2, 3, 4, 5, 8	Left trisectionectomy/extended left hepatectomy

posterolateral (posterior). The right hepatic vein runs within the right scissura. The sectors are further divided into segments by the branches of portal veins. The right anterior sector is composed of Couinaud segment V and VIII. The right posterior sector is composed of Couinaud segment VI and VII.

The left portal scissura divides the left liver into two sectors, but the left portal scissura is not within the umbilical fissure because this fissure is not a portal scissura, and instead it contains a portal pedicle. The left portal scissura is located posterior to the ligamentum teres and within the left liver, along the course of the left hepatic vein.

Couinaud gave numbers to the segments in a clockwise manner starting from I to VIII. Couinaud's sectors are referred to as section in Brisbane terminology [11] (Table 3.1).

3.3.2 Bismuth's Liver Segmentation

He described the three fissures (scissurae) containing the hepatic veins and a transverse fissure passing through the right and left portal branches. The median fissure containing the MHV divides the whole liver into right and left hemiliver, with each hemiliver having anterior (topographically medial) and posterior (topographically lateral) sectors (segments) [12]. He took into specific consideration the caudate lobe (segment 1). The left lobe is thus divided into three segments: II (left lateral superior subsegment), III (left lateral inferior subsegment), and IV (left medial subsegment). The right lobe has four segments: V (right anterior inferior subsegment), VI (right anterior superior subsegment), VII (right posterior inferior subsegment), and VIII (right posterior superior subsegment).

3.4 Caudate Lobe

The caudate lobe or segment I is the dorsal portion of the liver between the portal vein bifurcation and the IVC (Fig. 3.6a *Caudate Lobe*). The caudate lobe is divided into right and left portions and a caudate process. The caudate lobe is intimately related to major vascular structure. On the left, caudate lies between the IVC posteriorly, left portal triad inferiorly, and IVC and MHV and LHV superiorly. The caudate lobe (segment I) lies mostly on the left side (Fig. 3.6b). The caudate lobe is supplied by blood vessels and drained by biliary tributaries from both the right and left portal triad. In 44% of individuals, three separate ducts drain these three parts of the lobe, whereas in another 26%, a common duct lies between the right portion of the caudate lobe proper and the caudate process and an independent duct that drains the left part of the caudate lobe. The biliary drainage of the caudate (segment I) enters both the right and the left hepatic duct systems in 80% of individuals [13]. In 15% of cases the caudate lobe drains only into the left hepatic duct system, and in 5% it drains only in the right system [9]. The right portion of the caudate predominantly receives portal venous blood from the right portal vein or from the bifurcation of the main portal vein, whereas on the left side, the portal supply arises from the left branch of the portal vein almost exclusively. The number of

a

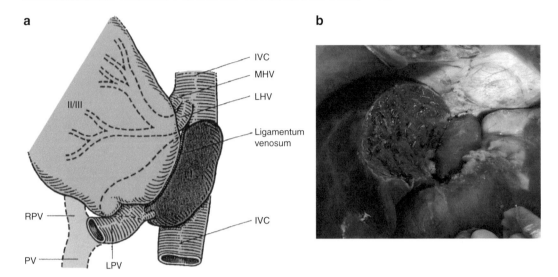

b

Fig. 3.6 (**a**) Caudate lobe anatomy (reprinted with permission from Blumgart's Surgery of the Liver, Biliary Tract and Pancreas, Sixth Edition, 2017). (**b**) Caudate lobe anatomy

portal branches to segment 1 varies from 1 to 6 (average 3) [14]. The hepatic venous drainage of the caudate is unique in that it is the only hepatic segment that drains directly into the IVC.

3.4.1 Hepatocaval Ligament (Makuuchi Ligament)

The posterior edge of the caudate on the left has a fibrous component (the hepatocaval ligament or dorsal ligament or Makuuchi ligament) that attaches to the crus of the diaphragm and extends posteriorly behind the vena cava to join segment VII on the right side of the IVC (Fig. 3.7). In a large proportion of patients, this fibrous tissue is replaced by hepatic parenchyma, in whole or in part, and the caudate may completely encircle the IVC and may contact segment VII on the right side; a significant retrocaval component may prevent a left-sided approach to the caudate veins.

In LDLT, during right hepatectomy, the caudate vein must be ligated and divided on the right side for looping the right portal vein. Failing to do so can lead to injury to the portal vein and hemorrhage while looping the right portal vein. Similarly, the hepatocaval ligament must be divided to get exposure to the RHV. While dividing the hepatocaval ligament, one must be careful

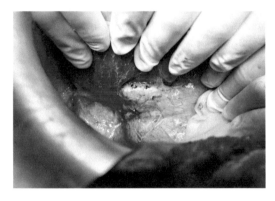

Fig. 3.7 Hepatocaval LIGAMENT

to ligate and divide the caudate vein draining into IVC in this ligament.

3.4.2 Riedel Lobe (Fig. 3.8)

Riedel lobe is a tongue-like, inferior projection of the right lobe of the liver beyond the level of the most inferior costal cartilage on cross-sectional images [15]. It is not considered a true accessory lobe of the liver but an anatomical variant of the right lobe of the liver. It can simulate a mass in the right hypochondrium and its misidentification as a pathologic abdominal mass has led to surgery in the past [16].

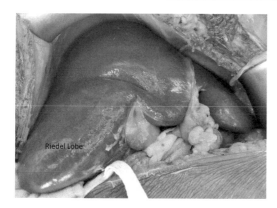

Fig. 3.8 Riedel lobe

3.5 Hepatic Veins (Venous Outflow)

The liver is drained by the three major hepatic veins (right, middle, and left) and around 10–50 smaller veins that open into the IVC [17]. The major hepatic veins lie within the three major scissura of the liver dividing the liver parenchyma into the right anterior and posterior sectors, and the right and left lobes.

The right hepatic vein is the largest among the three major hepatic veins and has a short extrahepatic course of approximately 1–2 cm and drains directly into suprahepatic IVC. The right hepatic vein lies within the right scissura (or segmental fissure) and divides the right lobe into a posterior (segments VI and VII) and anterior (segments V and VIII) sector. The RHV mainly drains the right posterior sector and part of the right anterior sector.

The middle hepatic veins lie within the main hepatic scissura (or main lobar fissure) separating the right anterior sector (segments V and VIII) from the quadrate lobe (segment IV). The MHV drains both the part of right anterior sector (segments V and VIII) and segment IV.

The Umbilical Fissural Vein is a tributary flowing into the LHV, the middle hepatic vein (MHV), or the confluence of the LHV and MHV; it runs along the umbilical fissure and drains segments III and IV [17–19]. In a study of 358 RT-LDLT by Soin et al. [20], UFV (or fissural vein) was seen on CT scan in 233 (65.2%) patients. Of these, fissural vein was seen to drain

both segments IVA and IVB in 92 (39.5%), IVA alone in 11 (4.7%), and IVB alone in 130 (55.8%) patients. Fissural vein was found to cranially drain into the LHV in 179 (76.8%), MHV in 30 (12.8%), and into the LHV–MHV junction in 23 (9.8%) patients. Although segments IVA and IVB predominantly drained into the MHV, their alternative drainage into the LHV, either directly or through the fissural vein, was found in 288 (80.3%) and 332 (92.8%) patients, respectively.

The left hepatic vein lies within the left scissura (or the left segmental fissure) in line with or just to the right of the falciform ligament and drain the left lateral segment of the liver (II and III). In about 60% of individuals, the left and middle veins unite to form a common venous channel of approximately 2 cm in length that traverses to the left part of the anterior surface of the IVC below the diaphragm to enter the IVC as a single vein [17]. In the rest, MHV and LHV may drain separately into IVC.

The branching pattern of MHV is important in LDLT as it drains both the right liver (V and VIII) and the left liver (Segment IV). MHV main stem is usually formed by two main branches of segment V and IVb. In some cases, the middle hepatic vein was formed by a single strong vessel that received smaller branches from adjacent tissue to the left and right. MHV anatomy has been defined by Neumann [21], Hwang [22], and Nakamura [17].

We have classified the MHV anatomy by modifying the Neumann classification into four types [23] as opposed to three types by Neumann et al. with type 4 being a mirror image of type 3 or what we call double or bifid MHV (Fig. 3.9a–d).

The MHV (Neumann Type 1) was formed by two equally sized secondary vessels that originated in segments 5 and 4b (Fig. 3.2a). Above this junction, venous branches from segments VIII and IVa joined the main stem on both sides. This type of MHV anatomy is suitable for modified right lobe graft (MRLG). The MHV (Neumann Type 2) can be described as a single, strong vessel that receives branches from adjacent tissue throughout its complete course. This type of MHV anatomy is suitable for partial right

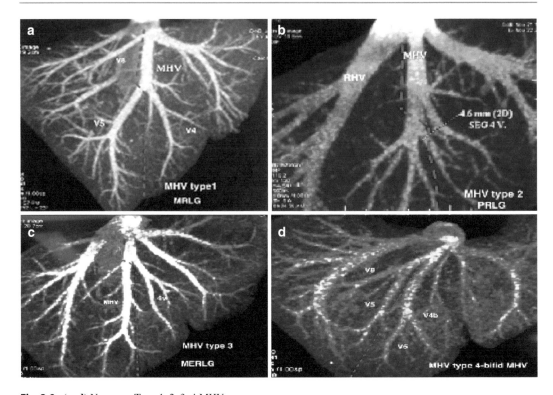

Fig. 3.9 (a–d) Neumann Type 1, 2, 3, 4 MHV

lobe graft (PRLG). The MHV Neumann type III is similar to type I in its overall configuration, but the main stem branches unequally with the right branch extending far into Segments V and VI. The Neumann type 3 and 4 anatomy is suitable for modified extended right lobe graft (MERLG) [21, 23].

The hepatic venous drainage of segment IV is of utmost important in RL LDLT. Hwang et al. [22] have classified segment IV drainage as type A (middle hepatic vein [MHV] dominant), type B (middle hepatic vein dominant, but enabling preservation of dorsal V4 branch), type C (mixed), and type D (left hepatic vein [LHV] dominant). Segment 4 venous drainage was classified as favorable or unfavorable as it shifted from predominantly into the left hepatic vein (LHV) to the proximal MHV, the same as the Nakamura/Hwang classification. The LHV dominant (Nakamura type 1, Hwang type C, D) type was considered favorable for a MERLG, whereas a MRLG was chosen for Nakamura 3, Hwang A. A PRLG was selected for partially favorable

(Nakamura 2, Hwang B) venous anatomy (Fig. 3.10a–c) [21–23].

3.5.1 Right Inferior Hepatic Veins: RIHV (Fig. 3.11)

One or more accessory right inferior hepatic vein(s) is the most common variation in the hepatic venous system. It is present in 48–55% of the population and drains mainly the right posterior sector (segments VI and VII) directly into the IVC [24–26]. The size of RIHVs is related to the size of the right hepatic vein, i.e., the larger the diameter of the right hepatic vein, the smaller the diameter of the RIHV, and vice versa. The RIHVs are divided into the superior, medial, and inferior right hepatic veins according to the position of the RIHV entering the inferior vena cava. The superior right hepatic vein mainly drains the superior part of segment VII, and the medial right hepatic vein drains the middle part of segment VII [27]. RIHV >5 mm in diameter must be

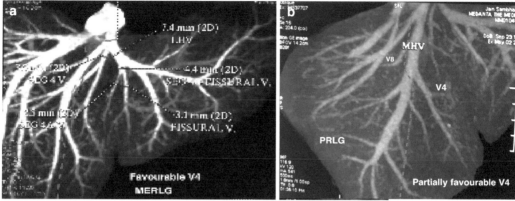

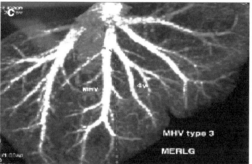

Fig. 3.10 (a–c) Nakamura Type A, B, C MHV

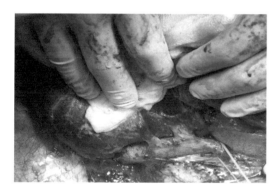

Fig. 3.11 Right inferior hepatic vein

reconstructed to avoid the congestion of right posterior sector in RL LDLT [28]. There may be more than one RIHV in an individual. During right hepatectomy, these veins must be dissected and ligated to avoid hemorrhage.

3.5.2 Inferior Phrenic Veins

The right and left inferior phrenic vein drains into the cranial most part of the RHV and common trunk of MHV and LHV respectively. These inferior phrenic veins must be ligated and divided to get better exposure of these major hepatic veins. Their stumps need ligation when the suprahepatic inferior vena cava is being prepared in a deceased donor liver graft on the bench prior to implantation.

3.6   Anatomical Relations Around the Hilum

A precise knowledge of the hilar anatomy and its variation is the key for portal dissection and division of hilar structures. Dissection, preparation,

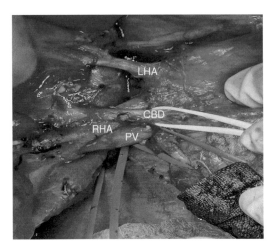

Fig. 3.12 Hepatic hilum

and division of the hilar structures are of vital importance in LDLT. The hepatic hilum and the hepatoduodenal ligament are composed of three main structures positioned in layers antero-posteriorly (Fig. 3.12).

The portal vein is located in the most dorsal aspect, hepatic artery is anterior to it in the middle layer, and the bile duct is located in the most ventral part.

3.6.1 Extrahepatic and Intrahepatic Vasculature

The liver has a dual blood supply from the portal vein [29, 30] and common hepatic artery. The portal vein is responsible for approximately 70% and the hepatic artery for 30% of the blood flow of the liver. Although 70% of the blood supplied to the liver comes from the portal vein, it only supplies 50% of the oxygen supply to the liver, and the hepatic artery the remaining half. In the liver, arteries, portal veins, and bile ducts are surrounded by a fibrous sheath, the Glissonian sheath [23]. Hepatic veins in the hepatic parenchyma lack such protection [2].

3.7 Portal Vein

The portal vein (Fig. 3.13) is 7–10 cm long, 0.8 and 1.4 cm in diameter, and is without valves. It is formed by the confluence of the superior mesenteric vein and the splenic vein behind the neck of the pancreas [3]. There are anterior and posterior and superior and inferior pancreaticoduodenal veins that drain to the portal vein and the SMV. The left gastric vein and the inferior mesenteric vein (IMV) usually drain into the splenic vein, but they can drain directly into the portal vein, whereas the various small splenic tributaries drain directly to the splenic vein. At the porta hepatis, the portal vein bifurcates into right and left branches before entering the liver.

The right branch of the portal vein is located anterior to the caudate process and is shorter than LPV. Near its origin it gives off 1–3 branches for the caudate lobe. The right portal vein divides into anterior (supplying segments V and VIII) and posterior (supplying segments VI and VII) branches. Each segmental branch further divides into inferior and superior subsegmental branches for its respective parenchymal subsegments.

The left portal vein may be divided into transverse and umbilical portions, as delineated by the ligamentum venosum, and is mostly extrahepatic in course. It begins in the porta hepatis as the transverse part [12], which gives off a caudate branch, and travels to the left. At the level of the umbilical fissure, the umbilical part turns sharply. It courses anteriorly in the direction of the round ligament and terminates in a *cul-de sac* proximally to the inferior border of the liver. Further on, the left portal vein divides into medial and lateral segmental branches, each with superior and inferior subsegmental branches [2].

Portal vein (PV) variations are one of the common vascular variations (incidence up to 22%) in RL grafts and usually associated with a high rate of anatomical biliary variations [31–34]. The clinical implications of PV and biliary variations

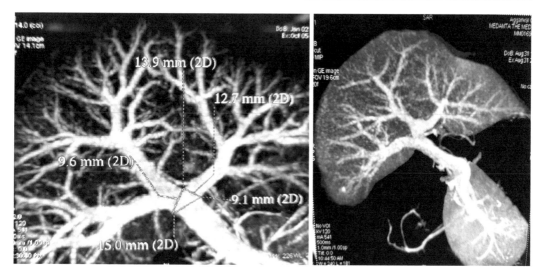

Fig. 3.13 Portal Vein (PV)

include technically challenging operations with complex reconstructions, as well as the rejection of potential donors.

Nakamura et al. [31] have classified the branching pattern of the portal vein to the right lobe into five types, which were defined by branches to the anterior segment.

3.8 Hepatic Artery

The usual classic description of the arterial blood supply of the liver and biliary system is found in only approximately 55% of patients [35] (Fig. 3.14). Aberrant hepatic arteries are a common variation of the hepatic vascular anatomy and can be classified as either accessory (occurring in addition to the normal arterial supply) or replaced (representing the primary arterial supply to the lobe). The incidences of aberrant left and right hepatic arteries are 12–22% and 13–25%, respectively [35–38].

The celiac trunk divides into three major arterial branches, i.e., left gastric artery, splenic artery, and common hepatic artery immediately after its origin from the aorta. The common hepatic artery usually takes origin from the celiac trunk (86%); however it may take origin from other sources like the superior mesenteric artery

(2.9%), the aorta (1.1%), and, very rarely, the left gastric artery [39].

The common hepatic artery then runs horizontally along the upper border of the head of the pancreas covered by the peritoneum of the posterior wall of the omental bursa. The gastroduodenal artery that supplies the proximal duodenum and pancreas is typically the first branch of the common hepatic artery. The right gastric artery takes off shortly thereafter and continues within the lesser omentum along the lesser curve of the stomach. The common hepatic artery continues as the proper hepatic artery which soon divides into the right and left hepatic arteries.

While coursing through the hepatoduodenal ligament, the proper hepatic artery, common bile duct, and portal vein are enveloped in a peritoneal sheath within the hepatoduodenal ligament. The proper hepatic artery bifurcates earlier than the common bile duct and portal vein. In 80% of cases the right hepatic artery courses posterior to the common hepatic duct before entering the hepatic parenchyma. In 20% of cases, the right hepatic artery may lie anterior to the common hepatic duct. Before entering the liver, the right hepatic artery gives off the cystic artery in the hepato-cystic triangle located between the cystic duct and the common hepatic duct (Fig. 3.15). Upon reaching the hepatic

Fig. 3.14 Classical
hepatic artery branches

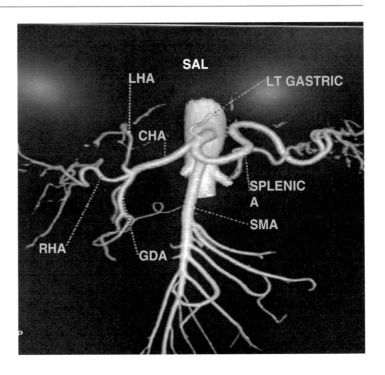

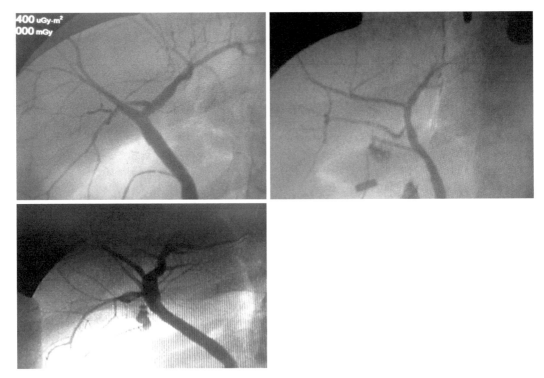

Fig. 3.15 Variation in right hepatic duct

parenchyma, the right hepatic artery branches into right anterior (segments V and VIII) and right posterior sectoral branches (segments VI and VII) [40]. An artery for the caudate lobe also originates from the right hepatic artery and supplies the caudate process and the right side of the caudate lobe. These arteries are found under the respective bile duct branches [12].

In case of replaced RHA or accessory RHA from SMA, the hepatic artery passes posterior and then lateral to the portal vein while it ascends and lies posterolateral to the CBD in the hepato-duodenal ligament, where it is susceptible to operative injury if not recognized.

The left hepatic artery runs vertically towards the umbilical fissure where it gives off a small branch (often called the middle hepatic artery or segment 4 artery) to segment IV, before continuing on to supply segments II and III. In 25–30% of cases, the left hepatic artery arises from the left gastric artery. In 40% of subjects the left hepatic artery branches into a median and a lateral segmental artery [35, 39, 40]. Additional small branches of the left hepatic artery supply the caudate lobe (segment I), although caudate arterial branches may also arise from the right hepatic artery.

Careful identification of multiple hepatic arteries and their source [41], as well as their preservation is essential in retrieval of deceased donor liver grafts. The multiple arteries can be taken on one stem of the celiac artery or SMA by anastomosing the separate stumps on the bench. Alternatively, two separate anastomoses can be performed in the recipient. Restoring complete arterial supply to both partial and full grafts is vital in liver transplantation to avoid both parenchymal necrosis and biliary complications.

Segment IV artery usually arises from the LHA; however, in approximately 11% of patients, it arises from the RHA (Fig. 3.16) and may traverse the transection plane to ascend into the left lobe [42, 43]. The segment 4 artery may arise from RAHA or RPHA or very rarely from GDA. Similarly, there may be two segment IV artery one each from RHA and LHA. Similarly the identification of the dominant

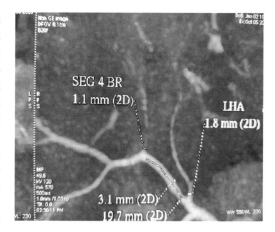

Fig. 3.16   Segment 4 HA arising from RHA

arterial supply to segment IV is very important because its integrity is indispensable for the regeneration of remnant donor liver. In such cases, RHA is divided distal to the origin of segment IV artery. It is important to ensure preoperatively that the RHA segment distal to segment IV artery is of sufficient length to permit anastomosis. Similarly, for the left-sided liver graft, the origin of segment 4 artery plays a major role in deciding the number of arterial stump in the graft. If the segment 4 artery arises from the LHA, then there will be single arterial stump in the graft. However, if the segment IV artery arises from other than the LHA, there can be more than one arterial stump depending on the origin of segment IV and if any accessory or replaced LHA.

Michels et al. [35] first reported ten basic types of hepatic arterial supply (Table 3.2). However, the classical hepatic arterial anatomy was seen in approximately 55% of the population, while the remaining have a variant arterial anatomy. Since then, common and rare hepatic artery variants have been reported. Most of these studies, however, focused only on replaced or accessory arterial branches that are helpful for whole-liver harvesting and transplantation. However, in LDLT the number of hepatic artery orifice in the graft is more important than the origin of the artery.

Table 3.2 Micheles classification

Type	Description	Michels's series ($n = 200$)
1	Normal	55%
2	Replaced LHA from LGA	10
3	Replaced RHA and MHA from SMA	11
4	Replaced LHA from LGA, and replaced RHA from SMA	1
5	Accessory LHA	8
6	Accessory RHA	7
7	Accessory LHA and accessory RHA	1
8	Accessory LHA and replaced RHA, or replaced LHA and accessory RHA	2
9	PHA from SMA	4.5
10	PHA from LGA	0.5

Based on the number of hepatic artery stumps in right liver LDLT, the anatomy of RHA can be classified into four types [44].

1. Single Arterial Orifice—Type 1
2. Multiple Arterial Orifice—Type 2, 3, and 4

- Single Arterial Orifice
  - Type 1: single artery in the right liver graft
  - Type 1A, normal anatomy in which RHA originates from the common hepatic artery and the middle hepatic artery (MHA/A4) originates from the LHA
  - Type IB, similar as Type IA, but MHA/A4 originates from RHA
  - Type IC, replaced RHA from superior mesenteric artery (SMA)
  - Type ID, replaced RHA and MHA from the SMA
  - Type IE, entire common hepatic artery from the SMA and the MHA from the LHA
  - Type IF, same as with Type IE except for the MHA originated from the RHA
- Multiple Arterial Orifice
  The hepatic arterial bifurcations that might provide multiple orifices in the right liver graft were divided into three types.
  Multiple orifices
  - Type II
    MHA/A4 originates from the paramedian (Type IIA) or lateral branch (Type IIB) of the RHA (from RPHA/RAHA).

- Type III: the right paramedian and lateral branch of the RHA has separate origin.
  IIIA—right lateral branch from the LHA
  IIIB—right lateral branch from the SMA
- Type IV: accessory branch from segment VI (A6). This type was divided into three subtypes according to the root of A6 as follows:
  Type IVA, from the hepatic artery proper
  Type IVB, from the celiac trunk
  Type IVC, from the superior pancreaticoduodenal artery

Although multiple hepatic arteries are more common in left lobe graft, up to 5% of right lobe graft can have multiple arteries [45, 46]. Dilemma exists whether to reconstruct all or perform partial reconstruction, sacrificing smaller less conspicuous one. The proponents suggest that all the hepatic arteries need to be reconstructed to minimize the risk of biliary complications [47, 48] whereas several other studies mainly in L-LDLT with multiple graft had shown that partial reconstruction of multiple hepatic arteries did not increase the biliary complication rate and possibly decreased hepatic artery complication [49, 50]. We recommend reconstruction of the second or even a third artery in right- and left-sided living donor grafts if they do not have a pulsatile backflow after reconstruction of the first artery.

3.9   Biliary Anatomy

Understanding the surgical anatomy of the biliary ductal system along with its variations at porta is of great surgical important in the LDLT during the donor hepatectomy. Anomalies of the bile duct are more common than those of the portal vein [9]. Preoperative MRCP is done to know the biliary anatomy of the potential donor. Intraoperative cholangiogram is usually done to visualize the biliary anatomy and to identify the precise site of bile duct division.

3.9.1   Intrahepatic Bile Duct Anatomy

Bile canaliculi are formed by parts of the membrane of adjacent parenchymal cells, and they are isolated from the perisinusoidal space by the junctions. Bile flows from the canaliculi through ductules (canals of Hering) into the interlobular bile ducts found in portal pedicles.

3.9.2   The Right Hepatic Duct

The right hepatic duct has short extrahepatic course formed by the union of right anterior and right posterior sectoral ducts. The right posterior sectional duct is formed by the confluence of the duct of segments VI and VII and has an almost horizontal course. The right anterior sectional duct is formed by the confluence of the ducts draining segments V and VIII (Fig. 3.17). The RPSD then runs to join the right anterior sectional duct, as it descends in a vertical manner [13]. The junction of these two RASD and RPSD usually occurs above the right branch of the portal vein. The right hepatic duct is short and joins the left hepatic duct to constitute the confluence lying in front of the right portal vein and forming the common hepatic duct.

3.9.3   The Left Hepatic Duct

The left hepatic duct drains the three segments—II, III, and IV—that constitute the left liver. The segment III is joined by the tributary from segment IVb to form the left duct, which is similarly joined by the duct of segment II and the duct of segment IVa. The left hepatic duct traverses beneath the left liver at the base of segment IV, just above and behind the left branch of the portal vein; it crosses the anterior edge of that vein and joins the right hepatic duct to constitute the hepatic ductal confluence.

Fig. 3.17 Normal biliary anatomy. (Reprinted with permission from Blumgart's Surgery of the Liver, Biliary Tract and Pancreas, Sixth Edition, 2017)

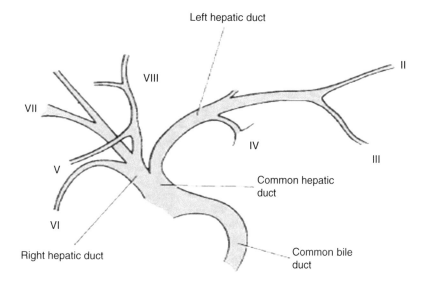

3.9.4 Extrahepatic Biliary Anatomy

The extrahepatic bile ducts represent the extrahepatic segments of the right and left hepatic ducts which join to form the biliary confluence, CHD and CBD. The cystic duct joins the CHD to form the CBD (average diameter 6 mm) draining to the duodenum. The confluence of the right and left hepatic ducts occurs at the right of the hilar fissure of the liver, anterior to the portal venous bifurcation and overlying the origin of the right branch of the portal vein. The biliary confluence is separated from the posterior aspect of segment IVB of the liver by the hilar plate, which is the fusion of connective tissue enclosing the biliary and vascular elements with the Glisson capsule. The common bile duct courses downward anterior to the portal vein, in the free edge of the lesser omentum while the HAP runs in upward direction on the left side of the CBD and give rise to RHA which crosses the CBD usually posteriorly. In around 20% of the case, RHA runs anterior to CBD. The cystic artery, arising from the RHA, may cross the common hepatic duct posteriorly or anteriorly.

3.9.5 Biliary Ductal Anomalies

The normal biliary confluence formed by union of the right and left hepatic ducts is reported in only 72% of patients [9]. There is trifurcation of biliary confluence into the right anterior and posterior sectional ducts and the left hepatic duct in 12% of individuals, and a right sectional duct joins the main bile duct directly in 20%. In 16% the right anterior sectional duct, and in 4% the right posterior sectional duct, may approach the main bile duct in this fashion. In 6%, a right sectional duct may join the left hepatic duct (the posterior duct in 5% and the anterior duct in 1%). In 3%, there is an absence of the hepatic duct confluence, and the right posterior sectional duct may join the neck of the gallbladder, or it may be entered by the cystic duct in 2% [10] (Fig. 3.15). All these biliary ductal variations are important to recognize during cholecystectomy and donor hepatectomy.

In around 20–50% of cases, there may be a subvesical duct embedded in the cystic plate which joins either common hepatic duct or RHD. It does not drain any specific liver territory and never communicates with the gall bladder. The importance of this variant anatomy lies in the fact that it may get injured during cholecystectomy if the cystic plate is not preserved and may lead to postoperative bile leak [13].

In 67% of patients [9] a classic distribution of the main left intrahepatic biliary ductal system exists. The main variation in this region is represented by a common union between the ducts of segments III and IV in 25%, and in only 2% does the duct of segment IV join the common hepatic duct independently.

The mode of union of the cystic duct with the common hepatic duct may be angular, parallel, or spiral. An angular union is the most frequent and is found in 75% of patients. The cystic duct may run a parallel course to the common hepatic duct in 20%, with connective tissue ensheathing both ducts. Finally, the cystic duct may approach the CBD in a spiral fashion [13, 51]. The absence of a cystic duct is probably an acquired anomaly, representing a cholecystocholedochal fistula.

Although several other classifications of variation in hilar biliary anatomy exist, the Huang Classification [52] of variation in hilar biliary anatomy is simple to comprehend and helpful to predict the number of graft bile duct orifice in procurement of right lobe graft in LDLT. In LDLT, recognition of such biliary anatomy is important to procure the graft without compromising the donor safety and optimal biliary outcomes in recipient.

3.9.6 Bile Duct Blood Supply

The bile duct may be divided into three segments to simplify the blood supply of the bile duct: hilar, supraduodenal, and retropancreatic. The blood supply of the supraduodenal duct is mainly arterial, essentially axial, and runs along the lateral borders of the bile duct at 3 o'clock and 9 o'clock position [53] (Fig. 3.18). Most vessels to the supraduodenal duct arise from the superior

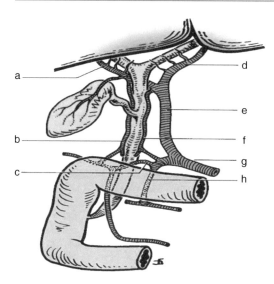

Fig. 3.18 The bile duct blood supply (reprinted with permission from Blumgart's Surgery of the Liver, Biliary Tract and Pancreas, Sixth Edition, 2017). Note the axial arrangement of the vasculature of the supraduodenal portion of the main bile duct and the rich network enclosing the right and left hepatic ducts: right branch of the hepatic artery (**a**), 9 o'clock artery (**b**), retroduodenal artery (**c**), left branch of the hepatic artery (**d**), hepatic artery (**e**), 3 o'clock artery (**f**), common hepatic artery (**g**), gastroduodenal artery (**h**)

The source of blood supply to the retropancreatic CBD is from the retroduodenal artery, which provides multiple small vessels running around the duct to form a mural plexus.

To avoid bile duct ischemia, the RHA should be divided to the right of bile duct during harvesting of a right lobe graft, especially if it is closely adherent to the undersurface of the CBD. Similarly the RHA should not be dissected from the bile duct during recipient hepatectomy, and the RHA should be divided to the left of bile duct during recipient hepatectomy, unless its anterior/posterior branch(es) are needed for later graft arterial reconstruction. In the latter instance, care should be taken not to bare the CBD while separating the artery from it.

The veins draining the bile ducts are satellites to the corresponding described arteries, draining into 3 o'clock and 9 o'clock veins along the borders of the common biliary channel. Veins draining the gallbladder empty into this venous system, not directly into the portal vein, and the biliary tree seems to have its own portal venous pathway to the liver.

pancreaticoduodenal artery, right hepatic artery, cystic artery, gastroduodenal artery, and retroduodenal artery. On average, eight small arteries supply the supraduodenal bile duct. Of the blood vessels vascularizing the supraduodenal duct, 60% run upward from the major inferior vessels, and only 38% of arteries run downward, originating from the right hepatic artery and other vessels. Only 2% of the arterial supply is nonaxial, arising directly from the main trunk of the hepatic artery, as it courses up parallel to the main biliary channel [13].

The hilar ducts receive a copious supply of arterial blood from surrounding vessels, forming a rich network on the surface of the ducts in the sub-Glissonian plane, underneath the hilar sheath, in continuity with the plexus around the supraduodenal duct [54]. To avoid biliary stricture in LDLT, we follow a strict protocol of harvesting the graft hepatic duct along with its hilar plate Glissonian sheath (HPGS) covering during living donor hepatectomy [55].

3.10 Gallbladder and Cystic Duct

The gallbladder is a reservoir located on the undersurface of the right lobe of the liver (segments V and IVB) within the cystic fossa. GB is separated from the hepatic parenchyma by the cystic plate which is composed of connective tissue that extends to the left as the hilar plate.

The gallbladder is divided into a fundus, a body, and a neck. The fundus usually reaches the free edge of the liver and is closely applied to the cystic plate. The cystic fossa is a precise anterior landmark to the main liver incisura. The neck of the gallbladder makes an angle with the fundus and creates Hartmann's pouch, which may obscure the common hepatic duct and constitute a real danger point during cholecystectomy. The cystic duct arises from the neck or infundibulum of the gallbladder and extends to join the common hepatic duct.

The cystic duct has a diameter of approximately 1–3 mm, and its length varies, depending on the type of union with the common hepatic duct and cystic duct. The mucosa of the cystic duct is arranged in spiral folds known as the valves of Heister. The cystic duct usually joins the CHD in supraduodenal part (in 80% cases); it may extend downward to the retroduodenal or retropancreatic area. Occasionally, the cystic duct may join the right hepatic duct or a right hepatic sectional duct.

3.10.1 The Calot's Triangle (Fig. 3.19)

The Calot's triangle has the following boundaries:

- Upper border—inferior surface of the right lobe of the liver
- Lower border—cystic duct
- Base—CHD
- Content—Cystic artery, or RHA

Dissection of the triangle of Calot is of key significance during cholecystectomy to avoid the injury of RHA. In case of replaced or accessory common or right hepatic artery, it usually runs behind the cystic duct to enter the triangle of Calot (Fig. 3.19).

When freely patent, the cystic duct is occasionally used for biliary reconstruction in RL LDLT in case the liver graft has multiple hepatic ducts.

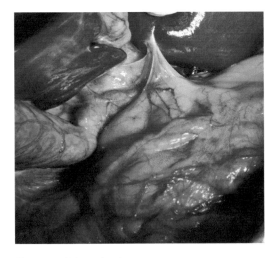

Fig. 3.19 Calots triangle

References

1. Mirilas P, Skandalakis JE. Benign anatomical mistakes: right and left coronary ligaments. Am Surg. 2002;68(9):832–5.
2. Ger R. Surgical anatomy of the liver. Surg Clin North Am. 1989;69(2):179–92.
3. Skandalakis JE, Skandalakis LJ, Skandalakis PN, Mirilas P. Hepatic surgical anatomy. Surg Clin North Am. 2004;84(2):413–35, viii.
4. Meyer WW, Lind J. The ductus venosus and the mechanism of its closure. Arch Dis Child. 1966;41(220):597–605.
5. Asuncion ZG, Silva YJ. Surgical significance of the ductus venosus Arantii. Am J Surg. 1971;122(1):109–11.
6. Majno PE, Mentha G, Morel P, Segalin A, Azoulay D, Oberholzer J, et al. Arantius' ligament approach to the left hepatic vein and to the common trunk. J Am Coll Surg. 2002;195(5):737–9.
7. Cantlie J. On a new arrangement of the right and left lobes of the liver. J Anat Physiol. 1898;32:4–10.
8. Bradley OC. A contribution to the morphology and development of the mammalian liver. J Anat Physiol. 1908;43(Pt 1):1–42.
9. Healey JE, Schroy PC. Anatomy of the biliary ducts within the human liver; analysis of the prevailing pattern of branchings and the major variations of the biliary ducts. AMA Arch Surg. 1953;66(5):599–616.
10. Couinaud C. [Liver lobes and segments: notes on the anatomical architecture and surgery of the liver]. Presse Med. 1954;62(33):709–12.
11. Strasberg SM. Nomenclature of hepatic anatomy and resections: a review of the Brisbane 2000 system. J Hepato-Biliary-Pancreat Surg. 2005;12(5):351–5.
12. Bismuth H. Surgical anatomy and anatomical surgery of the liver. World J Surg. 1982;6(1):3–9.
13. Jarnagin WR. Blumgart's surgery of the liver, biliary tract and pancreas, vol. 2. 6th ed. Amsterdam: Elsevier; 2016. https://www.elsevier.com/books/blumgarts-surgery-of-the-liver-biliary-tract-and-pancreas-2-volume-set/jarnagin/978-0-323-34062-5. Accessed 11 Oct 2020.
14. Kogure K, Kuwano H, Fujimaki N, Makuuchi M. Relation among portal segmentation, proper hepatic vein, and external notch of the caudate lobe in the human liver. Ann Surg. 2000;231(2):223–8.
15. Kudo M. Riedel's lobe of the liver and its clinical implication. Intern Med. 2000;39(2):87–8.
16. Gillard JH, Patel MC, Abrahams PH, Dixon AK. Riedel's lobe of the liver: fact or fiction? Clin Anat. 1998;11(1):47–9.
17. Nakamura S, Tsuzuki T. Surgical anatomy of the hepatic veins and the inferior vena cava. Surg Gynecol Obstet. 1981;152(1):43–50.
18. Tani K, Shindoh J, Akamatsu N, Arita J, Kaneko J, Sakamoto Y, et al. Venous drainage map of the liver for complex hepatobiliary surgery and liver transplantation. HPB. 2016;18(12):1031–8.

19. Kawasaki S, Makuuchi M, Miyagawa S, Matsunami H, Hashikura Y, Ikegami T, et al. Extended lateral segmentectomy using intraoperative ultrasound to obtain a partial liver graft. Am J Surg. 1996;171(2):286–8.

20. Soin AS, Mohanka R, Singla P, Piplani T, Menon B, Kakodkar R, et al. Segment IV preserving middle hepatic vein retrieval in right lobe living donor liver transplantation. J Am Coll Surg. 2011;213(2):e5–16.

21. Neumann JO, Thorn M, Fischer L, Schöbinger M, Heimann T, Radeleff B, et al. Branching patterns and drainage territories of the middle hepatic vein in computer-simulated right living-donor hepatectomies. Am J Transplant. 2006;6(6):1407–15.

22. Hwang S, Lee S-G, Choi S-T, Moon D-B, Ha T-Y, Lee Y-J, et al. Hepatic vein anatomy of the medial segment for living donor liver transplantation using extended right lobe graft. Liver Transpl. 2005;11(4):449–55.

23. Goja S, Yadav SK, Soin AS. Readdressing the middle hepatic vein in right lobe liver donation: triangle of safety. Liver Transpl. 2018;24(10):1363–76.

24. Kalaycı TÖ, Kutlu R, Karasu Ş, Yılmaz S. Investigation of right lobe hepatic vein variations of donor using 64-detector computed tomography before living donor liver transplantation. Turk J Gastroenterol. 2014;25(Suppl 1):9–14.

25. Ahmed A, Hafeez-Baig A, Sharif MA, Ahmed U, Gururajan R. Role of accessory right inferior hepatic veins in evaluation of liver transplantation. Ann Clin Gastroenterol Hepatol. 2017;1(1):012–6.

26. Radtke A, Sotiropoulos GC, Molmenti EP, Nadalinl S, Schroeder T, Schenk A, et al. The influence of accessory right inferior hepatic veins on the venous drainage in right graft living donor liver transplantation. Hepato-Gastroenterology. 2006;53(70):479–83.

27. Xing X, Li H, Liu W-G. Clinical studies on inferior right hepatic veins. Hepatobiliary Pancreat Dis Int. 2007;6(6):579–84.

28. Soin AS, Yadav SK, Saha SK, Rastogi A, Bhangui P, Srinivasan T, et al. Is portal inflow modulation always necessary for successful utilization of small volume living donor liver grafts? Liver Transpl. 2019;25(12):1811–21.

29. Sakamoto Y, Takayama T, Nakatsuka T, Asato H, Sugawara Y, Sano K, et al. Advantage in using living donors with aberrant hepatic artery for partial liver graft arterialization. Transplantation. 2002;74(4):518–21.

30. Ahn C-S, Lee S-G, Hwang S, Moon D-B, Ha T-Y, Lee Y-J, et al. Anatomic variation of the right hepatic artery and its reconstruction for living donor liver transplantation using right lobe graft. Transplant Proc. 2005;37(2):1067–9.

31. Nakamura T, Tanaka K, Kiuchi T, Kasahara M, Oike F, Ueda M, et al. Anatomical variations and surgical strategies in right lobe living donor liver transplantation: lessons from 120 cases. Transplantation. 2002;73(12):1896–903.

32. Yaprak O, Demirbas T, Duran C, Dayangac M, Akyildiz M, Tokat Y, et al. Living donor liver hilar variations: surgical approaches and implications. Hepatobiliary Pancreat Dis Int. 2011;10(5):474–9.

33. Hwang S, Lee S-G, Ahn C-S, Kim K-H, Moon D-B, Ha T-Y, et al. Technique and outcome of autologous portal Y-graft interposition for anomalous right portal veins in living donor liver transplantation. Liver Transpl. 2009;15(4):427–34.

34. Cheng YF, Huang TL, Lee TY, Chen TY, Chen CL. Variation of the intrahepatic portal vein; angiographic demonstration and application in living-related hepatic transplantation. Transplant Proc. 1996;28(3):1667–8.

35. Michels NA. Newer anatomy of the liver and its variant blood supply and collateral circulation. Am J Surg. 1966;112(3):337–47.

36. Soin AS, Friend PJ, Rasmussen A, Saxena R, Tokat Y, Alexander GJ, et al. Donor arterial variations in liver transplantation: management and outcome of 527 consecutive grafts. Br J Surg. 1996;83(5):637–41.

37. Hiatt JR, Gabbay J, Busuttil RW. Surgical anatomy of the hepatic arteries in 1000 cases. Ann Surg. 1994;220(1):50–2.

38. Suzuki T, Nakayasu A, Kawabe K, Takeda H, Honjo I. Surgical significance of anatomic variations of the hepatic artery. Am J Surg. 1971;122(4):505–12.

39. Vandamme JP, Bonte J. The branches of the celiac trunk. Acta Anat (Basel). 1985;122(2):110–4.

40. International Anatomical Nomenclature Committee. International Congress of Anatomists. Nomina anatomica: sixth edition authorised by the Twelfth International Congress of Anatomists in London, 1985: together with Nomina histologica, third edition, and Nomina embryologica. 3rd ed. Edinburgh; New York, NY: Churchill Livingstone; 1989.

41. Soin AS, Friend PJ, Rasmussen A, Saxena R, Tokat Y, Alexander GJ, Jamieson NV, Calne RY. Donor arterial variations in liver transplantation: management and outcome of 527 consecutive grafts. Br J Surg. 1996;83:637–41.

42. Couinaud C. [A "scandal": segment IV and liver transplantation]. J Chir (Paris). 1993;130(11):443–6.

43. Marcos A, Fisher RA, Ham JM, Olzinski AT, Shiffman ML, Sanyal AJ, et al. Selection and outcome of living donors for adult to adult right lobe transplantation. Transplantation. 2000;69(11):2410–5.

44. Kishi Y, Sugawara Y, Kaneko J, Akamatsu N, Imamura H, Asato H, et al. Hepatic arterial anatomy for right liver procurement from living donors. Liver Transpl. 2004;10(1):129–33.

45. Ikegami T, Kawasaki S, Matsunami H, Hashikura Y, Nakazawa Y, Miyagawa S, et al. Should all hepatic arterial branches be reconstructed in living-related liver transplantation? Surgery. 1996;119(4):431–6.

46. Tanaka K, Uemoto S, Tokunaga Y, Fujita S, Sano K, Nishizawa T, et al. Surgical techniques and innovations in living related liver transplantation. Ann Surg. 1993;217(1):82–91.

47. Uchiyama H, Harada N, Sanefuji K, Kayashima H, Taketomi A, Soejima Y, et al. Dual hepatic artery reconstruction in living donor liver transplanta-

tion using a left hepatic graft with 2 hepatic arterial stumps. Surgery. 2010;147(6):878–86.

48. Suehiro T, Ninomiya M, Shiotani S, Hiroshige S, Harada N, Ryosuke M, et al. Hepatic artery reconstruction and biliary stricture formation after living donor adult liver transplantation using the left lobe. Liver Transpl. 2002;8(5):495–9.

49. Lee KW, Lee S, Oh DK, Na BG, Choi JY, Cho W, et al. Outcome of partial reconstruction of multiple hepatic arteries in pediatric living donor liver transplantation using left liver grafts. Transpl Int. 2016;29(8):890–6.

50. Sugawara Y, Tamura S, Kaneko J, Iida T, Mihara M, Makuuchi M, et al. Single artery reconstruction in left liver transplantation. Surgery. 2011;149(6):841–5.

51. Mortelé KJ, Ros PR. Anatomic variants of the biliary tree: MR cholangiographic findings and clinical applications. AJR Am J Roentgenol. 2001;177(2):389–94.

52. Huang TL, Cheng YF, Chen CL, Chen TY, Lee TY. Variants of the bile ducts: clinical application in the potential donor of living-related hepatic transplantation. Transplant Proc. 1996;28(3):1669–70.

53. Northover JM, Terblanche J. A new look at the arterial supply of the bile duct in man and its surgical implications. Br J Surg. 1979;66(6):379–84.

54. Gunji H, Cho A, Tohma T, Okazumi S, Makino H, Shuto K, et al. The blood supply of the hilar bile duct and its relationship to the communicating arcade located between the right and left hepatic arteries. Am J Surg. 2006;192(3):276–80.

55. Soin AS, Kumaran V, Rastogi AN, Mohanka R, Mehta N, Saigal S, et al. Evolution of a reliable biliary reconstructive technique in 400 consecutive living donor liver transplants. J Am Coll Surg. 2010;211(1):24–32.

Pathophysiology of Chronic Liver Disease

Anjan Trikha and Bikash Ranjan Ray

4.1 Introduction

The liver being the largest solid organ in the human body is affected by many different pathogenic agents and processes. Increasing incidence of liver disease is primarily driven by lifestyle factors (alcohol, obesity) and infection of the liver parenchyma. Liver diseases can be manifested in a number of ways, which may be acute or chronic, focal or diffuse, mild or severe. Acute liver disease is a self-limiting disease in which symptoms do not persist beyond 6 months. Most cases are due to episodes of hepatocyte inflammation or damage, which resolve without causing any further complications. Mostly the manifestation of acute liver disease (e.g., viral hepatitis) is so mild that they never come to medical attention. However the entire liver may be affected in few cases leading to fulminant liver failure, which is a life-threatening condition. In chronic liver disease the symptoms persist for more than 6 months. It occurs because of permanent structural damage to the liver architecture as a result of continued inflammation of the hepatocytes after the primary insult. Cirrhosis is the ultimate consequence of progressive liver injury. Cirrhosis develops in a subset of cases of chronic liver disease and may be a consequence of repeated episodes of acute liver injury. Cirrhosis is manifested as a grossly impaired liver function due to decrease amount of functional liver tissue. Change in liver architecture leads to change in the physics of blood flow in and around the liver. Elevation in portal vein pressure diverts blood away from the liver causing portosystemic shunting, which has a profound effect on functioning of various organ systems.

Understanding of the liver parenchymal arrangement and blood flow is critical to the understanding of the liver inflammation.

4.2 Cellular Anatomy of the Liver

The liver is the largest organ in the human body and is located in the right upper quadrant of the abdomen. The liver receives around 25% of the cardiac output from the portal vein and the hepatic artery [1]. The blood flow exits the liver via the central veins which drains into the hepatic vein and finally to the inferior vena cava [2].

The liver parenchyma consists of hepatocytes, which are organized into plate of hepatocytes, and is supported by reticuloendothelial cells. These one-cell-thick plates of hepatocytes are separated from each other by vascular spaces called sinusoids. The blood from the portal vein and the hepatic artery is mixed in these sinusoids while flowing toward the central vein. The reticuloendothelial cells, which consist approximately 30% of

A. Trikha (✉) · B. R. Ray
Department of Anaesthesiology, Pain Medicine and Critical Care, All India Institute of Medical Sciences, New Delhi, India

all cells of the liver, have diverse types of cells [2]. Endothelial cells (makes the boundary of the sinusoids), Kupffer cells (specialized macrophages), and stellate cells (fat storing cells) are the most important cell types in the reticuloendothelial cell meshwork. These cells perform specific functions by communicating with each other and with the hepatocytes. Dysfunction of these cells leads to different grades of inflammations, starting from necrosis of hepatocytes in acute liver diseases to fibrosis in chronic liver disease and cirrhosis.

Liver architecture has been traditionally described in terms of the lobule. In a lobule arrays of hepatocyte plates are organized in the form of a hexagon around a central vein with portal triads at the corners of the hexagon. The portal triad consists of a bile canaliculus, portal venule, and hepatic arteriole. The hepatocytes adjacent to the portal triad consist of the limiting plate and disruption of this is a significant marker of some immune-mediated liver disease [2].

4.3   Etiology of Chronic Liver Disease

Many different pathogenic agents and processes cause chronic liver disease. These etiologies can be simply classified as per Table 4.1.

Although many factors contribute toward the development of chronic liver disease, they ulti-

Table 4.1 Chronic liver failure etiology

Etiology of chronic liver failure	
Common causes:	Lesser common causes:
• Alcohol	• Drug and toxin induced
• Chronic viral hepatitis (B and C)	• Autoimmune chronic hepatitis (1, 2, and 3)
• Biliary obstruction	• Genetic and metabolic disease
– Biliary atresia	• Infection
– Cystic fibrosis	• Idiopathic
• Primary and secondary biliary cirrhosis	• Veno-occlusive disease
• Nonalcoholic fatty liver diseases (NAFLD)	• Vascular abnormalities
• Hemochromatosis	• Miscellaneous

mately lead to development of cirrhosis. The three common model of hepatic injury are the: alcoholic-induced model, post viral hepatitis model, and drugs- and toxin-induced model.

4.4   Pathophysiology of Chronic Liver Disease

Irrespective of the etiology the path of progression of a liver injury to chronic liver injury follows a similar flow, which is demonstrated in Flow Diagram 4.1.

4.4.1   Basics of Liver Inflammation

The classical picture of any insult to the liver is inflammation and damage leading to production of stressed hepatocytes. Persistent and recurrent injuries ultimately lead to hepatic fibrosis, which is the common end point for most of the chronic liver disease. Normally the liver eliminates the cellular debris produced by the inflammation and tries to restitute the cellular integrity by regeneration. However when the liver fails to maintain this sequence of elimination and regeneration, inflammation continues and fibrosis follows. When the fibrosis becomes an irreversible process, then the cirrhosis sets in.

Different types of disease may lead to different patterns of fibrosis during disease progression. Histology shows predominance of different fibrogenic cells in different types of fibrosis [3, 4]. Chronic infection of the liver caused by hepatotropic viruses follows a classic pattern of inflammation, the death of hepatocytes, and finally liver fibrosis [5] whereas alcoholic hepatitis and nonalcoholic steatohepatitis are associated with a change in hepatocyte lipids on histology, hepatocyte ballooning/necrosis, neutrophil infiltration, and the development of a particular type of fibrosis. Chronic or persistent obstruction of the biliary tree leads to hepatocyte necrosis and to lobular bile infarcts due to extensive proliferation of periductular fibroblasts [6].

Flow Diagram 4.1 Pathophysiology of chronic liver disease

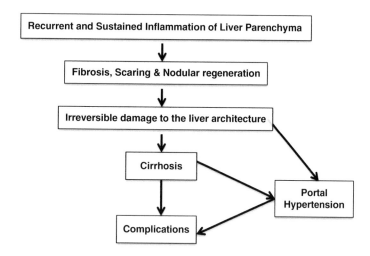

4.4.2 Cells Involved in Liver Inflammation

Hepatocytes constitute 70–80% of the cytoplasmic mass of the liver and have an average life span of 5 month, with the ability to regenerate [7]. Hepatocytes are responsible for most of the functions of the liver. They are also responsible for the synthesizing cytokines, acute phase proteins like C-reactive protein (CRP) or serum amyloid A (SAA), and many others during an acute phase [8, 9]. These cells also possess different intracellular defense mechanism to combat any acute insult. However when these defense mechanisms are not sufficient to withstand, the damaging cells start to synthesize chemokines, which are supposed to be responsible for attraction of inflammatory cells like granulocytes and mononuclear phagocytes and activation of resident macrophages. In this attempt to eliminate the damage, the defense response however leads to death of the stressed hepatocyte.

Hepatic stellate cells (HSC) have a very important role as they modulate the inflammatory conditions, based on their capability of cytokine and chemokine production.

Hepatic stellate cells might also play a role during liver inflammation by modulating the recruitment and migration of mononuclear cells within the perisinusoidal space of diseased livers.

Sinusoids display a discontinuous, fenestrated endothelial cell lining. The sinusoidal "wall" does not possess a basement membrane and the endothelial cells are separated from the hepatocytes by the space of Disse which drains lymph into the portal tract lymphatics [7]. During inflammation the chemokine expression profile of the normal hepatic endothelium changes. Similarly to the chemokine profile the expression pattern of adhesion molecules also changes in the endothelial cells.

Kupffer cells are scattered within the liver sinusoid; they are a major part of the reticuloendothelial system and phagocytose spent erythrocytes. Kupffer cells are the specialized macrophages of the liver that form a major part of the reticuloendothelial system (mononuclear phagocyte system) [10].

Activation of Kupffer cells results in secretion of a large number of chemical mediators, most of which can induce liver injury either by acting directly on the liver cells or via chemoattraction of extrahepatic cells (e.g., neutrophils and lymphocytes). The chemical mediators released by Kupffer cells and by hepatocytes attract extrahepatic cells to the liver. Neutrophils (PMN) are the characteristic cellular compound of the chemoattracted cells and are involved in acute inflammation. They are always present in the inflammatory infiltrate of chronic liver disease. However, neutrophil infiltration is most prominent in alcoholic hepatitis. Up to now the role of T lymphocytes in liver disease is still ill-understood.

Hepatocellular stress (induced by toxins or infections) leads to activation of macrophages in the liver parenchyma and release of proinflammatory chemokines and cytokines from various cell types in the liver. This leads to recruitment and sinusoidal transmigration of inflammatory cells toward the target hepatocyte. Inflammation persists as long as the damaging stimulus persists or are repeatedly exposed. The hepatic infiltrate includes granulocytes, macrophages, T lymphocytes, B lymphocytes, and plasma cells. The inflammatory macrophages activate the mesenchymal cells and stimulate the synthesis of matrix with the help of cytokines and growth factors.

4.4.3   Repair of the Damaged Liver

The processes of liver repair and fibrogenesis resemble that of a wound-healing process. Following injury and acute inflammation response takes place resulting in moderate cell necrosis and extracellular matrix damage. After that tissue repair takes place where dead cells are replaced by normal tissue with regeneration of specialized cells by proliferation of surviving ones or generation from stem cells, formation of granulation tissue, and tissue remodeling with scar formation [4].

Recurrent or chronic, injury or insult give way to excess matrix deposition as a result of an imbalance between fibrogenesis and fibrolysis leading to scar formation. The high rate of tissue destruction with slow regeneration also provides the space for matrix deposition. Liver fibrosis is a common sequel to diverse liver injuries such as chronic viral hepatitis, ethanol, biliary tract diseases, iron or copper accumulation. As scarring progresses from bridging fibrosis to the formation of complete nodules it results in an architectural distortion and ultimately in liver cirrhosis [11].

Liver fibrosis is defined as an abnormal accumulation of extracellular matrix in the liver. Its end point is liver cirrhosis which is responsible for significant morbidity and mortality. Cirrhosis is an advanced stage of fibrosis, characterized by the formation of regenerative nodules of liver parenchyma separated by fibrotic septa, which result from cell death, aberrant extracellular matrix deposition, and vascular reorganization. Advanced liver fibrosis results in cirrhosis, liver failure, and portal hypertension and often requires liver transplantation [11].

Accumulating data from clinical and laboratory studies demonstrate that even advanced fibrosis and cirrhosis are potentially reversible. The hepatic stellate cells have been identified as the pivotal effector cells orchestrating the fibrotic process and, furthermore, reversibility appears to hinge upon their elimination. Removing the insult and stopping the persistent inflammatory stimuli is probably the best way to prevent progression of fibrosis; nevertheless, prevention of the progression of fibrosis to cirrhosis remains the major clinical goal. The poor prognosis of cirrhosis is aggravated by the frequent occurrence of hepatocellular carcinoma.

4.5   Cirrhosis and Portal Hypertension

Cirrhosis is the end product of steady or recurrent episode of liver parenchymal inflammation leading to necrosis and disruption of normal hepatic architecture. The normal liver is replaced by advanced fibrosis, scaring, and formation of regenerative nodules. These changes in liver architecture lead to change in blood flow in and around the liver. Increase resistance to blood flow results in the formation of shunts between the afferent and efferent vessels and increase in portal venous pressure. The resulting portal hypertension can be quantified by measuring the hepatic venous pressure gradient (HVPG). Portal hypertension is present if HVPG is >5 mmHg; however it is clinically significant if it is >10–12 mmHg. The buildup of portal hypertension is a turning point in the pathophysiology of CLD as at this point the CLD becomes a systemic disease, affecting other organ systems as well. Portal hypertension contributes to the pathogenesis of cirrhosis and its complications by formation of venous collaterals, increase production of bio-chemical (vasoconstrictors, splanchnic vasodila-tors, nitric oxide and others) and other functional abnormalities (expansion of plasma volume, increased cardiac output, etc.) [12, 13].

The complications of cirrhosis occur second-ary to portal hypertension, abnormal synthetic function, or combination of both. Major compli-cations of cirrhosis and portal hypertension include changes in hemostasis and coagulation, ascites, pulmonary involvement, renal involve-ment, hepatic encephalopathy, and varices (Flow Diagram 4.2).

4.5.1 Hemostasis

Chronic liver disease leads to a form of "rebal-anced" hemostasis. This is due to diminished hepatic function leading to both procoagulant and anticoagulant effects. All stages of the hemo-static process may be abnormal, including pri-mary hemostasis (platelet adhesion and activation), coagulation (generation and cross-linking of fibrin), and fibrinolysis (clot dissolu-tion). Risk of bleeding and thrombosis in an individual depends upon the balance or imbal-ance between altered blood flow, qualitative and quantitative dysfunction of platelets, and endo-thelial cell dysfunction [14, 15].

Coagulation factor defects Almost all of the coagulation factors (Factor I, II, V, VII, IX, X, and XI) except factor VIII (produced by endothe-lial cells) are produced by hepatocytes [16, 17]. Additionally, hepatocytes also help in post-translational modification (glycosylation, gamma-carboxylation) of certain factors, which is crucial for the activation of these factors. Chronic liver disease impairs both synthesis and post-translational modifications of clotting fac-tors affecting coagulation in cirrhosis. In some liver disease (alcoholics), deficiency of vitamin K further exacerbates the deficiency and modifica-tion of vitamin K dependent factors (factor II, VII, IX, and X) [18, 19]. Qualitative defects in fibrinogen also contribute to the coagulopathy of cirrhosis.

Thrombocytopenia and platelet dysfunc-tion Patients with cirrhosis have both qualita-tive and quantitative defects in platelet functions. The correlation between platelet count and clini-cal bleeding is weak [20]. Thrombocytopenia in liver diseases has multiple mechanisms, which includes impaired platelet production (due to decreased hepatic synthesis of thrombopoi-etin), bone marrow suppression (alcohol use, HCV infection, drugs), and sequestration plate-lets in the spleen due to portal hypertension induced hypersplenism. Also, coexisting uremia,

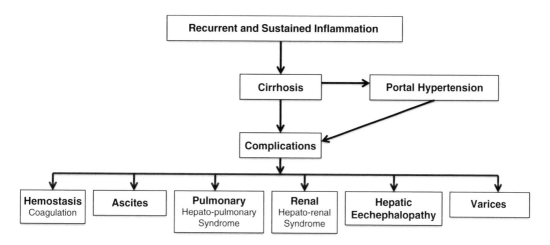

Flow Diagram 4.2 Complications of cirrhosis and portal hypertension

infection, and endotoxemia of sepsis contribute to thrombocytopenia.

Altered fibrinolytic system The fibrinolytic system is altered in patients with cirrhosis. Often fibrinolysis (dissolution of fibrin clot) is increased in chronic liver disease; however clinically significant hyperfibrinolysis is less commonly found in decompensated cirrhosis [21]. Hyperfibrinolysis promotes premature clot dissolution and interferes with clot formation due to the consumption of clotting factors. Hyperfibrinolysis in cirrhosis is associated with multiple mechanisms, which include: increased levels of tissue plasminogen activator (tPA) (which generates plasmin), decreased levels of alpha 2 antiplasmin, factor XIII and thrombin-activatable fibrinolysis inhibitor (TAFI) [22–24].

Prothrombotic changes The liver is the primary producer of endogenous inhibitors of coagulation (e.g., protein S, protein C, antithrombin) and fibrinolytic factors. Reduced level of these natural inhibitors in cirrhosis is responsible for the prothrombotic state [25, 26]. Also, elevated levels of Von Willebrand factor (VWF) and certain acute phase reactants (plasminogen activator inhibitor 1 (PAI-1)) may contribute to prothrombotic state [27, 28]. Reduced vascular flow also contributes to local prothrombotic tendencies.

Hemostatic abnormalities in chronic liver disease are similar regardless of the underlying cause. However, some differences have been noted, such as cholestatic liver diseases [primary biliary cholangitis (PBC) and primary sclerosing cholangitis (PSC)] appear to have a less pronounced effect on anticoagulant than procoagulant mechanisms and may be at higher risk for portal vein thrombosis. Nonalcoholic fatty liver disease (NAFLD) may confer a greater prothrombotic risk whereas acute-on-chronic liver failure (ACLF) may present with unique coagulopathies.

4.5.2 Cardiac Manifestations

Hyperdynamic circulation is the hallmark of cirrhosis which is characterized by a high cardiac output, low arterial blood pressure, and low systemic vascular resistance. Although these patients have an increased intravascular volume, most of this volume is sequestered in the dilated and collateralized splanchnic circulation. Thus the effective circulating volume is reduced. The root cause of these changes is the portal hypertension, which is responsible for production of many vasodilators (natriuretic peptides, vasoactive intestinal peptide, endotoxin, glucagon) especially nitric oxide [29, 30]. Furthermore excessive production of vasodilators also leads to diminished circulatory responsivity to sympathetic stimulation.

Individuals with cirrhosis often have combinations of other cardiac abnormalities apart from hyperdynamic circulation which is termed as "cirrhotic cardiomyopathy" [1]. The four key components of this are (1) increase in cardiac output and decrease in systemic vascular resistance, (2) systolic and diastolic dysfunction, (3) reduced cardiac responsiveness to adrenergic stimulation, and (4) electrophysiologic abnormalities. The severity of cardiac dysfunction is directly correlated with the severity of liver disease.

4.5.3 Renal Dysfunction

Renal dysfunction is an important factor in the prediction of mortality and prognosis in cirrhosis. Renal dysfunction in cirrhosis is mainly caused by inappropriate retention of sodium and free water, together with renal hypoperfusion, which leads to a decrease in glomerular filtration rate (GFR) [31–33]. The hepatorenal syndrome (HRS) is one of the extreme manifestations of the renal response to the circulatory abnormalities of advanced cirrhosis. HRS is a diagnosis of exclu-

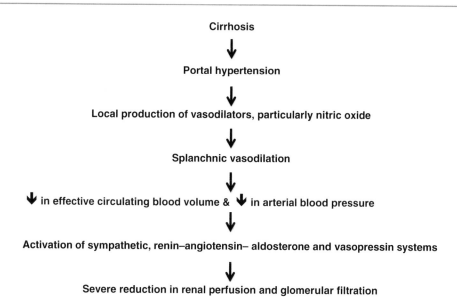

Cirrhosis

↓

Portal hypertension

↓

Local production of vasodilators, particularly nitric oxide

↓

Splanchnic vasodilation

↓

↓ in effective circulating blood volume & ↓ in arterial blood pressure

↓

Activation of sympathetic, renin–angiotensin– aldosterone and vasopressin systems

↓

Severe reduction in renal perfusion and glomerular filtration

Flow Diagram 4.3 Pathophysiology of HRS

sion and is associated with a poor prognosis [32, 33]. The pathophysiology of HRS is shown in Flow Diagram 4.3.

Arterial vasodilatation in the splanchnic circulation, triggered by excessive production of nitric oxide (vasodilator), plays a central role in the hemodynamic changes and decline in renal function and perfusion. Elevated levels of renal prostaglandins help in maintaining renal perfusion.

Although HRS is the most common differential diagnosis of acute renal dysfunction in cirrhotic, it only accounts for 23% of the cases of acute kidney injury in hospitalized cirrhotic patients. Thus, cirrhotic patients are also at high risk of other causes of renal dysfunction, such as parenchymal renal disease, sepsis, nephrotoxicity, and hypovolemia. In addition possibilities of co-existence of other comorbidities (glomerulonephritis, diabetic nephropathy, immunonephropathies associated with hepatitis C, amyloidosis, SLE, etc.) should be kept in mind. Individuals with cirrhosis are also at high risk for hypovolemia from other causes like gastrointestinal bleeding, use of diuretic and diarrhea resulting from lactulose or rifaximin administration.

HRS is classified into two types (Type 1 and Type 2) as per its presentation; however the

Table 4.2 Classification of HRS

Type-1 HRS	Type-2 HRS
• Rapidly progressive renal failure, typically represented by at least a doubling of serum creatinine over the course of 2 weeks	• Renal impairment that is less severe than that observed with type 1 disease
• More serious, median survival of 2–4 weeks without therapy	• Median survival is about 6 months
• Associated with failure of other organ system	• Presents with ascites that is resistant to diuretics

mechanism and pathophysiology remain the same in both the types (Table 4.2).

4.5.4 Pulmonary Complications

No risk factor other than presence of portal hypertension is associated with the presence of pulmonary complications in chronic liver disease and cirrhosis. The presence of vascular abnormalities in the setting of portal hypertension is the hallmark of pulmonary complications in cirrhosis [34, 35]. Two distinct types of vascular abnormalities have been recognized which affect the morbidity and mortality. These are named as hepatopulmonary syndrome (HPS) and portopulmonary hypertension (PPHTN). When these pulmonary complications are present in a patient, they overshadow the symptoms of liver disease.

HPS is defined by a triad of liver dysfunction, unexplained hypoxemia, and intrapulmonary vascular dilatation (IPVD). The diagnostic criteria are mentioned in Table 4.3.

Table 4.3 Diagnostic criteria for HPS

1. **Liver dysfunction**: Presence of portal hypertension
2. **Hypoxemia**: Room air partial pressure of oxygen (PO_2) <80 mmHg or alveolar–arterial oxygen gradient ($P_AO_2 - PaO_2$) ≥15 mmHg
3. **Pulmonary vascular dilatation**: Positive contrast echocardiography

The pathogenesis of HPS is not clearly defined. However various factors have been implicated as per different experimental studies [36–39]. The pathogenesis is shown in the Flow Diagram 4.4.

Pulmonary capillary dilation and less commonly direct arteriovenous connections are the pathogenic process of HPS, regardless of the mechanism. The resulting IPVDs are associated with HPS-related hypoxemia via ventilation-perfusion mismatch and oxygen diffusion limitation and rarely via shunt [35, 37].

PPHTN is defined as pulmonary hypertension that exists in a patient who has portal hypertension with no other known cause. The diagnostic criteria for PPHTN are mentioned in Table 4.4.

PPHTN occurs only in 2% of individuals with portal hypertension [1]. PPHTN is not related to the severity of the underlying liver disease or por-

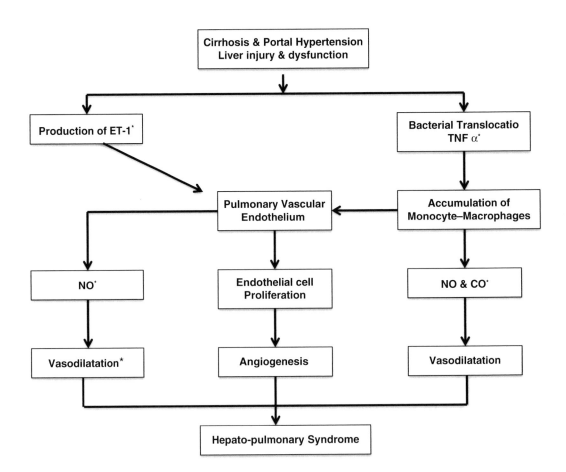

Flow Diagram 4.4 Pathogenesis of HPS. *ET 1* endothelin 1, *TNF α* tissue necrosis factor, *NO* nitric oxide, *CO* carbon monoxide

Table 4.4 Diagnostic criteria for PPHTN

1. Clinical evidence of portal hypertension
2. Mean pulmonary artery pressure (PAP) >25 mmHg at rest or >30 mmHg during exercise
3. Mean pulmonary artery occlusion pressure (PAOP) <15 mmHg
4. Pulmonary vascular resistance (PVR) >240 dynes/s/cm^5

tal hypertension. Female patients, autoimmune hepatitis, and chronic hepatitis C are the risk factors for the development of PPHTN.

Vascular proliferation as a reaction to the shear stress of chronically elevated cardiac output has been described as the most common theory regarding the pathophysiology of PPHTN. However increased association with female gender and autoimmune hepatitis suggest humoral and immunogenic mechanisms. Also, increased level of endothelin has been associated with PPHTN.

4.5.5 Hepatic Encephalopathy

Hepatic encephalopathy (HE) is a spectrum of potentially reversible neuropsychiatric abnormalities that can be associated with both acute and chronic liver failure. The manifestations varies from subclinical abnormalities to gross neurologic and behavioral derangements. The exact mechanism of brain dysfunction is still not known. However, it is not a single clinical entity and may be manifested as a result of a reversible metabolic encephalopathy, brain atrophy, brain edema, or any combination of these conditions.

HE is often associated with features of advanced and end-stage liver disease like ascites, hypoalbuminemia, hyperbilirubinemia, and coagulopathy. Failure of the diseased liver to adequately metabolize certain substances leads to accumulation of these neurotoxic substances responsible for neuropsychiatric abnormalities. Among the metabolic factors, ammonia is most commonly implicated; however there may be a role of inhibitory neurotransmission through gamma-aminobutyric acid (GABA) receptors in

the central nervous system and changes in central neurotransmitters and circulating amino acids [40].

4.5.5.1 Ammonia Hypothesis

The pathophysiology of how ammonia causes encephalopathy is illustrated in Flow Diagram 4.5.

Elevated levels of glutamate are responsible for the neuroexcitatory signs of HE whereas the neuroinhibitory state is due to the downregulation of glutamate receptors and inactivation of astrocyte glutamate transporters [40–42].

Although historically hyperammonemia has been attributed as the main cause of HE, severity of HE does not correlate with ammonia levels. Thus several other hypotheses are used to explain the mechanism of HE.

4.5.5.2 Impaired Neurotransmission Hypothesis

Increased tone of the inhibitory gamma-aminobutyric acid (GABA)A-benzodiazepine neurotransmitter system has been implicated in the development of HE; however contributing evidence are lacking to prove this hypothesis [43, 44]. Other endogenous GABA receptor agonists, oxidative stress, inflammatory mediators, and abnormal serotonin and histamine neurotransmission have been proposed to have a role in the pathogenesis of HE, but lack significant evidence.

4.5.6 Ascites

Ascites (defined as the pathologic accumulation of fluid in the peritoneal cavity) is the most common complication of cirrhosis. Portal hypertension is essential for the development of ascites. A portal pressure of >12 mmHg has been implicated in the pathogenesis of ascites. Various anatomical, biochemical, and pathophysiological abnormalities are responsible for the development of ascites in cirrhosis. Previously, underfill theory and overfill theory were popular for understanding the mechanism of ascites [45, 46]. However nowadays the arterial dilatation theory

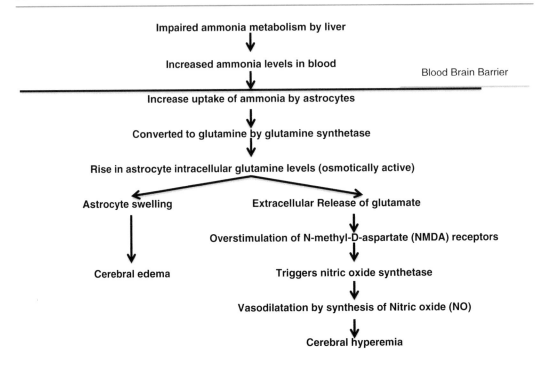

Flow Diagram 4.5 Pathogenesis of HE

is most popular and accepted theory explaining the formation of ascites [47, 48]. The various factors responsible for ascites in cirrhosis are mentioned in Table 4.5.

4.5.7 Varices

Varices, particularly esophageal varices, are one of the end results of portal hypertension. In cirrhosis, increases in portal pressure result from distorted hepatic architecture left in the wake of inflammatory insults. Fibrosis and regenerative nodules cause impedance to splanchnic flow through the liver and lead to the formation of portosystemic collaterals, particularly with the gastric and esophageal venous systems [49–51]. Rupture of the high-pressure collaterals that are formed is a highly lethal and feared complication of portal hypertension.

Chronic liver disease may be caused by varied etiologies but persistent or recurrent insult leading to inflammation remains the core stone of pathophysiology. Cirrhosis represents the last stage of this inflammation, where progressive

Table 4.5 Factors responsible for ascites

Circulatory factors	Vascular factors
• Reduced SVR	• Splanchnic vasodilatation
• Reduced arterial pressure	• Pulmonary vasodilatation
• Increased heart rate	
• Increased plasma volume	
• Reduced renal blood flow	
Functional factors	Biochemical factors
• Activation of systemic and renal vasodilator	• Sodium retention
• Activation of systemic vasoconstrictor	• Water retention
• Reduction in GFR	• Increased systemic nitric oxide
	• Increased systemic prostaglandin
	• Increased renal nitric oxide and prostaglandins

hepatic fibrosis causes distortion of the hepatic architecture and the formation of regenerative nodules. Initially these changes may be reversible; however it is irreversible in its advanced stages. Patients with cirrhosis are susceptible to a variety of complications due to the anatomical and physiological changes in the liver. The prognosis of cirrhosis is highly variable since it is influenced by a number of factors, including etiology, severity, presence of complications, and comorbid diseases.

References

1. Barash PG, Cullen BF, Stoelting RK, Chalan MK, Stock MC, Ortega R. Clinical anaesthesia. 7th ed. Philadelphia, PA: Lippincott Williams & Wilkins; 2013. p. 1294–325, Chapter 45.
2. McCuskey R. Anatomy of the liver. In: Boyer TD, et al., editors. Zakim and Boyer's hepatology: a textbook of liver disease. 6th ed. Philadelphia, PA: Elsevier Saunders; 2012, Chapter 1, Figures 1–11.
3. Ramadori G, Saile B. Portal tract fibrogenesis in the liver. Lab Investig. 2004;84:153–9.
4. Saile B, Ramadori G. Inflammation, damage repair and liver fibrosis-role of cytokines and different cell types. Z Gastroenterol. 2007;45:77–86.
5. Cassiman D, Libbrecht L, Desmet V, et al. Hepatic stellate cell/myofibroblast subpopulations in fibrotic human and rat livers. J Hepatol. 2002;36:200–9.
6. Gall EA, Dobrogorski O. Hepatic alterations in obstructive jaundice. Am J Clin Pathol. 1964;41:126–39.
7. Grisham JW, Nopanitaya W, Compagno J, Nägel AE. Scanning electron microscopy of normal rat liver: the surface structure of its cells and tissue components. Am J Anat. 1975;144:295–321.
8. Sambasivam H, Rassouli M, Murray RK, et al. Studies on the carbohydrate moiety and on the biosynthesis of rat C-reactive protein. J Biol Chem. 1993;26:10007–16.
9. Ramadori G, Rieder H, Sipe J, Shirahama T, Meyer, Büschenfelde KH. Murine tissue macrophages synthesize and secrete amyloid proteins different to amyloid A (AA). Eur J Clin Investig. 1989;19:316–22.
10. Stachura J, Galazka K. History and current status of Polish gastroenterological pathology. J Physiol Pharmacol. 2003;54:183–92.
11. Ramadori G, Moriconi F, Malik I, Dudas J. Physiology and pathophysiology of liver inflammation, damage and repair. J Physiol Pharmacol. 2008;59(Suppl 1):107–17.
12. Pinzani M, Rosselli M, Zuckermann M. Liver cirrhosis. Best Pract Res Clin Gastroenterol. 2011;25:281.54.
13. Ripoll C, Groszmann R, Garcia-Tsao G, et al. Hepatic venous pressure gradient predicts clinical decompensation in patients with compensated cirrhosis. Gastroenterology. 2007;133:481.
14. Tripodi A, Mannucci PM. The coagulopathy of chronic liver disease. N Engl J Med. 2011;365:147.
15. Intagliata NM, Argo CK, Stine JG, et al. Concepts and controversies in haemostasis and thrombosis associated with liver disease. Proceedings of the 7th International Coagulation in Liver Disease Conference. Thromb Haemost. 2018;118:1491.
16. Marks PW. Hematologic manifestations of liver disease. Semin Hematol. 2013;50:216.
17. Wölpl A, Lattke H, Board PG, et al. Coagulation factor XIII A and B subunits in bone marrow and liver transplantation. Transplantation. 1987;43:151.
18. Shah NL, Intagliata NM, Northup PG, et al. Procoagulant therapeutics in liver disease: a critique and clinical rationale. Nat Rev Gastroenterol Hepatol. 2014;11:675.
19. Hugenholtz GC, Macrae F, Adelmeijer J, et al. Procoagulant changes in fibrin clot structure in patients with cirrhosis are associated with oxidative modifications of fibrinogen. J Thromb Haemost. 2016;14:1054.
20. Qamar AA, Grace ND, Groszmann RJ, et al. Incidence, prevalence, and clinical significance of abnormal hematologic indices in compensated cirrhosis. Clin Gastroenterol Hepatol. 2009;7:689.
21. Fisher C, Patel VC, Stoy SH, et al. Balanced haemostasis with both hypo- and hyper-coagulable features in critically ill patients with acute-on-chronic-liver failure. J Crit Care. 2018;43:54.
22. Van Thiel DH, George M, Fareed J. Low levels of thrombin activatable fibrinolysis inhibitor (TAFI) in patients with chronic liver disease. Thromb Haemost. 2001;85:667.
23. Bedreli S, Sowa JP, Malek S, et al. Rotational thromboelastometry can detect factor XIII deficiency and bleeding diathesis in patients with cirrhosis. Liver Int. 2017;37:562.
24. Agarwal S, Joyner KA Jr, Swaim MW. Ascites fluid as a possible origin for hyperfibrinolysis in advanced liver disease. Am J Gastroenterol. 2000;95:3218.
25. Sinegre T, Duron C, Lecompte T, et al. Increased factor VIII plays a significant role in plasma hypercoagulability phenotype of patients with cirrhosis. J Thromb Haemost. 2018;16:1132.
26. Lisman T, Bos S, Intagliata NM. Mechanisms of enhanced thrombin-generating capacity in patients with cirrhosis. J Thromb Haemost. 2018;16:1128.
27. Lisman T, Bongers TN, Adelmeijer J, et al. Elevated levels of von Willebrand Factor in cirrhosis support platelet adhesion despite reduced functional capacity. Hepatology. 2006;44:53.
28. Palyu E, Harsfalvi J, Tornai T, et al. Major changes of von Willebrand factor multimer distribution in cirrhotic patients with stable disease or acute decompensation. Thromb Haemost. 2018;118:1397.
29. Moller S, Henriksen JH. Cardiovascular complications of cirrhosis. Gut. 2008;57:268.
30. Schepke M, Heller J, Paschke S, et al. Contractile hyporesponsiveness of hepatic arteries in humans with cirrhosis: evidence for a receptor-specific mechanism. Hepatology. 2001;34:884.

31. Ginès P, Schrier RW. Renal failure in cirrhosis. N Engl J Med. 2009;361:1279.

32. Ginès P, Guevara M, Arroyo V, Rodés J. Hepatorenal syndrome. Lancet. 2003;362:1819.

33. Wadei HM, Mai ML, Ahsan N, Gonwa TA. Hepatorenal syndrome: pathophysiology and management. Clin J Am Soc Nephrol. 2006;1:1066.

34. Rodríguez-Roisin R, Krowka MJ. Hepatopulmonary syndrome--a liver-induced lung vascular disorder. N Engl J Med. 2008;358:2378.

35. Grace JA, Angus PW. Hepatopulmonary syndrome: update on recent advances in pathophysiology, investigation, and treatment. J Gastroenterol Hepatol. 2013;28:213.

36. El-Shabrawi MH, Omran S, Wageeh S, et al. (99m) Technetium-macroaggregated albumin perfusion lung scan versus contrast enhanced echocardiography in the diagnosis of the hepatopulmonary syndrome in children with chronic liver disease. Eur J Gastroenterol Hepatol. 2010;22:1006.

37. Fussner LA, Iyer VN, Cartin-Ceba R, et al. Intrapulmonary vascular dilatations are common in portopulmonary hypertension and may be associated with decreased survival. Liver Transpl. 2015;21:1355.

38. Nunes H, Lebrec D, Mazmanian M, et al. Role of nitric oxide in hepatopulmonary syndrome in cirrhotic rats. Am J Respir Crit Care Med. 2001;164:879.

39. Carter EP, Hartsfield CL, Miyazono M, et al. Regulation of heme oxygenase-1 by nitric oxide during hepatopulmonary syndrome. Am J Physiol Lung Cell Mol Physiol. 2002;283:L346.

40. James JH, Ziparo V, Jeppsson B, Fischer JE. Hyperammonaemia, plasma amino acid imbalance, and blood-brain amino acid transport: a unified theory of portal-systemic encephalopathy. Lancet. 1979;2:772.

41. Sawhney R, Jalan R. Liver: the gut is a key target of therapy in hepatic encephalopathy. Nat Rev Gastroenterol Hepatol. 2015;12:7.

42. Vogels BA, van Steynen B, Maas MA, et al. The effects of ammonia and portal-systemic shunting on brain metabolism, neurotransmission and intracranial hypertension in hyperammonaemia-induced encephalopathy. J Hepatol. 1997;26:387.

43. Schafer DF, Jones EA. Hepatic encephalopathy and the gamma-aminobutyric-acid neurotransmitter system. Lancet. 1982;1:18.

44. Ferenci P, Püspök A, Steindl P. Current concepts in the pathophysiology of hepatic encephalopathy. Eur J Clin Investig. 1992;22:573.

45. Sherlock S, Shaldon S. The aetiology and management of ascites in patients with hepatic cirrhosis: a review. Gut. 1963;4:95.

46. Lieberman FL, Denison EK, Reynolds TB. The relationship of plasma volume, portal hypertension, ascites, and renal sodium retention in cirrhosis: the overflow theory of ascites formation. Ann N Y Acad Sci. 1970;170:292.

47. Solà E, Ginès P. Renal and circulatory dysfunction in cirrhosis: current management and future perspectives. J Hepatol. 2010;53:1135.

48. Ginès P, Fernández-Esparrach G, Arroyo V, Rodés J. Pathogenesis of ascites in cirrhosis. Semin Liver Dis. 1997;17:175.

49. Garcia-Tsao G, Groszmann RJ, Fisher RL, et al. Portal pressure, presence of gastroesophageal varices and variceal bleeding. Hepatology. 1985;5:419.

50. Lebrec D, De Fleury P, Rueff B, et al. Portal hypertension, size of esophageal varices, and risk of gastrointestinal bleeding in alcoholic cirrhosis. Gastroenterology. 1980;79:1139.

51. Garcia-Tsao G, Sanyal AJ, Grace ND, et al. Prevention and management of gastroesophageal varices and variceal hemorrhage in cirrhosis. Hepatology. 2007;46:922.

Pharmacokinetics and Pharmacodynamics of Drugs in Liver Disease

5

Aparna Pande, Rashmi Ramachandran, and Vimi Rewari

5.1 Introduction

Any therapeutic substance that is administered to the body undergoes metabolism and elimination. Metabolism is the biotransformation of all the endogenous and exogenous compounds within our body which converts them into water soluble substances which may be readily eliminated.

Pharmacokinetics is a term used to denote the fate of the drug in the body. This refers to the absorption, distribution, metabolism, and elimination of a drug as it passes through the human body. All these factors influence the final available concentration of the drug at the site of action. To make it simpler, it is termed as "what the body does to the drug." Pharmacodynamics refers to the effect of the drug on the body which is affected by the drugs affinity and action at its receptors. In general, it refers to "what the drug does to the body." First-pass metabolism refers to the metabolism of the drug before its entry into the systemic circulation, thereby reducing its bioavailability. The liver is an important site for first-pass metabolism.

Understanding clinical pharmacokinetics is important to enhance the efficacy and reduce the toxicity of the drug therapy while pharmacodynamic principles would help in understanding the interplay between the concentration of the drug at its receptor site and its pharmacological effect.

5.2 The Normal Liver

The liver is an intraperitoneal organ located in the right upper quadrant of the abdomen. It consists of a right and a left lobe. The liver has a dual blood supply by the hepatic artery and the portal vein. The portal blood flow is the major regulator of the vascular tone of the hepatic artery—a phenomenon termed as the "Hepatic arterial Buffer response" [1]. The hepatic arteries and portal veins divide to supply each lobe of the liver and converge at the sinusoids of the liver to supply blood to the hepatocytes. The hepatic sinusoids are low pressure vascular channels which consist of fenestrated endothelium which is essential for influx and efflux of various molecules into the perisinusoidal space of Disse. After draining the liver, the blood enters a central vein via the hepatic lobule, which eventually drains into the hepatic vein.

5.3 Role of Liver in Drug Metabolism

Disposition of most of the drugs relies on the functioning of the liver, which may be altered to varying extent in hepatic dysfunction. In order to

A. Pande · R. Ramachandran · V. Rewari (✉)
Department of Anesthesiology, Pain Medicine and Critical Care, All India Institute of Medical Sciences, New Delhi, India

understand the effect of hepatic impairment on drug xenobiotics, it is prudent to understand the basic role of the liver in metabolism as well as the factors affecting liver metabolism. The liver is the most metabolically active tissue in the human body. At physiological pH, most of the therapeutic agents are non-ionized or partially ionized. They undergo reactions in a phased manner which converts them into polar substances, which may then be excreted from the body. The endoplasmic reticulum of the hepatocytes is the major site of this biotransformation of drugs. It is abundant in microsomes, which contains the enzymes necessary for this process. The cytochrome P450 (CYP) system is one such membrane-bound oxidative enzymatic system, which is essentially a heme-containing protein [2]. The iron in this heme protein is the active site for binding with the drugs, which then undergo a series of reactions ultimately leading to the metabolism of the therapeutic substance. The human genome sequencing revealed the presence of 58 genes coding for the CYP proteins, and these genes are polymorphic in nature. These genetic polymorphisms are responsible for significant variations in drug metabolisms between individuals [3]. Many isoenzymes of the cytochrome P-450 exist, which have different activities, different tissue distribution, and variable drug affinities [4, 5]. Drugs undergo phase 1 and phase 2 reactions, either sequentially or only one and subsequently are excreted by transporters which are present on the membranes of canaliculi or hepatic sinusoids. This transport via canaliculi is often termed as the phase 3 reactions of xenobiotics [6].

Phase 1 reactions are essentially functionalization reactions. Lipophilic molecules undergo oxidation, reduction, or hydrolysis reactions via the mixed function oxygenases and are converted into hydrophilic moieties. Oxidation reaction involves insertion of a single molecule of oxygen within the parent compound. Examples of oxidative reactions include deamination, hydroxylation, dealkylation, dehalogenation, and epoxidation. This phase is also responsible for the generation of electrophilic substances and toxic-free radicals which may lead to cellular injury.

In phase 2 reactions, a parent drug can undergo phase 2 reactions directly or after it has been processed via the phase 1 pathway. These reactions are popularly termed as the "conjugation" reactions. These are responsible for addition of a polar ligand such as glucuronide, sulfate, glutathione, methyl group, acetate etc. Conjugation reactions occur within the cytosol of the hepatocytes and are mediated by transferases—enzymes which transfer the conjugating polar ligand to the compound undergoing the biotransformation [7].

Phase 3 reactions are responsible for the transport of the end products of metabolism into the bile [7]. These transporters are termed as ATP-binding cassettes (ABCs) [8]. The drug transport is mediated by ATP-hydrolysis, hence the name. The clinically important ABCs include the P-glycoprotein, the Bile Salt Exporter protein (BSEP), and the Multidrug Resistant proteins (MRP). The genes encoding for these transporter proteins are also susceptible to genetic polymorphisms, and variations of these proteins may play a role in the development of adverse drugs reactions as well as drug-drug interactions [9]. Some drugs are excreted in the bile initially but are reabsorbed from the small intestine—a phenomenon termed as "enterohepatic circulation" [10]. Enterohepatic circulation may lead to prolonged duration of actions of some drugs. Enterohepatic circulation may alter the bioavailability, volume of distribution, and clearance of a given drug. Furthermore, the liver being one of the important sites of first-pass metabolism, the amount of drug available at the receptor site is ultimately dependent on the functioning of the liver in case of drugs which have a high first-pass metabolism [11].

Hepatic drug clearance is defined as the volume of blood from which a drug is removed entirely by the liver per unit time. This is depended on two factors—the hepatic blood flow and the hepatic extraction ratio (Clearance = Blood flow × Extraction ratio) [12, 13]. Hepatic extraction ratio is the fraction of the drug which is "extracted" or removed during one pass of blood through the liver [14]. This is governed by the amount of unbound drug available and the intrinsic clearance of the liver. The effect of the hepatic blood flow on clearance of the drug depends on its hepatic extraction ratio. With increases in the blood flow to the liver, the extraction ratio declines for all drugs. Since the extraction ratio also depends on the amount of unbound drug available to the hepatocytes, the extraction ratio is also affected by the protein binding. Increasing hepatic blood flow causes a more rapid fall in the extraction ratios of drugs with low intrinsic clearance. On the basis of the efficiency of the liver in removing substances from the circulation, the extraction ratio is classified as high when it is more than 0.7 and low when it is less than 0.3. An extraction ratio of 0.3–0.7 is termed as intermediate. The hepatic clearance of drugs with high extraction ratios is limited by the blood flow and is indifferent to alterations in enzymatic activity or drug binding.

5.4 Consequences of Liver Disease on Pharmacokinetics

Pharmacokinetics of a drug broadly consists of drug absorption, distribution, and metabolism. The ability of the liver to metabolize a drug is dependent on both—hepatic blood flow and the enzymatic activity of the liver enzyme [15]. Hepatic dysfunction would impact both ultimately altering the drug disposition and its therapeutic effect. In hepatic dysfunction, both the hepatic blood flow and the activity of the cytochrome P-450 enzymes may be altered, and the effect of the two together may be synergistic. Acute liver insults primarily effect the hepatic blood flow while chronic liver diseases usually involve the enzymatic systems of the liver.

5.5 Drug Absorption

Patients with liver impairment have co-existing gastrointestinal dysfunction. Cirrhotic patients are known to have altered intestinal permeability which may have a bearing on the absorption

of orally administered drugs [16]. Furthermore, patients with severe hepatic dysfunction also exhibit delayed gastric emptying and abnormal intestinal motility which may influence the absorption of drugs administered enterally [17, 18]. The liver being the major determinant of the pre-systemic metabolism, drugs which are subjected to a high first-pass metabolism are invariably affected. However, this would not be applicable to drugs with low extraction ratio as the fraction of these drugs that is taken up by the liver from the blood during a single pass is already insignificant. Liver cirrhosis may lead to reduced activity of the enzymes involved in the first-pass metabolism. This in conjunction with portosystemic shunts would lead to reduced first-pass metabolism, thereby increasing the bioavailability of the drugs. Furthermore, in cirrhosis, there would be a decline in the clearance of the "flow-limited" drugs, thereby increasing the concentration of these drugs substantially. Therefore, such drugs need to have their dose modified in patients with hepatic dysfunction [19]. A classic example of this would be reduced oral dosing of labetalol and carvedilol in patients with liver cirrhosis due to decreased first-pass metabolism and reduced clearance [20, 21]. Another example is midazolam which has an oral bioavailability ranging from 34% to 68% as it is dose-dependent [22]. It undergoes first-pass metabolism by CYP3A enzymes and is 95% plasma protein bound. In advanced liver disease, there is more unbound form of the drug available due to reduced protein binding, greater oral bioavailability due to reduced pre-systemic metabolism, and increased half-life due to reduced clearance [23]. Pre-systemic metabolism is the major determinant of the oral bioavailability of midazolam. Gorski et al. showed that interindividual variations in the first-pass extraction of drugs such as midazolam which have a very high affinity for the CYP3A enzyme are basically a function of the intestinal enzyme activity [24].

5.6 Plasma Protein Binding and Drug Distribution

The distribution of a therapeutic substance within the body depends on the fraction of unbound form available. This in turn depends upon the binding of the drug in a reversible fashion with various macromolecules like blood cells and plasma proteins. The unbound fraction of drugs which have a high plasma protein binding to albumin or alpha-1 glycoprotein may change in advanced hepatic impairment. The reduced plasma protein binding may be multifactorial in origin—due to reduced protein synthesis, due to synthesis of altered proteins in liver disease, and due to presence of endogenous inhibitors of plasma protein binding like elevated bilirubin [25]. Increased unbound fraction due to reduced binding to plasma proteins may in turn affect the volume of distribution of these drugs. Increased unbound fraction is also the fraction which being pharmacologically active is cleared more rapidly through the liver or kidney. Therefore, hypoproteinemic patients may have increased proportion of drug which distributes into the tissues and does not stay within the circulation, thereby decreasing its therapeutic levels.

Liver cirrhosis predisposes the patient to development of anasarca—particularly ascites. This would significantly increase the volume of distribution of hydrophilic agents. For these drugs, in case a rapid action is desired, it may be achieved by increasing the loading doses as is seen in the case of antimicrobials belonging to beta-lactam and aminoglycoside classes [26]. Simultaneously, the increased volume of distribution translates into increased elimination half-life of the drug [27]. This increased half-life predisposes to the development of drug toxicity due to accumulation [14].

All these factors help in understanding the possible influence of hepatic dysfunction on drug pharmacokinetics but, owing to the variable extent of liver impairment and change in the pharmacodynamics of the drug as well along with extrahepatic mechanisms, contribute to an unpredictable drug effect and complicate the drug dose adjustments in patients with liver dysfunction.

5.7 Metabolism

The intrinsic hepatic clearance is primarily regulated by two factors—the efficacy of the hepatic enzymatic systems and the activity of the transporter proteins present in hepatic sinusoidal and canalicular membranes. Intrinsic hepatic clearance could be defined as the capability of the liver to remove unbound fraction of a drug from the blood in the absence of any blood flow limitations [7, 13]. However, with the onset of liver cirrhosis, even the blood flow to the liver gets impeded. This results in reduced presentation of the drugs to the liver, and drugs which predominantly dependent on hepatic clearance would be prone to accumulation.

Of the various pathways of drug metabolism, some are more affected than the others in liver disease. With the loss of functionally intact hepatocytes in liver disease, the synthesis of enzymes is also reduced. The cytochrome (CYP) mixed function oxygenases are affected more than those involved in the phase 2 reactions of the metabolism in an inconsistent and nonuniform way not in correlation with the hepatic blood flow [28].

Caffeine being completely metabolized by the hepatic CYP1A2 is used as a probe to evaluate the decline in the activity of this enzyme in hepatic derangements [29]. Furthermore, it has been demonstrated that the extent of hepatic impairment correlates well with the degree of decline in the activity of this enzyme [30]. Similarly, coumarin is utilized as a metabolic probe for evaluating the activity of the CYP2A6 which hydroxylates the parent compound [31]. After oral administration of coumarin, decreased urinary concentration of the hydroxylated metabolite was observed in patients with liver cirrhosis, which inversely correlated with their Child-Pugh scores [32]. Four isoenzymes have been identified in the CYP2C class which include CYP2C8, CYP2C9, CYP2C10, and CYP2C19. Metabolic probes for

CYP2C9 and CYP2C10 include Irbesartan, tolbutamide, and mephenytoin [33]. The study with these probes revealed that CYP2C9 is not affected significantly in patients with hepatic impairment. Mephenytoin is a racemic drug—with R-enantiomer being metabolized by the CYP2C9 and the S-enantiomer being metabolized by the CYP2C19 [34]. After oral administration of mephenytoin to patients with liver cirrhosis, there was a simultaneous decrease in oral clearance of its S-enantiomer along with reduced urinary excretion of its hydroxylated metabolite [35]. Again, this decline was associated with the extent of liver disease with patients with moderate cirrhosis exhibiting greater reductions in their clearance. The specific probe for evaluating CYP2D6 is debrisoquine. When the same group of patients were administered debrisoquine per orally, the metabolism was not altered significantly in hepatic impairment [35]. This further corroborates the fact that various enzyme systems are altered to varying extent in hepatic impairment, and extrapolating this knowledge to clinical circumstances may be very intricate. CYP3A activity is also reduced to varying extents in patients with liver disease—reduction of up to 30–50% has been reported in patients with nonalcoholic fatty liver disease [36]. Many drugs have been used as probes for this particular enzyme—commonly used one being MEGX (monoethylglycinexylidide) [37]. Huang YS injected intravenous lignocaine to patients with liver cirrhosis and chronic hepatitis and measured the concentration of its metabolite—MEGX. They found that the serum MEGX concentrations were inversely proportional to the Child-Pugh severity [38].

Subsequently a "sequential progressive model of hepatic dysfunction" was suggested [14, 29]. This model used the activity of various CYP enzymes to assess qualitative hepatic impairment. This model suggests that in mild degrees of hepatic impairment, only the activity of CYP2C19 will be impaired and the metabolites of CYP1A2, CYP2D6, and CYP2E1 would remain unaltered. But with progressive hepatic dysfunction as seen in decompensated cirrhotics, the clearance of drugs by all of these would be hampered. With intermediate level of liver dysfunction, the clearances would be dependent upon the extent to which the enzyme systems are affected. It is also important to remember that most of the genes coding for these enzymes are polymorphic in nature, and interindividual variation would be present to varying extents in patients with liver disease as well as healthy individuals [3].

That the impact of liver disease is primarily on the mixed function oxygenases or the phase 1 reactions and phase 2 reactions are not affected significantly is demonstrated by the clearance of various benzodiazepines. Midazolam and diazepam undergo phase 1 metabolism and their clearance is affected, whereas oxazepam, temazepam, and lorazepam undergo glucuronidation directly (phase 2 metabolism) and their clearance is not decreased in patients with liver cirrhosis [22, 39, 40]. The selective sparing of glucuronidation in liver dysfunction may be partially explained by upregulation of this enzyme in patients with liver disease, or by increased extrahepatic glucuronidation [41, 42]. However, of late this theory has also been questioned as patients with end-stage liver disease demonstrated impaired glucuronidation of many drugs including morphine, oxazepam, mycophenolate among others [43]. But the plausible explanation of this is that genetic polymorphism is seen in genes coding for UDP-glucuronyltransferases and various isoforms of this enzyme have also been identified [44]. Another possibility is that different isoforms of this enzyme may be affected to different extents in liver injury [45, 46].

Apart from enzyme inhibition, even enzyme induction may be altered in patients with liver disease. However, the number of human studies performed in this regard is limited, and animal studies conclude that the inducibility of enzymes would be affected both by the type of isoform under question and the nuclear receptor being evaluated [47].

The effect of transporter proteins on the disposition of drugs metabolized by the liver has been researched recently. The transported proteins are responsible for substances within the hepatocytes, as well as their efflux against a concentration gradient into the bile by ATP hydrolysis [8]. Due to fibrosis occurring within the space of

Disse in liver cirrhosis, the microvascular bed of the liver is occluded which impairs the uptake of macromolecules and drugs into the hepatocytes. This would be more applicable to drugs which are highly plasma protein bound as is seen in the case of propranolol [48]. Liver biopsy samples of patients with nonalcoholic steatohepatitis revealed altered expression and internalization of some of the transporter proteins which can possibly impair elimination of drugs predisposing the patient to adverse drug reactions [49].

5.8 Biliary Excretion

Cholestasis may be intra- or extrahepatic in nature. Intrahepatic cholestasis occurs due to functional impairment of the canalicular transport mechanisms. This is seen in cases of drugs like erythromycin and phenothiazines [50, 51]. Due to reduced secretion of bile, the elimination of drugs by the hepatobiliary route will decline, which has been observed in patients undergoing surgery for common biliary duct obstruction [52]. These patients demonstrated decreased biliary secretion of beta-lactams antibiotics, clindamycin, cephalosporins, and ciprofloxacin. Cholestasis may predispose to drug accumulation of such drugs. Additionally, the accumulation of these drugs may also indirectly lead to hepatocyte injury further aggravating the liver damage [53]. Simultaneously, cholestasis also has an inhibitory effect on some liver enzymes like the CYP2C and CYP2E1—thereby necessitating dose modification of drugs metabolized by these pathways in patients with cholestasis [54]. Pharmacokinetics of antineoplastic agents has been studied extensively in patients with cholestasis and dose adjustment for vinca alkaloids and doxorubicin is suggested in accordance with the bilirubin levels [55].

5.9 Drugs Undergoing Renal Excretion

Hepatorenal syndrome is a type of functional renal failure complicating the course of disease of patients with end-stage liver disease. It occurs due to abnormal circulatory and neurohormonal mechanisms. Splanchnic vasodilation mediated by nitric oxide and other vasodilators leads to reduced effective blood volume. This reduced effective blood volume leads to activation of the renin-angiotensin-aldosterone system (RAAS), release of arginine vasopressin, and stimulation of sympathetic nervous system. These neurohormonal vasoconstrictors increase the renal vasomotor tone leading to a dramatic decline in the glomerular filtration rate which leads to the pathogenesis of the hepatorenal syndrome [56]. Reduced renal excretion of some drugs which are otherwise excreted in an unchanged form by the kidneys has been reported in patients with decompensated liver cirrhosis—examples include diuretics and levetiracetam [57, 58]. The creatinine clearance estimated by the Cockcroft-Gault equation is also inaccurate due to cachexia in patients with cirrhosis as well as due to impaired creatinine synthesis; and cystatin-c may be a better marker in this cohort of patients [59, 60]. Thus, it would be prudent to remember that even drugs undergoing renal elimination may require dose modifications while administering them to a patient with severe hepatic insufficiency.

5.10 Consequences of Liver Disease on Pharmacodynamics

Pharmacokinetics and pharmacodynamics are not isolated processes and in clinical practice, both are inter-related and influence each other. Plasma protein binding has a significant effect on the pharmacodynamics of any drug as ultimately it is the unbound fraction which exerts pharmacological effects. Nonetheless, a significant number of alterations in drug effects are observed in patients with cirrhosis which cannot be explained by changes in pharmacokinetics alone. This deviation in drug behavior may be explained by altered receptor interactions, altered receptor affinity, and transformed intrinsic activity in diseased states. However, this is insufficient research on pharmacodynamic deviations in hepatic insufficiency. Altered receptor sensitivity is commonly observed in patients with liver disease. The two organ systems specifically prone to pharmacodynamic alteration include the brain and the kidney [15]. Patients with moderate to severe degrees of hepatic insufficiency are more sensitive to the psychoactive actions of opioids and benzodiazepines [61, 62]. Benzodiazepines and opioids are common precipitating factors of hepatic encephalopathy in patients with severe liver disease [63]. The concurrent administration of more than one class of sedative agents may therefore be hazardous to patients with significant liver pathology. Increased number of GABA receptors, altered GABA-ergic tone, and increased permeability to the blood-brain barrier are the postulated mechanisms of increased sensitivity to these agents. Accumulation of endogenous GABA-mimetic agents in patients with hepatic decompensation may also play a role as patients with hepatic encephalopathy demonstrate neurological improvement with the administration of flumazenil [64].

The response to diuretics in a cirrhotic patient is not so well elucidated. Diuretic resistance has been observed commonly in patients with cirrhosis—more so with furosemide [65]. When compared to healthy population, cirrhotics require a greater diuretic concentration to excrete similar amount of sodium. This alteration in their natriuretic potency could be due to reduced number of nephrons as well as due to the extent of response of each nephron to diuretic [66, 67]. Diuretic use in patients of cirrhotic ascites has also been associated with the development of hepatorenal syndrome [56]. The nephrotoxicity of aminoglycoside group of antibiotics is also enhanced in patients with severe liver derangements—the plausible explanation of this phenomenon being altered pharmacodynamics [68]. Cirrhotics are more prone to the renal toxicity of nonsteroidal anti-inflammatory drugs than the usual population [69]. Not only can they precipitate acute renal failure in these patients, but they can also cause gastrointestinal bleed, thereby predisposing the patient to development of hepatic encephalopathy.

The therapeutic effect of beta blockers is attenuated in patients with ascites and cirrhosis.

Cirrhotic patients exhibit downregulation of beta-adrenergic receptors which is also implicated in the development of cirrhotic cardiomyopathy [70]. It may be surmised that advanced liver disease results in reduced sensitivity of the beta-adrenergic receptors as is observed in the case of propranolol [71].

5.11 Assessment of Liver Function

The functional impairment of liver is difficult to assess. Various scores have been suggested to this effect [72]. The Child-Pugh scoring system is one such widely accepted tool which is used to assess the prognosis of chronic liver disease—specifically liver cirrhosis [73]. It incorporates five clinical variables which are assigned into three risk levels—and the final score is amalgamated into three clinical classes. The Child-Pugh score has been validated for prediction of mortality in patients with liver cirrhosis undergoing surgery [74]. It has also been validated as a prediction tool for survival in nonsurgical cirrhotic patients [75].

5.12 Child-Pugh Scoring System

Clinical/ biochemical indicator	Score 1	Score 2	Score 3
Serum bilirubin (mg/dL)	<2	2–3	>3
Serum albumin (g/dL)	>3.5	3.5–2.8	<2.8
Prothrombin time (s > control)	<4	4–6	>6
Encephalopathy grade	Absent	1 or 2	3 or 4
Ascites	Absent	Slight	Moderate

Total score according to severity is classified as:

- Group A—Mild—Total score of 5–6
- Group B—Moderate—Total score of 7–9
- Group C—Severe—Total score of 10–15

The MELD (Model for End-stage Liver Disease) score has also been used to prognosticate patients with liver cirrhosis. It comprises bilirubin concentration, serum creatinine values, coagulation parameter in the form of INR (International Normalized Ratio), and the cause of cirrhosis. The original score was used to predict 3-month survival in cirrhotics [76]. Subsequently the etiology of liver disease was dropped from the score as it was spurious or multifactorial in many patients [77]. Due to its accuracy in predicting short-term survival in chronic liver disease, it was adopted for use in prioritizing patients awaiting orthotopic hepatic transplantation. Subsequently the MELD-Na or the MELD-sodium score was developed to include serum sodium which is a marker of the severity of liver cirrhosis [78].

Dynamic tests to assess the liver function to predict the effect of various drugs in liver disease have also been suggested [79]. These tests involve administration of an exogenous substance which depends solely on the liver for its elimination. The concentration of the exogenous substrate in blood or of its metabolite in urine, serum, or exhaled breath is measured. The exogenous substrates with high extraction ratios would be flow-limited and those with low extraction ratios would be capacity-limited. These test compounds with high extraction ratio include indocyanine green (ICG), sorbitol, and galactose [80–82]. Co-administration of indocyanine green and sorbitol helps in approximating the extent of hepatic sinusoidal shunting [83]. The metabolic elimination of caffeine, midazolam, and antipyrine is exclusively dependent on the CYP isoenzymes and is not affected by hepatic blood flow or portosystemic shunting. These tests constitute "Dynamic Liver Function" tests and can be used to evaluate the metabolic hepatocellular dysfunction. Caffeine being primarily metabolized by the CYP1A2, the ratio of caffeine metabolite paraxanthine to caffeine is reduced in patients with liver disease in linear correlation with Child-Pugh scores [28, 84].

Breath tests have been used to assess the hepatic mitochondrial function [85]. The test compound in these tests incorporates isotopes of carbon—a ^{14}C atom or a ^{13}C atom which undergoes metabolism and the amount of the isotope is measured in the exhaled breath [86].

The ^{14}C-erythromycin breath test and ^{13}C-Methacetin breath tests are a few tests which have been used in research practice for this purpose [87–89]. More recently, nuclear imaging techniques have been suggested for the assessment of dynamic liver function [90]. ^{99m}Technetium labeled iminodiacetic acid (IDA) is frequently employed for this technique. These scintigraphic techniques provide information about global and regional hepatic blood flow and functioning. The liver is the sole site for ^{99m}Tc galactosyl human albumin (GSA), thereby making it a suitable agent to assess hepatic function [91]. Its uptake is not influence by elevated bilirubin concentration further promoting its applicability in cholestatic liver pathologies also.

The results of dynamic tests for liver function exhibit a linear correlation with the severity of Child-Pugh classification. However, these tests are not widely used in clinical practice owing to cost implications and requirement of specialized assessment techniques which may not be available in out of research situation. Furthermore, no test has been designated as the "gold standard" of dynamic liver function which is analogous to creatinine clearance in renal pathologies. The need of the hour is to develop such a dynamic test which measures the residual eliminating capacity of the diseased liver so that the drug dose modification could be done accordingly. Hence, clinical methods rely on the more readily available scoring systems like the Child-Pugh system to decide the dosage of drugs in hepatic disease. In such circumstances, due to lack of a model predicting dose modifications in hepatic insufficiency, therapeutic drug monitoring may be suggested for drugs with narrow therapeutic index [92]. This would be beneficial particularly when sicker patients may be exposed to a number of drugs, thereby increasing the potential for drug-drug interactions as well which cannot be predicted by a simplified pharmacokinetic-pharmacodynamic interaction model in diseased state [93]. Furthermore, despite recommendation by the US-FDA (Food and Drugs Administration) and the EMA (European Medical Agency), information about altered pharmacokinetics in liver disease is lacking [94]. Therefore, safe administration and optimal usage of drugs in hepatic insufficiency may be guided by therapeutic drug monitoring.

5.13 Conclusion

- Liver cirrhosis is characterized by reduced hepatic blood flow, portosystemic shunting of blood, decreased number and activity of functional hepatocytes, and hepatic sinusoidal capillarization.
- Liver disease reduces the pre-systemic metabolism, thereby warranting a dose reduction of drugs administered orally.
- Reduced uptake of drugs may occur into the liver due to reduced hepatic blood flow in patients with liver cirrhosis.
- Drugs with high extraction ratios are blood flow-limited and are insensitive to plasma protein binding or enzyme activity.
- Drugs with low extraction ratios are enzyme activity-limited and are dependent on protein binding along with intrinsic hepatic clearance.
- Drug metabolizing enzymes are not only polymorphic in nature accounting for the interindividual variations but are also affected differentially in liver disease.
- Volume of distribution of polar drugs may be altered in liver disease due to ascites and anasarca. This should be accounted for, particularly while administering loading doses of drugs like antimicrobials.
- Creatinine clearance is not a reliable marker for glomerular filtration in patients with hepatic pathologies as it overestimates the GFR.
- End-stage liver disease patients may be suffering from hepatorenal syndrome in which the excretion of the renally eliminated drugs will also be hampered, thereby necessitating appropriate dose adjustments for this phenomenon.
- The interplay between pharmacokinetic and pharmacodynamic interactions is complex, heterogenous, unpredictable, and drug specific; hence estimation of drug dose modification becomes difficult.

- Extreme vigilance is warranted while prescribing drugs with narrow therapeutic index to patients with severe degrees of hepatic insufficiency.
- Therapeutic drug monitoring could be utilized in patients with severe liver disease to ensure adequate drug exposure along with avoidance of drug toxicity.

Key Points
- Drug disposition depends on adequate functioning of the liver as it is the major site for metabolism of endogenous as well as exogenous substrates.
- Pharmacokinetics refers to the series of processes that a drug undergoes to reach its fate in the body. Pharmacodynamics is the effect of the drug on the body.
- Various steps of drug metabolism include uptake of drugs in the liver, phase 1 and 2 reactions, and transport into the bile followed by elimination.
- The impairment of drug metabolism usually correlates well with the extent of hepatocellular damage.
- Liver disease may lead to reduced hepatic blood flow, flow diversion in the form of portosystemic anastomosis, reduced first-pass metabolism, reduced metabolism and clearance, altered secretion, and prolonged half-life of drugs.
- Liver diseases are associated with varied and nonuniform reductions in activities of drug-metabolizing enzymes. Some enzymes are more affected than others.
- Pharmacodynamic alterations in liver disease are commonly manifested in the central nervous system and the kidney.
- Patients with end-stage liver disease may have concomitant renal dysfunction, necessitating dose adjustments for renally eliminated drugs as well.
- The complexities of the pharmacokinetic and pharmacodynamic interactions make it difficult to predict the therapeutic effect of drugs in diseased states.

References

1. Lautt WW. Mechanism and role of intrinsic regulation of hepatic arterial blood flow: hepatic arterial buffer response. Am J Physiol Gastrointest Liver Physiol. 1985;249(5):G549–56.
2. Nelson DR. The cytochrome P450 homepage. Hum Genomics. 2009;4(1):59–65.
3. Preissner SC, Hoffmann MF, Preissner R, Dunkel M, Gewiess A, Preissner S. Polymorphic cytochrome P450 enzymes (CYPs) and their role in personalized therapy. PLoS One. 2013;8(12):e82562.
4. Rendic S, Carlo FJD. Human cytochrome P450 enzymes: a status report summarizing their reactions, substrates, inducers, and inhibitors. Drug Metab Rev. 1997;29(1–2):413–580.
5. Guengerich FP. Human cytochrome P450 enzymes. In: Ortiz Montellano PR, editor. Cytochrome P450. Springer; 1995. p. 473–535.
6. Testa B, Krämer SD. The biochemistry of drug metabolism–an introduction: part 1. principles and overview. Chem Biodivers. 2006;3(10):1053–101.
7. Almazroo OA, Miah MK, Venkataramanan R. Drug metabolism in the liver. Clin Liver Dis. 2017;21(1):1–20.
8. Faber KN, Müller M, Jansen PL. Drug transport proteins in the liver. Adv Drug Deliv Rev. 2003;55(1):107–24.
9. Chandra P, Brouwer KL. The complexities of hepatic drug transport: current knowledge and emerging concepts. Pharm Res. 2004;21(5):719–35.
10. Roberts MS, Magnusson BM, Burczynski FJ, Weiss M. Enterohepatic circulation: physiological, pharmacokinetic and clinical implications. Clin Pharmacokinet. 2002;41(10):751–90.
11. Blaschke TF, Rubin PC. Hepatic first-pass metabolism in liver disease. Clin Pharmacokinet. 1979;4(6):423–32.
12. Wilkinson GR, Shand DG. A physiological approach to hepatic drug clearance. Clin Pharmacol Ther. 1975;18(4):377–90.
13. Rowland M, Benet LZ, Graham GG. Clearance concepts in pharmacokinetics. J Pharmacokinet Biopharm. 1973;1(2):123–36.
14. Verbeeck RK. Pharmacokinetics and dosage adjustment in patients with hepatic dysfunction. Eur J Clin Pharmacol. 2008;64(12):1147–61.
15. Blaschke TF. Effect of liver disease on dose optimization. International congress series. Amsterdam: Elsevier; 2001. p. 247–58.
16. Zuckerman MJ, Menzies IS, Ho H, Gregory GG, Casner NA, Crane RS, et al. Assessment of intestinal permeability and absorption in cirrhotic patients with ascites using combined sugar probes. Dig Dis Sci. 2004;49(4):621–6.
17. Verne GN, Soldevia-Pico C, Robinson ME, Spicer KM, Reuben A. Autonomic dysfunction and gastroparesis in cirrhosis. J Clin Gastroenterol. 2004;38(1):72–6.
18. Roland BC, Garcia-Tsao G, Ciarleglio MM, Deng Y, Sheth A. Decompensated cirrhotics have slower intestinal transit times as compared with compensated cirrhotics and healthy controls. J Clin Gastroenterol. 2013;47(10):888–93.
19. Delco F, Tchambaz L, Schlienger R, Drewe J, Krahenbuhl S. Dose adjustment in patients with liver disease. Drug Saf. 2005;28(6):529–45.
20. Homeida M, Jackson L, Roberts CJ. Decreased first-pass metabolism of labetalol in chronic liver disease. Br Med J. 1978;2(6144):1048–50.
21. Neugebauer G, Gabor M, Reiff K. Pharmacokinetics and bioavailability of carvedilol in patients with liver cirrhosis. Drugs. 1988;36(6):148–54.
22. Pentikäinen PJ, Välisalmi L, Himberg J-J, Crevoisier C. Pharmacokinetics of midazolam following intravenous and oral administration in patients with chronic liver disease and in healthy subjects. J Clin Pharmacol. 1989;29(3):272–7.
23. Trouvin J-H, Farinotti R, Haberer JP, Servin F, Chauvin M, Duvaldestin P. Pharmacokinetics of midazolam in anaesthetized cirrhotic patients. Br J Anaesth. 1988;60(7):762–7.
24. Gorski JC, Jones DR, Haehner-Daniels BD, Hamman MA, O'Mara EM Jr, Hall SD. The contribution of intestinal and hepatic CYP3A to the interaction between midazolam and clarithromycin. Clin Pharmacol Ther. 1998;64(2):133–43.
25. Delco F, Tchambaz L, Schlienger R, Drewe J, Krähenbühl S. Dose adjustment in patients with liver disease. Drug Saf. 2005;28(6):529–45.
26. Bartoletti M, Giannella M, Lewis RE, Viale P. Bloodstream infections in patients with liver cirrhosis. Virulence. 2016;7(3):309–19.
27. Roberts JA, Lipman J. Pharmacokinetic issues for antibiotics in the critically ill patient. Crit Care Med. 2009;37(3):840–51.
28. Villeneuve J-P, Pichette V. Cytochrome P450 and liver diseases. Curr Drug Metab. 2004;5(3):273–82.
29. Frye RF, Zgheib NK, Matzke GR, Chaves-Gnecco D, Rabinovitz M, Shaikh OS, et al. Liver disease selectively modulates cytochrome P450–mediated metabolism. Clin Pharmacol Ther. 2006;80(3):235–45.
30. Jodynis-Liebert J, Flieger J, Matuszewska A, Juszczyk J. Serum metabolite/caffeine ratios as a test for liver function. J Clin Pharmacol. 2004;44(4):338–47.
31. Pelkonen O, Rautio A, Raunio H, Pasanen M. CYP2A6: a human coumarin 7-hydroxylase. Toxicology. 2000;144(1–3):139–47.
32. Sotaniemi EA, Rautio A, Backstrom M, Arvela P, Pelkonen O. CYP3A4 and CYP2A6 activities marked by the metabolism of lignocaine and coumarin in patients with liver and kidney diseases and epileptic patients. Br J Clin Pharmacol. 1995;39(1):71–6.
33. Relling MV, Aoyama T, Gonzalez FJ, Meyer UA. Tolbutamide and mephenytoin hydroxylation by human cytochrome P450s in the CYP2C subfamily. J Pharmacol Exp Ther. 1990;252(1):442–7.

34. Brøsen K, Meyer UA, Goldstein JA. A multifamily study on the relationship between CYP2C19 genotype and s-mephenytoin oxidation phenotype. Pharmacogenetics. 1995;5(5):312–7.

35. Adedoyin A, Arns PA, Richards WO, Wilkinson GR, Branch RA. Selective effect of liver disease on the activities of specific metabolizing enzymes: investigation of cytochromes P450 2C19 and 2D6. Clin Pharmacol Ther. 1998;64(1):8–17.

36. Woolsey SJ, Mansell SE, Kim RB, Tirona RG, Beaton MD. CYP3A activity and expression in nonalcoholic fatty liver disease. Drug Metab Dispos. 2015;43(10):1484–90.

37. Oellerich M, Armstrong VW. The MEGX test: a tool for the real-time assessment of hepatic function. Ther Drug Monit. 2001;23(2):81–92.

38. Huang Y-S, Lee S-D, Deng J-F, Wu J-C, Lu R-H, Lin Y-F, et al. Measuring lidocaine metabolite—monoethylglycinexylidide as a quantitative index of hepatic function in adults with chronic hepatitis and cirrhosis. J Hepatol. 1993;19(1):140–7.

39. Ochs HR, Greenblatt DJ, Verburg-Ochs B, Matlis R. Temazepam clearance unaltered in cirrhosis. Am J Gastroenterol. 1986;81(1):80–4.

40. Kim JW, Phongsamran PV. Drug-induced liver disease and drug use considerations in liver disease. J Pharm Pract. 2009;22(3):278–89.

41. George J. Elevated serum β-glucuronidase reflects hepatic lysosomal fragility following toxic liver injury in rats. Biochem Cell Biol. 2008;86(3):235–43.

42. Tanaka Y, Kobayashi Y, Gabazza EC, Higuchi K, Kamisako T, Kuroda M, et al. Increased renal expression of bilirubin glucuronide transporters in a rat model of obstructive jaundice. Am J Physiol Gastrointest Liver Physiol. 2002;282(4):G656–62.

43. Hoyumpa AM, Schenker S. Is glucuronidation truly preserved in patients with liver disease? Hepatology. 1991;13(4):786–95.

44. Sugatani J. Function, genetic polymorphism, and transcriptional regulation of human UDP-glucuronosyltransferase (UGT) 1A1. Drug Metab Pharmacokinet. 2013;28:83.

45. Lin JH, Wong BK. Complexities of glucuronidation affecting in vitro-in vivo extrapolation. Curr Drug Metab. 2002;3(6):623–46.

46. Furlan V, Demirdjian S, Bourdon O, Magdalou J, Taburet A-M. Glucuronidation of drugs by hepatic microsomes derived from healthy and cirrhotic human livers. J Pharmacol Exp Ther. 1999;289(2):1169–75.

47. Palatini P, De Martin S, Pegoraro P, Orlando R. Enzyme inhibition and induction in liver disease. Curr Clin Pharmacol. 2008;3(1):56–69.

48. Gariépy L, Fenyves D, Kassissia I, Villeneuve J-P. Clearance by the liver in cirrhosis. II. Characterization of propranolol uptake with the multiple-indicator dilution technique. Hepatology. 1993;18(4):823–31.

49. Hardwick RN, Fisher CD, Canet MJ, Scheffer GL, Cherrington NJ. Variations in ATP-binding cassette transporter regulation during the progression of human nonalcoholic fatty liver disease. Drug Metab Dispos. 2011;39(12):2395–402.

50. Klaassen CD, Watkins JB. Mechanisms of bile formation, hepatic uptake, and biliary excretion. Pharmacol Rev. 1984;36(1):1–67.

51. Elferink RPO, Meijer DK, Kuipers F, Jansen PL, Groen AK, Groothuis GM. Hepatobiliary secretion of organic compounds; molecular mechanisms of membrane transport. Biochim Biophys Acta Rev Biomembr. 1995;1241(2):215–68.

52. Padda MS, Sanchez M, Akhtar AJ, Boyer JL. Drug-induced cholestasis. Hepatology. 2011;53(4):1377–87.

53. Pauli-Magnus C, Meier PJ. Hepatobiliary transporters and drug-induced cholestasis. Hepatology. 2006;44(4):778–87.

54. Bramow S, Ott P, Thomsen Nielsen F, Bangert K, Tygstrup N, Dalhoff K. Cholestasis and regulation of genes related to drug metabolism and biliary transport in rat liver following treatment with cyclosporine A and sirolimus (Rapamycin). Pharmacol Toxicol. 2001;89(3):133–9.

55. Tchambaz L, Schlatter C, Jakob M, Krähenbühl A, Wolf P, Krahenbuhl S. Dose adaptation of antineoplastic drugs in patients with liver disease. Drug Saf. 2006;29(6):509–22.

56. Erly B, Carey W, Kapoor B, McKinney J, Tam M, Wang W. Hepatorenal syndrome: a review of pathophysiology and current treatment options. Semin Interv Radiol. 2015;32(4):445–54.

57. Brockmöller J, Thomsen T, Wittstock M, Coupez R, Lochs H, Roots I. Pharmacokinetics of levetiracetam in patients with moderate to severe liver cirrhosis (Child-Pugh classes A, B, and C): characterization by dynamic liver function tests. Clin Pharmacol Ther. 2005;77(6):529–41.

58. Brater DC. Update in diuretic therapy: clinical pharmacology. Seminars in nephrology. Amsterdam: Elsevier; 2011. p. 483–94.

59. Woitas RP, Stoffel-Wagner B, Flommersfeld S, Poege U, Schiedermaier P, Klehr H-U, et al. Correlation of serum concentrations of cystatin C and creatinine to inulin clearance in liver cirrhosis. Clin Chem. 2000;46(5):712–5.

60. Caregaro L, Menon F, Angeli P, Amodio P, Merkel C, Bortoluzzi A, et al. Limitations of serum creatinine level and creatinine clearance as filtration markers in cirrhosis. Arch Intern Med. 1994;154(2):201–5.

61. Bergasa NV, Rothman RB, Mukerjee E, Vergalla J, Jones EA. Up-regulation of central mu–opioid receptors in a model of hepatic encephalopathy: a potential mechanism for increased sensitivity to morphine in liver failure. Life Sci. 2002;70(14):1701–8.

62. Hasselstrom J, Eriksson S, Persson A, Rane A, Svensson JO, Sawe J. The metabolism and bioavailability of morphine in patients with severe liver cirrhosis. Br J Clin Pharmacol. 1990;29(3):289–97.

63. Vilstrup H, Amodio P, Bajaj J, Cordoba J, Ferenci P, Mullen KD, et al. Hepatic encephalopathy in chronic liver disease: 2014 Practice Guideline by the American Association for the Study of Liver Diseases

and the European Association for the Study of the Liver. Hepatology. 2014;60(2):715–35.

64. Laccetti M, Manes G, Uomo G, Lioniello M, Rabitti PG, Balzano A. Flumazenil in the treatment of acute hepatic encephalopathy in cirrhotic patients: a double blind randomized placebo controlled study. Dig Liver Dis. 2000;32(4):335–8.

65. Keller E, Hoppe-Seyler G, Mumm R, Schollmeyer P. Influence of hepatic cirrhosis and end-stage renal disease on pharmacokinetics and pharmacodynamics of furosemide. Eur J Clin Pharmacol. 1981;20(1):27–33.

66. Schwartz S, Brater DC, Pound D, Green PK, Kramer WG, Rudy D. Bioavailability, pharmacokinetics, and pharmacodynamics of torsemide in patients with cirrhosis. Clin Pharmacol Ther. 1993;54(1):90–7.

67. Gentilini P, La Villa G, Marra F, Carloni V, Melani L, Foschi M, et al. Pharmacokinetics and pharmacodynamics of torasemide and furosemide in patients with diuretic resistant ascites. J Hepatol. 1996;25(4):481–90.

68. Moore RD, Smith CR, Lietman PS. Increased risk of renal dysfunction due to interaction of liver disease and aminoglycosides. Am J Med. 1986;80(6):1093–7.

69. Imani F, Motavaf M, Safari S, Alavian SM. The therapeutic use of analgesics in patients with liver cirrhosis: a literature review and evidence-based recommendations. Hepat Mon. 2014;14(10):e23539.

70. Møller S, Henriksen JH. Cirrhotic cardiomyopathy: a pathophysiological review of circulatory dysfunction in liver disease. Heart. 2002;87(1):9–15.

71. Caujolle B, Ballet F, Poupon R. Relationship among beta-adrenergic blockade, propranolol concentration, and liver function in patients with cirrhosis. Scand J Gastroenterol. 1988;23(8):925–30.

72. Forman LM, Lucey MR. Predicting the prognosis of chronic liver disease: an evolution from Child to MELD. Hepatology. 2001;33(2):473–5.

73. Child CG. The liver and portal hypertension. Philadelphia, PA: Saunders; 1967.

74. Garrison RN, Cryer HM, Howard DA, Polk HC. Clarification of risk factors for abdominal operations in patients with hepatic cirrhosis. Ann Surg. 1984;199(6):648–55.

75. Albers I, Hartmann H, Bircher J, Creutzfeldt W. Superiority of the Child-Pugh classification to quantitative liver function tests for assessing prognosis of liver cirrhosis. Scand J Gastroenterol. 1989;24(3):269–76.

76. Malinchoc M, Kamath PS, Gordon FD, Peine CJ, Rank J, ter Borg PC. A model to predict poor survival in patients undergoing transjugular intrahepatic portosystemic shunts. Hepatology. 2000;31(4):864–71.

77. Wiesner RH, McDiarmid SV, Kamath PS, Edwards EB, Malinchoc M, Kremers WK, et al. MELD and PELD: application of survival models to liver allocation. Liver Transpl. 2001;7(7):567–80.

78. Leise MD, Kim WR, Kremers WK, Larson JJ, Benson JT, Therneau TM. A revised model for end-stage liver disease optimizes prediction of mortality among patients awaiting liver transplantation. Gastroenterology. 2011;140(7):1952–60.

79. Rassam F, Olthof PB, Bennink RJ, van Gulik TM. Current modalities for the assessment of future remnant liver function. Visc Med. 2017;33(6):442–8.

80. Herold C, Heinz R, Niedobitek G, Schneider T, Hahn EG, Schuppan D. Quantitative testing of liver function in relation to fibrosis in patients with chronic hepatitis B and C. Liver. 2001;21(4):260–5.

81. Clemmesen JO, Tygstrup N, Ott P. Hepatic plasma flow estimated according to Fick's principle in patients with hepatic encephalopathy: evaluation of indocyanine green and d-sorbitol as test substances. Hepatology. 1998;27(3):666–73.

82. Marchesini G, Bua V, Brunori A, Bianchi G, Pisi P, Fabbri A, et al. Galactose elimination capacity and liver volume in aging man. Hepatology. 1988;8(5):1079–83.

83. Molino G, Avagnina P, Ballarè M, Torchio M, Niro AG, Aurucci PE, et al. Combined evaluation of total and functional liver plasma flows and intrahepatic shunting. Dig Dis Sci. 1991;36(9):1189–96.

84. Fuhr U, Rost KL. Simple and reliable CYP1A2 phenotyping by the paraxanthine/caffeine ratio in plasma and in saliva. Pharmacogenetics. 1994;4(3):109–16.

85. Wagner DA, Woolf GM. Breath test for assessing hepatic function. 1999.

86. Bonfrate L, Grattagliano I, Palasciano G, Portincasa P. Dynamic carbon 13 breath tests for the study of liver function and gastric emptying. Gastroenterol Rep. 2015;3(1):12–21.

87. Schmidt LE, Olsen AK, Stentoft K, Rasmussen A, Kirkegaard P, Dalhoff K. Early postoperative erythromycin breath test correlates with hepatic cytochrome P4503A activity in liver transplant recipients. Clin Pharmacol Ther. 2001;70(5):446–54.

88. Braden B, Lembcke B, Kuker W, Caspary WF. 13C-breath tests: current state of the art and future directions. Dig Liver Dis. 2007;39(9):795–805.

89. Petrolati A, Festi D, De Berardinis G, Colaiocco-Ferrante L, Di Paolo D, Tisone G, et al. 13C-methacetin breath test for monitoring hepatic function in cirrhotic patients before and after liver transplantation. Aliment Pharmacol Ther. 2003;18(8):785–90.

90. de Graaf W, Bennink RJ, Vetelainen R, van Gulik TM. Nuclear imaging techniques for the assessment of hepatic function in liver surgery and transplantation. J Nucl Med. 2010;51(5):742–52.

91. Kokudo N, Vera DR, Makuuchi M. Clinical application of TcGSA. Nucl Med Biol. 2003;30(8):845–9.

92. Sonne J. Drug metabolism in liver disease: implications for therapeutic drug monitoring. Ther Drug Monit. 1996;18(4):397–401.

93. Guaraldi G, Cocchi S, Codeluppi M, Di Benedetto F, Bonora S, Pecorari M, et al. Role of therapeutic drug monitoring in a patient with human immunodeficiency virus infection and end-stage liver disease undergoing orthotopic liver transplantation. Transplant Proc. 2005;37(6):2609–10.

94. Weersink RA, Bouma M, Burger DM, Drenth JPH, Hunfeld NGM, Kranenborg M, et al. Evaluating the safety and dosing of drugs in patients with liver cirrhosis by literature review and expert opinion. BMJ Open. 2016;6(10):e012991.

Viral Markers and Their Relevance in Liver Disease and Transplantation

Manav Wadhawan and Saurabh Argal

6.1 Introduction

Hepatitis is an inflammation of the liver, mainly caused by a viral infection. There are five principal hepatitis viruses, namely types A, B, C, D, and E. These viruses are quite divergent in their structure, epidemiology, route of transmission, incubation period, clinical presentations, natural history, diagnosis, and preventive and treatment options (Table 6.1). HAV and HEV are important because of the burden of illness they cause and the potential for outbreaks and epidemic spread. Hepatitis B and C are especially prevalent and lead to chronic hepatitis—the most important cause of liver cirrhosis and cancer [1]. Currently 240 million people are chronically infected with hepatitis B and 184 million people have antibodies against hepatitis C [1, 2].

The epidemiology, impact, and duration of the infection vary according to the type of virus as well as the route of transmission. Most people are asymptomatic and are unaware of having an infection that can result in liver cirrhosis and liver cancer.

The most common clinical consequence of infection with HAV or HEV is acute hepatitis and rarely acute liver failure (ALF). Patients with ALF have a high case-fatality rate, in the absence of liver transplantation.

Infections with HBV, HCV, or HDV viruses have the potential to cause chronic persistent infection, which may progress to liver cirrhosis or liver cancer and can become life-threatening. The risk of chronic infection with HBV is determined primarily by the age of acquisition of infection, being much higher when the infection occurs in infancy or early childhood and below 5% when it occurs in adults.

Liver transplantation (LT) is now a widely accepted lifesaving therapy for the complications of cirrhosis and acute liver failure. Before the availability of LT, medical management provided a temporizing measure but not a definitive cure for the complications of end-stage liver disease (ESLD). Cirrhosis resulting from chronic hepatitis C virus (HCV) infection remains one of the leading indications for LT. Without curative treatment before transplant, graft failure resulting from recurrent hepatitis B or C represents a major source of morbidity and mortality [3]. In this chapter we focus on hepatitis viruses and their implications on causation of liver disease as well as considerations for and after liver transplant.

M. Wadhawan · S. Argal (✉)
Institute of Digestive and Liver Diseases, BLK
Hospital, Delhi, India

© The Author(s), under exclusive license to Springer Nature Singapore Pte Ltd. 2023
V. Vohra et al. (eds.), *Peri-operative Anesthetic Management in Liver Transplantation*,
https://doi.org/10.1007/978-981-19-6045-1_6

Table 6.1 Nomenclature and features of hepatitis viruses

Hepatitis type	Size (nm)	Morphology	Genome	Classification	Antigen
HAV	27	Icosahedral, nonenveloped	ss linear RNA	Picornavirus	HAV Ag
HBV	42	Double shelled virion	Partially ds circular DNA	Hepadnavirus	HBsAgHBcA gHBeAg
	27	Nucleocapsid core			HBcAgHBeAg
	22	Virus coat material (spherical/filamentous)			HBsAg
HCV	40–60	Enveloped	ss linear RNA	Flavivirus	HCV C100-3 C33c C22-3 NS5
HDV	35–37	Enveloped hybrid (HBsAg coat + HDV core)	ss circular RNA	Defective virus (Delta agent)	HBsAg HDV Ag
HEV	32–34	Icosahedral, non-enveloped	Linear RNA	Hepevirus	HEV Ag

6.2 Hepatitis A Virus (HAV)

Hepatitis A virus is a 27 nm single-stranded RNA virus that belongs to the Picorna family of viruses and is the exclusive member of the genus *Hepatovirus* [4]. The viral particle is a non-lipid envelope structure that is resistant to ether, chloroform, and alcohol. HAV remains infectious after refrigeration and freezing and is resistant to heating at 60 °C for 30 min. However, it is inactivated by phenol, ionizing radiation, and formaldehyde. There is only one serotype of HAV and a single infection confers lifelong immunity. Genetic heterogeneity has resulted in seven different HAV genotypes (I to VII), where types I, II, III, and VII have been associated with human disease.

Symptomatology The majority of acute HAV infections are subclinical [5]. When symptoms do appear, they tend to be mild and nonspecific in nature. Most commonly they include fever, general malaise, fatigue, abdominal discomfort, and change in bowel habits. When severe, dark urine, pale stool, and jaundice may appear. The severity of acute HAV infections is proportional to the age of the patient, with younger patients tending to have milder disease than the elderly [6]. The overall mortality rates are only 0.1% in the general population as opposed to 1–2% in the elderly [7]. Hepatitis A infections do not progress to chronic hepatitis (defined as hepatitis persisting beyond 6 months) or cirrhosis [8].

Transmission HAV is an enterically transmitted disease, usually through the fecal-oral route, either through person-to-person contact or contaminated water or food (e.g., salad, fruits, shellfish). Person-to-person contact is the main route of spread of the virus, especially in children, adolescents, and young adults [9]. Foodborne outbreaks have been associated with uncooked food (usually related to shellfish ingestion) and contaminated water. Although the virus is present in blood, the limited amount of circulating virus and short duration of viremia render parenteral transmission of this virus extremely uncommon. Feces of infected individuals tend to contain the virus for a 2-week period prior to the onset of illness and for at least 2 weeks and perhaps as long as 3 months thereafter [10]. There are several reports of patients in pediatric hospitals and neonatal nurseries in particular who have transmitted HAV to health care workers [11–14].

Serology The serologic diagnosis of an acute hepatitis A infection is relatively straightforward. A positive IgM antibody to hepatitis A virus (IgM anti-HAV) indicates that infection with this virus has taken place within the past 3–6 months [15]. Shortly after the appearance of the IgM anti-HAV, IgG anti-HAV appears in the circulation. Unlike IgM anti-HAV, the IgG antibody persists for decades and indicates long-standing immunity against future HAV infections. Thus, individuals with acute HAV infections are IgM anti-HAV positive. There is very effective vaccine available against HAV. Those who are IgG

Fig. 6.1 Course of
acute hepatitis A

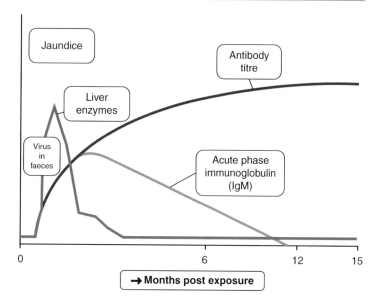

anti-HAV negative are susceptible to HAV and therefore candidates for vaccination.

Treatment of acute HAV infections is supportive, as the majority of cases resolve spontaneously without residual damage or sequelae. In those rare cases that progress to fulminant hepatic failure, liver transplantation should be considered (Fig. 6.1).

6.3 Hepatitis E Virus (HEV)

The hepatitis E virus is a single-stranded RNA virus belonging to the Calici virus family [16]. A positive anti-HEV test is used to establish the diagnosis [17]. Like HAV, HEV does not cause chronic liver disease and is spread by fecal/oral transmission [18–20]. Unlike HAV and other hepatotropic viruses, the mortality of acute HEV infections in pregnant women is high (15–20%) [21]. Phylogenetic analysis of human HEV isolates reveals 4 geographically distinct genotypes (genotypes 1 to 4) [22]. Genotype 1 includes isolates from Asia and Africa, and genotype 2 includes 1 strain from Mexico and some isolates from western Africa; both of these genotypes are restricted to humans and have been associated with waterborne disease outbreaks. On the other hand, genotype 3 and 4 cases account for less than 1% of cases of acute viral hepatitis.

Epidemiology and Transmission Two distinct epidemiologic patterns of infection and human disease caused by HEV are observed: (1) genotype 1 or 2 HEV disease in areas of high endemicity and (2) genotype 3 or 4 disease in areas of lower endemicity. Genotypes 1 and 2 are frequent in developing countries of Asia (Indian subcontinent, southeast and central Asia), the Middle East, Africa, parts of South America and Mexico [23, 24]. In these areas, human HEV infection occurs in the form of disease outbreak [24–26] and frequent cases of sporadic disease. Characteristically, with genotype 1 and 2 infection, the rates of disease and mortality are high in pregnant women. Hepatitis E virus (usually genotype 1 and 2) is transmitted mainly via fecal-oral route, with fecally contaminated water providing the most common route of transmission.

The cases in low-endemicity areas have mostly been related to HEV genotype 3. The source and route of infection in hepatitis E in areas of low endemicity remain unclear. The available evidence suggests that most such cases are related to zoonotic transmission from pigs (or other animals) by the oral route. Such transmission could occur through consumption of undercooked animal meat, close contact with infected animals, or contamination of water supplies from animal feces.

Symptomatology The most common recognizable form of HEV genotype 1 and 2 infection is **acute** icteric hepatitis, with clinical features resembling acute hepatitis A or B. Acute hepatitis E is usually self-limited. A few patients have a prolonged course with marked cholestasis (cholestatic hepatitis), including persistent jaundice lasting 2 to 6 months, prominent itching, and marked elevation of the serum alkaline phosphatase level, ultimately with spontaneous resolution. In a small proportion of patients, the disease is severe and associated with subacute or fulminant hepatic failure. **Pregnant women**, particularly those in the second or third trimester, are affected more frequently during hepatitis E outbreaks than are others in the population and have a worse outcome, with mortality rates of 5% to 25%. In an epidemic in Kashmir, India, clinical hepatitis E developed in 17.3% of pregnant women (8.8%, 19.4%, and 18.6% of those in trimesters 1, 2, and 3, respectively), compared with 2.1% of nonpregnant women and 2.8% of men of similar age [27]. Fulminant hepatic failure developed in approximately 22% of the affected pregnant women, with an increased frequency of abortions, stillbirths, and neonatal deaths. **Chronic Hepatitis E** infection, with persistent viremia and fecal excretion lasting for several months to years, can occur in areas of low endemicity and have been associated with HEV genotype 3 infection [28]. Such persistent infection is seen commonly (but not exclusively) in immunosuppressed patients, including organ transplant recipients, those receiving cancer chemotherapy, and HIV-infected persons.

Serology The diagnosis of human HEV infection is based either on detection of HEV RNA in stool and serum specimens using a reverse transcription-PCR assay [29]. IgM anti-HEV is a surrogate marker of acute infection and is more commonly used to diagnose acute HEV hepatitis (Fig. 6.2). The presence in serum of IgM anti-HEV strongly suggests acute infection, whereas detection of IgG anti-HEV indicates the convalescent phase or past infection. IgM anti-HEV appears in the early phase of clinical illness, lasts 4 to 5 months, and can be detected in 80% to 100% of cases during

Fig. 6.2 Course of acute hepatitis E

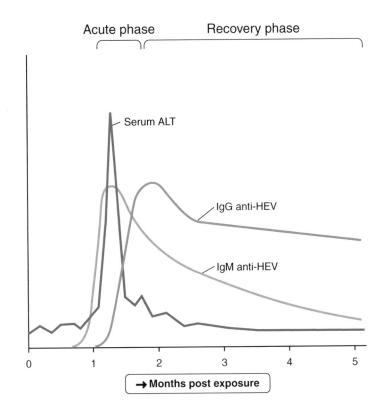

outbreaks. IgG anti-HEV appears a few days after IgM anti-HEV and remains detectable for at least one to several years. In contrast to HAV, IgM HEV does not provide immunity against subsequent infections. Also currently, there is no vaccine available for hepatitis E.

Treatment of acute HAV infections is supportive, as the majority of cases resolve spontaneously without residual damage or sequelae. In those rare cases that progress to fulminant hepatic failure, liver transplantation should be considered.

6.4   Hepatitis B Virus (HBV)

The hepatitis B virus is a 42 nm, double-stranded DNA virus that belongs to the Hepadnaviridae (Hepatitis DNA) family of viruses [30]. HBV is a small (3.2-kilobase [kb]) virus with a DNA genome that has a relaxed, circular, partially double-stranded configuration. It has an incubation period of 40–160 days (75 days on average).

6.4.1   Epidemiology

The prevalence of infection varies geographically and can be divided into areas of low (less than 2%), intermediate (2–8%), and high (more than 8%) endemicity (Fig. 6.3).

6.4.2   Transmission

Perinatal transmission and horizontal spread among children are the major means of transmission in high-risk areas while sexual transmission and injection drug abuse are common means of transmission in low-risk areas.

The epidemiology, impact, and duration of the infection vary according to the type of virus as well as the **route of transmission**. The main routes are blood transfusion, injection with contaminated material, iv drug abuse, transmission from mother to child at birth, and sexual activity. Most people are asymptomatic and are unaware of having an infection that can result in liver cirrhosis and liver cancer.

HBV infection (Table 6.2; Fig. 6.4) in adults can present as acute hepatitis, chronic hepatitis, and an "inactive disease" state. By definition, the acute hepatitis phase represents the first 6 months of the infection. During this phase, patients are often asymptomatic or have nonspecific complaints similar to those described with mild HAV infections [31, 32]. HBsAg, IgM anti-HBc, and HBeAg testing are frequently positive during this phase of the illness. If the infection is contracted in adulthood, in 90–95% cases acute hepatitis resolves spontaneously and patients develop natural immunity (seroconvert from HBsAg to anti-HBs positive). The more severe the acute hepatitis, the more likely this is to occur [31]. Unfortunately, if infection is contracted in

Fig. 6.3 Prevalence of HBV infection worldwide

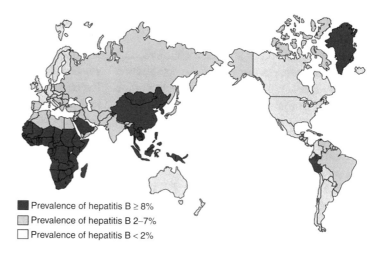

- Prevalence of hepatitis B ≥ 8%
- Prevalence of hepatitis B 2–7%
- Prevalence of hepatitis B < 2%

Table 6.2 Natural history of viral hepatitis

Features	HAV	HBV	HCV	HDV	HEV
IP (mean)	30 days	60–90 days	50 days	60–90 days	40 days
Onset	Acute	Insidious	Acute	Insidious	Acute
Age	Child and young	Young adults	Any age	Any age	Young adults
Severity	Mild	Occ severe	Moderate	Occ severe	Mild
Fulminant	0.1%	0.1–1%	0.1%	5–20%	1–2%
Chronicity	None	1–10%	85%	Common	None
Cancer	None	+	+	±	None
Prognosis	Excellent	Worse with age	Moderate	Acute-good chronic-poor	Good

	CHRONIC INFECTION		CHRONIC HEPATITIS	
	HBeAg Positive	HBeAg Negative	HBeAg Positive	HBeAg Negative
HBsAg	High	Low	High/ Intermediate	Intermediate
HBeAg	Positive	Negative	Positive	Negative
HBV DNA	$>10^7$ IU/ml	<2000 IU/ml	10^4-10^7 IU/ml	>2000 IU/ml
ALT	Normal	Normal	Elevated	Elevated
Liver Disease	None/Minimal	None	Moderate/Severe	Moderate/Severe

Fig. 6.4 Natural course of patients with chronic HBV infection based upon HBV and liver disease markers

infancy or childhood, only 5–10% of patients resolve their infection (>90% continuing to develop chronic infection). Adolescents have an intermediate likelihood of spontaneously resolving their infection. If the HBsAg remains positive for 6 months after the onset of the illness or is documented to be positive on two occasions 6 months apart, the individual almost certainly has a chronic HBV infection.

Chronic HBV infection, once established, is a dynamic process reflecting the interaction between HBV replication and the host immune response. Chronic HBV infection is not synonymous with chronic hepatitis B (CHB), as will be clear from the following discussion. The natural history of chronic HBV infection has been divided into five phases, taking into account the presence of HBeAg, HBV DNA levels, alanine aminotransferase (ALT) values, and eventually the presence or absence of liver inflammation (Fig. 6.1). The new nomenclature is based on the description of the two main characteristics of chronicity: infection vs. hepatitis.

The first phase is **Immune Tolerant phase** also known as Replicative phase, characterized by HBsAg and HBeAg positivity, normal or near-normal enzymes with high HBV DNA levels. This is followed by **Immune Clearance/reactive phase**, also known as Immunoactive phase, characterized by HBsAg and HBeAg positivity, elevated enzymes with elevated HBV DNA levels. Eventually, symptoms resolve, liver enzymes return to normal or near-normal values, and the patient seroconverts from HBeAg to anti-HBe positive, indicating entry into the third phase of the infection, the **"inactive disease" state**. The inactive disease state tends to last from years to decades. During this phase, patients are largely asymptomatic, have normal or near-normal liver enzyme levels, are HBeAg negative, have low or undetectable levels of HBV DNA in the blood, and, if biopsied, have little evidence of active inflammation. The major complications of the hepatitis B carrier state—cirrhosis and hepatocellular carcinoma—tend to occur in approximately 30% and 15% of cases respectively [33, 34]. The inactive carrier state may either result in clearance of HBsAg or more commonly may progress to reactivation of HBV replication leading to chronic hepatitis and further liver damage. When cirrhosis does develop, it is often present during the chronic hepatitis phase, whereas hepatocellular carcinoma tends to be diagnosed during the late chronic hepatitis or inactive disease phase of the infection. In a small proportion of patients with inactive disease (around 5%), HBsAg disappears and anti-HBs appears marking resolution of the infection.

Maternal–infant transmission is the most common route of HBV infections in the world at the present time, in industrialized nations, parenteral drug abuse and needle stick exposures represent significant high-risk activities [35]. Needle stick exposures involving blood from an individual with high levels of viral replication (HBeAg positive or high HBV DNA levels) tend to result in HBV infections occurring in approximately 60% of cases. When the infection in the source is not actively replicating (HBeAg negative or low HBV DNA levels), the figure falls to approximately 30% [36]. In addition to the size of the inoculum, features of the needle itself, hollow or solid, appear to be important factors influencing the risk of viral transmission [37, 38]. The prevalence of HBV infection among health care workers is threefold to fivefold higher than the general population, with surgeons (particularly orthopedic surgeons and gynecologists) and dentists having the highest reported rates [39, 40].

6.4.3 Serology/Serological Markers

HBV diagnosis is accomplished by testing for a series of serological markers of HBV and by additional testing to exclude alternative etiological agents such as hepatitis A and C viruses. Serological tests are used to distinguish acute, self-limited infections from chronic HBV infections and to monitor vaccine-induced immunity.

The various serological markers for diagnosis of hepatitis B are:

1. **HBsAg (Hepatitis B surface antigen)**
   HBsAg is the **first serological** marker after infection (HBV DNA is the first marker). The antigen is detectable before the liver enzymes elevation and onset of clinical illness. In the typical case of acute hepatitis, it disappears within 2 months of start of clinical illness. If it lasts for more than 6 months, the infection is defined as chronic infection.

2. **Anti-HBs (Antibody to HBV surface antigen)**
   This antibody appears when HBsAg is no longer detectable. It is a protective antibody and **indicates immunity to HBV** either through past infection or through vaccination. The protective level of anti-HBs antibodies is defined as ≥ 10 mIU/ml.

3. **Anti-HBc (Antibody to HBV core antigen)**
   The anti-HBc **IgM** appears in the serum a week or two after the appearance of HBsAg and is therefore the **earliest antibody marker to be seen in blood.** The anti-HBc**IgG** antibody possibly persists for life and is therefore a useful indicator of prior infection with HBV. **IgM anti-HBc is seen in acute infections** but is replaced by IgG HBc in 6 months after HBV infection. **IgG anti-HBc is the most reliable marker for previous HBV infection;** it persists when anti-HBs titers decline to undetectable levels many years following recovery from HBV infection.

4. **HBeAg**
   It appears in the blood concurrently with HBsAg, or soon afterwards and generally disappears within several weeks in acute, resolving cases. It is an **indicator of active intrahepatic viral replication;** therefore its presence in blood means that the **person is highly infectious.** Its disappearance is followed by appearance of anti-HBe. Testing for HBeAg is not necessary in most cases of acute hepatitis B; however, testing of HBeAg is of value in chronic hepatitis B (where HBeAg is an important marker of viral replication). However, the **absence of HBeAg does not preclude active viral replication.**

5. **Anti-HBe**

Its presence in blood **denotes low infectivity.** It has **prognostic implication** as appearance of anti-HBe in acute hepatitis B implies a high likelihood that HBV infection will resolve spontaneously.

6.4.4 Occult Hepatitis B Infection (OBI)

This refers to presence of HBV DNA in circulating blood without detectable HBsAg. Anti-HBe may disappear and the only detectable marker would be anti-HB core in addition to HBV DNA. The clinical implication of this fact is that anyone who is positive for anti-HBc antibody without any other serological markers for HBV should be tested with HBV DNA in transplant scenario (donor or recipient).

6.4.5 Transplantation for Hepatitis B

Hepatitis B virus (HBV) associated chronic or fulminant liver disease is a common indication for LT across the world [41, 42].

Historically, the risk of HBV reactivation after liver transplant for HBV-related liver disease was >80% (in the absence of prophylaxis with antivirals) [43, 44]. Over the last 2 decades there have been major advances in the management of HBV transplant candidates. With the combination prophylaxis of hepatitis B immune globulin (HBIg) and nucleos(t)ide analogs, administered before and after transplantation, post-transplant survival in patients with hepatitis B has risen to more than 80% at 5 years and recurrence rates below 5% [45, 46]. However, HBIG is very expensive and inconvenient (intravenous or intramuscular use) for patients. This has led to the development of alternative strategies aiming to reduce the dose and duration of HBIG or recently to abolish HBIG use with monotherapy of nucleos(t)ide analogs having high barrier to resistance (Entecavir (ETV), Tenofovir (TDF), or Tenofovir Alafenamide).

6.4.5.1 Risk Factors for HBV Recurrence after Liver Transplant

The main risk factors for HBV recurrence are as follows:

- High pretransplant HBV viral load (i.e., HBV DNA > 10^3 IU/mL) [8, 19–23].
- Infection with LAM-resistant HBV virions (YMDD variants) increases the risk for recurrence regardless of viral load [47, 48].
- HCC at LT.
- Chemotherapy used for HCC is independently associated with an increased risk for HBV recurrence [48–51].

Factors associated with **low rates of recurrence are** surrogate markers for low levels of viral replication and include:

- Negative hepatitis B e antigen (HBeAg) status at listing.
- Low HBV DNA $\leq 10^3$
- Fulminant HBV
- HDV coinfection

6.4.5.2 Prophylaxis for Prevention of Hepatitis B Virus (HBV) Graft Recurrence Following Liver Transplantation

Antiviral Monotherapy

Entecavir (ETV) and Tenofovir (TDF), antivirals with high barrier to resistance, have been evaluated as a prophylactic therapy. The drug should be started before transplantation to achieve an undetectable HBV DNA before transplant and continued after transplantation without HBIg with excellent 1, 3, and 5 years outcome in terms of recurrence rate as well as survival [53]. Nucleos(t)ide monotherapy is the standard of care for prophylaxis of patients at low risk of HBV recurrence after liver transplant.

Fung et al. [60] investigated the efficacy of ETV as monoprophylaxis in 80 patients with chronic hepatitis B who received a liver transplant. A total of 18 patients (22.5%) had persistent HBsAg positivity after transplant without seroclearance (n = 8) or reappearance of HBsAg after initial seroclearance ($n = 10$). Seventeen patients had undetectable levels of HBV DNA at the time of last follow-up. The remaining patient had a very low HBV DNA level of 217 copies/mL at 36 months after LT.

6.4.5.3 Prophylaxis for Prevention of Hepatitis B Virus (HBV) Graft Recurrence Following Liver Transplantation (LT)

Combination Prophylaxis

The use of antivirals with high resistance barrier before transplantation followed by a combination of antivirals and HBIG after LT minimizes risk for reinfection (Fig. 6.5). With this combination approach the HBV recurrence rate at 1–2 years after transplantation has been reduced to <10%. Combination prophylaxis is currently recommended for patients at high risk of recurrence after liver transplant. Originally, HBIG used to be given intraoperatively during the anhepatic phase, followed postoperatively as intravenous injections to be continued lifelong. A combination of high potency oral antivirals with HBIG has been recommended based on various meta-analysis [52–54]. However, all these meta-analyses have mostly included studies where lamivudine and/or adefovir have been used. With the currently available evidence, it is safe to recommend usage of low-dose HBIG (800 IU intraoperatively, followed by 400–800 IU daily for 7 days and then monthly) in patients who are DNA positive at the time of transplant [55, 56].

There is enough evidence now to discontinue HBIG shortly after liver transplant. HBIG withdrawal has been shown to be safe and does not increase recurrence of HBV infection [57–60]. HBIG withdrawal has been done as early as on first postoperative day after transplant. However, most centers would withdraw HBIG after 1 year provided the patients are HBsAg as well HBV DNA negative.

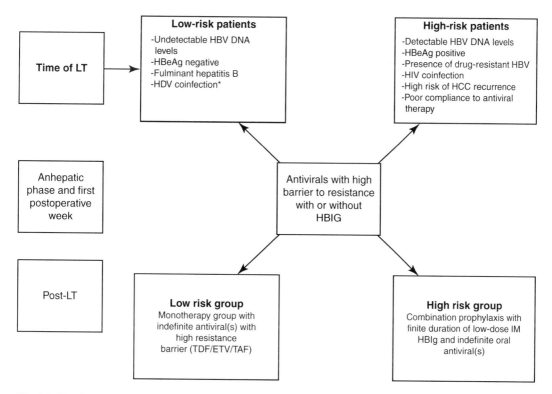

Fig. 6.5 Prophylaxis for prevention of HBV graft recurrence following liver transplantation

6.4.6 Antiviral Monotherapy

With the use of high potency antivirals like tenofovir and entecavir, the need for HBIg in the immediate post-transplant period has been questioned. There are many studies that have not used HBIg at all in the immediate post-transplant period [61–63]. All these studies have reported HBV recurrence rates of <10% which are comparable to HBIG regimens. With the available evidence, we would recommend that HBIG could be omitted in patients who are at low risk of recurrence (low or negative HBV DNA at the time of transplant).

With the excellent outcomes and cost effectiveness of antiviral monotherapy (Entecavir (ETV) and/or Tenofovir), it has become standard treatment in many transplant centers across the world.

6.5 Hepatitis D Virus (HDV)

Delta hepatitis agent or HDV, the only member of the genus Deltavirus, is a **defective RNA virus** that co-infects with and requires the helper function of HBV (or other hepadnaviruses) for its replication and expression. Slightly smaller than HBV, delta is 35- to 37-nm virus with a hybrid structure. Its nucleocapsid expresses delta antigen. The delta core is "encapsidated" by an outer envelope of HBsAg. **Chronicity**: There are 100% chances **of chronicity** in patients with **HDV superinfection over HBV** (HBV-HDV coinfection have **1–10% chances**), while perinatal HBV and HCV have 90% and 85% chances of chronicity, respectively. The highest chances of viral hepatitis to culminate into FHF (fulminant hepatic failure) are with HDV superinfection over preexisting HBV infection while HBV-HDV coinfection has 5% chances for FHF.

6.5.1 Laboratory Diagnosis

The diagnosis of HDV infection is done by antibody to HDV antigen (**anti-HDV**), detected by EIA or RIA. The presence of IgM anti-HDV does not distinguish acute from chronic HDV infection, as IgM anti-HDV also persists in chronic infection and high titers are often found in patients with severe liver inflammation. HBV-HDV **coinfection** is diagnosed on the **detection of anti-HDV** in serum in association **with HBsAg or IgM anti-HBc** (as IgM anti-HBc may sometimes be the only marker of HBV infection in this setting as HDV suppresses HBV replication).

HDV **superinfection** in chronic hepatitis B is diagnosed by presence of anti-HDV in a patient who harbors HBsAg and IgG anti-HBc. HDV antigen in the liver (by IEM) and HDV RNA in serum and liver can be detected during HDV replication but are not routinely used for diagnosis.

6.5.2 Liver Transplantation in Patients with Hepatitis D Virus Liver Cirrhosis

Around 5% of the chronic carriers of HBV worldwide have serological evidence of exposure to HDV. HDV coinfection is associated with more severe disease and a higher incidence of cirrhosis than HBV monoinfection [64, 65]. Some European studies have demonstrated a threefold and twofold risk increase, respectively, for developing HCC and for death in HDV patients compared with HBV monoinfected patients [66]. Patients chronically infected with HBV and HDV are less at risk for HBsAg reappearance after transplantation than patients infected with HBV alone and have better post-transplant survival (with or without HBV prophylaxis) [67]. The lower risk for recurrence among the patients with HDV cirrhosis could be explained by the fact that 70% to 90% of patients with HDV coinfection are HBeAg negative, and most have low serum HBV DNA levels because of the inhibitory effect of HDV on HBV replication.

Prevention of Recurrence After LT   The strategies for prevention of HBV + HDV recurrence are same as those for HBV recurrence (discussed in the previous section). In view of low risk of recurrence after LT, potent nucleos(t)ide mono-therapy is preferred over HBIG combination.

6.6 Hepatitis C Virus (HCV)

HCV belongs to the Flaviviridae family of viruses and is an enveloped RNA virus 50 nm in diame-ter. There are currently six described genotypes (types 1–6).

6.6.1 Epidemiology

According to **WHO estimates** the global preva-lence of HCV is 3%, with 170 million people infected worldwide. African countries (especially Egypt) have the highest prevalence of HCV (approximately 13% of the population), while it ranges between 2% and 5% in Asia and 1% and 2% in Europe and USA.

Transmission Exposure to blood products, especially from contaminated syringes or needles is the most common mode of transmission of HCV. Sexual contact and vertical transmission are other less clearly defined modes.

6.6.2 Clinical Features

The incubation period for hepatitis C is between 2 weeks and 6 months. HCV has a high (>approx. 80%) propensity to progress to **chronicity** [68, 69]. Since most of infections are subclinical (>75% of people are asymptomatic), the only way to detect HCV infection early is by screen-ing the high-risk population. Symptomatic indi-viduals can have a wide range of clinical presentations including fever, jaundice, dark urine, fatigue, nausea, vomiting, loss of appetite, and abdominal pain.

6.6.3 Diagnosis

By convention, acute hepatitis C virus (HCV) infection refers to the presence of clinical signs or symptoms of hepatitis within 6 months of pre-sumed HCV exposure. Patients infected with hep-atitis C virus may spontaneously clear the virus or develop chronic infection. Approximately 10–40% spontaneously clear the virus within 3 months (no later than 20 weeks after the onset of signs or symptoms). Symptomatic acute HCV infection is associated with a higher rate of spontaneous clear-ance than asymptomatic infection. The diagnosis of **chronic hepatitis C** is based on the detection of both HCV antibodies and HCV RNA in the pres-ence of signs of chronic hepatitis, either by ele-vated aminotransferases or by histopathology. Spontaneous viral clearance is very rare beyond 6 months of infection; the diagnosis of chronic hepatitis C can be made after that time period.

6.6.4 Screening Test: (Anti-HCV Antibody)

Anti-HCV antibody detection by **ELISA**, a third-generation immunoassay, is a standard method of diagnosis. This test has a sensitivity of 97% although the positive predictive value may be low. It detects antibodies within 6–8 weeks of infection, i.e., during the initial phase of elevated aminotransferases. This is only a screening test; results have to be confirmed by a HCV RNA PCR test. Infants should not be tested for anti-HCV antibodies before 12 months of age as anti-HCV from the mother may last until this age. The diagnosis of HCV in infants depends on the pres-ence of HCV RNA in baby blood after the second month of life.

Chronic HCV infection rarely clears sponta-neously. Chronic hepatitis C causes continuous liver damage, resulting in liver cirrhosis and HCC (Fig. 6.6). The rate of progression of fibrosis to cirrhosis and HCC is highly variable. Host fac-tors (alcohol, obesity, metabolic syndrome, etc.) have a significant role to play in its progression. In studies published till lately, cirrhosis devel-oped in around 16% of patients within 20 years after the onset of HCV infection [70]. Longer duration of infection may result in higher inci-dence of cirrhosis and HCC.

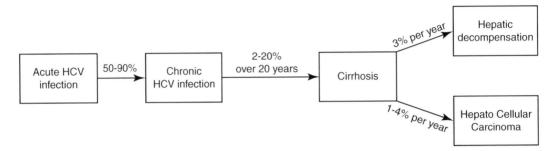

Fig. 6.6 Natural history of hepatitis C infection

6.6.5 Treatment Strategies and End-Stage Liver Disease

The most challenging HCV treatment candidates are individuals with cirrhosis. With the advent of newer Directly Acting Antivirals (DAAs) like pangenotypic Velpatasvir with Sofosbuvir combination a SVR of >90% is achievable in compensated cirrhotics in 12 weeks regimen and with addition of Ribavirin in Decompensated cirrhotics a SVR of >70% is achievable. Though the definitive management is Liver Transplantation in Decompensated cirrhotics, an undetectable RNA level with DAA before transplantation almost negates chances of post-transplant recurrence, which historically was a major issue post-transplantation.

6.6.6 Liver Transplantation for HCV-Related Liver Disease

If patient is HCV RNA positive at the time of transplant, recurrence of HCV infection in the allograft post-transplant is universal. Recurrent hepatitis C is significantly more aggressive in liver transplant recipients than in patients whose immunity is intact, with progression to cirrhosis reported in about one third of patients by the end of fifth year after transplant. Antiviral therapy with DAAs before transplant to achieve SVR (if possible) is a good way to improve outcomes and to prevent HCV reinfection.

6.6.6.1 Hepatitis C Virus Infection After Liver Transplantation

With the advances in medical management (i.e., DAAs) and increase in number of living donor liver transplants (with advantage of using antiviral therapy pretransplantation, shorter cold ischemic time, and a younger donor age), chances of post-transplant recurrent HCV infection have reduced significantly. However, in today's era the HCV treatment after transplant has also become very straightforward. Unlike in interferon era, the treatment with DAAs after transplant is done as early as 3 months after transplant.

6.6.6.2 Treatment Strategies for HCV

Antiviral therapy with clearance of HCV improves prognosis after transplant. Sustained viral eradication is associated with a decreased risk for fibrosis progression, hepatic decompensation, and graft loss, ultimately resulting in enhanced survival [71, 72]. Three approaches to antiviral therapy can be used in HCV-positive recipients:

1. Treatment before transplantation, with the goal of suppressing viral replication so that viral reinfection is prevented—This most preferred approach as lesser duration (12 weeks) of therapy with newer DAAs achieves >90% SVR.
2. Preemptive early post-transplant antiviral therapy—In some cases, treatment of HCV before transplant is not possible (e.g., DDLT,

ALF/ACLF setting, high MELD before transplant). This strategy attempts to treat HCV early after transplant before histological damage has occurred. Usually treatment is started 3–6 months after transplant. However, it can be earlier also if graft injury occurs.

3. Treatment of established disease—This used to be the predominant approach when only treatment option was interferon with ribavirin. Currently this is not widely practiced.

6.7 Donors with Viral Hepatitis

6.7.1 Hepatitis B Virus

Hepatitis B virus is widely prevalent with approximately one third of the world population having current or previous infection [73]. Thus the proportion of donors with HBcAb positivity is substantial; up to 57% in southeast Asia, 8% in India, and 2–5% in the United States. Management of HBV transmission risks is critical for safely expanding the donor pool. Patients with prior exposure to HBV (positive HbcAb) have lifelong hepatocyte infection due to covalently closed circular DNA (cccDNA) in the hepatocyte nucleus that cannot be cleared by the host immune response [72]. Even HbcAb-positive donors with negative serum HBV DNA can transmit HBV to the recipient [73]. All organ donors (whether LDLT or DDLT) should be tested for surface antigen (HbsAg) and HbcAb. Potential living kidney or liver donors are also tested for surface antibody (hepatitis B surface antibody [HbsAb]) [75, 76].

6.7.2 Approach to the Isolated HbcAb-Positive Donor

In donors who are HbsAg negative and HbcAb positive, transmission of HBV is expected, and preventative approaches with antiviral treatment for the recipient can minimize the risk of disease transmission [75–80]. Without prophylaxis, non-immune liver recipients (HbsAb negative) have the highest rates (77%) of HBV infection from HbcAb-positive donors [81]. In successfully vaccinated recipients (HbcAb negative, HbsAb positive), HBV transmission can rarely occur. For recipients who had isolated HbcAb positivity, transmission occurred in 13%. No HBV transmission occurred in naturally immune (HbcAb positive, HBSAg negative, HbsAb positive) recipients. **Current guidelines** recommend recipients of organs from isolated HbcAb+ donors receive prophylaxis with oral antivirals. In the era of effective antivirals, hepatitis B immune globulin is no longer needed for recipients getting HBcAb-positive grafts [74, 80]. Vaccinated liver transplant recipients should receive antiviral prophylaxis for at least 1 year, and if the levels of HbsAb are greater than 10 IU/mL at 1 year, withdrawal of prophylaxis can be considered [74]. In patients (receiving HBcAb-positive grafts) who are HbsAb negative and HbcAb negative, prophylaxis is recommended indefinitely. For liver recipients who are naturally immune (HbcAb positive and HbsAb positive), prophylaxis is not generally required. In all liver recipients, HBV DNA and/or HBSAg should be monitored every 3 months for the first year and every 3–6 months indefinitely. Prophylaxis is suggested if rituximab is given to recipients getting HBcAb-positive grafts (irrespective of immunity status of the recipient) [82, 83].

6.7.3 Approach to Use of HbsAg or HBVNAT-Positive Donors

In DDLT setting, donors who are HbsAg or HBV NAT positive are infrequently used out of safety concerns. Active HBV infection leads to unacceptably high rates of HBV transmission to the recipient. When used, these grafts are typically donated to recipients with active HBV infection themselves or after meticulous informed consent for urgent situations [75]. Any liver graft from a donor who is HbsAg positive should be evaluated for histological evidence of liver disease before transplantation. On the other hand, HBsAg-positive donors are not used in LDLT scenario (for the fear of reactivation of HBV in the donor after hepatectomy).

In liver transplant recipients, without prophylaxis, HBV infection occurs in nearly 100% of all recipients of HBSAg-positive donors [84]. Current guidelines recommend any cadaveric organ recipients from HbsAg-positive donors receive indefinite prophylaxis with entecavir or tenofovir [75]. Also HBsAg-positive living donors should be rejected for donation.

Hepatitis C Virus The newer direct-acting antiviral agents (DAAs) have revolutionized the treatment of HCV. The high efficacy (cure rates, >95%) and minimal side effect profile of DAAs make treatment of HCV simpler than interferon-based regimens. In addition, recipients with pre-existing HCV can be successfully treated with DAAs before or after transplantation. Testing of donors for HCV traditionally was limited to serology (anti-HCV antibody), the presence or absence of which labeled a donor HCV positive or negative [85]. However, in 2014, OPTN policy mandated that in addition to HCV antibody all donors must also undergo HCV NAT [85]. Use of NAT not only reduces the likelihood of missing a window period infection but also helps to discriminate between a viremic donor and ones who have either spontaneously cleared the virus or achieved cure after treatment. **Donors with active infection** (NAT positive and anti-HCV positive) clearly represent a risk of potential donor-to-recipient transmission. In contrast, patients who are **NAT negative and anti-HCV positive** have prior HCV exposure but no current infection (either treatment cure or spontaneous clearance), or possibly have a false-positive anti-HCV. Those who are NAT positive and anti-HCV negative may have acute infections in the window period, or possibly false-positive NAT. The term "**HCV viremic donor**" has been proposed rather than "HCV-positive donor" to more accurately identify the donors with documented active infection [85].

Traditionally, HCV "positive" organs (previously defined only by positive anti-HCV) were only transplanted into HCV-positive recipients [85]. Current data supports the safety of this practice in liver recipients, with no differences in graft or patient survival if the donor liver has no greater than stage 2 fibrosis [86–94]. Donors who are NAT negative and anti-HCV positive represent an exceptionally low risk of donor-derived HCV transmission (hence acceptable as grafts). Transplantation of hepatic allografts from anti-HCV-positive donors to recipients with HCV-related liver disease has not resulted in differences in graft and patient survival, compared with HCV recipients of grafts from HCV-negative donors.

However, it should be noted that this practice of using NAT-positive donors is only limited to DDLT setting. In LDLT scenario, all NAT-positive donors should be rejected. If there is a prior history of treatment for HCV, LDLT donor can be accepted if SVR has been achieved and there is no evidence of fibrosis in the donor liver.

6.8   Hepatitis A and E Virus

Hepatitis A and E virus is most commonly encountered in underdeveloped countries where transmission is largely fecal-oral [95] and is traditionally characterized as causing acute hepatitis. Because of the acute self-limited course of infection, HEV and HAV are not routinely tested for in organ donors. HEV/HAV RNA usually becomes undetectable in the serum approximately 3 weeks after the onset of symptoms, but can persist in stool for 2 additional weeks in immunocompetent patients [96] and for prolonged periods in the immunocompromised patients [97, 98].

There are no data or guidelines for use of donor livers with past HAV or HEV infection. Donors with ongoing acute hepatitis will obviously be rejected for donation. It is important to remember that liver inflammation may persist in patients with acute hepatitis A or E for many months after acute infection. Hence donation in such case should be postponed for at least 3–6 months. Moreover, if it is decided to take the person as a donor, we recommend liver biopsy to document normal liver in such cases (specially if the acute hepatitis was within 1 year of proposed donation).

6.9 Conclusion

Viral hepatitis, caused by hepatitis viruses A through E, is a major public health problem. Whereas HAV and HEV are known to cause acute hepatitis with spontaneous recovery and rarely acute liver failure (ALF), infection with HBV, HCV, or HDV is responsible for chronic hepatitis, leads to End-Stage Liver Disease, and is the main cause of Liver Transplantation.

Serological tests/biomarkers are used to distinguish acute, self-limited infections from chronic infections, to monitor vaccine-induced immunity, response to treatment, and determine the prognosis. Many serological tests are available, most common being Enzyme Immunoassays.

Liver transplantation (LT) is now a widely accepted lifesaving therapy for the complications of cirrhosis and acute liver failure due to infectious hepatitis (Hepatitis A through E). HBV and HCV are likely to recur after transplant if adequate treatment is not instituted. Graft failure resulting from recurrent hepatitis represents a major source of morbidity and mortality. Fortunately, effective treatment options for HBV as well as HCV are available (for treatment before as well as after transplant). With judicious use of currently available antiviral therapy, graft reinfection and failure can be successfully prevented.

Donors with HBV or HCV (past or current) need proper evaluation and strict adherence to guidelines before accepting them as donors. The criteria are different for LDLT and DDLT and should be carefully followed.

References

1. Alter MJ. Epidemiology of hepatitis B in Europe and worldwide. J Hepatol. 2003;39:S64–9.
2. Armstrong GL, Wasley A, Simard EP, McQuillan GM, Kuhnert WL, Alter MJ. The prevalence of hepatitis C virus infection in the United States, 1999 through 2002. Ann Intern Med. 2006;144:705–14.
3. Garcia-Retortillo M, Forns X, Feliu A, et al. Hepatitis C virus kinetics during and immediately after liver transplantation. Hepatology. 2002;35:680–7.
4. Siegl G. Virology of hepatitis. In: Zuckerman AJ, editor. Viral hepatitis and liver disease. New York: Alan R Liss; 1988. p. 3–7.
5. Dienstag JL, Szmuness W, Stevens CE, Purcell RH. Hepatitis A virus infection: new insights from seroepidemiologic studies. J Infect Dis. 1978;137:328–40.
6. Wright R, Millward-Salder GH, Bull FG. Acute viral hepatitis. In: Wright R, Millward-Sadler GH, Alberti KGMM, Karran S, editors. Liver and biliary disease. London: Bailliere Tindall; 1985. p. 677–767.
7. Lemon SM. Type A viral hepatitis. New developments in an old disease. N Engl J Med. 1985;313:1059–67.
8. Gust ID, Feinstone SM. Clinical features. In: Hepatitis A. Florida: CRC Press; 1988. p. 145–62.
9. Coulepis AG, Locarnini SA, Lehmann NI, Gust ID. Detection of hepatitis A virus in the feces of patients with naturally acquired infections. J Infect Dis. 1980;141:151–6.
10. Yotsuyanagi H, Koike K, Yasuda K, et al. Prolonged fecal excretion of hepatitis A virus in adult patients with hepatitis A as determined by polymerase chain reaction. Hepatology. 1996;24:10–3.
11. Reed C, Gustafson T, Siegel J, Duer P. Nosocomial transmission of hepatitis A from a hospital acquired case. Pediatr Infect Dis. 1984;3:300–3.
12. Krober MS, Bass JW, Brown JD, Lemon SM, Rupert KJ. Hospital outbreak of hepatitis A: risk factors for spread. Pediatr Infect Dis. 1984;3:296–9.
13. Drusin LM, Sohmer M, Groshen SL, Spiritos MD, Senterfit LB, Christenson WN. Nosocomial hepatitis A infection in a pediatric intensive care unit. Arch Dis Child. 1987;62:690–5.
14. Burkholder BT, Coronado VG, Brown J, et al. Nosocomial transmission of hepatitis A in a pediatric hospital traced to an anti-hepatitis A virus negative patient with immunodeficiency. Pediatr Infect Dis J. 1995;14:261–6.
15. Bradley DW, Maynard JE, Hindman SH, et al. Serodiagnosis of viral hepatitis A: detection of acute-phase immunoglobulin M anti-hepatitis A virus by radioimmunoassay. J Clin Microbiol. 1977;5:521–30.
16. Krawczynski K. Hepatitis E. Hepatology. 1993;17:932–41.
17. Goldsmith R, Yarbough PO, Reyes GR, et al. Enzyme-linked immunosorbent assay for diagnosis of acute sporadic hepatitis E in Egyptian children. Lancet. 1992;339:328–31.
18. Balayan MS, Andjaparidze AG, Savinskaya SS, et al. Evidence for a virus in non-A, non-B hepatitis transmitted via the fecal-oral rout. Intervirology. 1983;20:23–31.
19. Bradley DW, Krawczynski K, Kane MA. Hepatitis E. In: Belshe RB, editor. Textbook of human virology. 2nd ed. St Louis; 1991. p. 781–90.
20. Khuroo MS, Duermeyer W, Zargar SA, et al. Acute sporadic non-A, non-B hepatitis in India. Am J Epidemiol. 1983;118:360–4.
21. Kane MA, Bradley DW, Shretha SM, et al. Epidemic non-A, non-B hepatitis in Nepal. JAMA. 1984;252:3140–5.
22. Lu L, Li C, Hagedorn CH. Phylogenetic analysis of global hepatitis E virus sequences: genetic diversity, subtypes and zoonosis. Rev Med Virol. 2006;16:5–36.

23. Aggarwal R, Jameel S. Hepatitis E. Hepatology. 2011;54:2218–26.
24. Aggarwal R, Naik S. Epidemiology of hepatitis E: current status. J Gastroenterol Hepatol. 2009;24:1484–93.
25. Naik S, Aggarwal R, Salunke P, et al. A large waterborne viral hepatitis E epidemic in Kanpur, India. Bull WHO. 1992;70:597–604.
26. Zhuang H. Hepatitis E and strategies for its control. Basel: Karger; 1992.
27. Khuroo M, Teli M, Skidmore S, et al. Incidence and severity of viral hepatitis in pregnancy. Am J Med. 1981;70:252–5.
28. Kamar N, Garrouste C, Haagsma EB, et al. Factors associated with chronic hepatitis in patients with hepatitis E virus infection who have received solid organ transplants. Gastroenterology. 2011;140:1481–9.
29. Aggarwal R. Diagnosis of hepatitis E. Nat Rev Gastroenterol Hepatol. 2013;10:24–33.
30. Tiollais P, Charnay P, Vyas GN. Biology of hepatitis B virus. Science. 1981;213:406–11.
31. McMahon BJ, Alward WLM, Hall DB, et al. Acute hepatitis B virus infection. Relation of age to the clinical expression of disease and subsequent development of the carrier state. J Infect Dis. 1985;151:599–603.
32. Hall AJ, Winter PD, Wright R. Mortality of hepatitis B positive blood donors in England and Wales. Lancet. 1985;1:91–3.
33. Weissberg JI, Andres LL, Smith CI, et al. Survival in chronic hepatitis B: an analysis of 379 patients. Ann Intern Med. 1984;101:613–6.
34. Beasley RP, Hwang LY. Epidemiology of hepatocellular carcinoma. In: Vyas GN, Dienstag JL, Hoofnagle JH, editors. Viral hepatitis and liver disease. Orlando: Grune & Statton; 1984. p. 209.
35. Francis DP, Favero MS, Maynard JE. Transmission of hepatitis B virus. Semin Liver Dis. 1981;1:27–32.
36. Seeff LB, Wright EC, Zimmerman HJ, et al. Type B hepatitis after needle-stick exposures: prevention with hepatitis B immunoglobulin. Final report of the Veterans Administration Cooperative Study. Ann Intern Med. 1978;88:285.
37. Scott RM, Snitbhan D, Bancroft WH, et al. Experimental transmission of hepatitis B virus by semen and saliva. J Infect Dis. 1980;142:67–71.
38. Shikata T, Karasawa T, Abe K, et al. Hepatitis B antigen and infectivity of hepatitis B virus. J Infect Dis. 1977;136:571–6.
39. Denes AE, Smith JL, Maynard JE, et al. Hepatitis B infection in physicians: results of a nation-wide seroepidemiology survey. JAMA. 1978;239:210–2.
40. Olubuyide IO, Ola SO, Aliyu B, et al. Hepatitis B and C in doctors and dentists in Nigeria. Q J Med. 1997;90:417–22.
41. Kim WR, Terrault NA, Pedersen RA, et al. Trends in waiting list registration for liver transplantation for viral hepatitis in the United States. Gastroenterology. 2009;137(5):1680–6.
42. European liver transplant registry. Available at http://www.eltr.org.
43. O'Grady JG, Smith HM, Davies SE, et al. Hepatitis B virus reinfection after orthotopic liver transplantation. Serological and clinical implications. J Hepatol. 1992;14(1):104–11.
44. Todo S, Demetris AJ, Van Thiel D, et al. Orthotopic liver transplantation for patients with hepatitis B virus-related liver disease. Hepatology. 1991;13(4):619–26.
45. Steinmuller T, Seehofer D, Rayes N, et al. Increasing applicability of liver transplantation for patients with hepatitis B-related liver disease. Hepatology. 2002;35(6):1528–35.
46. Kim WR, Poterucha JJ, Kremers WK, et al. Outcome of liver transplantation for hepatitis B in the United States. Liver Transpl. 2004;10(8):968–74.
47. Xie SB, Zhu JY, Ying Z, et al. Prevention and risk factors of the HBV recurrence after orthotopic liver transplantation: 160 cases follow-up study. Transplantation. 2010;90(7):786–90.
48. Chun J, Kim W, Kim BG, et al. High viremia, prolonged lamivudine therapy and recurrent hepatocellular carcinoma predict posttransplant hepatitis B recurrence. Am J Transplant. 2010;10(7):1649–59.
49. Faria LC, Gigou M, Roque-Afonso AM, et al. Hepatocellular carcinoma is associated with an increased risk of hepatitis B virus recurrence after liver transplantation. Gastroenterology. 2008;134(7):1890–9. quiz 2155
50. Yi NJ, Suh KS, Cho JY, et al. Recurrence of hepatitis B is associated with cumulative corticosteroid dose and chemotherapy against hepatocellular carcinoma recurrence after liver transplantation. Liver Transpl. 2007;13(3):451–8.
51. Saab S, Yeganeh M, Nguyen K, et al. Recurrence of hepatocellular carcinoma and hepatitis B reinfection in hepatitis B surface antigen-positive patients after liver transplantation. Liver Transpl. 2009;15(11):1525–34.
52. Cholongitas E, Goulis J, Akriviadis E, Papatheodoridis GV. Hepatitis B immunoglobulin and/or nucleos(t)ide analogues for prophylaxis against hepatitis B virus recurrence after liver transplantation: a systematic review. Liver Transpl. 2011;17:1176–90.
53. Rao W, Wu X, Xiu D. Lamivudine or lamivudine combined with hepatitis B immunoglobulin in prophylaxis of hepatitis B recurrence after liver transplantation: a meta-analysis. Transpl Int. 2009;22:387–94.
54. Cholongitas E, Papatheodoridis GV. High genetic barrier nucleos(t)ide analogue(s) for prophylaxis from hepatitis B virus recurrence after liver transplantation: a systematic review. Am J Transplant. 2013;13:353–62.
55. Angus PW, McCaughan GW, Gane EJ, Crawford DH, Harley H. Combination low-dose hepatitis B immune globulin and lamivudine therapy provides effective prophylaxis against posttransplantation hepatitis B. Liver Transpl. 2000;6:429–33.
56. Degertekin B, Han SH, Keeffe EB, et al. Impact of virologic breakthrough and HBIG regimen on hepatitis B recurrence after liver transplantation. Am J Transplant. 2010;10(8):1823–33.

57. Wong SN, Chu CJ, Wai CT, Howell T, Moore C, Fontana RJ, Lok AS. Low risk of hepatitis B virus recurrence after withdrawal of long-term hepatitis B immunoglobulinin patients receiving maintenance nucleos(t)ide analogue therapy. Liver Transpl. 2007 Mar;13(3):374–81.

58. Singer GA, Zielsdorf S, Fleetwood VA, et al. Limited hepatitis B immunoglobulin with potent nucleos(t) ide analogue is a cost-effective prophylaxis against hepatitis B virus after liver transplantation. Transplant Proc. 2015 Mar;47(2):478–84.

59. Cholongitas E, Vasiliadis T, Antoniadis N, Goulis I, Papanikolaou V, Akriviadis E. Hepatitis B prophylaxis post liver transplantation with newer nucleos(t)ide analogues afterhepatitis B immunoglobulin discontinuation. Transpl Infect Dis. 2012 Oct;14(5):479–87.

60. Buti M, Mas A, Prieto M, Casafont F, Gonzalez A, Miras M, et al. A randomized study comparing lamivudine monotherapy after a short course of hepatitis B immune globulin (HBIg) and lamivudine with long-term lamivudine plus HBIg in the prevention of hepatitis B virus recurrence after liver transplantation. J Hepatol. 2003;38:811–7.

61. Fung J, Cheung C, Chan SC, Yuen MF, Chok KS, Sharr W, et al. Entecavir monotherapy is effective in suppressing hepatitis B virus after liver transplantation. Gastroenterology. 2011;141:1212–9.

62. Wadhawan M, Gupta S, Goyal N, Taneja S, Kumar. Living related liver transplantation for hepatitis b–related liver disease without hepatitis b immune globulin prophylaxis. Liver Transpl. 2013;19:1030–5.

63. Gane EJ, Patterson S, Strasser SI, McCaughan GW, Angus PW. Combination of lamivudine and adefovir without hepatitis B immune globulin is safe and effective prophylaxis against hepatitis B virus recurrence in hepatitis B surface antigen-positive liver transplant candidates. Liver Transpl. 2013;19(3):268–74.

64. Rizzetto M. Hepatitis D: thirty years after. J Hepatol. 2009;50(5):1043–50.

65. Hughes SA, Wedemeyer H, Harrison PM. Hepatitis delta virus. Lancet. 2011;378(9785):73–85.

66. Fattovich G, Giustina G, Christensen E, et al. Influence of hepatitis delta virus infection on morbidity and mortality in compensated cirrhosis type B. The European Concerted Action on ViralHepatitis (Eurohep). Gut. 2000;46(3):420–6.

67. Samuel D, Muller R, Alexander G, et al. Liver transplantation in European patients with the hepatitis B surface antigen. N Engl J Med. 1993;329(25):1842–7.

68. Tong MJ, El-Farra NS, Reikes AR, Co RL. Clinical outcomes after transfusion-associated hepatitis C. N Engl J Med. 1995;332:1463–6.

69. Minuk G, Assy N. The consequences of hepatitis C viral infection in humans. Can J Gastroenterol. 1995;9:373–6.

70. Thein HH, Yi Q, Dore GJ, et al. Estimation of stage-specific fibrosis progression rates in chronic hepatitis C virus infection: a meta-analysis and meta-regression. Hepatology. 2008;48:418–31.

71. Berenguer M, Ferrell L, Watson J, et al. HCV-related fibrosis progression following liver transplantation: increase in recent years. J Hepatol. 2000;32:673–84.

72. Berenguer M, Aguilera V, Prieto M, et al. Delayed onset of severe hepatitis C-related liver damage following liver transplantation: a matter of concern? Liver Transpl. 2003;9(11):1152–8.

73. Liaw YF, Chu CM. Hepatitis B virus infection. Lancet. 2009;373:582–92.

74. Cholongitas E, Papatheodoridis GV, Burroughs AK. Liver grafts from anti-hepatitis B core positive donors: a systematic review. J Hepatol. 2010;52:272–9.

75. Huprikar S, Danziger-Isakov L, Ahn J, et al. Solid organ transplantation from hepatitis B virus-positive donors: consensus guidelines for recipient management. Am J Transplant. 2015;15:1162–72.

76. Lucey MR, Terrault N, Ojo L, et al. Long-term management of the successful adult liver transplant: 2012 practice guideline by the American Association for the Study of Liver Diseases and the American Society of Transplantation. Liver Transpl. 2013;19:3–26.

77. Skagen CL, Jou JH, Said A. Risk of de novo hepatitis in liver recipients from hepatitis-B core antibody-positive grafts—a systematic analysis. Clin Transpl. 2011;25:E243–9.

78. Chang MS, Olsen SK, Pichardo EM, et al. Prevention of de novo hepatitis B in recipients of core antibody-positive livers with lamivudine and other nucleos(t)ides: a 12-year experience. Transplantation. 2013;95:960–5.

79. MacConmara MP, Vachharajani N, Wellen JR, et al. Utilization of hepatitis B core antibody-positive donor liver grafts. HPB (Oxford). 2012;14:42–8.

80. Saab S, Waterman B, Chi AC, et al. Comparison of different immunoprophylaxis regimens after liver transplantation with hepatitis B core antibody-positive donors: a systematic review. Liver Transpl. 2010;16:300–7.

81. Yen RD, Bonatti H, Mendez J, et al. Case report of lamivudine-resistant hepatitis B virus infection post liver transplantation from a hepatitis B core antibody donor. Am J Transplant. 2006;6:1077–83.

82. Hwang JP, Lok AS. Management of patients with hepatitis B who require immunosuppressive therapy. Nat Rev Gastroenterol Hepatol. 2014;11:209–19.

83. FDA Hepatitis Update - Hepatitis B reactivation with certain immunesuppressing and anti-cancer drugs. Infectious Diseases Society of America (IDSA). Updated 29 Oct 2013. Accessed 22 Mar 2018.

84. Saidi RF, Jabbour N, Shah SA, et al. Liver transplantation from hepatitis B surface antigen-positive donors. Transplant Proc. 2013;45:279–80.

85. Levitsky J, Formica RN, Bloom RD, et al. The American Society of transplantation consensus conference on the use of hepatitis C viremic donors in solid organ transplantation. Am J Transplant. 2017;17:2790–802.

86. Saab S, Chang AJ, Comulada S, et al. Outcomes of hepatitis C- and hepatitis B core antibody-positive

grafts in orthotopic liver transplantation. Liver Transpl. 2003;9:1053–61.

87. Burr AT, Li Y, Tseng JF, et al. Survival after liver transplantation using hepatitis C virus-positive donor allografts: case-controlled analysis of the UNOS database. World J Surg. 2011;35:1590–5.

88. Northup PG, Argo CK, Nguyen DT, et al. Liver allografts from hepatitis C positive donors can offer good outcomes in hepatitis C positive recipients: a US National Transplant Registry analysis. Transpl Int. 2010;23:1038–44.

89. Alvaro E, Abradelo M, Fuertes A, et al. Liver transplantation from anti hepatitis C virus-positive donors: our experience. Transplant Proc. 2012;44:1475–8.

90. Ballarin R, Cucchetti A, Spaggiari M, et al. Long-term follow-up and outcome of liver transplantation from anti-hepatitis C virus-positive donors: a European multicentric case-control study. Transplantation. 2011;91:1265–72.

91. Saab S, Ghobrial RM, Ibrahim AB, et al. Hepatitis C positive grafts may be used in orthotopic liver transplantation: a matched analysis. Am J Transplant. 2003;3:1167–72.

92. Marroquin CE, Marino G, Kuo PC, et al. Transplantation of hepatitis C-positive livers in hepatitis C-positive patients is equivalent to transplanting hepatitis C-negative livers. Liver Transpl. 2001;7:762–8.

93. Vargas HE, Laskus T, Wang LF, et al. Outcome of liver transplantation in hepatitis C virus-infected patients who received hepatitis C virus-infected grafts. Gastroenterology. 1999;117:149–53.

94. Testa G, Goldstein RM, Netto G, et al. Long-term outcome of patients transplanted with livers from hepatitis C-positive donors. Transplantation. 1998;65:925–9.

95. Kamar N, Legrand-Abravanel F, Izopet J, et al. Hepatitis E virus: what transplant physicians should know. Am J Transplant. 2012;12:2281–7.

96. Dalton HR, Bendall R, Ijaz S, et al. Hepatitis E: an emerging infection in developed countries. Lancet Infect Dis. 2008;8:698–709.

97. Dalton HR, Bendall RP, Keane FE, et al. Persistent carriage of hepatitis E virus in patients with HIV infection. N Engl J Med. 2009;361:1025–7.

98. Ollier L, Tieulie N, Sanderson F, et al. Chronic hepatitis after hepatitis E virus infection in a patient with non-Hodgkin lymphoma taking rituximab. Ann Intern Med. 2009;150:430–1.

Indication and Contraindications for Liver Transplantation

7

Naimish N. Mehta and Srinivas Bojanapu

Patients undergoing liver transplantation should benefit from the extension of life expectancy beyond the natual course of survival or should have an improved quality of life.

Liver transplantation is the treatment of choice for patients with decompensated liver disease, cirrhosis with liver cancer, liver-based metabolic conditions causing systemic disease.

Since the time, liver transplantation was first attempted, continuous refinements in surgical techniques and an in-depth understanding of the immunological role in the rejection and discovery of newer effective immunosuppressants have changed the perception of liver transplantation to a comparatively safer and standard procedure for patients with end-stage liver failure.

Acceptance of liver transplantation as a treatment of choice has broadened the indications for liver transplantation and an increase in referrals [1].

Graft liver can be obtained from either a living donor (LD) or deceased donor (DD). Rationing of the scarce resource is vital as also the requirement of a replacement in the affected patient.

7.1 Indications

Indications can be classified into end-stage liver disease, fulminant liver failure, benign and malignant liver tumour [2] (Table 7.1).

7.1.1 Acute Liver Failure

Acute liver failure (ALF) is a potentially reversible, often sudden, persistent and progressive liver dysfunction characterized by the occurrence of encephalopathy within 4 weeks of symptoms in the absence of pre-existing liver disease [3]. ALF is relatively rare, but carries a short-term (3 week) mortality above 40%. However, if the patient survives, typically the liver recovers fully, both structurally and functionally (except in autoimmune hepatitis and Wilson's cases) [4].

Assessment is required to segregate patients who can survive with supportive measures alone or require liver transplantation (LT). Several models have been proposed to prognosticate patients with ALF. These include King's College Hospital (KCH) criteria, Clichy criteria, serum Group-specific component protein levels, liver volume on CT scanning, blood lactate levels, hyperphosphataemia, Acute Physiology and Chronic Health Evaluation II score, etcetera. Dynamic models like ALF early dynamic model (ALFED) [5] can also be used to stratify patients needing LT and to pre-

N. N. Mehta (✉) · S. Bojanapu
Department of Surgical Gastroenterology, HPB Surgery and Liver Transplantation, Sir Ganga Ram Hospital, New Delhi, India

Table 7.1 Indications for liver transplantation

Acute liver failure	
Hepatitis A/B	
Drug induced (eg. Paracetamol, Anti- Tuberculosis therapy, etc)	
Wilson's disease	
Budd–Chiari syndrome	
Chronic liver failure	
Noncholestatic cirrhosis	**Cholestatic cirrhosis**
Hepatitis B/C	Primary biliary cirrhosis (PBC)
Autoimmune hepatitis	Primary sclerosing cholangitis (PSC)
Alcohol-induced cirrhosis	Secondary biliary cirrhosis
Metabolic	**Vascular**
Wilson's disease	Budd–Chiari syndrome
Hemochromatosis	
α-1 Antitrypsin deficiency	
Amyloidosis	
Cystic fibrosis	
Other indications	**Malignant disease**
Primary oxalosis	Hepatocellular carcinoma (HCC)
Glycogen storage diseases	Fibrolamellar carcinoma (FLC)
Hyperlipidaemia	Hepatoblastoma
Polycystic liver disease	Epithelioid haemangioendothelioma
	Cholangiocellular adenocarcinoma
	Neuroendocrine liver metastases
Liver transplantation in paediatric patients	**Chronic liver failure**
Biliary atresia	Tyrosinemia
Byler's disease	**Benign liver tumours**
Alagille's syndrome	Adenomatosis
Neonatal hepatitis/neonatal viral hepatitis	
Autoimmune hepatitis	
Hepatoblastoma	

Table 7.2 King's College Hospital (KCH) criteria [6]

Paracetamol-induced ALF	Non-Paracetamol-induced ALF
Arterial blood pH < 7.30 (irrespective of the grade of encephalopathy)	Prothrombin time >100 s (INR > 6.5) (irrespective of the grade of encephalopathy)
OR	OR
All of the following	Any 3 of the following (irrespective of the grade of encephalopathy)
• Prothrombin time >100 s (INR >6.5)	• Age <10 or >40 years
• Serum creatinine >3.4 mg/dl	• Aetiology: non-A/non-B hepatitis, drug-induced
• Grade III or IV hepatic encephalopathy	• Duration of jaundice to encephalopathy >7 days
	• Prothrombin time >50 (INR > 3.5)
	• Serum bilirubin >18 mg/dl

dict mortality. Among the above, the King's College hospital criteria are the most validated and widely practiced guidelines across the world (Table 7.2).

The King's college criteria have a high positive predictive value (around 80% in paracetamol-induced ALF, 70–90% in non-paracetamol cases). Their negative predictive value is, however, lower (70–90% in paracetamol-induced ALF, 25–50%, only, in non-paracetamol induced cases) [4]. Nevertheless, the criteria will select around 20% of patients for OLT, who might have survived without LT. More importantly, perhaps, not meeting the criteria does not guarantee survival without a transplant, particularly in non-paracetamol cases [4].

Aetiologically, variations occur featuring a high incidence with paracetamol (acetaminophen) induced ALF in the West as compared to hepatitis viruses, specifically hepatitis E and B in Southeast Asia including India [5, 7]. Establishing an aetiologic diagnosis accurately is vital in the management of ALF as the diagnosis impacts scoring as well as therapeutic strategy and prognostication. Any patient meeting the above criteria should be offered LT as a treatment option.

Table 7.3 The Child-Pugh score

Parameter	Score		
	1	2	3
Ascites	None	Controlled	Refractory
Encephalopathy (grade)	None	1–2 (minimal)	3–4 (coma)
Bilirubin (micromol/L)	<34	35–50	>51
Albumin (g/L)	>35	28–35	<28
INR	<1.7	1.8–2.3	>2.3

7.1.2 Chronic Liver Disease

How to assess and determine the candidature for liver transplantation in patients with chronic liver disease.

Tools:

MELD (Model for End-stage Liver Disease)
CTP (Child Turcotte Pugh) score
UKELD (United Kingdom model for End stage Liver disease)
Disease-specific indices for primary biliary cirrhosis and sclerosing cholangitis
UNOS System

Referral for transplantation to be done for patients with cirrhosis when they develop evidence of hepatic dysfunction (CTP ≥ 7 and MELD ≥ 10) or when they experience their first major complication (ascites, variceal bleed or hepatic encephalopathy). Expedited referral for LT if a patient is diagnosed with type I hepatorenal syndrome [8] (Tables 7.3 and 7.4).

Table 7.4 Old UNOS system—classification of candidates [9]

Status	Characteristics
Status 1	Fulminant liver failure with life expectancy <7 days: 1. Fulminant hepatic failure as traditionally defined 2. Primary graft nonfunction <7 days of transplantation 3. Hepatic artery thrombosis <7 days of transplantation 4. Acute decompensated Wilson's disease
Status 2a	Hospitalized in ICU for chronic liver failure with life expectancy <7 days, with a Child-Pugh score of ≥10 and one of the following: 1. Unresponsive active variceal haemorrhage 2. Hepatorenal syndrome 3. Refractory ascites/hepatic hydrothorax 4. Stage 3 or 4 hepatic encephalopathy
Status 2B	Requiring continuous medical care, with a Child-Pugh score of ≥10, or a Child-Pugh score ≥7 and one of the following: 1. Unresponsive active variceal haemorrhage 2. Hepatorenal syndrome 3. Spontaneous bacterial peritonitis 4. Refractory ascites/hepatic hydrothorax, or presence of hepatocellular carcinoma
Status 3	Requiring continuous medical care, with a child-Pugh score of ≥7, but not meeting criteria for Status 2B
Status 7	Temporary inactive

MELD score equation = 9.57 × loge(creatinine) + 3.78 × Loge(total bilirubin) + 11.2 × Loge(INR) + 6.43 [10].

The Child-Pugh score should be reassessed periodically since the patient's clinical condition may improve or deteriorate with time (Table 7.5).

UKELD = [5.395 × INR] + [1.485 × Creatinine(micromol/L)] + [3.13 × Bilirubin(micromol/L)] − [81.565 × Sodium (mmol/L)] + 435

Table 7.5 Percentage of survival in cirrhotic liver disease

Child-Pugh grade	Child-Pugh score	1-Year survival (%)	5-Year survival (%)	10-Year survival (%)
A	5–6	84	44	27
B	7–9	62	20	10
C	10–15	42	21	0

7.1.2.1 Viral Hepatitis

Chronic liver disease secondary to infection with hepatitis C virus (HCV) and hepatitis B virus (HBV) is the most common indication for liver transplantation in the West. Listing in HBV infections for Liver Transplantation is done for patients with hepatocellular carcinoma (HCC) and well compensated Liver function and decompensated liver function with or without HCC [11]. Survival rates once decompensation (ascites, bleeding, hepatic encephalopathy, spontaneous bacterial peritonitis, hepatorenal syndrome) occurs falls to 50% at 5 years [12]. Chronic alcohol abuse accelerates the process. HCC develops at a rate of 3.4% per year in patients with HCV infection [13].

HBV infection acquired during birth or early life is a risk factor for developing cirrhosis and HCC.

7.1.2.2 Alcoholic Liver Disease

There is a reluctance for LT in alcoholic liver disease since patients themselves are responsible for their illness and are likely to resume alcohol after LT.

Severe alcoholic hepatitis which is nonresponsive to medication (Lille score ≥0.45) has a survival rate of 30% at 6 months. Hence LT is

indicated after careful assessment of patient's addiction profile, though studies show recidivism up to 35% [14].

Alcoholic liver cirrhosis is one of the leading causes for end-stage liver disease and the most common indication for liver transplantation around the world. Broad consensus but though not a rule is for abstinence from alcohol for a duration of 6 months preceding LT, though there is a relapse in alcohol abuse even after 2 years of abstinence with geographical differences existing [15].

LT benefits most when a patient with alcoholic cirrhosis with Child's C status undergoes LT with a 5-year survival of 58% compared to 35% in patients without LT [16]. It is much more liberal when an alcoholic recipient is receiving a graft from a related living donor and not from the pool of deceased donors.

7.1.2.3 Cholestatic Liver Disease

These are a heterogeneous disorder group which can progress to biliary cirrhosis and LT is the only definitive therapy for patients in whom condition has progressed to end-stage liver disease.

Primary Sclerosing Cholangitis (PSC)

Primary Sclerosing Cholangitis is a rare disease with an estimated 10-year survival approximating 65%. There is geographical variation in the number of LTs being done for PSC with highest done in Scandinavian and Nordic regions. The American Association for Study of Liver Disease recommends against using disease-specific models for predicting outcomes in individual patients [17]. Two unique indications for LT in PSC apart from indications of chronic liver disease are cholangiocarcinoma (CCA) and recurrent bacterial cholangitis. About 25–50% of PSC patients waitlisted for LT may not have radiographic and/or histologic evidence of cirrhosis or complications of portal hypertension [18]. Patients with PSC may also develop longstanding cholestasis including weight loss, metabolic bone disease and refractory pruritus which resultantly lead to significant morbidity, which uniquely affects this group of patients [18].

Inclusion Criteria for Liver Transplantation in PSC
- Intraluminal brush or biopsy showing evidence of positive tumour cells or cells strongly suspicious for CCA, or
- Radiographically malignant appearing stricture, and one of the following criteria:

  - Ca 19–9 > 100 U/mL in the absence of acute bacterial cholangitis
  - Polysomy on fluorescence in situ hybridization (FISH)
  - Well-defined mass on cross-sectional imaging

Exclusion criteria for Liver Transplantation in PSC
- Evidence of extrahepatic disease or regional lymph node involvement
- Previous malignancy (excluding skin or cervical cancer) within the 5 years before a diagnosis of CCA
- Previous abdominal radiotherapy
- Uncontrolled infection before treatment
- A prior attempt at the surgical resection of the tumour leading to violation of the tumour plane
- Any medical condition precluding transplantation
- Any transperitoneal biopsy, including percutaneous and/or endoscopic ultrasound-guided FNA

Primary Biliary Cirrhosis (PBC)

PBC is a disorder of unknown aetiology and believed to have a genetic susceptibility, with a female predominance. PBC is characterized by fatigue and pruritis, which are common initial symptoms. Pathologically ductopenia is a characteristic feature of PBC. PBC is considered one of the best indicators for LT. EASL guideline suggests referral of patients to LT when serum bilirubin reaches 6 mg/dl, a Mayo risk score ≥7.8 and/or MELD score of 12 or higher is calculated. Exceptions to these are when a patient concomi-

tantly has associated HCC, which develops in patients with cirrhosis (PBC 4–12% at 10 years) [19].

7.1.2.4 Malignancy
Hepatocellular Cancer (HCC)

Evolution of multidisciplinary approaches has resulted in a new era of Transplant Oncology, with the amalgamation of surgical oncology and transplant surgery. Substantial risk exists in patients with cirrhosis for development of hepatocellular malignancy which reaches up to 3% incidence per year and carries a dismal prognosis. Mazzaferro et al. in 1996 laid down Milan criteria in their original study and found that patients meeting the criteria (*patients with a single tumour ≤5 cm in diameter, or no more than three tumours ≤3 cm,*) had 4-year overall and recurrence-free survival of 85 and 92 per cent respectively. The Milan criteria are presently well-accepted and recommended guidelines for LT in HCC [20].

A considerable subset of patients who were excluded from strict Milan criteria would have had a better prognosis with LT; hence several extended criteria have been reported with acceptable outcomes. In acceptable outcomes such as Pittsburg criteria, University of California at San Francisco (UCSF) criteria and Up to 7 criteria (Table 7.6).

Downstaging of advanced HCC to reduce and comply within Milan or UCSF criteria with Transarterial Chemoembolization, Transarterial Radioembolization, and Radiofrequency ablation can achieve similar outcomes as those primarily fulfilling Milan/UCSF criteria.

Due to social and cultural practices existing in the East, there is a shortage of deceased donation and hence approximately 70% of LDLT recipients are from Asian countries, indirectly bearing advantages by reducing pre-transplantation waiting time for patients with HCC, alleviating ischaemic reperfusion injury and providing an optimal donor graft for those with end-stage liver disease [21].

Cholangiocarcinoma
Intrahepatic Cholangiocarcinoma
Intrahepatic cholangio carcinoma is currently not an accepted standard indication, but as part of clinical trials with neoadjuvant chemotherapy and LT.

Table 7.6 Extended criteria for transplant in patients with HCC [21]

UCSF	Tumour ≤6.5 cm, or ≤3 nodules with the largest ≤4.5 cm and a total tumour ≤8 cm
Up-to-7	The sum of the tumour number and the size of the largest tumour no larger than 7 cm
Tokyo	Tumours no larger than 5 cm and no more than 5 nodules
Kyoto	Tumour ≤10 nodules, all ≤5 cm, and a serum DCP level ≤400 mAU/mL
Shanghai	Tumour ≤9 cm, or ≤3 lesions with the largest ≤5 cm, tumour ≤9 cm without macrovascular and lymph node invasion and extrahepatic metastasis
ASAN	Tumour ≤5 cm in diameter, ≤6 in nodule number, and free of gross vascular invasion

Table 7.7 New Wilson Index for predicting mortality [26]

Score	Bilirubin (μmol/L)	INR	AST (IU/L)	White cell count (10^9/L)	Albumin (g/L)
0	0–100	0–1.29	0–100	0–6.7	>45
1	101–150	1.3–1.6	101–150	6.8–8.3	34–44
2	151–200	1.7–1.9	151–300	8.4–10.3	25–33
3	201–300	2.0–2.4	301–400	10.4–15.3	21–24
4	>301	>2.5	>401	>15.4	<20

Hilar Cholangiocarcinoma (H-CCA)

Surgical resection is the standard care with the primary goal of R0 resection, in the absence of metastatic or locally advanced disease or PSC. Negative margins are obtained only in 60–80% of patients with long-term survival ranging from 20% to 40% at 5 years. Investigators from Mayo Clinic reported a 5-year survival of 82% after transplantation in selected patients including unresectable, solitary tumours, less than 3 cm in radial diameter, without evidence of lymph node metastases, and resectable disease in the setting of PSC [22].

Metastatic Neuroendocrine Tumours

Though there are multeity of choices for managing patients with metastatic neuroendocrine tumours including somatostatin or radioactive metaiodo-benzyl-guanidine therapy, surgical excision, radiofrequency ablation among others, LT is primarily indicated in scenarios where (1) nonaccessible tumour for curative surgery or major tumour reduction, (2) tumours not responding to medical or interventional treatment and (3) tumours causing life-threatening hormonal symptoms [23].

7.1.2.5 LT in Metabolic Liver Disease

Wilson's disease (WD) is due to mutations which encode copper-transporting ATPase, resulting in accumulation of copper in affected tissues. Presentation varies widely with key features being liver disease and cirrhosis, neuropsychiatric disturbances and Kayser–Fleischer rings. The affected liver may present as acute or in chronic forms. Acute liver failure predominantly affects young females. Many patients may present with signs of chronic liver disease with decompensation. Neurological and psychiatric symptoms usually follow. Wilson's disease is universally fatal if untreated. Since biochemical defect lies in the liver itself, orthotopic liver transplantation corrects the underlying problem. Patients with revised WD prognostic index (RWPI)/revised King's College score for WD of >11 should be referred for LT in an acute setting. In chronic cases, LT is indicated as per MELD scores [24, 25] (Table 7.7).

7.1.2.6 Vascular Causes

Budd–Chiari syndrome (BCS) consists of a group of disorders characterized by hepatic venous outflow obstruction at the level of hepatic venules, large hepatic veins, inferior vena cava or right atrium. Characteristic features include abdominal pain, hepatomegaly and ascites. LT is indicated in likely situations of fulminant BCS, BCS with cirrhosis and failure of a portosystemic shunt. The five-year survival rate among patients with LT for BCS is as high as 95%. Complications after LT in BCS involve arterial and venous thrombosis and bleeding due to anticoagulation. However, multiple aetiologic factors may be present and therefore the recommendation is for long-term anticoagulation after LT [27].

7.2 Liver Transplantation in Paediatric Patients

Most common indications for LT in the paediatric age group include (1) Extrahepatic biliary atresia, (2) Intrahepatic cholestasis: sclerosing cholangitis; Alagille's syndrome; progressive familial intrahepatic cholestasis, (3) Metabolic diseases: Wilson's disease; α1 antitrypsin deficiency; Crigler–Najjar syndrome, (4) Acute liver failure, (5) Others; primary liver tumour and cystic fibrosis.

Biliary Atresia Single most common cause of liver failure in infancy and childhood. Kasai procedure is successful in one-half of all patients if jaundice is fully relieved. Primary LT is routinely not indicated unless the patient has signs of severe liver damage like coagulopathy, hypoalbuminemia and ascites.

Progressive Familial Intrahepatic Cholestasis (PFIC) This is a chronic cholestasis syndrome which begins in infancy and usually progresses to cirrhosis within the first decade of life.

Liver Tumours in Children Hepatoblastoma is the most common liver tumour in children and when non-resectable, transplantation is the treatment of choice [28, 29].

7.3 Contraindication

Contraindication, can be divided into relative and absolute [30] (Table 7.8).

Obesity Obesity Patients with BMI ≥ 40 (severe obesity) tend to have adverse outcomes post LT; hence it is a relative contraindication [31].

Age In the absence of significant comorbidities, the older recipient (>70 years) is not a contraindication for LT.

Portopulmonary hypertension (POPH) Mild and moderate POPH if controlled with medication are not contraindication for LT but severe POPH with pulmonary systolic arterial pressure ≥60 mm of Hg is considered a contraindication for LT in most centres.

Extrahepatic Malignancy Having an extrahepatic malignancy is a contraindication for liver transplantation. Having a tumour-free period of 2–5 years is accepted in general as a requirement before LT. Benten et al. [32] in their series of 37 patients with a history of various solid tumours and myeloproliferative disease and who underwent OLT, the overall recurrence rate was 2.8%. Such series have

Table 7.8 Contraindications for Liver Transplant

Absolute contraindications	Relative contraindications
• Brain death	Advanced age
• Extrahepatic malignancy	Cholangiocarcinoma
• Active uncontrolled infection	HIV infection
• Active alcoholism and substance abuse	Portal vein thrombosis
• AIDS	Psychologic instability
• Severe cardiopulmonary disease	
• Uncontrolled sepsis	
• Inability to comply with medical regimen	
• Lack of psychosocial support	
• Anatomic abnormalities precluding liver transplantation	
• Compensated cirrhosis without complications (Child-Turcotte-Pugh score, 5–6)	

been published more often now questioning the past wisdom of absolute contraindication in patients with extrahepatic malignancy. In the coming times, extrahepatic malignancy may not be an absolute contraindication when an appropriate selection of such patients is done and subjected to OLT.

Active Uncontrolled Infection Any sort of ongoing active infection in the body is an absolute contraindication for LT. LT may proceed after adequate control of infection.

HIV Infection HIV infection per se is not a contraindication for LT, in the era of highly active antiretroviral treatment (HAART). Though it requires well-coordinated team management by the transplant and HIV teams [8].

Anatomical Causes LT requires a viable mesenteric venous circulation; portal vein thrombosis is no more a contraindication. Portal vein thrombosis may be addressed with either thrombectomy or jump grafts.

Active Alcohol and Substance Abuse Ongoing alcohol or substance abuse is an absolute contraindication for LT. Existing shortage of organs and potentially harmful effects of alcohol relapse posttransplant necessitate providing LT only for deserving candidates. One of the risk factors for relapse is the shorter duration of pretransplant abstinence, hence the recommendation of 6 months minimum abstinence before LT.

Inability to Comply with Medical Regimen and Lack of Psychosocial Support Post LT complying with regular follow-up and investigations are mandatory for long-term survival of the graft and patient. Patients need psychosocial support for this lifelong compliance within the recommended lifestyle changes and adherence to the same [33].

7.4 Contraindications for Live Liver Donors as per OPTN (Organ Procurement and Transplantation Policy) [34]

Age less than 18 years with a lack of mental capacity for informed decision-making

HIV infection, unless the requirements for a variance are met

Active malignancy

High suspicion of donor coercion

High suspicion of illegal financial exchange between the donor and recipient

Evidence of acute symptomatic infection

Active mental illness requiring treatment before donation, including any evidence of suicidality

HCV RNA positivity

HBsAg positivity

Donors with ZZ, Z-null, null-null, and S-null alpha-1-antitrypsin phenotypes

Expected donor remnant volume less than 30 per cent of native liver volume

Prior living liver donation

In India, only a related donor will be considered for donation.

7.5 Summary

Organ availability is scarce and rationing the resource to suitable and eligible candidates is of prime importance. Patients should meet the recommended minimum criteria for LT and not have any of the absolute contraindications. The recommendations and guidelines are dynamic and with gradually increasing indications and declining contraindications. The King's College Hospital criteria are used globally for assessing the need for LT in acute Fulminant Liver failure. MELD and CTP score are used for non-malignant aetiology of cirrhosis for LT. The Milan criteria are presently used for eligibility in HCC patients.

References

1. Gordon RD, Shaw BW, Iwatsuki S, Esquivel CO, Starzl TE. Indications for liver transplantation in the Cyclosporine Era. Surg Clin North Am. 1986;66:541–56.
2. Farkas S, Hackl C, Schlitt HJ. Overview of the indications and contraindications for liver transplantation. Cold Spring Harb Perspect Med. 2014;4:a015602.
3. Tandon B, Bernauau J, O'Grady J, Gupta S, Krisch R, Liaw Y-F, et al. Recommendations of the International Association for the Study of the liver subcommittee on nomenclature of acute and subacute liver failure. J Gastroenterol Hepatol. 2002;14:403–4.
4. Renner EL. How to decide when to list a patient with acute liver failure for liver transplantation? Clichy or King's College criteria, or something else? J Hepatol. 2007;46:554–7.
5. Kumar R, Shalimar, Sharma H, Goyal R, Kumar A, Khanal S, et al. Prospective derivation and validation of early dynamic model for predicting outcome in patients with acute liver failure. Gut. 2012;61:1068–75.
6. O'Grady JG, Alexander GJM, Hayllar KM, Williams R. Early indicators of prognosis in fulminant hepatic failure. Gastroenterology. 1989;97:439–45.
7. Bernal W, Lee WM, Wendon J, Larsen FS, Williams R. Acute liver failure: a curable disease by 2024? J Hepatol. 2015;62:S112–20.
8. Murray KF, Carithers RL. AASLD practice guidelines: evaluation of the patient for liver transplantation. Hepatology. 2005;41:1407–32.
9. Varma V, Mehta N, Kumaran V, Nundy S. Indications and contraindications for liver transplantation. Int J Hepatol. 2011;2011:1–9.
10. Durand F, Valla D. Assessment of the prognosis of cirrhosis: child–Pugh versus MELD. J Hepatol. 2005;42:S100–7.
11. Ferrarese A. Liver transplantation for viral hepatitis in 2015. World J Gastroenterol. 2016;22:1570.
12. Fattovich G, Giustina G, Degos F, Tremolada F, Diodati G, Almasio P, et al. Morbidity and mortality in compensated cirrhosis type C: a retrospective follow-up study of 384 patients. Gastroenterology. 1997;112:463–72.
13. Sangiovanni A, Del Ninno E, Fasani P, De Fazio C, Ronchi G, Romeo R, et al. Increased survival of cirrhotic patients with a hepatocellular carcinoma detected during surveillance. Gastroenterology. 2004;126:1005–14.
14. Philippe M, Christophe M, Didier S, Jérôme D, Julia S, François D, et al. Early liver transplantation for severe alcoholic hepatitis. N Engl J Med. 2011;365:1790–800.
15. Vaillant GE. The natural history of alcoholism and its relationship to liver transplantation. Liver Transpl Surg. 1997;3:304–10.
16. Poynard T, Naveau S, Doffoel M, Boudjema K, Vanlemmens C, Mantion G, et al. Evaluation of efficacy of liver transplantation in alcoholic cirrhosis using matched and simulated controls: 5-year survival. J Hepatol. 1999;30:1130–7.
17. Carrion AF, Bhamidimarri KR. Liver transplant for cholestatic liver diseases. Clin Liver Dis. 2013;17:345–59.
18. Khungar V, Goldberg DS. Liver transplantation for cholestatic liver diseases in adults. Clin Liver Dis. 2016;20:191–203.
19. Schöning W, Schmeding M, Ulmer F, Andert A, Neumann U. Liver transplantation for patients with cholestatic liver diseases. Visc Med. 2015;31:194–8.
20. Mazzaferro V, Regalia E, Doci R, Andreola S, Pulvirenti A, Bozzetti F, et al. Liver transplantation for the treatment of small hepatocellular carcinomas in patients with cirrhosis. N Engl J Med. 1996;334:693–700.
21. Xu D-W, Wan P, Xia Q. Liver transplantation for hepatocellular carcinoma beyond the Milan criteria: a review. World J Gastroenterol. 2016;22:3325–34.
22. Ethun CG, Lopez-Aguiar AG, Anderson DJ, Adams AB, Fields RC, Doyle MB, et al. Transplantation versus resection for hilar cholangiocarcinoma: an argument for shifting treatment paradigms for resectable disease. HPB. 2017;19:S1–2.
23. Olausson M, Friman S, Cahlin C, Nilsson O, Jansson S, Wängberg B, et al. Indications and results of liver transplantation in patients with neuroendocrine tumors. World J Surg. 2002;26:998–1004.
24. European Association for the Study of the Liver. EASL clinical practice guidelines: Wilson's disease. J Hepatol. 2012;56:671–85.
25. Petrasek J, Jirsa M, Sperl J, Kozak L, Taimr P, Spicak J, et al. Revised King's College score for liver transplantation in adult patients with Wilson's disease. Liver Transpl. 2007;13:55–61.
26. Dhawan A, Taylor RM, Cheeseman P, De Silva P, Katsiyiannakis L, Mieli-Vergani G. Wilson's disease in children: 37-year experience and revised King's score for liver transplantation. Liver Transpl. 2005;11:441–8.
27. Menon KVN. The Budd–Chiari syndrome. N Engl J Med. 2004;350(6):578–85.
28. Spada M, Riva S, Maggiore G, Cintorino D, Gridelli B. Pediatric liver transplantation. World J Gastroenterol. 2009;15:648.
29. Engelmann G, Schmidt J, Oh J, Lenhartz H, Wenning D, Teufel U, et al. Indications for pediatric liver transplantation. Data from the Heidelberg pediatric liver transplantation program. Nephrol Dial Transplant. 2007;22:viii23–8.

30. Ahmed A, Keeffe EB. Current indications and contra-indications for liver transplantation. Clin Liver Dis. 2007;11:227–47.

31. Martin P, DiMartini A, Feng S, Brown R, Fallon M. Evaluation for liver transplantation in adults: 2013 practice guideline by the American Association for the Study of Liver Diseases and the American Society of Transplantation: Martin et al. Hepatology. 2014;59:1144–65.

32. Benten D, Sterneck M, Panse J, Rogiers X, Lohse AW. Low recurrence of preexisting extrahepatic malignancies after liver transplantation. Liver Transpl. 2008;14:789–98.

33. Carbonneau M, Jensen LA, Bain VG, Kelly K, Meeberg G, Tandon P. Alcohol use while on the liver transplant waiting list: a single-center experience. Liver Transpl. 2010;16:91–7.

34. Organ Procurement and Transplantation Network [Internet]. [cited 2019 July 7]. Available from: https://optn.transplant.hrsa.gov/media/1200/optn_policies.pdf#nameddest=Policy_14%20(Accessed%20on%20March%2002,%202017.

Disease Severity Scoring System in Chronic Liver Disease

8

Neeraj Saraf and Swapnil Dhampalwar

8.1 Introduction

Cirrhosis is the result of the progression of a chronic necro-inflammatory liver disease leading to fibrosis and vascular remodelling leading to development of portal hypertension. When established, cirrhosis remains compensated for a variably long time.

The earliest consequence of cirrhosis is a progressive increase in portal pressure up to the Clinically Significant Portal Hypertension (CSPH) threshold of ≥ 10 mmHg. Bleeding, ascites, encephalopathy and jaundice indicate decompensated cirrhosis. Renal function impairment, refractory ascites, infections and circulatory dysfunction indicate more advanced decompensation and are associated with very poor survival.

Acute-on-chronic liver failure (ACLF) may occur either in decompensated or in compensated cirrhosis and is associated with a high short-term (28-day) mortality. Systemic inflammatory response to several critical events is the most important mechanism activating ACLF.

8.2 Clinical States in Cirrhosis

A patient with cirrhosis may have different clinical morbidities with significantly different outcomes in the course of disease. A comprehensive multistate model for the clinical course of cirrhosis as proposed by D'Amico et al. [1] has been shown in Fig. 8.1. These clinical states enable the classification of patients according to increasing mortality risk. However, there is no predictable sequence of such clinical states and that they may not be considered as progressive disease stages.

N. Saraf (✉) · S. Dhampalwar
Institute of Digestive and Hepatobiliary Sciences,
Medanta The Medicity, Gurgaon, India

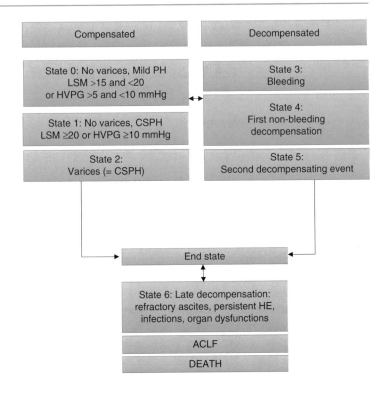

Fig. 8.1 Comprehensive multistate model of natural history of cirrhosis adapted from D'Amico et al. [1]

8.3   Different Scoring Systems in Cirrhosis

8.3.1 CTP Score

The Child-Pugh scoring system [also known as the Child-Turcotte-Pugh (CTP) score] was designed to predict mortality in patients with cirrhosis. It was originally conceptualised by Child and Turcotte [2] in 1964 to guide the selection of patients who would benefit from elective surgery for portal decompression. Their original scoring system used 5 clinical and laboratory criteria to categorise patients: serum bilirubin, serum albumin, ascites, neurological disorder and clinical nutrition status.

The scoring system was modified later by Pugh et al. [3] substituting prothrombin time for clinical nutrition status (Table 8.1). CTP score is obtained by adding the score for each parameter. CTP class A = 5–6 points, B = 7–9 points, C = 10–15 points.

However, there are limitations to the use of CTP score. It has subjective assessment of ascites and encephalopathy; it does not account for renal

function (creatinine and sodium) and has only ten different scores (based on points) available.

8.3.2 Modified CTP Score

In 2006, Huo et al. [4] proposed modified CTP (mCTP) score. It was obtained by assigning an additional point in patients whose serum bilirubin was >8 mg/dL, prothrombin time prolongation >11 s or albumin <2.3 g/dL; accordingly, a mCTP score of 16–18 was defined as mCTP class D, which identified severely decompensated cirrhosis.

8.3.3 MELD Score and Its Modifications

The Model for End-Stage Liver Disease (MELD) score was first described in 2000 to predict 3-month survival rates in patients with chronic liver disease undergoing transjugular intrahepatic portosystemic shunt [5]. At present, MELD is widely used for organ allocation.

Table 8.1 Child-Turcotte-Pugh score

	Points		
	1	2	3
Encephalopathy	None	Grade 1–2 (or precipitant-induced)	Grade 3–4 (or chronic)
Ascites	None	Mild/moderate (diuretic-responsive)	Severe (diuretic-refractory)
Bilirubin (mg/dL)	<2	2–3	>3
Albumin (g/dL)	>3.5	2.8–3.5	<2.8
PT (sec prolonged) or INR	<4 <1.7	4–6 1.7–2.3	>6 >2.3

Table 8.2 MELD score and its modifications

MELD	$(3.78 \times \log_e (\text{bilirubin})) + (11.2 \times \log_e (\text{INR})) + (9.57 \times \log_e (\text{creatinine})) + 6.43$
iMELD	$\text{MELD} + (\text{age} \times 0.3) - (0.7 \times \text{Na}) + 100$
MELD Na	$\text{MELD} + 1.32 \times (137-\text{Na}) - [0.033 \times \text{MELD} \times (137-\text{Na})]$
MELD sarcopenia	$\text{MELD} + 10.35 \times \text{sarcopenia}$
MELD L3-SMI	$\text{MELD} - 0.3065 \times \text{L3 SMI}$

Table 8.3 MELD score and probability of mortality

MELD score	Mortality probability
40	71.3% mortality
30–39	52.6% mortality
20–29	19.6% mortality
10–19	6.0% mortality
9 or less	1.9% mortality

MELD score (Table 8.2) is calculated using the patient's bilirubin level, creatinine level and INR. Lower limit of Serum Sodium (Na) is capped at 125, and upper limit is capped at 137. Upper limit of serum creatinine is capped at 4; in addition, if the patient had dialysis at least twice in the past week, the value for serum creatinine will be automatically adjusted to 4. The maximum MELD score is 40. Three-month survival rates as per MELD score have been shown in Table 8.3.

MELD also has some limitations. MELD benefits patients with cholestasis or renal failure and is not directly influenced by other complications of cirrhosis associated with poor survival (such as persistent ascites and hyponatremia). For this reason, many recent studies have evaluated the effect of incorporating other variables into the model, such as serum sodium and age (Table 8.2) to give other variables such as integrated MELD [6] and MELD sodium [7].

Loss of skeletal muscle mass, i.e. sarcopenia, is associated with higher mortality independent of MELD score in cirrhotic patients on waiting list. There are two modifications of MELD considering muscle mass with two different variables. Addition of sarcopenia (a dichotomous variable) to MELD; MELD-sarcopenia model [8] has shown to improve predictive value at 1 year in patients with MELD score < 15, who are traditionally deemed to have a low risk of death. The addition of L3 Skeletal Muscle Index (as a continuous variable) to MELD; MELD-L3 SMI [9] yielded inferior performance compared with MELD-sarcopenia. This is probably because sarcopenia as a dichotomous variable is corrected to gender and height and has more statistical strength.

8.3.4 Alcoholic Liver Disease

Alcoholic hepatitis (AH) is caused by acute inflammation of the liver in patients that consume excessive amounts of alcohol, usually in a background of cirrhosis. AH can range from mild to severe, life-threatening disease with a high short-term mortality. Different prognostic models have been used to stratify severity and estimate mortality in order to identify those that may benefit from corticosteroids (Table 8.4).

Maddrey et al. [10] in 1978 first yielded the Discriminant Function, later modified DF [11], based on prothrombin time (PT) and serum bilirubin that identified patients with a significant risk for early mortality. Those patients with mDF >32 were considered to have severe AH. Patients with an elevated mDF and/or with encephalopathy that received corticosteroid therapy showed a 28-day mortality of 6% in the treatment group compared to 35% in the placebo group.

Dunn et al. [12] showed that MELD score of 21 was the only independent predictor of mortality in patients with AH. Forrest et al. [13] used 5 variables including age, blood urea, peripheral blood leukocyte count, serum bilirubin and INR PT, expressed as a ratio of the control value to develop a new prognostic scoring system, Glasgow alcoholic hepatitis score (GAHS), for AH. Values obtained ranged from 5 to 12, separated into those with value <9 or ≥9 points. Corticosteroids therapy was associated with better survival in those with GAHS ≥9 compared to no treatment.

Dominguez et al. [14] advised a predictive score from multivariate analysis of variables

Table 8.4 Severity scores in alcoholic hepatitis

Scoring system	Formula				Severe disease
mDF	4.6 (patient's PT in seconds − control PT in seconds) + total bilirubin (mg/dL)				≥32
MELD	See Table 8.2				≥21
GAHS	**Points**	**1**	**2**	**3**	≥9
	Age	<50	≥50	–	
	WBC (10⁹/l)	<15	≥15	–	
	Urea (mg/dl)	<14	≥14	–	
	INR	<1.5	1.5–2.0	>2.0	
	Bilirubin (mg/dl)	<7.3	7.3–14.6	>14.6	
Lille score	3.19–0.101 × (age in years) + 0.147 × (albumin day 0 in g/L) + 0.0165 × (evolution in bilirubin level in μM) − (0.206 × renal insufficiency) − 0.0065 × (bilirubin day 0 in μM) − 0.0096 × (INR or prothrombin time in seconds)				≥0.45
ABIC score	(age × 0.1) + (serum bilirubin × 0.08) + (serum creatinine × 0.3) + (INR × 0.8)				>9.0
AHHS	**Histopathology**	**Points**			
	Stage of fibrosis				Mild (0–3)
	No fibrosis or portal fibrosis	0			Moderate (4–5)
	Expansive fibrosis	0			Severe (6–9)
	Bridging fibrosis or cirrhosis	3			
	Bilirubinostasis				
	No	0			
	Hepatocellular only	0			
	Canalicular or ductular	1			
	Canalicular or ductular plus hepatocellular	2			
	PMN infiltration				
	No/Mild	2			
	Severe	0			
	Megamitochondria				
	No megamitochondria	2			
	Megamitochondria	0			

identified during admission, the ABIC score. Using a cut-off value of 6.71 and 9, the score identified patients with AH that have a low (100% survival), intermediate (70% survival), and high risk (25% survival) of death at 90 days.

Louvet et al. [15] generated a prognostic model, the Lille model, to identify "non-responders" to corticosteroid therapy in patients with severe AH. The model combined six objective variables (age, renal insufficiency, albumin, PT, bilirubin and evolution of bilirubin at day 7) which were highly predictive of death at 6 months in patients treated with corticosteroids ($p < 0.000001$). A cut-off value of 0.45 was determined to be the best identifier of patients at high risk of death. Patients receiving corticosteroids after 7 days with a score ≥ 0.45 may be futile and alternative treatments should be considered.

Altamirano et al. [16] developed a histologic scoring system based on liver biopsy findings to predict short-term (90-day) mortality in AH patients. AHHS cut-off score categorised patients as low 0–3 (97% survival), intermediate 4–5 (81% survival), and high risk 6–9 (49% survival)

of death. When combing the AHHS with analytical scoring systems, the AHHS was able to refine the prognostic stratification of those with a MELD score <21 (low risk group) with different 90-day survival using a cut-off of 5 points (94% vs. 72%; $p = 0.001$).

Louvet et al. [17] evaluated the prognostic value of combining static models for AH, such as mDF, MELD score and ABIC score with dynamic models, such as the Lille score. This joint effect model was able to predict survival after 2 and 6 months significantly better than either the static or dynamic models alone ($p < 0.01$). The MELD + Lille combination model predicted survival better than the mDF + Lille or ABIC + Lille models.

8.3.5 Primary Biliary Cirrhosis

The Mayo risk score (MRS) was first described by Dickson et al. [18] and includes five variables which predict survival in PBC without transplantation. The prognostic index is calculated using the following equation:

$$0.871 \times \log_e (\text{bilirubin in mg} / \text{dL} - 2.53 \times \log_e (\text{albumin in g} / \text{dL}) + 0.039 \times \text{age}(\text{years})$$
$$+ 2.38 \times \log_e (\text{prothrombin time in seconds}) + 0.859 \, \text{edema}^*$$

$^*0 =$ no oedema, no diuretic therapy; $0.5 =$ oedema, no diuretic therapy or no oedema, diuretic therapy; $1 =$ oedema and diuretic therapy.

A MRS of 7.8 was identified as optimal for liver transplantation.

8.3.6 Primary Sclerosing Cholangitis

Mayo PSC Risk Score was described by Kim et al. [19] based on Natural history survival model. The prognostic index R is calculated using the following equitation:

$$0.03 \times (\text{age in years}) + 0.54 \times \log_e (\text{total bilirubin in mg} / \text{dL}) - 0.84 \times (\text{serum albumin in g} / \text{dL})$$
$$+ 0.54 \times \log_e (\text{AST in IU} / \text{L}) + 1.24 \times (\text{points for variceal bleeding})$$

If Mayo Risk Score (R) is greater than 2, patient is in the "high" risk group.

8.4 Acute on Chronic Liver Failure

Acute on Chronic Liver Failure (ACLF) is a syndrome characterised by acute hepatic insult in patients with underlying chronic liver disease leading to organ failures and high short-term mortality. The syndrome is varyingly defined by different working groups given its inherent heterogeneity and dynamicity. Two important definitions of ACLF which differ between Eastern (Asian Pacific Association for the Study of the Liver [APASL]–ACLF Research Consortium, AARC [20]) and Western countries (European Association for the Study of the Liver [EASL]–Chronic Liver Failure Consortium, CLIF-C [21]) are discussed here.

8.4.1 APASL AARC Definition

As per APASL [20], ACLF is defined as an acute hepatic insult manifesting as jaundice (serum bilirubin level of ≥5 mg/dL) and coagulopathy (INR of ≥1.5 or prothrombin activity of <40%), complicated within 4 weeks by ascites and/or

encephalopathy in patients with previously diagnosed or undiagnosed chronic liver disease (including cirrhosis) and is associated with high 28-day mortality.

Definitions of organ failures as per these two consortia are summarised in Table 8.5 [22]. APASL analyses severity of disease by liver failure-based variables, namely serum bilirubin, INR, serum lactate, serum creatinine and grade of encephalopathy. The AARC ACLF score is calculated based on these variables (range 5 to 15) and liver failure is graded into 3 grades (Table 8.6). These grades show a potentially recoverable group (Grade I), a group that needs special monitoring (Grade II) and a group that demands immediate interventions for improved outcome (Grade III) [23].

The AARC score can be calculated at bedside. It is dynamic in nature. It can predict 28-day survival at presentation (score of ≤9) and at day 7 (score of ≤9). For a score of ≥10, with each unit increase, mortality increases sharply compared with those <10 at initial presentation (20 vs. 4%). A shift from Grade I to Grade III liver failure at day 4 and 7 increases mortality. Persistence of Grade I or II until 7 days predicted improved survival, whereas persistence in Grade III failure carries grave prognosis and warrants early consideration for transplantation.

Table 8.5 Definitions of organ failures (OFs) as per different consortia

Failing organ	APASL definition	EASL-CLIF definition
Liver	Total bilirubin ≥5 mg/dL and INR ≥1.5	Bilirubin level of >12 mg/dL
Kidney	Acute Kidney Injury Network criteria	Creatinine level of ≥2.0 mg/dL or renal replacement
Brain	Hepatic encephalopathy grade III-IV (West Haven)	Hepatic encephalopathy grade III-IV (West Haven)
Coagulation	INR ≥1.5	INR ≥2.5 OR Platelet <20,000
Circulation	–	Use of vasopressor (terlipressin and/or catecholamines)
Respiration	–	PaO2/FiO2 of ≤200 OR SpO2/FiO2 of ≤214 OR Need for mechanical ventilation

Table 8.6 AARC score and ACLF grade

AARC score						ACLF grade		
Points	Total bilirubin (mg/dL)	HE grade	PT-INR	Lactate (mmol/L)	Creatinine (mg/dL)	Grade	Score	28-day mortality
1	<15	0	<1.8	<1.5	<0.7	I	5–7	12.7%
2	15–25	I–II	1.8–2.5	1.5–2.5	0.7–1.5	II	8–10	44.5%
3	>25	III–IV	>2.5	>2.5	>1.5	III	11–15	85.9%

8.4.2 EASL CLIF-C Definition

As per EASL-CLIF Consortium [21], ACLF is defined as acute decompensation (AD) of cirrhosis associated with Organ Failure (OF) and high short-term mortality (28-day mortality ≥15%).

Definitions of organ failures are based on CLIF-Sequential Organ Failure Assessment (CLIF-SOFA) score [24] (modified SOFA score used in critically ill patients) which was later simplified to CLIF Consortium Organ Failure score (CLIF-C OFs) as shown in Table 8.7.

Since presence of mild renal or brain dysfunction in the presence of another organ failure is associated with a significant short-term mortality, these two organs received special attention. Classification and grades of ACLF as per EASL CLIF Consortium are summarised in Table 8.8. Data from the CANONIC study showed overall 28-day mortality of 33% of all cases of ACLF, and specific 28-day mortality rates in patients with ACLF grade 1, 2 and 3 were 22%, 32% and 73%, respectively [21].

Whenever a patient with cirrhosis with acute decompensation is admitted, CLIF-C OF score should be calculated. This score will divide patients according to the presence or absence of ACLF. If patient has ACLF, CLIF-C AD score [25] is calculated. If ACLF is absent, CLIF-C ACLF score [26] is calculated. These scores predict mortality in patients with ACLF and without ACLF, respectively.

Table 8.7 CLIF Consortium Organ Failure score: simplified version

Organ/system	Variable	Score = 1	Score = 2	Score = 3
Liver	Bilirubin (mg/dL)	<6	6 to ≤12	>12
Kidney	Creatinine (mg/dL)	<2	2 to <3.5	≥3.5 or RRT
Brain	Encephalopathy grade (West-Haven)	0	I–II	III–IV
Coagulation	INR	<2	2 to <2.5	≥2.5
Circulation	MAP (mm Hg)	≥70	<70	Vasopressors
Respiratory	PaO_2/FiO_2 or SpO_2/FiO_2	>300 >357	≤300 and >200 >214 and ≤357	≤200 ≤214

Table 8.8 Classification and grades of ACLF

Grades of ACLF	Clinical characteristics	28-day mortality	90-day mortality
No ACLF	No organ failure, OR Single non-kidney organ failure, creatinine <1.5 mg/dL, no HE, OR Single cerebral failure, creatinine <1.5	4.7%	14%
ACLF Ia	Single renal failure	22.1%	40.7%
ACLF Ib	Single non-kidney organ failure, creatinine 1.5–1.9 mg/dL and/or HE grade 1–2, OR Single cerebral failure, creatinine 1.5–1.9		
ACLF II	Two organ failures	32%	52.3%
ACLF III	Three or more organ failures	76.7%	79.1%

8.4.3 CLIF-C AD Score

$$10 \times \left[\begin{array}{l} 0.03 \times \text{Age} + 0.66 \times \log_e (\text{Creatinine}) + 1.71 \\ \times \log_e (\text{INR}) + 0.88 \times \log_e (\text{WBC}) 0.05 \times \text{Sodium} + 8 \end{array} \right]$$

Although ACLF grade at diagnosis correlates with prognosis, clinical course of the syndrome during hospitalisation is the most important determinant of short-term mortality. Majority of patients achieve their final grade of ACLF within the first week; therefore, the assessment of ACLF grade at days 3–7 after diagnosis predicted 28-day and 90-day mortality more accurately than ACLF grade at diagnosis.

8.4.4 CLIF-C ACLF Score

$$10 \times \left[\begin{array}{l} 0.033 \times \text{CLIF OFs} + 0.04 \\ \times \text{Age} + 0.63 \times \log_e (\text{WBC}) 2 \end{array} \right]$$

The final score ranges from 0 to 100. CLIF-C ACLF score showed a significantly higher accuracy for predicting mortality than MELD, MELD-Na and Child-Pugh-Turcotte score at all main time points after ACLF diagnosis (28, 90, 180 and 365 days) with 7–11% improvement in the discrimination ability. Presence of ≥4 organ failures and CLIF-C ACLF >64 at day 7 have been shown to predict poor survival and futility of liver transplantation.

8.5 Conclusion

The clinical spectrum of cirrhosis encompasses several clinical states. The progression across such states does not occur through a predictable sequence, because of the variable interplay between pathophysiological mechanisms. Therefore, a multistate, multi-model approach provides a more realistic description of the disease course. These models should be considered for when planning clinical research either of prognosis or of treatment efficacy in cirrhosis.

References

1. D'Amico G, Morabito A, D'Amico M, Pasta L, Malizia G, Rebora P, et al. Clinical states of cirrhosis and competing risks. J Hepatol. 2018;68(3):563–76.
2. Child CG, Turcotte JG. Surgery and portal hypertension. Major Probl Clin Surg. 1964;1:1–85.

3. Pugh RN, Murray-Lyon IM, Dawson JL, Pietroni MC, Williams R. Transection of the oesophagus for bleeding oesophageal varices. Br J Surg. 1973;60(8):646–9.

4. Huo TI, Lin HC, Wu JC, Lee FY, Hou MC, Lee PC, et al. Proposal of a modified Child-Turcotte-Pugh scoring system and comparison with the model for end-stage liver disease for outcome prediction in patients with cirrhosis. Liver Transpl. 2006;12:65–71.

5. Malinchoc M, Kamath PS, Gordon FD, Peine CJ, Rank J, ter Borg PC. A model to predict poor survival in patients undergoing transjugular intrahepatic portosystemic shunts. Hepatology. 2000;31(4):864–71.

6. Luca A, Angermayr B, Bertolini G, Koenig F, Vizzini G, Ploner M, et al. An integrated MELD model including serum sodium and age improves the prediction of early mortality in patients with cirrhosis. Liver Transpl. 2007;13:1174–80.

7. Kim WR, Biggins SW, Kremers W, Wiesner R, Kamath PS, Benson JT, et al. Hyponatremia and mortality among patients on the liver-transplant waiting list. N Engl J Med. 2008;359:1018–26.

8. van Vugt J, Laurens A, et al. A model including sarcopenia surpasses the MELD score in predicting waiting list mortality in cirrhotic liver transplant candidates: a competing risk analysis in a national cohort. J Hepatol. 2018;68(4):707–14.

9. Montano-Loza AJ, Duarte-Rojo A, Meza-Junco J, Baracos VE, Sawyer MB, Pang JX, et al. Inclusion of sarcopenia within MELD (MELD-sarcopenia) and the prediction of mortality in patients with cirrhosis. Clin Transl Gastroenterol. 2015;16(6):e102.

10. Maddrey WC, Boitnott JK, Bedine MS, Weber FL, Mezey E, White RI. Corticosteroid therapy of alcoholic hepatitis. Gastroenterology. 1978;75(2):193–9.

11. Carithers RL, Herlong HF, Diehl AM, Shaw EW, Combes B, Fallon HJ, et al. Methylprednisolone therapy in patients with severe alcoholic hepatitis. A randomized multicenter trial. Ann Intern Med. 1989;110(9):685–90.

12. Dunn W, Jamil LH, Brown LS, Wiesner RH, Kim WR, Menon KV, et al. MELD accurately predicts mortality in patients with alcoholic hepatitis. Hepatology. 2005;41(2):353–8.

13. Forrest EH, Evans CD, Stewart S, Phillips M, Oo YH, McAvoy NC, et al. Analysis of factors predictive of mortality in alcoholic hepatitis and derivation and validation of the Glasgow alcoholic hepatitis score. Gut. 2005;54(8):1174–9.

14. Dominguez M, Rincón D, Abraldes JG, Miquel R, Colmenero J, Bellot P, et al. A new scoring system for prognostic stratification of patients with alcoholic hepatitis. Am J Gastroenterol. 2008;103(11):2747–56.

15. Louvet A, Naveau S, Abdelnour M, Ramond MJ, Diaz E, Fartoux L, et al. The Lille model: a new tool for therapeutic strategy in patients with severe alcoholic hepatitis treated with steroids. Hepatology. 2007;45(6):1348–54.

16. Altamirano J, Miquel R, Katoonizadeh A, Abraldes JG, Duarte-Rojo A, Louvet A, et al. A histologic scoring system for prognosis of patients with alcoholic hepatitis. Gastroenterology. 2014;146(5):1231–9.

17. Louvet A, Labreuche J, Artru F, Boursier J, Kim DJ, O'Grady J, et al. Combining data from liver disease scoring systems better predicts outcomes of patients with alcoholic hepatitis. Gastroenterology. 2015;149(2):398–406.

18. Dickson ER, Grambsch PM, Fleming TR, Fisher LD, Langworthy A. Prognosis in primary biliary cirrhosis: model for decision making. Hepatology. 1989;10:1–7.

19. Kim WR, Therneau TM, Wiesner RH, Poterucha JJ, Benson JT, Malinchoc M, et al. A revised natural history model for primary sclerosing cholangitis. Mayo Clin Proc. 2000;75:688–94.

20. Sarin SK, Kedarisetty CK, Abbas Z, et al. Acute-on-chronic liver failure: consensus recommendations of the Asian Pacific Association for the Study of the Liver (APASL) 2014. Hepatol Int. 2014;8:453–71.

21. Moreau R, Jalan R, Gines P, et al. Acute-on-chronic liver failure is a distinct syndrome that develops in patients with acute decompensation of cirrhosis. Gastroenterology. 2013;144:1426–37.

22. Hernaez R, Solà E, Moreau R, Ginès P. Acute-on-chronic liver failure: an update. Gut. 2017;66:541–53.

23. Choudhury A, Jindal A, Maiwall R, Sharma MK, Sharma BC, Pamecha V, et al. Liver failure determines the outcome in patients of acute-on chronic liver failure (ACLF): comparison of APASL ACLF research consortium (AARC) and CLIF-SOFA models. Hepatol Int. 2017;11(5):461–71.

24. Jalan R, Saliba F, Pavesi M, et al. Development and validation of a prognostic score to predict mortality in patients with acute-on-chronic liver failure. J Hepatol. 2014;61:1038–47.

25. Jalan R, Pavesi M, Saliba F, Amoros A, Fernandez J, Holland-Fischer P, et al. The CLIF consortium acute decompensation score (CLIF-C ADs) for prognosis of hospitalised cirrhotic patients without acute-on-chronic liver failure. J Hepatol. 2015;62:831–40.

26. Jalan R, Saliba F, Pavesi M, Amoros A, Moreau R, Gines P, et al. Development and validation of a prognostic score to predict mortality in patients with acute-on-chronic liver failure. J Hepatol. 2014;61:1038–47.

Preoperative Assessment and Optimization of Liver Transplant Patient: Ascites and Hydrothorax

9

Archna Koul and Jayashree Sood

9.1 Introduction

The word "ascites" is derived from the Greek Word "askos" meaning a "leather bag for carrying wine, water or oil" [1] and in the context of liver disease it refers to abnormal accumulation of fluid in the peritoneal cavity. It is the most common complication of cirrhosis followed by hepatic encephalopathy and variceal bleeding [2].

The onset of ascites is associated with a poor prognosis as it heralds the progression of the natural history of cirrhosis from an asymptomatic to a decompensated stage.

About 50% of patients with compensated disease develop ascites during an observation period of 10 years [2, 3].

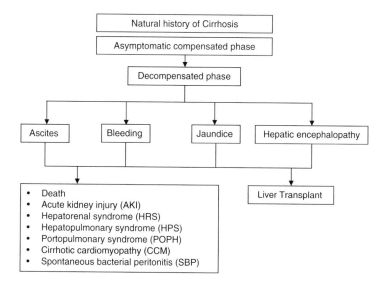

A. Koul (✉) · J. Sood
Institute of Anaesthesiology, Pain and Perioperative
Medicine, Sir Ganga Ram hospital, New Delhi, India

Liver transplantation is the ultimate treatment option in these patients, but it should be contemplated before the occurrence of renal dysfunction [2].

9.2 Pathophysiology of Ascites in Cirrhosis [4, 5]

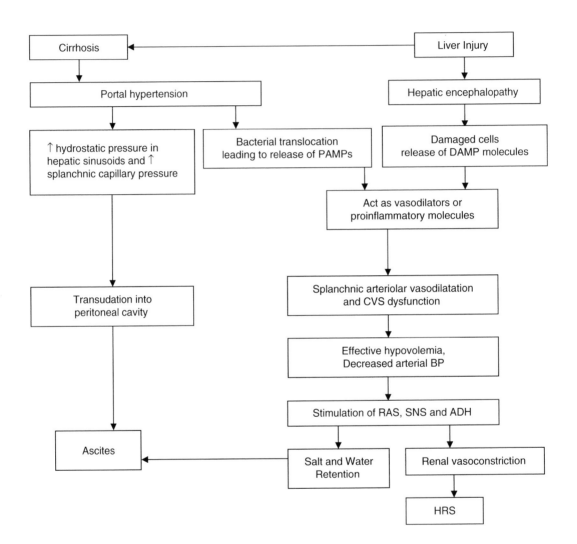

PAMP Pathogen-Associated Molecular Pattern (proinflammatory cytokines and chemokines).
DAMP Damage-Associated Molecular Patterns.

RAS Renin Angiotensin System.
SNS Sympathetic Nervous System.
ADH Antidiuretic hormone.

9.3   Standard Diagnostic Steps

These are followed in all patients who present with ascites

- History.
- Physical examination.
- Blood tests.
- Abdominal ultrasound.
- Paracentesis (diagnostic).
- Ascitic fluid analysis.

9.3.1   History

Although present in 85% [6] of all liver disease patients cirrhosis is the commonest cause of ascites, and other nonhepatic causes of ascites should also be ruled out by taking history from the patients. History of alcohol consumption, blood transfusion, hepatitis in the past, drug abuse, dietary indiscretion, or fever should be taken to ascertain the cause of cirrhosis.

9.3.2   Physical Examination

On visual inspection, bulging flanks can be detected. Flank dullness is the most sensitive physical sign present in 90% of the patients with ascites [7]. Shifting dullness becomes evident when there is at least 1500 mL of ascitic fluid collection; it is a more specific, but less sensitive, physical sign. Other signs of cirrhosis like palmar erythema, spider naevi, and jaundice can also be looked for.

9.3.3   Laboratory Assessment

In the meantime, laboratory assessment should be carried out by sending blood samples for liver function tests, complete blood count, renal function tests, coagulation profile, electrolytes, and viral serology.

9.3.4   Abdominal Ultrasound

The findings of history and physical examination should be confirmed by an abdominal ultrasound. The imaging confirms the presence as well as the quantity of ascitic fluid. Even small amount of ascitic fluid (as little as 100 mL) can be detected.

9.3.5   Diagnostic Paracentesis

Diagnostic paracentesis should be carried out in all patients presenting with ascites for the first time and also whenever there is clinical deterioration in a cirrhotic patient with known ascites. Paracentesis is a safe procedure with a very low risk of serious complications. There is no need for patient to be empty stomach before the procedure. Blood or blood products are not required for paracentesis [8]. It should however be avoided when DIC or hyperfibrinolysis is documented. Inferior epigastric artery and any visible collateral in the abdominal wall should be avoided during puncture of peritoneum. Care should be taken not to puncture an enlarged liver or spleen. The preferred sites for paracentesis are either midline caudal to umbilicus or either of lower quadrants. The left lower quadrant is the preferred site, as the abdominal wall is thin here and it is easy to locate the ascitic fluid in this quadrant.

9.3.6   Analysis of Ascitic Fluid in a Cirrhotic Patient

Ascitic fluid is sent for analysis of

1. Neutrophil count
   WBC count of more than 500 cell/mm^3 and neutrophil count of more than 250 cell/mm^3 indicate SBP.
2. Total protein concentration
   The cirrhotic ascitic fluid is a transudate, so has a total protein concentration of less than 1.5 g/dL. Low protein indicates a high risk of SBP.

Total protein of more than 2.5 g/dL is more in favor of cardiac causes, malignancy, or tuberculosis.

3. Albumin concentration and serum ascites albumin gradient (SAAG):

SAAG of >1.1 g/L indicates portal hypotension.

SAAG of >1.1 g/L with portal hypertension has an accuracy of 97% for detection of cirrhosis [9].

A SAAG of less than 1.1 is indicative of tuberculous or malignant ascites.

4. Cytology to differentiate malignant and non malignant causes of ascites.

Other optional tests are

- Gram stain and culture.
- AFB smear and culture.
- Glucose estimation.
- Amylase levels.
- LDH levels.

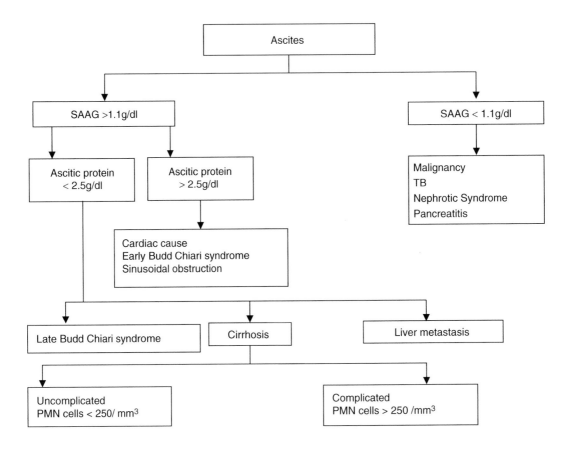

9.4   Management: Depends on the Grade of Ascites

On the basis of amount of fluid, ascites is graded as [10]:

Grade I—mild ascites detected only by ultrasound examination, does not require treatment.

Grade II—moderate ascites, causing moderate symmetrical abdominal distension.

Grade III—large or gross ascites leading to marked abdominal distension.

9.5   Management of Patient with Grade II Ascites [5, 6]

Management of Patient with Grade II ascites [5,6]

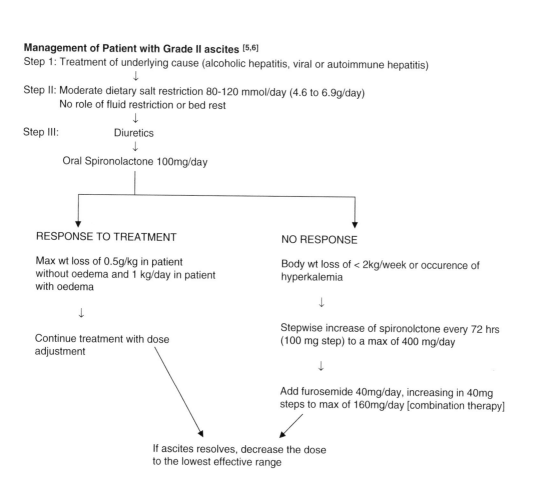

Step 1: Treatment of underlying cause (alcoholic hepatitis, viral or autoimmune hepatitis)
↓
Step II: Moderate dietary salt restriction 80-120 mmol/day (4.6 to 6.9g/day)
No role of fluid restriction or bed rest
↓
Step III: Diuretics
↓
Oral Spironolactone 100mg/day

RESPONSE TO TREATMENT

Max wt loss of 0.5g/kg in patient without oedema and 1 kg/day in patient with oedema
↓
Continue treatment with dose adjustment

NO RESPONSE

Body wt loss of < 2kg/week or occurence of hyperkalemia
↓
Stepwise increase of spironolctone every 72 hrs (100 mg step) to a max of 400 mg/day
↓
Add furosemide 40mg/day, increasing in 40mg steps to max of 160mg/day [combination therapy]

If ascites resolves, decrease the dose to the lowest effective range

9.5.1 Diuretics

In patients with ascites diagnosed for the first time, antimineralocorticoids (spironolactone) alone should be started.

The disadvantage in starting spironolactone alone is delay in the onset of action and probability of occurrence of hyperkalemia [11]. Patients with long-standing and recurrent ascites should be started on combination therapy with aldosterone antagonists and loop diuretics.

Patients on combination therapy require frequent clinical and biochemical assessment like S.Cr, Na, K, body weight, 24 h urine Na, and assessment of orthostatic symptoms.

Loop diuretics should not be used as sole agents as their antinatriuretic effect can be negated by unopposed hyperaldosteronism.

Diuretics should be stopped if serum Na < 125 mmol/L or there is evidence of acute kidney injury, worsening of hepatic encephalopathy (HE), painful muscle cramps, painful gynecomastia, and hyperkalemia.

Drugs that are contraindicated in patients with ascites are.

NSAIDs—due to risk of reduced urinary sodium excretion and renal failure.
ACE inhibitors and Angiotensin II antagonists due to risk of hypotension.

$\alpha 1$ Adrenergic receptor blockers.
Aminoglycosides and contrast media.

9.6 Management of Grade III Ascites/Tense Ascites

Large volume paracentesis (LVP) (removal of large volume of ascitic fluid) which is the treatment of choice is effective and a safe procedure [12]. However it can lead to depletion of effective central blood volume and subsequent stimulation for compensatory vasoconstrictor mechanism leading to a condition called post-paracentesis circulatory dysfunction (PPCD). PPCD, if uncorrected, can precipitate HRS in up to 20% patients [13]. LVP of more than 5 Lshould be supplemented with intravenous albumin (8 g/L of ascitic fluid removed) to prevent PPCD, given usually at the end of the procedure, while LVP of less than 5 L, though a low risk for PPCD, is still supplemented with alb 8 g/L of ascitic fluid removed.

To prevent reaccumulation of ascites, dietary Na restriction should be followed and diuretics should be started.

A meta-analysis of randomized trials has shown that albumin is preferable to all other plasma expanders as it is effective and prevents PPCD and complications like hypernatremia [14, 15].

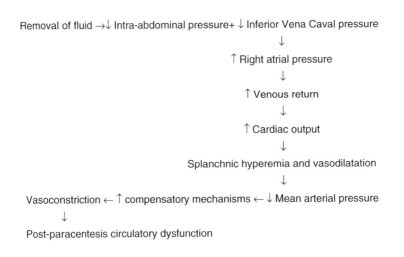

9.6.1 Refractory Ascites (RA)

RA occurs in 5–10% of patients with ascites every year [15]. Presence of refractory ascites is associated with poor survival and poor quality of life. Refractory ascites is of two types:

- Diuretic resistant—No response of the patient to maximal diuretic therapy with spironolactone 400 mg/day and furosemide 160 mg/day for at least 1 week with salt-restricted diet and early recurrence within 4 weeks of initial mobilization [EASL + AASLD guideline].
- Diuretic intractable—Complications prevent the use effective dosage of diuretics. These complications could be hepatic encephalopathy (HE), renal impairment, hyponatremia, hypo or hyperkalemia.

9.6.1.1 Management of Patient Refractory Ascites

- Definitive—liver transplant.
- Palliative—to improve the quality of life.
  - Serial therapeutic paracentesis.
  - Transjugular intrahepatic portosystemic shunt (TIPS).
  - Peritoneovenous shunt (PVS).
- Newer interventions.
  - Indwelling peritoneal catheter.
  - Peritoneal urinary drainage.
  - Cell free and concentrated ascites reinfusion therapy [CART].
- New experimental medical management.
  - Vasoconstrictors.
  - Vasopressin V2 receptor antagonists.
  - Gut microbiome-based therapies.

9.6.1.2 Large Volume Paracentesis (LVP)

In refractory ascites, LVP along with intravenous albumin administration is the first-line treatment. Diuretics should be stopped if the patient does not excrete sodium of more than 30 mmol/day [16]. In patients with refractory ascites with SBP, high doses of nonselective beta blockers (NSBB) should be avoided till the circulatory dysfunction recovers [17].

9.6.1.3 Transjugular Intrahepatic Portosystemic Shunt (TIPS)

TIPS insertion is recommended in patients with recurrent and refractory ascites. This is a side-to-side shunt between high-pressure portovenous system and low-pressure hepatic venous system. Stent placed in the tract between [18] portal and hepatic veins decompresses the portal system. The stent should not extend beyond portal bifurcation [19].

It is indicated for RA and variceal bleeding and is useful when portal hypertension is not associated with advanced liver failure. After insertion of the stent, there is increase in right atrial and pulmonary artery pressure, decrease in portal pressure, and secondary decrease in activation of RAAS leading to increased RBF, increased GFR, and increased renal Na excretion. In about 30–50% patients, TIPS insertion is followed by HE [20] while other late complications are shunt thrombosis and stenosis [21]. Polytetrafluoroethylene (PTFE)-covered stents are associated with low incidence of shunt dysfunction as compared to bare stents [22] Larger the diameter of stent more the incidence of HE; so small diameter stents are recommended. TIPS leads to significant reduction in hepatic venous pressure gradient (HVPG) [23] and actually acts like a bridge, allowing time for preparation of the patient for liver transplant. In patients with serum bilirubin >3 mg/dL, platelet count <75,000 cell/mm^3, HE grade $\geq$ 2, and progressive renal failure, TIPS insertion is not justified.

Presence of CHF, severe TR, severe portal HT, and advanced liver failure are contraindications for the insertion of TIPS.

Meta-analysis of several RCTs conducted for evaluating the function of TIPS revealed that:

1. TIPS is more effective than LVP for control of ascites.
2. TIPS is associated with a higher incidence of HE.
3. Effects on survival as compared to LVP are not clear; while some studies showed no difference, others reported a better survival with LVP as compared to TIPS [24–30].

9.6.1.4 Peritoneovenous Shunt

It was used frequently in the 1970s for the treatment of refractory ascites and diuretic-resistant ascitic patients who were not fit for transplant, TIPS, or serial paracentesis. One end of the shunt is placed in the peritoneal cavity while the other end at the junction of SVC and right atrium with a valve at the venous end which prevents backflow of blood. The driving force is the peritoneal venous pressure gradient. It basically reinfuses the ascitic fluid into the systemic circulation—increasing plasma volume and inhibiting RAAS and ADH systems thus leading to increase GFR, diuresis, natriuresis, and free water clearance.

Complications—the shunt is prone to obstruction, and thus maintenance of long-term patency is a problem.

It does not decrease the hospital stay and does not increase survival, so paracentesis with albumin is a better alternative in a patient with refractory ascites [31].

Although it leads to rapid control of ascites as compared to TIPS, but TIPS has more long-term benefits [32].

Other complications—include sepsis, peritonitis, DIC, and variceal bleeding.

Other treatment modalities are the result of search for alternative treatment for those patients who do not respond to any treatment.

9.6.1.5 Pharmacological Therapies

These basically aim at preventing splanchnic vasodilatation and maintaining effective circulatory volume and renal perfusion and may be used with diuretic drugs. α1 Adrenergic agonists like midodrine [33], vasopressin analog—terlipressin [33], and α2 adrenergic agonist clonidine [34] have been investigated in patient with recurrent or refractory ascites. Though promising results were obtained, further investigations are required.

In cirrhotic patients, dilutional hyponatremia can occur due to arginine vasopressin which acts on V2 receptor in distal convoluted tubule (DCT) and induces water resorption. Vaptans are a group of drugs which block the V2 receptors and can be given for the management of dilutional hypona-

tremia [35]. Several V2 receptor antagonists have been tried: satavaptan [36] and Tolvaptan [37] have been studied; however large randomized trials are required before their use can be validated.

9.6.1.6 Indwelling Peritoneal Catheters

Tunneled indwelling catheters that drain 2 L per week to 1 L/day have been tried in patients who require repeated paracentesis and have complications due to multiple punctures, PICD, and renal failure [38].

However there is a high incidence of infection following a long-term drainage.

9.6.2 CART—Cell Free Concentrated Ascites Reinfusion Therapy

Ascitic fluid is reinfused into the patients after filtration and concentration, so that serum albumin levels are maintained; however high cost of instrument and frequent allergic reactions offset the benefits [39].

9.6.2.1 Peritoneal Urinary Drainage (Alfa Pump System)

It is a low flow pump that is implanted subcutaneously in the patient, is battery driven, and pumps ascitic fluid from the peritoneal cavity into the urinary bladder [40].

It reduces the frequency of paracentesis, improves quality of life, and provides nutritional benefits to the patient. However it can be associated with activation of endogenous vasoconstrictor systems leading to impairment of effective circulatory volume and renal impairment, apart from device- and procedure-related adverse effects [41].

Experimental strategies like diuretics with salt ingestion have been tried in cirrhotic patients with profound hyponatremia [42]. Antibiotics like rifaximin that reduce the bacterial endotoxins, induce splanchnic vasodilatation, and reduce SBP are also under investigation in patients with refractory ascites [43].

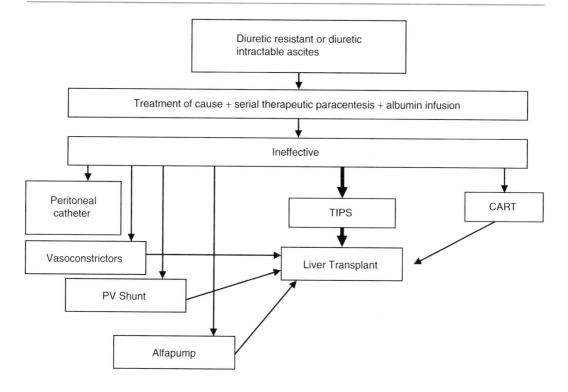

9.7   Hepatic Hydrothorax

Transudative pleural effusion in patients with cirrhosis and ascites is known as hepatic hydrothorax. Appearance of hepatic hydrothorax indicates poor prognosis with median survival ranging from 8 to 12 months [44, 45].

It occurs in 5–12% of patients with cirrhosis and portal hypertension and is usually >500 mL [46]. It is secondary to a diaphragmatic defect, usually right sided in 85% cases and left sided in approximately 13% and bilateral in 2% cases, and occurs in the absence of cardiac, pulmonary, or pleural disease. Negative intrathoracic pressure during inspiration facilitates the movement of ascitic fluid into pleural space, as the intra-abdominal pressure is high. The protein concentration of the pleural fluid is higher than ascitic fluid (serum to pleural fluid albumin gradient is >1.1 g/dL). The fluid can get infected leading to spontaneous bacterial empyema even in absence of SBP. Large pleural effusion can result in dyspnea, cough, respiratory compromise, and even cardiac tamponade.

During thoracocentesis, no more than 2 L should be removed at a time to prevent re-expansion pulmonary edema. Placement of chest drain is avoided due to volume and electrolyte disturbance and associated morbidity and mortality. Consider thoracoscopic mesh repair of diaphragm in very selected patients with nonadvanced cirrhosis and preserved renal function.

9.7.1   Uncomplicated Hepatic Hydrothorax [45]

Diagnostic criteria on analysis of pleural fluid

- WBC count: <250 cells/mm^3
- Total protein: <25 g/L
- Pleural effusion: <0.5
- Total protein/serum
- Total protein ratio
- Pleural effusion: >1.1
- Albumin/serum albumin ratio
- Effusion pleural glucose level is equal to serum glucose level.

9.7.2 Management

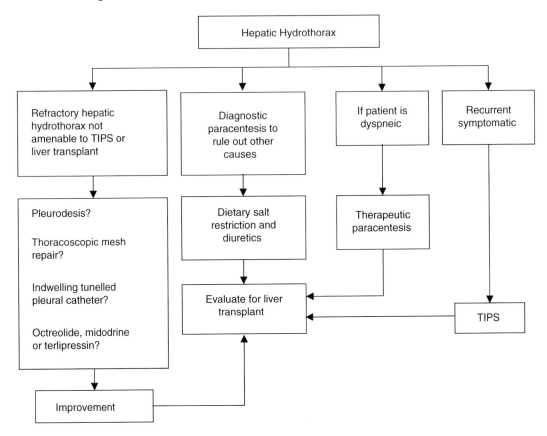

Key Points
- Paracentesis is mandatory in all patients at initial presentation.
- Serum ascites albumin gradient, ascitic protein content, neutrophil count, and culture of ascitic fluid should be done in all patients.
- Dietary sodium restriction should be up to 80–120 mmol/day.
- Spironolactone should be the first line of treatment increasing from 100 to 400 mg/day.
- Frusemide (40–160 mg/day) can be added in a stepwise manner.
- Careful biochemical and clinical monitoring is required for all ascitic patients on diuretics.
- LVP is the first-line treatment in patients with large or refractory ascites.
- LVP of more than 5 L of ascitic fluid drained should be supplemented with albumin 8 g/L of ascitic fluid drained.
- TIPS is preferred in patients with refractory ascites requiring frequent paracentesis or in whom paracentesis is ineffective.
- Liver transplant is definitive treatment in all patients with cirrhotic ascites or hepatic hydrothorax.
- Bed rest and very low sodium containing diets (<40 mmol/day) are not recommended.

References

1. D'Amico G, Garcia-Tsao G, Pagliaro L. Natural history and prognostic indicators of survival in cirrhosis: a systematic review of 118 studies. J Hepatol. 2006;44(1):217–31.
2. Ginès P, Quintero E, Arroyo V, Terés J, Bruguera M, Rimola A, Caballería J, Rodés J, Rozman C. Compensated cirrhosis: natural history and prognostic factors. Hepatology. 1987;7(1):122–8.
3. Fernández-Esparrach G, Sánchez-Fueyo A, Ginès P, Uriz J, Quintó L, Ventura PJ, Cárdenas A, Guevara M, Sort P, Jiménez W, Bataller R, Arroyo V, Rodés J. A prognostic model for predicting survival in cirrhosis with ascites. J Hepatol. 2001;34(1):46–52.
4. Bernardi M, Moreau R, Angeli P, Schnabl B, Arroyo V. Mechanisms of decompensation and organ failure in cirrhosis: from peripheral arterial vasodilation to systemic inflammation hypothesis. J Hepatol. 2015;63(5):1272–84.
5. European Association for the Study of the Liver. Electronic address: easloffice@easloffice.eu; European Association for the Study of the Liver. EASL clinical practice guidelines for the management of patients with decompensated cirrhosis. J Hepatol. 2018;69(2):406–60.
6. Runyon BA. AASLD. Introduction to the revised American Association for the Study of Liver Diseases practice guideline management of adult patients with ascites due to cirrhosis 2012. Hepatology. 2013;57(4):1651–3.
7. Cattau EL Jr, Benjamin SB, Knuff TE, Castell DO. The accuracy of the physical examination in the diagnosis of suspected ascites. JAMA. 1982;247(8):1164–6.
8. Runyon BA, AASLD Practice Guidelines Committee. Management of adult patients with ascites due to cirrhosis: an update. Hepatology. 2009;49(6):2087–107.
9. Runyon BA, Montano AA, Akriviadis EA, Antillon MR, Irving MA, McHutchison JG. The serum-ascites albumin gradient is superior to the exudate-transudate concept in the differential diagnosis of ascites. Ann Intern Med. 1992;117(3):215–20.
10. European Association for the Study of the Liver. EASL clinical practice guidelines on the management of ascites, spontaneous bacterial peritonitis, and hepatorenal syndrome in cirrhosis. J Hepatol. 2010;53(3):397–417.
11. Angeli P, Fasolato S, Mazza E, Okolicsanyi L, Maresio G, Velo E, Galioto A, Salinas F, D'Aquino M, Sticca A, Gatta A. Combined versus sequential diuretic treatment of ascites in non-azotaemic patients with cirrhosis: results of an open randomised clinical trial. Gut. 2010;59(1):98–104.
12. Pache I, Bilodeau M. Severe haemorrhage following abdominal paracentesis for ascites in patients with liver disease. Aliment Pharmacol Ther. 2005;21(5):525–9.
13. Ginès P, Titó L, Arroyo V, Planas R, Panés J, Viver J, Torres M, Humbert P, Rimola A, Llach J, et al. Randomized comparative study of therapeutic paracentesis with and without intravenous albumin in cirrhosis. Gastroenterology. 1988;94(6):1493–502.
14. Bernardi M, Caraceni P, Navickis RJ, Wilkes MM. Albumin infusion in patients undergoing large-volume paracentesis: a meta-analysis of randomized trials. Hepatology. 2012;55(4):1172–81.
15. Ginès P, Cárdenas A, Arroyo V, Rodés J. Management of cirrhosis and ascites. N Engl J Med. 2004;350(16):1646–54.
16. Moore KP, Wong F, Gines P, Bernardi M, Ochs A, Salerno F, Angeli P, Porayko M, Moreau R, Garcia-Tsao G, Jimenez W, Planas R, Arroyo V. The management of ascites in cirrhosis: report on the consensus conference of the international ascites Club. Hepatology. 2003;38(1):258–66.
17. Sersté T, Melot C, Francoz C, Durand F, Rautou PE, Valla D, Moreau R, Lebrec D. Deleterious effects of beta-blockers on survival in patients with cirrhosis and refractory ascites. Hepatology. 2010;52(3):1017–22.
18. Ochs A, Rössle M, Haag K, Hauenstein KH, Deibert P, Siegerstetter V, Huonker M, Langer M, Blum HE. The transjugular intrahepatic portosystemic stent-shunt procedure for refractory ascites. N Engl J Med. 1995;332(18):1192–7.
19. Guerrini GP, Pleguezuelo M, Maimone S, Calvaruso V, Xirouchakis E, Patch D, Rolando N, Davidson B, Rolles K, Burroughs A. Impact of tips preliver transplantation for the outcome posttransplantation. Am J Transplant. 2009;9(1):192–200.
20. Boyer TD, Haskal ZJ. American Association for the Study of Liver Diseases. The role of transjugular intrahepatic portosystemic shunt in the management of portal hypertension. Hepatology. 2005;41(2):386–400.
21. Riggio O, Angeloni S, Salvatori FM, De Santis A, Cerini F, Farcomeni A, Attili AF, Merli M. Incidence, natural history, and risk factors of hepatic encephalopathy after transjugular intrahepatic portosystemic shunt with polytetrafluoroethylene-covered stent grafts. Am J Gastroenterol. 2008;103(11):2738–46.
22. Bureau C, Garcia Pagan JC, Layrargues GP, Metivier S, Bellot P, Perreault P, Otal P, Abraldes JG, Peron JM, Rousseau H, Bosch J, Vinel JP. Patency of stents covered with polytetrafluoroethylene in patients treated by transjugular intrahepatic portosystemic shunts: long-term results of a randomized multicentre study. Liver Int. 2007;27(6):742–7.
23. Unger LW, Stork T, Bucsics T, Rasoul-Rockenschaub S, Staufer K, Trauner M, Maschke S, Pawloff M, Soliman T, Reiberger T, Berlakovich GA. The role of TIPS in the management of liver transplant candidates. United European Gastroenterol J. 2017;5(8):1100–7.
24. Albillos A, Banares R, Gonzalez M, Catalina MV, Molinero LM. A meta-analysis of transjugular intrahepatic portosystemic shunt vs. paracentesis for refractory ascites. J Hepatol. 2005;43:990–6.
25. Bai M, Qi XS, Yang ZP, Yang M, Fan DM, Han GH. TIPS improves liver transplantation-free survival in cirrhotic patients with refractory ascites: an updated meta-analysis. World J Gastroenterol. 2014;20:2704–14.

26. Chen RP, Zhu Ge XJ, Huang ZM, Ye XH, Hu CY, Lu GR, et al. Prophylactic use of transjugular intrahepatic portosystemic shunt aids in the treatment of refractory ascites: metaregression and trial sequential meta-analysis. J Clin Gastroenterol. 2014;48:290–9.

27. D'Amico G, Luca A, Morabito A, Miraglia R, D'Amico M. Uncovered transjugular intrahepatic portosystemic shunt for refractory ascites: a meta-analysis. Gastroenterology. 2005;129:1282–93.

28. Deltenre P, Mathurin P, Dharancy S, Moreau R, Bulois P, Henrion J, et al. Transjugular intrahepatic portosystemic shunt in refractory ascites: a meta-analysis. Liver Int. 2005;25:349–56.

29. Saab S, Nieto JM, Lewis SK, Runyon BA. TIPS vs. paracentesis for cirrhotic patients with refractory ascites. Cochrane Database Syst Rev. 2006;2006:CD004889.

30. Salerno F, Camma C, Enea M, Rossle M, Wong F. Transjugular intrahepatic portosystemic shunt for refractory ascites: a meta-analysis of individual patient data. Gastroenterology. 2007;133:825–34.

31. Ginès P, Arroyo V, Vargas V, Planas R, Casafont F, Panés J, Hoyos M, Viladomiu L, Rimola A, Morillas R, et al. Paracentesis with intravenous infusion of albumin as compared with peritoneovenous shunting in cirrhosis with refractory ascites. N Engl J Med. 1991;325(12):829–35.

32. Rosemurgy AS, Zervos EE, Clark WC, Thometz DP, Black TJ, Zwiebel BR, Kudryk BT, Grundy LS, Carey LC. TIPS versus peritoneovenous shunt in the treatment of medically intractable ascites: a prospective randomized trial. Ann Surg. 2004;239(6):883–9.

33. Rai N, Singh B, Singh A, Vijayvergiya R, Sharma N, Bhalla A, Singh V. Midodrine and tolvaptan in patients with cirrhosis and refractory or recurrent ascites: a randomised pilot study. Liver Int. 2017;37(3):406–14.

34. Singh V, Singh A, Singh B, Vijayvergiya R, Sharma N, Ghai A, Bhalla A. Midodrine and clonidine in patients with cirrhosis and refractory or recurrent ascites: a randomized pilot study. Am J Gastroenterol. 2013;108(4):560–7.

35. Schrier RW, Gross P, Gheorghiade M, Berl T, Verbalis JG, Czerwiec FS, Orlandi C, Investigators SALT. Tolvaptan, a selective oral vasopressin V2-receptor antagonist, for hyponatremia. N Engl J Med. 2006;355(20):2099–112.

36. Wong F, Watson H, Gerbes A, Vilstrup H, Badalamenti S, Bernardi M, Ginès P. Satavaptan Investigators group. Satavaptan for the management of ascites in cirrhosis: efficacy and safety across the spectrum of ascites severity. Gut. 2012;61(1):108–16.

37. Akiyama S, Ikeda K, Sezaki H, Fukushima T, Sorin Y, Kawamura Y, Saitoh S, Hosaka T, Akuta N, Kobayashi M, Suzuki F, Suzuki Y, Arase Y, Kumada H. Therapeutic effects of short- and intermediate-term tolvaptan administration for refractory ascites in patients with advanced liver cirrhosis. Hepatol Res. 2015;45(11):1062–70.

38. Reinglas J, Amjadi K, Petrcich B, Momoli F, Shaw-Stiffel T. The palliative Management of Refractory Cirrhotic Ascites Using the PleurX (©) catheter. Can J Gastroenterol Hepatol. 2016;2016:4680543.

39. Yamada Y, Harada M, Yamaguchi A, Kobayashi Y, Chino T, Minowa T, Kosuge T, Tsukada W, Hashimoto K, Kamijo Y. Technical performance and clinical effectiveness of drop type with adjustable concentrator-cell free and concentrated ascites reinfusion therapy. Artif Organs. 2017;41(12):1135–44.

40. Solà E, Sanchez-Cabús S, Rodriguez E, Elia C, Cela R, Moreira R, Pose E, Sánchez-Delgado J, Cañete N, Morales-Ruiz M, Campos F, Balust J, Guevara M, García-Valdecasas JC, Ginès P. Effects of alfapump™ system on kidney and circulatory function in patients with cirrhosis and refractory ascites. Liver Transpl. 2017;23(5):583–93.

41. Fukui H, Kawaratani H, Kaji K, Takaya H, Yoshiji H. Management of refractory cirrhotic ascites: challenges and solutions. Hepat Med. 2018;3(10):55–71.

42. Licata G, Tuttolomondo A, Licata A, Parrinello G, Di Raimondo D, Di Sciacca R, Cammà C, Craxì A, Paterna S, Pinto A. Clinical trial: high-dose furosemide plus small-volume hypertonic saline solutions vs. repeated paracentesis as treatment of refractory ascites. Aliment Pharmacol Ther. 2009;30(3):227–35.

43. Hanafy AS, Hassaneen AM. Rifaximin and midodrine improve clinical outcome in refractory ascites including renal function, weight loss, and short-term survival. Eur J Gastroenterol Hepatol. 2016;28(12):1455–61.

44. Badillo R, Rockey DC. Hepatic hydrothorax: clinical features, management, and outcomes in 77 patients and review of the literature. Medicine (Baltimore). 2014;93(3):135–42.

45. Garbuzenko DV, Arefyev NO. Hepatic hydrothorax: an update and review of the literature. World J Hepatol. 2017;9(31):1197–204.

46. Strauss RM, Boyer TD. Hepatic hydrothorax. Semin Liver Dis. 1997;17(3):227–32.

Preoperative Assessment and Optimization of Liver Transplant Patients: Cardiac Issues in Liver Disease

10

Annu Sarin Jolly ⓘ, Seema Bhalotra, and Munish Kumar

The heart and the liver are closely related organs in health and disease. Hemodynamic swings in liver transplantation (LT) surgery impose extreme stress on the cardiovascular system. It is hardly surprising that cardiovascular complications following liver transplant are the third leading cause of mortality, the first two being infection and multiorgan failure [1]. In fact, cardiac dysfunction in cirrhosis may contribute to 50% mortality [2]. Coronary artery disease (CAD) progresses with age, and as the median age of transplant candidates is progressively increasing with improvement in antiviral and overall medical therapy, the percentage of chronic liver disease (CLD) patients with significant cardiovascular disease too is rising. There is a 16.2% incidence of severe CAD (>70% stenosis) in patients with cirrhosis, and 13.3% of them are asymptomatic, despite angiographically evident severe CAD [3].

Though cardiovascular disease rises with age, liver disease itself may contribute to higher cardiovascular risk. Further the spectrum of cardiac disease in cirrhosis may range from diseases that affect both the heart and the liver to cardiac diseases unique to cirrhosis (Table 10.1).

Earlier liver disease was considered to confer protection from CAD, but this has been challenged by recent research [4], and liver disease patients are now considered to be at an equivalent or increased risk of cardiovascular disease. Many of the common symptoms of CAD like exertional dyspnea may be missed because of the restricted mobility of liver disease patients. Similarly elevated BP is infrequent in advanced liver diseases because of decreased systemic vascular resis-

Table 10.1 Spectrum of heart diseases in patients with cirrhosis

Systemic disease that affects both the heart and the liver
Chronic alcoholism
Hemochromatosis
Nonalcoholic fatty liver disease
Amyloidosis
Specific cardiac disease of cirrhosis
Cirrhotic cardiomyopathy
Porto-pulmonary hypertension
Pericardial effusion
Common cardiac disease
Coronary artery disease
Heart failure
Cardiomyopathy (LVOTO)
Arrhythmias
Patent foramen ovale

A. S. Jolly (✉)
Liver Transplant and General Anaesthesia, Narayana Super Speciality Hospital, Gurgaon, India
e-mail: ANNU.SARINJOLLY.DR@narayanahealth.org

S. Bhalotra
Liver Transplant, GI Anesthesia and Critical Care, Medanta the Medicity, New Delhi, India

M. Kumar
Command Hospital (CC), Lucknow, Uttar Pradesh, India

© The Author(s), under exclusive license to Springer Nature Singapore Pte Ltd. 2023
V. Vohra et al. (eds.), *Peri-operative Anesthetic Management in Liver Transplantation*,
https://doi.org/10.1007/978-981-19-6045-1_10

tance (SVR). Furthermore, reduced cholesterol synthesis in diseased liver states [5] coupled with cardio-protective protection of estrogens seen in ESLD was considered to reduce the cardiovascular diseases burden. Thus, many patients with advanced cardiovascular disease are likely to be missed on routine examination unless actively screened for the same.

Even after the diagnosis of cardiac disease is established the preoperative optimization of patients with stenotic lesions presents a challenge to the transplant team. Revascularization strategies with stenting necessitate antiplatelet therapy which enhance bleeding risk. On the other hand, surgical revascularization involving coronary artery bypass grafting (CABG) in advanced liver disease may carry unacceptable risk. Intraoperative management too would be a challenge and includes advanced cardiac monitoring to maintain stable hemodynamic parameters. Reperfusion injury may be graver in patients with compromised cardiovascular systems. Many patients decompensate in the postoperative period as the SVR increases to normal levels, and cardiovascular mortality is of significant concern in the postoperative period. A clear understanding of the pathophysiology, a protocol for screening, and perioperative optimization of these patients may improve the outcome in this fragile group of patients.

10.1 Hemodynamic Changes in Patients with Cirrhosis

The cardiovascular system is hyperdynamic in patients with portal hypertension secondary to cirrhosis [6]. The mean arterial pressure (MAP) and SVR are lower, whereas the cardiac output (CO) and heart rate are increased. However, there is blunted ventricular inotropic and chronotropic response to stressful stimuli like surgery, bleeding, or vasoactive drug administration [7], making these patients extremely frail candidates for liver transplantation. Decreased clearance of gut-derived or locally produced humoral factors like endogenous cannabinoids and nitric oxide (NO) has been implicated as the possible mechanism

behind peripheral vasodilatation leading to reduced vascular resistance [8].

The incompetence of the cardiovascular system in coping with the physiological stresses has been termed as "cirrhotic cardiomyopathy [9]." It is a distinct entity and the clinical features comprise blunted systolic and diastolic contractile response to stress, accompanied with signs of ventricular hypertrophy/chamber dilatation and electrophysiological abnormalities. Altered membrane fluidity, impaired beta-adrenergic receptor signaling pathway, and over-activity of NO, carbon monoxide, and endocannabinoid pathways have been implicated in the pathogenesis of cirrhotic cardiomyopathy [10].

CO decreases, and BP and SVR start rising after liver transplantation as liver functions normalize. This may be partly attributable to immune-suppressants like cyclosporin [1]. Many cardiac patients may not be able to cope with the rapidly changing milieu leading to decompensation and heart failure.

10.2 Preoperative Cardiac Evaluation of Liver Transplant Candidates

The preoperative assessment starts with clinical history and physical examination and includes some basic diagnostic screening tests. More specific tests are indicated on the basis of the clinical profile and preliminary cardiac screening.

History and physical examination—The patient is asked about any specific symptoms of breathlessness on exertion, angina, past history of hypertension or CAD, relevant family history, and effort tolerance which should be objectively documented as METs to allow for detection of any deterioration in clinical status in subsequent visits. Exercise capacity may be severely compromised because of severe ascites, poor nutrition, or lack of motivation necessitating other diagnostic modalities to assess the functional status of the heart. In addition, the presence of some risk factors warrants further investigations (Table 10.2). Diabetes is a significant independent risk factor for CAD in these patients [3, 11, 12].

Table 10.2 Coronary risk factors

Traditional risk factors	Nontraditional risk factors
1. Age > 60 years	1. Nonalcoholic steatohepatitis
2. Male gender	2. Concomitant renal failure
3. History of CAD	3. Elevated CRP and intracoronary calcium
4. Dyslipidemia	
5. Smoking	
6. Diabetes mellitus	

Lipid profile should be done for all patients apart from routine laboratory and biochemical profile.

Other important routine diagnostic screening tests include:

1. **Electrocardiogram** could help to detect any ischemic changes due to long-standing CAD, arrhythmias due to electrolyte disturbances, or signs of right heart dysfunction like right axis deviation or right ventricular strain pattern. Left ventricular hypertrophy, left axis deviation, or left bundle branch block may also be detected on routine 12-lead ECG. It is important to note any QT-interval prolongation, and a prolonged QTc >440 msec is associated with a significantly reduced survival [13].

2. **Echocardiography** is invaluable in the diagnostic screening of liver transplant recipients [14] as it can detect structural and functional abnormalities, which cannot be detected on ECG. It can indicate LV dysfunction, valvular defects, left ventricular outflow defects (LVOTO), right ventricle (RV) dysfunction, elevated pulmonary artery pressure (PAP), and pericardial fluid or intracardiac shunt. In fact Garg et al. [15] have suggested that even a mildly reduced left ventricular function should raise the suspicion of a cardiomyopathy. An additional advantage is that Bubble ECHO can be simultaneously performed, and delayed passage of bubbles to the left side may indicate hepatopulmonary syndrome. However, a **transthoracic echocardiogram (TTE)** does not detect the presence or severity

of CAD for which further screening is recommended.

3. **Stress tests**—Stress echocardiogram is a family of examinations in which 2-D echocardiographic monitoring is undertaken before, during, and after cardiovascular stress. Bedsides TTE provides the functional status of the heart at rest, but liver transplant is a major procedure, and these tests help to assess the functioning of the heart under stress provided in the form of exercise or pharmacological agents. Though exercise stress testing has the advantage of evaluating exercise capacity too, most patients with advanced cirrhosis have markedly reduced motivation and mobility and are unlikely to achieve target heart rate. This makes pharmacological testing with dobutamine necessary—**Dobutamine Stress Echocardiogram (DSE)**. Stress increases myocardial oxygen demand leading to imbalance in the supply-demand ratio. This leads to myocardial thickening and/or impaired motility which can be detected on the echocardiogram. Further testing may be warranted on the basis of stress echocardiogram reports necessitating medical therapy or intervention procedures for optimizing the heart before undertaking transplant surgery.

Varying reports on the predictive ability of DSE have been quoted in literature. While some authors have reported a high sensitivity [16] and a high negative predictive value (86–100%) [17, 18], a recent review by Hogan et al. [14] has suggested that overall DSE has a poor sensitivity for ruling out CAD, but is reliable at predicting post-LT CV events. They attributed this discordance to the fact that 19–50% of patients did not achieve the target heart rate, which is 85% of the maximal predicted. Many patients of cirrhosis are on β-blocker therapy or suffer from chronotropic incompetence and consequently may not reach their target heart rate [19]. Thus, the test may be inconclusive in 26–56% patients. Recent protocols suggest that β-blockers may be safely withdrawn without rebound hypertension or variceal bleeding [20]. However, DSE may require early termination in 28% of patients due to chest pain, arrhythmias, or marked changes in blood pressure [14].

4. **Nuclear myocardial perfusion imaging** is done with the administration of vasodilator drugs (such as adenosine or dipyridamole), but is not reliable in cirrhosis as they are already maximally vasodilated due to low SVR and further vasodilatation may not be a possibility.

5. **Functional testing**—Perioperative risk is increased in patients who are unable to perform at least 4 **METs** of work. Current UK guidelines consider NAFLD patients at low risk if they are able to climb 2 flights of stairs which is the equivalent of 4 METs [14].

   Cardiopulmonary exercise testing (CPET)—Maximum aerobic capacity measure as VO_2 max correlates with maximal fitness and is usually not possible in severe disease. Only 32% of ESLD patients achieve it, but ventilatory threshold or anaerobic threshold (AT) can be achieved in 90% of these patients. It is the physiological point at which oxygen supply is inadequate and muscles switch over to anaerobic glycolysis, and indicates cardiopulmonary reserve. The remainder patients can be motivated or functional reserves built up to achieve AT. Patients with cirrhosis have a reduced aerobic capacity and researchers from the UK reported that preoperative CPET is a specific predictor of 90-day survival following liver transplantation. In a study involving 182 patients followed over a 3-year period, the mean anaerobic threshold (AT) was significantly higher in survivors compared to nonsurvivors and AT <9.0 mL/minute/kg was associated with reduced 90-day survival [21].

   Though this is not routinely followed in transplant centers over the world Dr. James Findlay from the Mayo Clinic in Rochester, Minnesota, commented that CPET could be a promising modality in assessing risk-benefit ratio and merits further evaluation. He further advocated simpler tests like the **6-minute walk test (6MWT)**. Carey et al. [22] reported that each 100-m increase in the 6MWT was significantly associated with increased survival, with 6MWT < 250 m being associated with an increased risk of death on the waiting list. They observed that the 6MWT is significantly reduced in patients awaiting LT and is inversely correlated with the native MELD score.

6. **Cardiac MRI** provides detailed structural and functional evaluation of heart as well as its tissue characterization. It is useful in early recognition of cirrhotic cardiomyopathy and aids in evaluating cardiac iron overload in hemochromatosis. Gadolinium-enhanced cardiac MRI is used to detect cardiac involvement in amyloidosis. MRI is also used to evaluate the presence of myocardial scars and viable myocardium.

7. **Right cardiac catheterization** should be performed to characterize the pressure-resistance relationship in the pulmonary artery whenever there is clinical suspicion of pulmonary HTN or porto-pulmonary hypertension as indicated by elevated Right Ventricular Systolic Pressure >50 mmHg on routine echocardiography.

8. **Cardiac computed tomography angiography** may be done in patients with unclear or inconclusive stress test results. It is noninvasive, hence carries lower bleeding risks in coagulopathic ESLD patients. However, its utility is limited to patients with low to intermediate risk of CAD, and it cannot replace conventional coronary angiography in symptomatic patients with high probability of CAD. It is more sensitive but less specific than conventional angiography. However, contrast-induced nephropathy is a problem in patients with ESLD who have renal dysfunction. Candidates suitable for CT angiography

Table 10.3 Coronary artery calcium score and risk stratification

CCS (Agaston)	Risk	Description
0	Nonidentified	Negative test. Findings are consistent with a low risk of having a cardiovascular event in the next 5 years
1–10	Minimal	Minimum atherosclerosis is present. Findings are consistent with a low risk of having a cardiovascular event in the next 5 years
11–100	Mild	Mild coronary atherosclerosis is present. There is likely mild or minimal coronary stenosis. A mild risk of having CAD exists
101–400	Moderate	Moderate calcium is detected in the coronary arteries and confirms the presence of atherosclerotic plaques. A moderate risk of having a cardiovascular event exists
>400	High	A high calcium score may be consistent with significant risk of having a cardiovascular event within the next 5 years

should have normal renal function, nontachycardiac regular cardiac rhythm, normal body habitus, and the ability to lie still and perform breath holding maneuvers. The last may be problematic in patients with severe ascites.

9. **Coronary artery calcium score (CACS)** may be a useful noninvasive test in patients with liver disease as it measures the calcium deposits within coronary vasculature by CT [23, 24].

It is gaining popularity as an adjunct surveillance tool for screening CAD, but the study samples have been small, and are not considered conclusive.

Higher CACS suggests a greater degree of coronary artery stenosis but the score has limited predictive value as a single screening study for CAD. Patients with CACS >100 are five times more likely to have ischemic events than with CACS<100 (Table 10.3).

10. **Conventional cardiac angiography** continues being the gold standard for diagnosing CAD. It is an invasive technique but has the advantage that both diagnosis and treatment can be accomplished in a single session, thus avoiding the need for repeated contrast exposure in liver patients with vulnerable or damaged kidneys. Bleeding remains a significant risk, and procoagulant cover may be indicated during the procedure. Trans-radial approach may minimize bleeding complica-

tions in ESLD patients and may be indicated in suitable patients.

Although active screening for cardiac diseases is desirable a brief summary of common cardiac diseases associated with cirrhosis would further aid in the understanding and management of these patients.

10.3 Systemic Disease That Affect Both Heart and Liver

Alcoholic cirrhosis is seen in chronic alcoholics. It is characterized by nonischemic dilated cardiomyopathy. There is myocardial fibrosis, disruption of myofibrillary structure, and an increased risk for CAD. Ejection fraction is decreased and there is increased propensity for supraventricular arrhythmias.

Hemochromatosis is characterized by dilated or restrictive cardiomyopathy, cardiac arrhythmias, and heart failure. Cardiac MRI is especially useful in diagnosis.

Nonalcoholic fatty liver disease (NAFLD) is often associated with metabolic syndrome and atherosclerotic plaques, and fatty liver is a strong predictor for CAD [25].

Amyloidosis—Restrictive cardiomyopathy and arrhythmias are seen along with small vessel CAD.

Cirrhotic cardiomyopathy has a 40–50% incidence in cirrhotic patients [14] and is characterized by an abnormal cardiac response during transplant. There is a 3.3–7% incidence of severe left heart failure after transplant which carries a 45% mortality. Cirrhotic cardiomyopathy is defined as cardiac dysfunction in patients suffering from cirrhosis characterized by impaired contractile responsiveness to physical and pharmacological stress and/or altered diastolic relaxation with associated electrophysiological abnormalities in absence of other known cardiac disease. The pathogenesis of cirrhotic cardiomyopathy involves autonomic dysfunction, cardiodepressant substances, and abnormal plasma membrane fluidity.

There is reduced systolic as well as diastolic function. Systolic dysfunction may be revealed as reduced cardiovascular response to stress testing even though the resting cardiac output is high. Diastolic dysfunction is indicated by fibrosis, myocardial hypertrophy, and subendothelial edema leading to reduced compliance and relaxation [26]. Diagnosis involves diastolic dysfunction (E/A ratio < 1) on 2D-ECHO and systolic dysfunction (chronotropic incompetence) on Stress ECHO.

Electrophysiological abnormalities include prolonged QT interval, and the QT interval corrected for heart rate (QTc) is more than 440 ms. In cirrhosis, gender difference in QT interval length is abolished. There is a higher chance of *torsades de pointes* and other rhythm disturbances. Electromechanical dissociation may be seen and there could be failure to recruit the whole myocardium during contraction.

Pericardial effusion—Fluid retention during ESLD may cause pericardial effusion which may further lead to cardiac tamponade. It can be diagnosed by complete bedside examination but preoperative screening with transthoracic ECHO (TTE) is invaluable, though the sensitivity may be reduced in the setting of porto-pulmonary hypertension. Treatment with pericardiocentesis or a pericardial window may be indicated.

Heart failure—Preoperative assessment of cardiac function with TTE could rule out heart failure. This pretransplant heart failure may resolve or worsen postoperatively in this cohort of patients. Perioperative medical therapy for heart failure may help to optimize cardiac function.

Left ventricular outflow tract obstruction (LVOTO)—Left ventricular hypertrophy (LVH) with hyperdynamic systolic function in ESLD may result in LVOTO. These patients exhibit poor tolerance to hemodynamic stresses encountered in transplantation. LVOTO may be functional secondary to high flow state or mechanical secondary to septal hypertrophy. The risk of intraoperative hypotension is increased if LVOTO exceeds 36 mmHg [27]. Intraoperative strategies to minimize LVOTO include avoiding tachycardia, minimizing preload reduction, and limiting inotropic agents. TEE-guided volume replacement may be useful [28–30]. Alcohol septal ablation may be indicated in cases of symptomatic heart failure with underlying hypertrophic obstructive cardiomyopathy (HOCM) [31].

Structural heart diseases—Atrial septal defect (ASD) and patent foramen ovale (PFO) may be associated with a prevalence similar to that of the general population, and do not preclude transplant [26]. Long-term ASD leads to altered pulmonary vascular resistance which may precipitate right heart failure in the postoperative period. PFO has a prevalence of 4% and is associated with paradoxical embolism, though it is not a contraindication for transplantation. Extra care should be taken to prevent thrombus formation and air entry into the venous system during surgery. Further studies are needed to determine the potential role of percutaneous PFO closure in LT candidates.

A stepwise approach to diagnosing liver disease is described in Fig. 10.1 [14].

Optimization of cardiac issues—Screening measures may detect cardiac disease which needs to be optimized for successful outcome in LT.

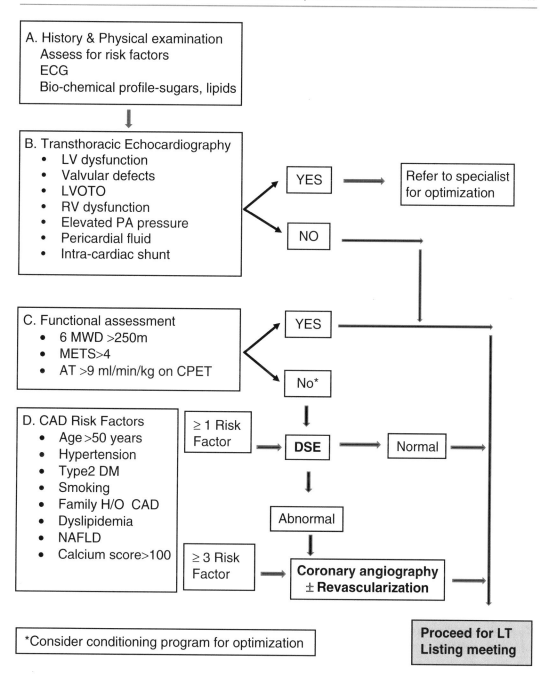

Fig. 10.1 Proposed algorithm for pretransplant cardiac evaluation of patient

10.4 Management of Stenotic CAD

Medical management—Patients with mild to moderate obstructive diseases should be aggressively managed medically. There are no separate guidelines for patients with cirrhosis and the general principles of risk reduction are followed. Abstinence from tobacco and lifestyle modifications as applicable are followed. Hb_1Ac levels should be aimed at less than 7 gm% as pretransplant diabetes carries significant risk. LDL levels should be kept below 100 mg% with lipid lowering drugs, and close monitoring of liver function tests is desirable as they may be hepatotoxic. Statins may have the dual advantage of lowering portal pressure in addition to their cardiovascular benefits [14]. Aspirin cannot be administered usually as there may be marked thrombocytopenia. β-blockers, ACE inhibitors, and aldosterone antagonists may be administered in the peri-transplant period. β-blockers attenuate both the sympathetic and neuro-endocrine response to stress. Perioperative β-blockers may be protective for death and improve perioperative cardiac outcome [32]. Among the β-blockers carvedilol may be preferred as it reduces splanchnic blood flow and porto-collateral resistance, thus reducing portal hypertension [33]. ACE-i and aldosterone antagonists may require dose reduction in the setting of renal dysfunction but are particularly indicated in patients who have suffered a myocardial infarction and have left ventricular dysfunction [34].

Preoperative revascularization strategies are indicated in patients with more severe obstruction to minimize the perioperative risk burden. There is a lack of consensus regarding the criteria of obstructive CAD in prospective liver transplant patients that need intervention. While traditional CAD is defined as >70% coronary stenosis or > 50% left main stenosis, experts have indicated that the threshold may be lowered in this cohort of patients considering the major hemodynamic swings integral to the surgery [4]. The choice for revascularization depends on the type and extent of occlusion. Most cardiologists favor **percutaneous intervention (PCI)** as the preferred therapy as it is less invasive and is successful in 93–94% of patients with ESLD [35–37].

Percutaneous transluminal coronary angioplasty **(PTCA)** either alone or with stenting is adequate in the majority of patients, and **Coronary Artery Bypass Grafting (CABG)** is reserved for the special group of patients whose anatomy is not favorable for PCI. However, PCI has its own risks in these patients with compromised renal function and coagulopathy. Carey et al. [3] observed a 5.5% rate of transient renal impairment in patients undergoing PCI secondary to contrast exposure. In addition, the antiplatelet medications increase the bleeding tendency. The new glycoprotein IIb/IIIa medications and even thienopyridine clopidogrel have not been adequately studied in ESLD patients. Bare Metal Stents are preferred as they need shorter dual antiplatelet therapy (DAPT) and may be switched over to aspirin alone after 1 month [38, 39]. This would expedite surgery in critical cases and minimize inherent bleeding risk. Drug eluting stents (DES) mandate longer DAPT and may delay transplant. Stopping DAPT before the recommended period carries a significant risk of stent thrombosis.

In the small subgroup of patients who cannot be treated by PCI techniques **CABG** may be considered; however, the risk of cardiac surgery in cirrhotic patients may be unacceptably high, and the one-year mortality in Child B & C has been reported between 45% and 80% [14]. CABG may only be indicated in the small subgroup of patients with anatomically unfavorable lesions which preclude stent placement, thereby denying the candidate a liver transplant.

Another important decision is regarding the **timing of CABG**—whether it should precede the transplant, follow the transplant, or be done alongside the transplant as a combined procedure. CABG before LT may be attempted in moderate ESLD, but there is a risk of postoperative liver decompensation and an urgent transplant may be needed in this period. Moreover, there is risk of acute liver decompensation intraoperatively which may hamper operative repair of CAD. CABG may be attempted after liver transplant if the cardiac disease is not deemed to be very severe and would permit the patient to tolerate the surgery without any major adverse cardiac event. An added theoretical advantage of

CABG after LT would be that normal liver function would reduce bleeding during CABG, but the majority of CAD patients with significant occlusion would not be able to tolerate a transplant surgery without adequate optimization of cardiac function. With advancement in surgical and anesthetic techniques a few case reports of combined CABG and liver transplant have been reported, although the decision is not to be taken lightly [40, 41]. Major complications included renal failure, massive blood loss, myocardial dysfunction, wound infection, and even one intraoperative death. Lebbinck et al. [42] used Offpump Coronary Artery Bypass Graft (OPCAB) sequential procedure in a patient with Child C and described it as a *"Good option for those in need of LT and coronary revascularization."* In the author's institute of current affiliation 5 combined CABG LT procedures have been conducted in the last decade with 100% 1 year graft and patient survival. All patients were managed off pump and had a pretransplant EF > 45%. OPCAB reduces bleeding as the equilibrium between procoagulant and anticoagulant activity is less disturbed. Moreover, there is lower inflammation, lower cardiac stunning, and reduced volume shifts. Besides these anesthetic modifications, organ quality is also important in combined procedure as graft dysfunction could predispose to increased bleeding and cardiac tamponade.

It needs to be emphasized that the decision for combined CABG-LT is not to be taken lightly and should be a multidisciplinary opinion. Main indication for combined procedure is the presence of significant, high-risk coronary lesions with preserved left ventricular function and very advanced liver disease.

Cirrhotic Cardiomyopathy—ESLD may be associated with cirrhotic cardiomyopathy and circulating inflammatory mediators with inherent cardio-depressant properties. There may be reduced sensitivity to beta-agonists, and such a heart may decompensate in the postoperative period, as preload reduces; and afterload normalizes with improved SVR.

No specific treatment can yet be recommended but caution is advised with respect to procedures that may stress the heart. Balance of myocardial oxygen supply and demand is critical in the perioperative period. Patients with heart failure should be treated following general guidelines.

An institution-specific protocol for cardiac screening is imperative for ruling out major cardiovascular diseases, which may otherwise be missed. Noninvasive tests should be a part of all screening processes, which may dictate further invasive tests [26]. The anesthesiologist must optimize the cardiac status before proceeding with the transplant. Revascularization by PCI is indicated in obstructive CAD, and stents which require minimal dual antiplatelet therapy are preferred. The risk of cirrhotic cardiomyopathy must always be kept in mind, and usually manifests in the postoperative period. Meticulous volume and hemodynamic management in the perioperative period and close invasive monitoring may minimize the risk.

A thorough understanding of the cardiovascular physiology in advanced liver disease combined with an awareness of diseases unique to this subset of population is necessary for successful optimization and perioperative management.

Key Points
- Cardiovascular physiology is considerably altered in liver disease.
- Cardiovascular diseases are a leading cause of post-transplant mortality.
- Active screening for cardiovascular disease should be a part of pretransplant workup.
- Revascularization with stenting is the preferred treatment modality in occlusive CAD.
- Stents which require minimal period of dual antiplatelet therapy are preferred.
- Cirrhotic cardiomyopathy is a distinct entity, and these patients may decompensate in the postoperative period.
- Close invasive monitoring with rapid response to hemodynamic swings may improve perioperative outcome.

References

1. Burroughs AK, et al. 3-month and 12-month mortality after first liver transplant in adults in Europe: predictive models for outcome. Lancet. 2006;367(9506):225–32. https://doi.org/10.1016/s0140-6736(06)68033-1.

2. Plotkin J, et al. Morbidity and mortality in patients with coronary artery disease undergoing orthotopic liver transplantation. Hepatol Res. 1997;7(2):136–7. https://doi.org/10.1016/s0928-4346(97)85773-8.

3. Carey WD, et al. The prevalence of coronary artery disease in liver transplant candidates over age 50. Transplantation. 1995;59(6):859–63. https://doi.org/10.1097/00007890-199503000-00010.

4. Keeffe B. Detection and treatment of coronary artery disease in liver transplant candidates. Liver Transpl. 2001;7(9):755–61. https://doi.org/10.1053/jlts.2001.26063.

5. Cicognani C. Serum lipid and lipoprotein patterns in patients with liver cirrhosis and chronic active hepatitis. Arch Intern Med. 1997;157(7):792–6. https://doi.org/10.1001/archinte.157.7.792.

6. Groszmann RJ. Hyperdynamic circulation of liver disease 40 years later: pathophysiology and clinical consequences. Hepatology. 1994;20(5):1359–63. https://doi.org/10.1002/hep.1840200538.

7. Lee SS, et al. Desensitization of myocardial β-adrenergic receptors in cirrhotic rats. Hepatology. 1990;12(3):481–5. https://doi.org/10.1002/hep.1840120306.

8. Carter EP, et al. Regulation of heme oxygenase-1 by nitric oxide during hepatopulmonary syndrome. Am J Phys Lung Cell Mol Phys. 2002;283(2):L346–53. https://doi.org/10.1152/ajplung.00385.2001.

9. Moller S. Cirrhotic cardiomyopathy: a pathophysiological review of circulatory dysfunction in liver disease. Heart. 2002;87(1):9–15. https://doi.org/10.1136/heart.87.1.9.

10. Rockey D. Vascular mediators in the injured liver. Hepatology. 2003;37(1):4–12. https://doi.org/10.1053/jhep.2003.50044.

11. Garcia-Compean D, et al. Liver cirrhosis and diabetes: risk factors, pathophysiology, clinical implications and management. World J Gastroenterol. 2009;15(3):280. https://doi.org/10.3748/wjg.15.280.

12. Rossetto A, et al. Cardiovascular risk factors and immunosuppressive regimen after liver transplantation. Transplant Proc. 2010;42(7):2576–8. https://doi.org/10.1016/j.transproceed.2010.05.160.

13. Bernardi M, et al. Q-T interval prolongation in cirrhosis: prevalence, relationship with severity, and etiology of the disease and possible pathogenetic factors. Hepatology. 1998;27(1):28–34. https://doi.org/10.1002/hep.510270106.

14. Hogan BJ, et al. Evaluation of coronary artery disease in potential liver transplant recipients. Liver Transpl. 2017;23(3):386–95. https://doi.org/10.1002/lt.24679.

15. Garg A, Armstrong WF. Echocardiography in liver transplant candidates. JACC Cardiovasc Imaging.

16. Geleijnse ML, et al. Methodology, feasibility, safety and diagnostic accuracy of dobutamine stress echocardiography. J Am Coll Cardiol. 1997;30(3):595–606. https://doi.org/10.1016/s0735-1097(97)00206-4.

17. Plotkin JS, et al. Dobutamine stress echocardiography for preoperative cardiac risk stratification in patients undergoing orthotopic liver transplantation. Liver Transpl Surg. 1998;4(4):253–7. https://doi.org/10.1002/lt.500040415.

18. Donovan CL, et al. Two-dimensional and dobutamine stress echocardiography in the preoperative assessment of patients with end-stage liver disease prior to orthotopic liver transplantation. Transplantation. 1996;61(8):1180–8. https://doi.org/10.1097/00007890-199604270-00011.

19. Findlay JY, et al. Preoperative dobutamine stress echocardiography, intraoperative events, and intraoperative myocardial injury in liver transplantation. Transplant Proc. 2005;37(5):2209–13. https://doi.org/10.1016/j.transproceed.2005.03.023.

20. Payancé A, et al. Lack of clinical or haemodynamic rebound after abrupt interruption of beta-blockers in patients with cirrhosis. Aliment Pharmacol Ther. 2016;43(9):966–73. https://doi.org/10.1111/apt.13577.

21. Prentis JM, et al. Submaximal cardiopulmonary exercise testing predicts 90-day survival after liver transplantation. Liver Transpl. 2012;18(2):152–9. https://doi.org/10.1002/lt.22426.

22. Carey EJ, et al. Six-minute walk distance predicts mortality in liver transplant candidates. Liver Transpl. 2010;16(12):1373–8. https://doi.org/10.1002/lt.22167.

23. Cassagneau P, et al. Prognostic value of preoperative coronary computed tomography angiography in patients treated by orthotopic liver transplantation. Eur J Gastroenterol Hepatol. 2012;24(5):558–62. https://doi.org/10.1097/meg.0b013e3283522df3.

24. Kemmer N, et al. The role of coronary calcium score in the risk assessment of liver transplant candidates. Transplant Proc. 2014;46(1):230–3. https://doi.org/10.1016/j.transproceed.2013.09.035.

25. Vanwagner LB, et al. Patients transplanted for non-alcoholic steatohepatitis are at increased risk for postoperative cardiovascular events. Hepatology. 2012;56(5):1741–50. https://doi.org/10.1002/hep.25855.

26. Raval Z, et al. Cardiovascular risk assessment of the liver transplant candidate. J Am Coll Cardiol. 2011;58(3):223–31. https://doi.org/10.1016/j.jacc.2011.03.026.

27. Maraj S, et al. Inducible left ventricular outflow tract gradient during dobutamine stress echocardiography: an association with intraoperative hypotension but not a contraindication to liver transplantation. Echocardiography. 2004;21(8):681–5. https://doi.org/10.1111/j.0742-2822.2004.03068.x.

2013;6(1):105–19. https://doi.org/10.1016/j.jcmg.2012.11.002.

28. Harley ID, et al. Orthotopic liver transplantation in two patients with hypertrophic obstructive cardiomyopathy. Br J Anaesth. 1996;77(5):675–7. https://doi.org/10.1093/bja/77.5.675.

29. Lim YC, et al. Intraoperative transesophageal echocardiography in orthotopic liver transplantation in a patient with hypertrophic cardiomyopathy. J Clin Anesth. 1995;7(3):245–9. https://doi.org/10.1016/0952-8180(94)00049-a.

30. Cywinski JB, et al. Dynamic left ventricular outflow tract obstruction in an orthotopic liver transplant recipient. Liver Transpl. 2005;11(6):692–5. https://doi.org/10.1002/lt.20440.

31. Paramesh AS, et al. Amelioration of hypertrophic cardiomyopathy using nonsurgical septal ablation in a cirrhotic patient prior to liver transplantation. Liver Transpl. 2005;11(2):236–8. https://doi.org/10.1002/lt.20327.

32. Safadi A, et al. Perioperative risk predictors of cardiac outcomes in patients undergoing liver transplantation surgery. Circulation. 2009;120(13):1189–94. https://doi.org/10.1161/circulationaha.108.847178.

33. Tripathi D, Hayes PC. The role of carvedilol in the management of portal hypertension. Eur J Gastroenterol Hepatol. 2010;22(8):905–11. https://doi.org/10.1097/meg.0b013e3283367a99.

34. Raval Z. Role of cardiovascular intervention as a bridge to liver transplantation. World J Gastroenterol. 2014;20(31):10651. https://doi.org/10.3748/wjg.v20.i31.10651.

35. Azarbal B, et al. Feasibility and safety of percutaneous coronary intervention in patients with end-stage liver disease referred for liver transplantation. Liver Transpl. 2011;17(7):809–13. https://doi.org/10.1002/lt.22301.

36. Pillarisetti J, et al. Cardiac catheterization in patients with end-stage liver disease: safety and outcomes. Catheter Cardiovasc Interv. 2010;77(1):45–8. https://doi.org/10.1002/ccd.22591.

37. Noureddin N, et al. Cardiac catheterization and percutaneous coronary intervention in patients with end stage liver disease. J Am Coll Cardiol. 2015;65(10):A1776. https://doi.org/10.1016/s0735-1097(15)61776-4.

38. Fleisher LA, et al. 2014 ACC/AHA guideline on perioperative cardiovascular evaluation and management of patients undergoing noncardiac surgery: executive summary. Circulation. 2014;130(24):2215–45. https://doi.org/10.1161/cir.0000000000000105.

39. Lentine KL, et al. Cardiac disease evaluation and management among kidney and liver transplantation candidates. Circulation. 2012;126(5):617–63. https://doi.org/10.1161/cir.0b013e31823eb07a.

40. Benedetti E, et al. Is the presence of surgically treatable coronary artery disease a contraindication to liver transplantation? Clin Transpl. 1999;13(1):59–61. https://doi.org/10.1034/j.1399-0012.1999.t01-1-130109.x.

41. Giakoustidis A, et al. Combined cardiac surgery and liver transplantation: three decades of worldwide result. J Gastrointestin Liver Dis. 2014;23(4):415–21. https://doi.org/10.15403/jgld.2014.1121.234.

42. Lebbinck H, et al. Sequential off-pump coronary artery bypass and liver transplantation. Transpl Int. 2006;19(5):432–4. https://doi.org/10.1111/j.1432-2277.2006.00298.x.

Preoperative Assessment and Optimisation of Liver Transplant Patients: Renal Issues

11

Nikunj Gupta

11.1 Introduction

The first successful human liver transplant was performed in 1969; since then liver transplant has evolved rapidly becoming the standard therapy for the acute and chronic liver failure of all aetiologies. The success has been attributed to several advances such as improvements in surgical techniques, the introduction of new immunosuppressants and preservative solutions and early diagnosis and management of complications [1]. Cirrhosis (57%) remains the most common cause for liver transplant followed by cancers (15%), cholestatic diseases (10%), acute hepatic failure (8%) and metabolic disorders (6%) [1].

Patients with liver pathology are susceptible to renal impairments due to pre-existing hormonal and circulatory imbalances or due to precipitating factors. Acute renal failure (ARF) is caused mainly by renal hypoperfusion and tubular necrosis. Haemorrhage, fluid loss due to the use of diuretics, sepsis and hepatorenal syndrome are the main causes of prerenal failure [2]. Liver disease and renal dysfunction can occur simultaneously as a result of a systemic condition affecting both these organs; however, renal dysfunction complicating primary disorders of the liver such as IgA nephropathy, cryoglobulinemia, membranous nephropathy and hepatorenal syndrome is much more common [3]. In 19% of cirrhotic patients awaiting a liver transplant, acute kidney injury is frequently developed during hospitalisation due to nephrotoxic drugs, diuretics and contrast dyes used in perioperative period [4–6] and approximately 1% of the patients develop chronic renal failure (CRF) [2–4]. In patients without renal impairment, acute kidney injury is diagnosed when serum creatinine level increases by more than 50% of the base value, to above 1.5 mg/dl [7]. It is imperative to assess and diagnose renal dysfunction early in patients with liver disease awaiting transplant. There has been an improvement in the understanding of renal complications in liver disease and the treatment options for the same. A thorough preoperative examination of all the systems is crucial and mandatory. Hemodynamic derangements and insults during the perioperative period are somewhat predictable based on the preoperative assessment of the patient and this is the time when preventive therapy can be initiated if the risk is aptly determined [8]. Anaesthetists play a pivotal role in identifying patients at risk for acute renal failure, optimising anaemia and treating hypovolemia in the preoperative period.

N. Gupta (✉)
Liver Transplant, GI Anesthesia and Critical Care,
Medanta the Medicity, Gurgaon, Haryana, India
e-mail: nikunj.gupta@medanta.org

© The Author(s), under exclusive license to Springer Nature Singapore Pte Ltd. 2023
V. Vohra et al. (eds.), *Peri-operative Anesthetic Management in Liver Transplantation*,
https://doi.org/10.1007/978-981-19-6045-1_11

11.2 Definition of Acute Kidney Injury

Comparison of the criteria for staging of AKI by three systems is tabulated in Table 11.1.

RIFLE (risk, injury, loss of kidney function, end-stage renal failure) system used serum creatinine and urine output to define adult kidney injury, the first-ever criterion for adult kidney injury to be published in 2004 [6].

A modification of RIFLE criteria was published by the Acute Kidney Injury Network (AKIN) in 2007 [9] AKIN criteria evolved from RIFLE criteria but with the understanding that smaller changes in concentration of serum creatinine are associated with morbidity and mortality [10]. AKIN criteria failed to define adult kidney injury without knowledge of baseline serum creatinine [6, 10, 11].

In 2012, the Kidney Disease: Improving Global Outcome (KIDGO) foundation proposed a clinical and practice guidelines of acute kidney injury. The guidelines included a comprehensive review of acute kidney injury definition, risk assessment, diagnosis, prevention, treatment and renal replacement therapy [12, 13]. The KIDGO criteria included absolute change in serum creatinine and accepted 48 hours and an extended 7-day time frame for diagnosis of acute kidney injury [12].

To define acute kidney injury based on serum creatinine levels would be flawed as it is influenced by [6] by overall nutrition state, volume overload, drugs especially steroids, muscle injury

Table 11.1 Comparison of RIFLE, AKIN and KIDGO criteria in the staging of acute injury [6, 9, 11, 13, 14]

Definition system	RIFLE 7 Days	AKIN 48 h	KIDGO
Staging	**Risk** Increased sCr × 1.5 or GFR decrease >25% or urine output <0.5 ml kg^{-1} h^{-1} for 6 h	**Stage 1** Increased sCr × 1.5–2 or sCr increase ≥0.3 mg dl^{-1} or urine output <0.5 ml kg^{-1} h^{-1} for >6 h	**Stage 1** Increased sCr × 1.5–1.9 that is known or presumed to have occurred within the preceding 7 days or sCr increase ≥0.3 mg dl^{-1} within 48 h or urine output <0.5 ml kg^{-1} h^{-1} for 6–12 h
	Injury Increased sCr × 2 or GFR decease >50% or urine output <0.5 ml kg^{-1} h^{-1} for 12 h	**Stage 2** Increased sCr × 2–3 or urine output <0.5 ml kg^{-1} h^{-1} for >12 h	**Stage 2** Increased sCr × 2–2.9 or urine output <0.5 ml kg^{-1} h^{-1} for ≥12 h
	Failure Increased sCr × 3 or GFR decrease 75% or sCr ≥ 4 mgdl−1 when sCr is in acute increase (≥0.5 mg dl^{-1}) or urine output <0.3 ml kg^{-1} h^{-1} for 24 h or anuria for 12 h	**Stage 3** Increased sCr × 3 or more or sCr ≥4 mg dl^{-1} when sCr is in acute increase (≥0.5 mg dl^{-1}) or urine output <0.3 ml kg^{-1} h^{-1} for >24 h or anuria for 12 h	**Stage 3** Increased sCr × 3 Or sCr ≥4 mg dl^{-1} or initiation of RRT or GFR decreases to <35 ml min^{-1} (1.73 m)$^{-2}$ in patients <18 years old or urine output <0.3 ml kg^{-1} h^{-1} for ≥24 h or anuria for ≥12 h

sCr serum creatinine, *GFR* glomerular filtration rate, *RIFLE* risk; injury; failure; loss of kidney function; end-stage renal failure, *AKIN* Acute Kidney Injury Network, *KIDGO* Kidney Disease: Improving Global Outcome, *RRT* renal replacement therapy and fluid overload. Over the last few years study in the field of acute kidney injury has expanded with identifying different molecules excreted from the injured kidney; these molecules have ranged from constitutive proteins released from the damaged kidney to molecules upregulated in response to injury or non-renal tissue products that are filtered, reabsorbed or secreted by the kidney. These biomarkers are proteins that can be found in urine exosomes and free filtered urine [15] and can be utilised to predict the nature, magnitude and site of injury based on their specificity. Biomarkers such as Cystatin C, Microalbumin, N-Acetyl-beta-d glucosaminidase, Neutrophil Gelatinase-associated lipocalin (NGAL) and Interleukin 18 have been used to detect early renal impairment [16].

Cystatin C is an endogenous inhibitor of cysteine proteinases, specifically cathepsin H, B, L and Calpains [16]. Cystatin C is produced in nucleated cells and is not bound to plasma proteins [37], hence freely filtered by the glomerulus and subsequently reabsorbed and degraded in the proximal tubules of the kidney and their appearance in the urine depends on the severity of AKI [38]. Cystatin C and albumin are both reabsorbed by megalin-facilitated endocytosis in the proximal tubule; hence albuminuria may inhibit reabsorption and increase urinary excretion of Cystatin C [17–20]. The blood concentration of Cystatin C depends on individual's GFR and the link between Cystatin C and GFR is evident even in ranges where serum creatinine cannot detect changes, GFR 60–90 ml/min [21]. Urine Cystatin C appears earlier and is a more sensitive marker in AKI. Use of Cystatin C as a biomarker in renal pathology is constantly evolving and it is unclear if the value of Cystatin C is generalizable to all forms of AKI [22].

Microalbumin is an inexpensive diagnostic tool in identifying the progression of renal diseases. Microalbumin detects urinary albumin below the threshold level by urinary dipstick (30–300 mg/l) [16, 22, 23]. Gene expressing albumin is increased in AKI and is more of a sensitive marker than previously thought [23]. Microalbumin as a marker fails to specify the site of injury and does not have the ability to separate CKD from AKI as albumin degrades with storage [24].

N-Acetyl-beta-d glucosaminidase (NAG) originates from lysosomes of the cells lining the proximal convoluted tube and can be measured using coulometry assay, hence is a sensitive marker for proximal tubule injury with loss of lysosome integrity. Critically ill patients awaiting liver transplant with elevated NAG levels have shown poor outcome. Urinary NAG is inhibited by urea and tends to degrade most appreciably over time compared with other biomarkers even when stored at extremely low temperature [25].

NGAL is a novel 25-kDa protein associated with gelatinase from human neutrophil [26]. NGAL is intensively upregulated in the condition of sepsis, suggesting that the release of NGAL into the urinary system is a major response of the kidney to systemic infection [27]. Clinical studies have shown that urinary and plasma NGAL are powerful and independent predictors of AKI when compared to serum creatinine [28].

IL-18 is expressed in human peripheral blood mononuclear cells, murine splenic macrophages and non-immune cells [29]. IL-18 levels in kidney double following AKI [30].

A recent study suggests two novel biomarkers—insulin-like growth factor binding protein 7 and tissue inhibitor of Metalloproteinases 2 which are sensitive in the early detection of acute kidney injury [15], but lack supporting data to standardise its efficacy.

11.3 Pathophysiology of Renal Dysfunction in Liver Impairments

Patients with liver pathology develop portal hypertension with splanchnic vasodilatation and pooling of blood secondary to increased resistance to portal flow [31]. Pooling of blood leads to decrease in circulatory blood volume in patients with cirrhosis [32]. Increase in cardiac output maintains sufficient renal perfusion, however with decompensation of the liver in cirrhosis and an increase in severity of portal hypertension, the compensatory increase in cardiac output is inadequate to maintain circulatory blood volume and adequate renal perfusion [32], and this causes activation of the renin-angiotensin-aldosterone system, resulting in sodium and water retention and extra-splanchnic vasoconstriction [33], causing ascites and explains the signs of adult kidney injury in liver pathologies.

11.4 Evaluating Criteria

Serum creatinine level is a variable in calculating the model for end-stage liver disease score, a recognised predictor of the three-month mortality risk and a method for allocating liver transplants [34, 35]; however, patients with compromised liver pathology show lower baseline serum creatinine as a result of liver dysfunction, drug-induced tubular secretion of creatinine, decreased conversion of creatine to creatinine as a consequence of reduced skeletal muscle mass from malnutrition and underestimation of serum creatinine in pre-existing hyperbilirubinemia in a laboratory setting [36, 37]. As mentioned earlier, Biomarker Cystatin C is the best alternative

method for estimating the glomerular filtration rate (GFR), and it has proven accurate in patients with liver pathologies as it is independent of hepatic function [14, 38].

Renal impairment in liver pathologies is usually hypovolemia-induced prenatal acute kidney injury, acute tubular necrosis and hepatorenal syndrome (HRS), with HRS being most fatal [37]. Hence a simplified algorithm in diagnosing renal impairments in patients with liver pathology can be adopted (Flow Chart 11.1) [37].

Prerenal impairment accounts for 68% of acute kidney impairment in patients with liver pathologies [31] due to underlying circulatory disturbances. Pathophysiological changes in the kidney are mild in prerenal impairment but severe in HRS due to neurohormonal activation [39]. The two main causes for prerenal impairment can be differentiated by the response to volume expansion - A) hypovolemia induced impairment responds whereas - B) HRS is insensitive to volume expansion [40]. The hypovolemia induced prerenal impairment results from excessive fluid loss due to diarrhoea, sodium and water restriction, gastrointestinal haemorrhage, large-volume

Flow Chart 11.1 Algorithm in diagnosing renal impairment in liver pathologies [37]

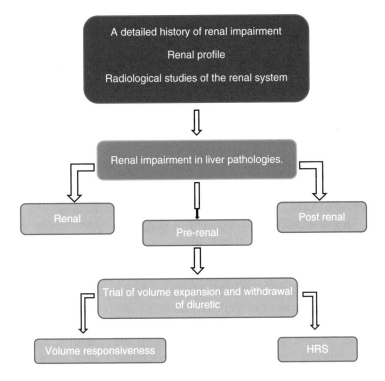

paracentesis and excessive diuretic therapy [41]. Measures should be taken to reduce and prevent intravascular volume depletion; and hence the risk of prerenal impairment which includes attaining fluid balance, judicious use of diuretics, avoidance of Reno toxic drugs, avoidance of lactose therapy and administration of intravenous albumin [42] Albumin is superior and safer to saline for volume expansion; the recommended dose of intravenous albumin is 1gm/kg of body weight/day up to a maximum of 100gm per day [39, 41, 42]. The incidence of renal impairment was 10% when albumin was added to antibiotic compared to renal impairment with antibiotic therapy alone which was 33% [7]; further, the 3-month mortality rate was lower with Albumin and Antibiotic combination compared to Antibiotic alone [32]. Albumin is suggested in patients with serum creatinine >88.4micro mol/l or bilirubin >68.4 micro mol/l and is not necessary for patients who do not meet this criterion [43]. The American Association for the Study of Liver Diseases suggests that patients with SBP who have serum creatinine >1 mg/dl, blood urea >30 mg/dl or total bilirubin >4 mg/dl should receive 1.5 g/kg of body weight within 6 hours of detection and 1gm/kg of body weight on day 3, and the European Association for the Study of the Liver recommends that the patient should be covered up with broad-spectrum antibiotics along with albumin [1, 37, 42].

Renal impairments due to acute tubular necrosis account for 41.7% to 44.4% of cases with liver pathologies [37, 43]. Hypovolemia-induced prerenal impairment may progress into renal impairment leading to severe ischemic acute tubular necrosis [37]. In acute tubular necrosis, reabsorption of sodium is hampered leading to increased concentration of sodium in urine (>40 mEq/L) and low urine osmolality (<35 mOsm/kg) [43] and vice versa in patients with HRS. This differentiation can be challenging in patients with liver pathologies on diuretic therapy which can hamper the results. Casts are seen both in acute tubular necrosis and HRS but epithelial casts are characteristic of acute tubular necrosis [44]. Renal biopsy is confirmatory for histological diagnosis in unresolved cases [45]

but carries the risk of internal bleeding due to coagulopathy and thrombocytopenia; hence it is rarely sought after in these instances [31].

Post-renal impairment due to urinary tract obstruction is uncommon and accounts for <1% of acute kidney injury in patients with liver pathology [46]. Imaging studies are most effective in differentiating hydronephrosis from pre- to post-renal causes.

11.5 Management

As per observations made by renowned authors, we would like to propose a working party algorithm in the management of renal issues in liver pathologies (Flow Chart 11.2).

Liver transplant is the ideal treatment for patients suffering from HRS with short-term survival rate. Systemic vasoconstrictor therapy with terlipressin and noradrenaline have proven beneficial in patients awaiting a liver transplant. MARS (molecular adsorbent recirculation system) and TIPS (Transjugular intrahepatic portosystemic shunt) improve renal function during the waiting period [1]. Additionally, the surgical and the anaesthetic team is advised to take measures to reduce blood loss and avoid unnecessary transfusion. Intraoperative hypotension should be avoided as it carries a risk of postoperative acute kidney injury. Normovolemia is of utmost importance [6]. Maintenance of higher blood pressure is required in hypertensive patients. Fluids in excess should not be administered to treat oliguria and administration of low chloride solution has shown beneficial effects [1, 3, 5].

Prognosis of transplant surgeries depends on the duration of renal failure before the surgery and appears to be a negative predictor of post-transplant renal function [47]. A retrospective study of patients undergoing liver transplant in regard to aetiology of renal dysfunction showed acute tubular necrosis as a cause of acute kidney injury with worst survival at 1 and 5 years after liver transplant compared to patients with hepatorenal syndrome [48]. Patients with hepatorenal syndrome recover their renal function after liver transplantation while patients with acute tubular

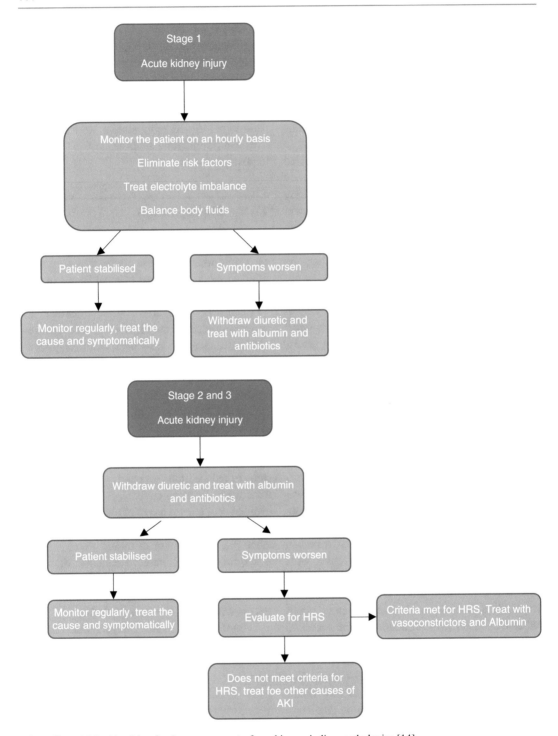

Flow Chart 11.2 Algorithm for the management of renal issues in liver pathologies [14]

necrosis (intrarenal causes) do not recover their renal functions post-liver transplant and would need simultaneous liver and kidney (SLK) transplant [31, 48]. Biomarkers such as NGAL, KIM-1, IL-18, ET-1 and FABP-2 have shown promise in making an early diagnosis of acute kidney injury and predicting reversal of acute kidney injury. Studies show that biomarkers have been successful in distinguishing acute tubular necrosis from prerenal aetiology of acute kidney injury [49]. The data on the use of biomarkers among patients with liver pathologies and receiving a liver transplant is limited. Conventional parameters such as serum creatinine, GFR and urine output along with biomarkers would be ideal for evaluation in patients with liver pathologies to avoid complications in all the phases of treatment.

References

1. European Association for Study of liver. Article in press: EASL clinical practice guidelines: liver transplantation. J Hepatol. 2016;64(2):433–85.
2. Choi YJ, Kim JH, Koo JK, Lee CI, Yang JH, et al. Prevalence of renal dysfunction in patients with cirrhosis according to ADQI-IAC working party proposal. Clin Mol Hepatol. 2014;20:185–91.
3. Wong F, Nadim MK, Kellum JA, Salerno F, Bellomo R, et al. Working party proposal for a revised classification system of renal dysfunction in patients with cirrhosis. Hepatology. 2011;60:702–9.
4. Moreau R, Lebrec D. Acute renal failure in patients with cirrhosis: perspectives in the age of MELD. Hepatology. 2003;37(2):233–43.
5. Marie Person J, Bureau C, Gonzalez L, Richard Garcia F, De Soyres O, et al. Treatment of hepatorenal syndrome as defined by the international ascites club by albumin and furosemide infusion according to the central venous pressure: a prospective pilot study. Am J Gastroenterol. 2005;100(12):2702–7.
6. Goren O, Matot I. Perioperative acute kidney injury. Br J Anaesth. 2015;115(S2):ii3–14.
7. Sort P, Navasa M, Arroyo V, Aldeguer X, Planas R, et al. Effect of intravenous Albumin on renal impairment and mortality in patients with Cirrhosis and spontaneous bacterial peritonitis. N Engl J Med. 1999;341(6):403–9.
8. Josephs SA, Thakar CV. Perioperative risk assessment, prevention, and treatment of acute kidney injury. Int Anesthesiol Clin. 2009;47(7):89–105.
9. Mehta RL, Kellum JA, Shah SV, Molitoris BA, Ronco C, et al. Acute kidney injury network: report of an ini-

10. Wang HE, Mutner P, Chertow CM, Warnock DG. Acute kidney injury and mortality in hospitalized patients. Am J Nephrol. 2012;35:349–55.
11. Lassnigg A, Schmidlin D, Mouheieddine M, Bachmann LM, Druml W, et al. Minimal changes of serum creatinine predict prognosis in patients after cardiothoracic surgery: a prospective cohort study. J Am Soc Nephrol. 2004;15:1597–605.
12. Kidney international supplement. Off J Int Soc Nephrol. 2012;2(1).
13. Machado MN, Nakazone MA, Maia LN. Acute kidney injury based on KDIGO (Kidney Disease Improving Global Outcomes) criteria in patients with elevated baseline serum creatinine undergoing cardiac surgery. Braz J Cardiovasc Surg. 2014;29(3):299–307.
14. Kashani K, Al-Khafaji A, Ardiles T, Artigas A, Bagshaw SM, et al. Discovery and validation of cell cycle arrest biomarkers in human acute kidney injury. Crit Care. 2013;17(25):1–12.
15. Murray PT, Mehta RL, Shaw A, Ronco C, Endre Z, et al. Current use of biomarkers in acute kidney injury: report and summary of recommendations from the 10th acute dialysis quality initiative consensus conference Patrick. Kidney Int. 2014;85(3):513–21.
16. Charlton JR, Portilla D, Okusa MD. A basic science view of acute kidney injury biomarkers. Nephrol Dialy Transpl. 2014;29:1301–11.
17. Kaseda R, Noriakilino, Hosojima M, Takeda T, Hosaka K, et al. Megalin-mediated endocytosis of cystatin C in proximal tubule cells. Biochem Biophys Res Commun. 2007;357(4):1130–4.
18. Vanmassenhove J, Vanholder R, Nagler E, Biesen WV. Urinary and serum biomarkers for the diagnosis of acute kidney injury: an in-depth review of the literature. Nephrol Dial Transplant. 2013;28:254–73.
19. Amsellem S, Gburek J, Hamard G, Nielsen R, Willnow TE, et al. Cubilin is essential for albumin reabsorption in the renal proximal tubule. J Am Soc Nephrol. 2010;21:1859–67.
20. Spanu S, Roeyen CR, Denecke B, Floege J, Muhlfeld AS, et al. Urinary exosomes: a novel means to non-invasively assess changes in renal gene and protein expression. PLoS One. 2014;9(10):1–8.
21. Rosenthal SH, Bokenkamp A, Hofmann W. How to estimate GFR-serum creatinine, serum cystatin C or equations? Clin Biochem. 2007;40(3):153–61.
22. Spahallari A, Parikh CR, Sint K, Koyner JL, Patel UD, et al. Serum cystatin C– versus creatinine-based definitions of acute kidney injury following cardiac surgery: a prospective cohort study. Am J Kidney Dis. 2012;60(6):922–9.
23. Zager RA. 'Biologic memory' in response to acute kidney injury: cytoresistance, toll-like receptor hyper-responsiveness and the onset of progressive renal disease. Nephrol Dial Transplant. 2013;28:1985–93.
24. Brinkman JW, Zeeuw D, Heerspink HJ, Gansevoort RT, Kema IP, et al. Apparent loss of urinary albumin

during long-term frozen storage: HPLC vs immu-nonephelometry. Clin Chem. 2007;53(8):1520–6.

25. Chew SL, Lins RL, Daelemans R, Nuyts GD, De Broe ME. Urinary enzymes in acute renal failure. Nephrol Dialy Transpl. 1993;8(6):507–11.

26. Kjeldsens L, Johnsen AH, Sengelba H, Borregaardll N. Isolation and primary structure of NGAL, a novel protein associated with human neutrophil gelatinase. J Biol Chem. 1993;268(14):10425–32.

27. Yan L, Borregaards N, Kjeldsen L, Moses MA. The high molecular weight urinary matrix metalloproteinase (MMP) activity is a complex of gelatinase B/MMP-9 and neutrophil gelatinase-associated lipocalin (NGAL) modulation of MMP-9 activity by NGAL. J Biol Chem. 2001;276(40):37258–65.

28. Paragas N, Qiu A, Hollmen M, Devrajan P, Barasch J. NGAL-siderocalin in kidney disease. Biochim Biophys Acta. 2012;1823(9):1451–8.

29. Puren AJ, Fantuzzi G, Dinarello CA. Immunology gene expression, synthesis, and secretion of interleukin 18 and interleukin 1b are differentially regulated in human blood mononuclear cells and mouse spleen cells. Proc Natl Acad Sci U S A. 1999;96:2256–61.

30. Melnikov VY, Ecder T, Fantuzzi G, Siegmund B, Lucia MS, et al. Impaired IL-18 processing protects caspase-1–deficient mice from ischemic acute renal failure. J Clin Invest. 2001;107(9):1145–52.

31. Russ KB, Stevens TM, Singal AK. Acute kidney injury in patients with cirrhosis. J Clin Transl Hepatol. 2015;3:195–204.

32. Bittencourt PL, Farias AQ, Terra C. Renal failure in cirrhosis: emerging concepts. World J Hepatol. 2015;7(21):2336–43.

33. Kashani A, Landaverde C, Medici V, Rossaro L. Fluid retention in cirrhosis: pathophysiology and management. Q J Med. 2008;101:71–85.

34. Belcher JM, Garcia-Tsao G, Sanyal AJ, Bhogal H, Lim JK, et al. Association of AKI with mortality and complications in hospitalized patients with cirrhosis. Hepatology. 2013;57(2):753–43.

35. Alessandria C, Ozdogan O, Guevara M, Restuccia T, Jimenez W, et al. MELD score and clinical type predict prognosis in hepatorenal syndrome: relevance to liver transplantation. Hepatology. 2015;41(6):1282–9.

36. Mindikoglu A, Dowling TC, Weir MR, Seliger SL, Christenson RH. Performance of chronic kidney disease epidemiology collaboration creatinine-cystatin c equation for estimating kidney function in cirrhosis. Hepatology. 2014;59(4):1532–42.

37. Low G, Alexander G, Lomas DJ. Renal impairment in cirrhosis unrelated to hepatorenal syndrome. Can J Gastroenterol Hepatol. 2015;29(5):253–7.

38. Mindikoglu A, Weir MR. Current concepts in the diagnosis and classification of renal dysfunction in cirrhosis. Am J Nephrol. 2013;38(4):345–54.

39. Salerno F, Gerbes A, Ginès P, Wong F, Arroyo V. Diagnosis, prevention and treatment of hepatorenal syndrome in cirrhosis. Gut. 2007;56:1310–8.

40. Schenker S, Martin RR, Hoyumpa AM. Antecedent liver disease and drug toxicity. J Hepatol. 1999;31:1098–105.

41. Runyon BA. Introduction to the revised American Association for the Study of Liver Diseases Practice Guideline management of adult patients with ascites due to cirrhosis 2012. Hepatology. 2013;57(4):1651–3.

42. Tsao-Garcia G, Parikh CR, Viola A. Acute kidney injury in cirrhosis. Hepatology. 2008;48(6):2064–77.

43. Suarez ML, Thomas DB, Barisoni L, Fornoni A. Diabetic nephropathy: is it time yet for routine kidney biopsy? World J Diabetes. 2013;4(6):245–55.

44. Hamid A, Hajage D, Glabeke EV, Belenfant X, Vincent F. Severe post-renal acute kidney injury, post-obstructive diuresis and renal recovery. BJU Int. 2012;110:E1027–34.

45. China L, Skene SS, Bennett K, Shabir Z, Hamilton R, et al. Albumin to prevent infection in chronic liver failure: study protocol for an interventional randomised controlled trial. BMJ Open. 2018;8(10):e023754.

46. Sigal SH, Stanca CM, Fernandez J, Arroyo V, Navasa M. Restricted use of albumin for spontaneous bacterial peritonitis. Gut. 2007;56:597–9.

47. Iglesias J, Frank E, Mehandru S, Davis JM, Levine JS. Predictors of renal recovery in patients with pre-orthotopic liver transplant (OLT) renal dysfunction. BMC Nephrol. 2013;141(47):1–12.

48. Nadim MK, Genyk YS, Tokin C, Fieber J, Ananthapanyasut W, et al. Impact of the etiology of acute kidney injury on outcomes following liver transplantation: acute tubular necrosis versus hepatorenal syndrome. Liver Transpl. 2012;18:539–48.

49. Hong G, Lee K-W, Suh S, Yoo T, Kim H, et al. The model for end-stage liver disease score-based system predicts short term mortality better than the current Child-Turcotte-Pugh score-based allocation system during waiting for deceased liver transplantation. J Korean Med Sci. 2013;28:1207–12.

Preoperative Assessment and Optimization of Liver Transplant Patients: Pulmonary Issues

12

Anjali Gera and Deepanjali Pant

12.1 Introduction

Chronic liver disease is one of the common causes of morbidity and mortality in adults. Liver transplant is the only management for end-stage liver disease (ESLD) and has evolved rapidly since the first successful transplant in 1967. The post-liver transplant survival rate has improved over last few decades, despite increasing donor and recipient age. For best possible outcomes, patients for liver transplant must be carefully evaluated and optimized.

Pulmonary disorders are the most commonly encountered comorbidities in liver transplant patients. Pulmonary disorders also have a significant impact on the prognosis of these patients. Respiratory symptoms may occur as a complication of chronic liver failure or may be seen in these patients due to coexisting respiratory illness. Smoking and chronic obstructive pulmonary diseases are very common in patients with liver failure. Moreover, certain liver diseases are associated with specific respiratory system abnormalities (like cystic fibrosis, sarcoidosis, $\alpha 1$ antitrypsin deficiency, primary biliary cirrhosis). Patients with end-stage liver disease with long-standing tense ascites may develop intercostal muscle wasting leading to restrictive respiration.

Respiratory complications are very common after liver transplantation and are associated with increased morbidity and mortality. A thorough preoperative evaluation of the pulmonary system and a good understanding of the pathophysiology of the disorders are necessary to optimize them before the transplant surgery.

The MELD system of scoring liver disease is used for ranking the patients awaiting deceased donor transplant, but the score does not have any respiratory parameter. Certain pulmonary disorders associated with liver failure affect the survival of these patients, so "standard MELD exceptions" have been made to upgrade the MELD score which include hepatopulmonary syndrome and portopulmonary hypertension.

Pulmonary disorders associated with liver failure and their management are discussed under the four main headings—hepatopulmonary syndrome (HPS), portopulmonary hypertension (PoPH), hydrothorax, and others.

12.2 Hepatopulmonary Syndrome

Hepatopulmonary syndrome is seen in advanced liver disease and is a clinical triad of hepatic disease, abnormal gas exchange, and intrapulmonary vasodilatation (IPVD). HPS can also occur with noncirrhotic portal hypertension, acute and chronic hepatitis, acute liver failure, and

A. Gera (✉) · D. Pant
Department of Anaesthesiology, Pain and Perioperative Medicine, Sir Ganga Ram Hospital, New Delhi, India

congenital vascular abnormalities like cavopulmonary shunts.

There are no specific symptoms of HPS but dyspnea, which is progressive, is the commonest complaint. Platypnea (dyspnea on standing and improved by lying supine) and orthodeoxia (decrease in arterial PO_2 by 5% or ≥ 4 mmHg from supine to upright) are the hallmarks of HPS. Other features that are seen in HPS are spider naevi, digital clubbing, cyanosis, nailbed telangiectasia, and hypoxemia (not responding to 100% O_2).

The diagnosis of HPS in the setting of liver disease is done by gas exchange analysis and documentation of intrapulmonary vasodilatation.

Arterial blood gas analysis is done while breathing ambient air and alveoloarterial gradient ≥ 15 mmHg (>20 mmHg in age >64 years), or $PaO_2 < 80$ mmHg is diagnostic of oxygenation defect. Pulse oximetry may be used as a noninvasive screening test for hypoxemia in sitting position. HPS may be classified as mild, moderate, or severe according to alveoloarterial pressure gradient (Table 12.1).

Intrathoracic vasodilatation may be diagnosed by transthoracic contrast echocardiography, radionuclide lung perfusion scan, pulmonary angiography, or high-resolution CT scan. The preferred method is transthoracic contrast echocardiography. In this technique, agitated saline (that creates microbubbles ≤ 10 μm in diameter) is injected intravenously and transthoracic echocardiography is done. Normally the bubbles are not seen as they get absorbed in the lung, but if pulmonary vasodilatation or shunts are present they come to the left side of the heart. If bubbles

appear within 3 heartbeats, it indicates intracardiac shunt and if it appears within 4–6 heartbeats it indicates intrapulmonary shunts (HPS).

Lung perfusion scanning using technetium-99-m labeled microaggregated albumin is another method of diagnosing HPS. Normally Tc^{99m} labeled albumin gets trapped in the lungs. In the presence of intrapulmonary shunts, it passes to systemic arteries and appears in the brain and kidneys. More than 6% uptake in the brain is significant. However, the scan cannot differentiate between intrapulmonary and intracardiac shunt.

Pulmonary angiography may also be done for diagnosis but is not routinely done because of its invasive nature.

High-resolution CT scan has been used for demonstrating dilatation of pulmonary arteries [1].

12.3 Epidemiology and Pathophysiology

HPS is found in 5–30% of liver transplant patients [2]. HPS is not related to severity of liver disease or its etiology. History of smoking is more common in liver transplant patient with HPS than those without HPS [3]. Some studies have observed an association between HPS and abnormal genes [4]. Since neither the etiology nor the severity of liver disease affects development of HPS, it contributes to the hypothesis of a genetic predisposition.

The hallmark of HPS is microvascular dilatation of pulmonary vasculature. This results in passage of mixed venous blood into systemic circulation and results in hypoxemia, ventilation–perfusion mismatch, shunting, and diffusion limitation. The exact cause of this vasodilatation is not clear and is multifactorial. Liver injury or portal hypertension triggers the release of vasoactive mediators like nitric oxide (NO), heme oxygenase-derived carbon monoxide, and tumor necrosis factor alpha which result in pulmonary vasodilatation or angiogenesis. Other mechanisms include failure of damaged liver to clear vasodilators (like vasoactive intestinal peptides and other substances synthesized by

Table 12.1 Classification of disease severity in hepatopulmonary syndrome

Disease severity	Alveolar arterial gradient (mmHg)	PaO2 (room air) (mmHg)	PaO2 (100% O2) (mmHg)
Mild	≥15 or >20 if age >64 years	≥80	
Moderate		60–79	
Severe		50–59	
Very severe		<50	<300

PaO2 partial pressure of oxygen in arterial blood

Fig. 12.1 (**a**) Chest PA view showing increased vascularity in the lung parenchyma. (**b**) Dilated pulmonary capillaries in hepatopulmonary syndrome

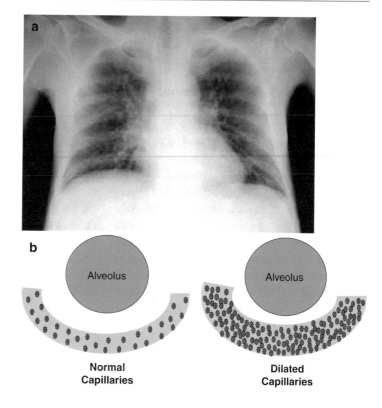

intestinal bacteria) or inhibition of circulating vasoconstrictors. Portal hypertension may decrease gut perfusion allowing translocation of bacteria and presence of endotoxin in portal blood. The key vasodilator involved in HPS is nitric oxide (NO). In a study on 45 patients with cirrhosis, those who met the diagnosis of HPS had high value of exhaled NO and there was correlation between exhaled NO and alveoloarterial oxygen difference [5, 6].

Regardless of the exact mechanism, these pathophysiological processes induce pulmonary capillary vasodilatation and direct arteriovenous connections. Increased blood flow through IPVDs with preserved alveolar ventilation results in ventilation–perfusion mismatch. At room air, partial pressure of oxygen is not sufficient for equilibrium with blood moving in the center of dilated capillary (because of increased diameter) resulting in hypoxia (Fig. 12.1a).

HPS-related hypoxemia is because of intrapulmonary shunting, ventilation–perfusion mismatch, impaired hypoxic pulmonary vasoconstriction (HPV), oxygen diffusion limitation, and atelectasis. Platypnea and orthodeoxia is caused by preferential perfusion of IPVDs, which occur disproportionately in lung bases (Fig. 12.1b) [6].

12.4 Portopulmonary Hypertension

Portopulmonary hypertension (PoPH) is characterized by pulmonary hypertension in a patient with coexisting portal hypertension and no alternative cause of pulmonary hypertension (like idiopathic heritable pulmonary hypertension, collagen vesicular disease, congenital heart disease, human immunodeficiency virus or drugs). The criteria for diagnosing this hemodynamic condition are [7]:

- Mean pulmonary arterial pressure (mPAP) > 25 mmHg at rest
- Pulmonary vascular resistance (PVR) >3 Wood units (240 dynes/s/cm^5)
- Pulmonary arterial wedge pressure (PAWP) <15 mmHg

The gold standard for diagnosing POPH is right heart catheterization. Excluding other causes of pulmonary arterial hypertension (PAH) like chronic thromboembolic pulmonary hypertension, sleep-disordered breathing, diastolic dysfunction, and significant obstructive and restrictive lung diseases is also important to make the diagnosis. An elevated PVR is important in making the diagnosis and to distinguish patients with precapillary disease from those who have passive elevation in mPAP due to hyperdynamic circulatory changes associated with chronic liver disease. It can be explained by the simple formula [8]:

$$mPAP = \left(CO \times PVR \right) + PAWP$$

PoPH always occurs in chronic liver disease with portal hypertension. A few cases have been reported in patients in absence of portal hypertension [9] and in patients without hepatitis [10]. Diagnosis of portal hypertension is usually clinical but it can be confirmed by hepatic venous catheterization, if necessary.

A PVR of 3 Wood units is used for diagnosing PoPH but in presence of hyperdynamic circulation, PVR between 2 and 3 Wood units is considered abnormal and has poor outcomes [11].

PoPH has been classified as mild, moderate, and severe based on the severity of pulmonary artery hypertension (Table 12.2).

Table 12.2 Classification of PoPH according to severity

Severity	mPAP (mmHg)	PVR (Wood unit)
Mild	25–34	>3
Moderate	35–44	
Severe	≥45	

12.5   Epidemiology

PoPH is seen in 5–6% of liver transplant patients [12]. Usually it is seen equally in males and females; some studies have shown higher incidence in females [13]. Autoimmune hepatitis is a clinical risk factor for PoPH [13]. Because of the infrequent or sporadic occurrence of this hemodynamic entity in patients with portal hypertension, genetic predisposition has been proposed. It has been found that mutations in the pathway involving estrogen signaling, cell growth, apoptosis, and oxidative stress play a role [14]. The prevalence of PoPH is not influenced by the severity of liver disease.

12.6   Pathophysiology

The exact cause of development of PoPH is not known although many theories have been proposed like:

1. A humoral substance with vasoactive property (which is normally metabolized in the liver) reaches pulmonary circulation through portosystemic circulation and causes pulmonary hypertension. These mediators are serotonin, interleukin 1, endothelin 1, glucagon, secretin, thromboxane β2, and vasoactive intestinal peptide [15].
2. Thromboembolism from portal venous system: according to this theory, blood clots pass from the portal system to pulmonary circulation through shunts [16].
3. The hyperdynamic circulation in chronic liver disease may cause PoPH. High cardiac output and increased blood flow through pulmonary vasculature cause sheer stress with vasoconstriction, hypertrophy, and proliferation of endothelial cells, resulting in pulmonary arterial hypertension [17]. However, this theory is not supported by studies that show increased blood flow is readily accommodated by pulmonary vasculature [18].

4. Certain inflammatory mediators like IL1 β, IL-6, and TNF-alpha are increased in cirrhotic patients [19].
5. For hereditary pulmonary hypertension, a specific gene has been identified. For PoPH, specific genetic defect has not been found but several pathways have been proposed that may cause vascular pathology in these cases.

Histopathological findings of PoPH are indistinguishable from pulmonary hypertension and include medial hypertrophy, remodeling of pulmonary arterial walls, and in situ thrombosis.

12.7 Diagnosis

These patients are asymptomatic at early stage of the disease. The most common symptoms are progressive dyspnea and worsening fatigue. They may have peripheral edema, chest pain, syncope, or near syncope. On physical examination they have raised jugular venous pressure, loud pulmonic component of second heart sound, a systolic murmur on left sternal border (because of tricuspid regurgitation), right ventricular heave,

and right-sided fourth heart sound. They may have ascites and peripheral edema. In PoPH patients, presence of peripheral edema and ascites is not indicative of its severity whereas in patients with idiopathic PH, these features reflect the severity of the disease.

The electrocardiogram reveals right axis deviation and right ventricular hypertrophy and may reveal right bundle branch block. Chest X-ray may demonstrate enlarged pulmonary arteries and cardiomegaly.

Patients with PoPH usually have mild hypoxia even when they have moderate to severe disease in contrast to HPS [20].

Transthoracic echocardiography is a specific test and is most commonly used in the diagnosis of PoPH and to rule out other causes of pulmonary hypertension. To exclude other causes of pulmonary hypertension like venous or arterial thromboembolism, ventilation–perfusion scan or computed tomography pulmonary angiography may be done. Right heart catheterization is the gold standard in the diagnosis and evaluation of PoPH.

Clinical features of HPS and PoPH are enumerated in Table 12.3.

Table 12.3 HPS versus PoPH

	HPS	PoPH
Diagnosis	Triad of	Pulmonary and portal hypertension
	Liver disease	$mPAP > 25$ mmHg
	Hypoxemia: $P(A-a) > 15$ mmHg	$PVR > 3$ Wood units
	IPVD	$PAWP < 15$ mmHg
Symptoms	Dyspnea, platypnea, orthodeoxia	Fatigue, dyspnea on exertion, orthopnea
	Clubbing, cyanosis, spider angiomas	Right heart failure (raised JVP, prominent P2, tricuspid regurgitation murmur, lower extremity edema)
Chest X-ray	Usually normal	Cardiomegaly
		Hilar enlargement
Diagnostic tools	Contrast echocardiography	Right heart catheterization
	Technetium-99 labeled macroaggregated albumin scan	Echocardiography
	Pulmonary angiography	
PFT	Decreased DLCO	Decreased DLCO
Treatment	Oxygen supplementation	Vasodilators (epoprostenol, iloprost, sildenafil)
	Liver transplant	Liver transplant (for mild to moderate)

12.8 Hepatic Hydrothorax

Hepatic hydrothorax (HH) is a manifestation of advanced liver disease and occurs in 5–12% of patients [21]. It is defined as accumulation of fluid in pleural space (usually >500 mL) in the absence of cardiac, pulmonary, or pleural diseases. It usually occurs in conjunction with ascites; however it may occur in the absence of ascites [22]. In the presence of ascites, the peritoneal fluid enters the thoracic cavity through microscopic openings in the tendinous part of the diaphragm. Cyclic negative intrathoracic pressure along with openings in diaphragm allows unidirectional passage of fluid from peritoneal to pleural cavity. HH becomes apparent when the absorptive capacity of pleural space is exceeded. It is usually right sided because congenital diaphragmatic fenestrations are more common in right hemidiaphragm, and left hemidiaphragm is thicker and muscular.

In the absence of ascites, the mechanism of fluid collection in the thoracic cavity is the same. In these cases, the reabsorption capacity of pleura is same as the accumulation of ascitic fluid, so ascites collection does not occur [23]. The mechanism of collection of fluid has been confirmed by demonstration of unidirectional passage of markers like 99mTc-human albumin or 99mTc-sulfur colloid from the peritoneal cavity to the pleural cavity [24, 25].

The fluid collected in HH is transudative in nature. Patients with HH may develop spontaneous bacterial empyema (SBE), similar to subacute bacterial peritonitis.

The symptoms of HH are nonspecific—dyspnea, nonproductive cough, and pleuritic chest pain and fatigue.

Thoracocentesis is done to establish the diagnosis and to exclude the other causes of pleural effusion, like infection, thromboembolic diseases, or metastatic carcinoma. Thoracocentesis also helps to relieve symptoms. Computed tomography is done to rule out lung or pleural lesion. Doppler ultrasonography may be done to evaluate portal and hepatic vessels patency.

Management of hepatic hydrothorax is similar to ascites. Diuretics and salt restriction are the first line of management. The aim of management is to relieve symptoms and to prevent infection and complications. Therapeutic thoracocentesis and paracentesis may be required before liver transplant surgery.

Refractory hydrothorax refers to persistent pleural effusion despite salt restriction <2 g/day and high-dose diuretic therapy and repeated thoracocentesis [26]. In these cases, transjugular intrahepatic portosystemic shunt (TIPS) may be considered to control pleural effusion.

Although hepatic hydrothorax is not an indication for liver transplant, it improves after the transplant surgery [26].

12.9 COPD and Smoking

Chronic obstructive pulmonary disease (COPD) is very common in patients undergoing liver transplantation. Old age and smoking are significant risk factors of COPD and have adverse consequences on the functional status and quality of life in these patients. Smoking is also commonly seen in patients undergoing liver transplant. According to a multicenter study, 60% of liver transplant candidates had a history of past or present smoking [27]. It is very important to optimize COPD and smoking in patients undergoing transplant because perioperative outcomes may be compromised. Moreover, smoking has been shown to increase the risk of malignancy [28].

COPD is characterized by progressive airflow limitation that is not fully reversible. These patients have dyspnea, exercise limitation, susceptibility to infections, and exacerbations. They have abnormal blood gases and pulmonary function tests. Patients with advanced liver disease also have abnormal pulmonary functions. Their lung volumes are decreased because of hepatomegaly, ascites, pleural effusion, and basal atelectasis. It is important to have prebronchodilator and postbronchodilator spirometry in patients suspected to have COPD to confirm the diagnosis. Postbronchodilator FEV1/FVC ratio less than 0.7 indicates airflow limitation.

The BODE index is a multidimensional system for the assessment of COPD severity and prognosis. This is calculated based on weight (BMI), airway obstruction (FEV1), dyspnea score (mMRC), and exercise capacity (6 min walk distance) and has been used to assess an individual's risk of death.

12.10 Obstructive Sleep Apnea

Obstructive sleep apnea (OSA) is a common disorder characterized by repetitive nocturnal breathing cessation due to upper airway collapse. Recent studies have demonstrated that OSA is associated with the development and evolution of nonalcoholic fatty liver disease (NAFLD), independent of obesity or other shared risk factors [29]. It is very important to properly diagnose and manage OSA before taking up these patients for surgery. Untreated OSA leading to hypoxia and hypercapnia may present challenges to postoperative weaning from ventilator.

Preoperative screening using STOP-BANG questionnaire and sleep study must be done in patients at risk for OSA. CPAP should be initiated from the preoperative period in patients with severe OSA, and sedative medications including opioids must be used carefully.

12.11 Interstitial Lung Disease

Interstitial lung disease (ILD) is a group of disorders that causes fibrosis of the lungs. ILD is characterized by four manifestations: (1) respiratory symptoms such as shortness of breath and cough, (2) specific chest radiographic abnormalities, (3) decreased lung capacity and restrictive PFT, (4) characteristic inflammation and fibrosis of interstitium.

ILD is associated with primary biliary cirrhosis and autoimmune hepatitis [26]. In telomerase mutations, ILD and cryptogenic CLD may occur concomitantly. Liver transplant does not improve ILD, rather it continues to progress after transplant. Antifibrotic drugs may improve ILD, but does not cure it completely. Liver transplant is contraindicated in moderate to severe ILD.

12.12 Alpha1 Antitrypsin Deficiency

Alpha1 antitrypsin deficiency (AAT) is a genetic disorder caused by the deficiency of alpha1 antitrypsin, a serine protease inhibitor. Individuals with this disorder develop obstructive pulmonary disease, liver disease (cirrhosis and hepatocellular carcinoma), and rarely skin lesions (panniculitis).

Individuals having 2 M alleles have normal AAT structure and function, whereas Z and S alleles have abnormal AAT [30]. The liver disease in this disorder occurs due to accumulation of abnormal AAT in the hepatocytes [31]. Emphysema results from an imbalance between neutrophil elastase in the lung that destroys elastin and the elastase inhibitor AAT that protects against proteolytic degradation of elastin [32].

Cigarette smoking and lung infections increase the elastase load in lungs further leading to lung degradation. The clinical features of AAT deficiency are similar to usual COPD except that its onset is at younger age and emphysema is panlobular or basilar and family history of emphysema may be present.

Liver transplant in these patients results in the normalization of AAT levels and function. However despite normal levels of AAT after liver transplant, FEV1 continues to decline unexpectedly in some ZZ or SZ patients [30].

12.13 Arteriovenous Malformations (AVM)

Hereditary hemorrhagic telangiectasia (Osler–Weber–Rendu syndrome) is an autosomal dominant disorder characterized by arteriovenous malformations in organs like liver, lung, brain, and gastrointestinal tract. It has a variety of clinical manifestations like epistaxis, gastrointestinal bleeding, iron deficiency anemia, and mucocutaneous telangiectasia.

Pulmonary AVM allow systemic venous blood to bypass pulmonary circulation and result in embolic stroke, brain abscess, and migraines. Cerebral AVMs can cause hemorrhagic stroke.

Hepatic AVMs can result in high output heart failure, portal hypertension, and biliary necrosis and require liver transplant. In patients with high output failure associated with hepatic AVM, **bevacizumab** has been shown to reduce cardiac output and quality of life [33]. Embolization of hepatic AVMs can also be done but may cause ischemic biliary necrosis.

12.14 Pulmonary Nodules

Pulmonary nodules may be detected during routine preoperative evaluation of liver transplant patients. A biopsy of the nodule is mandatory for diagnosis and further management. It can be primary lung malignancy or metastatic liver malignancy (HCC) or may represent granulomatous infection. In case it is granulomatous infection, it must be treated before transplant. However there is a possibility that the infection may be reactivated after transplant (immunosuppressive medication).

In metastatic HCC, liver transplant is contraindicated. In case nodules are >10 mm in diameter FDG-PET can be helpful in evaluation. If nodules are <10 mm in diameter, CT scan is preferable.

If pulmonary nodules are detected after the transplant surgery in HCC patients, they are managed with surgical excision of the nodules [26].

12.15 Preoperative Assessment

12.15.1 History

A carefully obtained detailed history from the patients scheduled for liver transplant is a must and helps in the diagnosis of diseases unrelated to liver failure. The most common pulmonary symptom in these patients is dyspnea, which can be multifactorial [8] (Table 12.4). It is important to ask the patient about the duration of symptoms and relieving or aggravating factors. Other associated symptoms like orthopnea, platypnea, cough, wheezing, chest pain, and edema should be asked for and should be characterized.

Table 12.4 Causes of dyspnea in patients with liver disease

Due to liver disease per se
1. Hepatopulmonary syndrome
2. Portopulmonary syndrome
3. Hepatic hydrothorax
4. Interstitial lung disease (associated with primary biliary cirrhosis)
5. Alpha1 antitrypsin deficiency (panlobular emphysema)
6. Arteriovenous malformations
7. Pulmonary nodules (metastatic)
8. Ascites (causes atelectasis and muscle wasting)
9. Cardiomyopathy (cirrhotic)
10. Severe anemia
Not related to liver disease
1. Chronic obstructive pulmonary disease
2. Restrictive pulmonary disease
3. Obstructive sleep apnea (OSA)
4. Cardiac disease

Dyspnea associated with cough with expectoration and wheezing indicates presence of COPD, bronchial asthma, or ILD. Dyspnea relieved with paracentesis is due to ascites. Dyspnea associated with platypnea suggests HPS. History of smoking should be elicited and if present, patient should be advised to quit before surgery.

Occupational hazards like exposure to asbestos may be present and can lead to ILD. These patients present with progressive dyspnea.

Symptoms like snoring, disturbed sleep, and daytime sleepiness suggest OSA, and appropriate measures should be taken to optimize the disorder. These patients may have difficulty in extubation during the postoperative period.

A positive family history helps in diagnosing α1 antitrypsin deficiency and hereditary hemorrhagic telangiectasia.

12.15.2 Physical Examination

A thorough physical examination of the patient provides clue to the diagnosis of pulmonary disorders. On general examination, patient's weight and BMI must be checked and recorded as it is important to screen for OSA [34]. If history of snoring and sleep breathing disorder is there,

STOP-BANG questionnaire helps in screening for OSA.

On general examination, finger clubbing, peripheral cyanosis, nail telangiectasia, and spider angiomatosis may be present and point towards presence of HPS. The presence of peripheral edema may be because of right heart failure.

Airway assessment and neck examination must be done to screen for difficult intubation. These patients have deranged coagulation, so intubation should be smooth and atraumatic.

In cardiovascular examination, the presence of systolic murmur at left sternal border, loud pulmonic component of second heart sound, right ventricular heave, and raised JVP suggests the presence of pulmonary hypertension.

In respiratory system examination, we should look for adventitious breath sounds like rhonchi, crepts, and crackles. These may suggest the presence of COPD and ILD.

Pulse oximetry shows decreased saturation in patients with liver failure and indicates hypoxemia. Fall in oxygen saturation with change in position from supine to upright is seen in HPS and requires further evaluation.

12.15.3 Laboratory Investigations

Laboratory investigations help us in the evaluation of disease and establishing the diagnosis. Although not directly affecting pulmonary assessment, MELD scoring helps us in staging the liver failure and urgency of liver transplantation. In patients with high MELD score requiring urgent liver transplantation, any concomitant pulmonary disease must be identified and optimized early for better outcome.

α1 antitrypsin levels and genotypic analysis (for M, S, Z alleles) must be done in patients with suspected α1 antitrypsin deficiency.

Patients with suspected OSA must undergo **overnight pulse oximetry**, which is a simple screening method [35]. It is important to identify this disorder, as this may delay extubation and will add to the pulmonary complications. These patients may have to undergo sleep study or polysomnography and may be advised noninvasive BiPAP/CPAP till they undergo transplantation.

ABG is done in patients with end-stage liver disease as a part of evaluation to look for hypoxia and hypercapnia, which may be due to hypoventilation. In case of HPS, orthodeoxia is present in which PaO_2 decreases by more than 5% or 4 mmHg in upright position. Although this is seen in only 25% of the patients, it is a significant finding [36]. ABG is also done to assess the severity of HPS.

NT-pro brain natriuretic peptide is a useful prognostic indicator in patients with PoPH [37].

Chest X-ray is done as a routine investigation in patients undergoing transplant. Hepatic hydrothorax, COPD, or any lung lesion may be diagnosed with chest X-ray. In a country like India where pulmonary tuberculosis is so common, chest X-ray may reveal old tubercular infection. Any active infection needs to be treated. In case any parenchymal lesion is found on chest X-ray, **computed tomogram** (CT) may be done to define the lesion.

Electrocardiogram (ECG) is another routine investigation done in all patients to assess cardiac rate, rhythm, and any ischemic changes. Any chamber enlargement or bundle branch block may be seen in ECG.

Pulmonary function test (PFT) is done in all the patients undergoing liver transplant as a part of pulmonary assessment. Interstitial fluid collection, pleural fluid, and liver cirrhosis all lead to abnormalities in PFT. All the parameters like FEV1, FVC, and FEV1/FVC and FEF 25–75% may be affected in these patients.

In case the patient has any respiratory symptom, PFT helps in evaluating whether it is restrictive or obstructive lesion. Moreover, it tells about bronchodilator responsiveness in obstructive lesion. Patients with ILD have restrictive defects and must undergo PFT to assess functional capacity of the lungs. These patients also have reduced diffusion capacity of CO.

Echocardiography is done in all patients undergoing transplant [38]. As regards pulmonary system evaluation, transthoracic echocardiography (TTE) is a screening test in PoPH for assessing right ventricular size and function and to evaluate right ventricular systolic pressure. Patients awaiting transplant with normal echocardiography must repeat TTE once a year. Various studies have given different threshold values of right ventricular systolic pressure (RVSP) which should prompt further investigation like right heart catheterization. A value of 38–50 mmHg in presence of right ventricular dilatation or dysfunction has been suggested as a cutoff value for further evaluation [39]. Recent guidelines by American Association for the study of Liver Diseases (AASLD) recommend right heart catheterization in patients with RVSP $\geq$ 45 mmHg [38].

Right heart catheterization is an invasive procedure that is done, when indicated, to confirm the diagnosis of PoPH. The prerequisite for this invasive procedure involves platelet counts $\geq$ 50,000 and INR < 1.5. It may be done as a day-care procedure. Swan-Ganz catheter is inserted into central vein and placed in pulmonary artery and is used to measure mPAP and PACW. Cardiac output is measured using thermodilution or Fick method, and pulmonary vascular resistance is measured using the formula:

$$PVR = (mPAP - PAWP) / CO$$

It is very important to calculate PVR in patients suspected to have PoPH. PVR reflects right heart afterload and if it is increased it means right heart failure is present and this will cause increased central venous pressure. This will be transmitted backward and will cause hepatic venous congestion and graft failure.

When PAP is >25 mmHg, PAWP is <15 mmHg, and PVR is >3 Wood units, diagnosis of PoPH is made.

Contrast echocardiography is a technique used to evaluate intracardiac or intrapulmonary shunting. Agitated saline is the most commonly used contrast. The gas microbubbles are short lived and diffuse into the lungs while traversing the pulmonary circulation. Whenever gas bubbles appear on the left side of the heart (visualized as opacification), it means either there is intracardiac shunt or intrapulmonary arteriovenous malformation leading to shunting. For detection of intrapulmonary shunt, the gas bubbles must be smaller in size (<10 µm diameter) [40]. The agitated saline is administered intravenously, and the appearance of bubbles on the left side within one or two cardiac cycles means presence of intracardiac shunt. If the bubbles are visualized after three or more cardiac cycles, it indicates intrapulmonary shunting [2]. According to American Society of Echocardiography guidelines, an alternative name for echocardiographic contrast agents as Ultrasound enhancing agents (UEAs) has been given [41].

Macroaggregated Albumin Technetium-99m-labeled macroaggregated albumin (99mTc MAA) lung perfusion scanning is an alternative method of confirming intrapulmonary shunt in HPS. 99mTcMAA is injected intravenously and in normal conditions it gets trapped in pulmonary circulation. The normal diameter of lung capillary vessel is less than 8–15 µm. Agitated saline creates bubbles greater than 10 µm in diameter that do not normally pass the lung capillaries. Scans showing radionuclide uptake by the brain or kidney indicate shunting and if the uptake is >6%, it is consistent with HPS. Unlike contrast echocardiograph, it does not differentiate between intracardiac and intrapulmonary shunts. However, concomitant transesophageal echocardiography may be used to visualize the source of microbubbles in the left heart [2]. 99mTc MAA may be used to quantify the shunt fraction in patients with HPS. Patients with shunt fraction more than 20% have higher perioperative mortality. This method is also useful to differentiate hypoxemia due to concomitant liver disease and due to intrapulmonary shunting (HPS) [42].

Another test used to assess pulmonary status in patients with liver disease is **6-min walk test**.

Although nonspecific, it indicates physical function and may be used for therapeutic response in patients with pulmonary dysfunction. During the 6-min walk test, a healthy individual can walk up to 400–700 m [43]. In patients undergoing transplant, the walk distance <250 m is associated with poor outcome [44].

12.16 Management

12.16.1 HPS

This life-threatening complication of advanced liver disease usually develops insidiously. However, this insidious progression with stable nature of CLD often leads to delay in diagnosis and listing for LT.

The definitive treatment of HPS is liver transplantation. For mild to moderate HPS, oxygen support to maintain saturation >89% is the most effective therapy. Otherwise once the diagnosis is made and till the patient undergoes transplantation supportive management is initiated.

Other therapies that have been tried with variable effect on improvement of gas exchange in HPS are spring coil embolization (to physically occlude shunts), octreotide, nitric oxide synthase inhibitors, indomethacin, almitrine bismesylate, methylene blue (inhibits NO stimulated guanylate cyclase), alum sativum (garlic), propranolol, plasma exchange, and pentoxifylline [7].

In patients with mild HPS with resting $PaO_2 > 55$ mmHg or $SpO_2 > 88\%$, oxygen support is not required unless they have exercise-induced or nocturnal hypoxemia. In these patients, 6-min walk test or nocturnal saturation monitoring may be done.

The prognosis of patients with HPS is poor with increased mortality, regardless of oxygenation status [3]. Due to poor quality of life and increased mortality, they should be considered for early liver transplantation, preferably before they have severe hypoxemia. Because of these reasons, HPS patients are eligible for "MELD exception policy." In case of $PaO_2 < 60$ mmHg on room air without clinical evidence of underlying pulmonary disease, presence of portal hyperten-

sion, and evidence of intrapulmonary vasodilatation by TTE, a score of 22 is assigned. The score increases by 10% mortality equivalent points if repeat ABG shows $PaO_2 < 60$ mmHg.

There is no lower cutoff limit of PaO_2 that would preclude liver transplant. However some studies have reported that severe hypoxemia ($PaO_2 < 50$ mmHg) and shunt fraction >20% are associated with increased mortality [45, 46].

The oxygenation usually improves after liver transplant, but the time course is variable. Some may improve within days after transplant; some may take 2–14 months. It may be related to the severity of pretransplant hypoxemia [45].

12.17 Portopulmonary Hypertension

Preoperative management of PoPH is complex and treatment should target portal hypertension as well as pulmonary hypertension. It should be done at experienced center with the goals to improve quality of life, exercise capacity, and survival of the patient. In liver transplant candidates, additional goals are improvement in pulmonary hemodynamics and right ventricular function to improve the outcomes of liver transplant.

General measures—like all patients with PAH, patients with PoPH should receive supportive measures like oxygen and diuretics. Oxygen is supplemented to maintain saturation >89%. They are counseled against smoking if positive history is there. They are encouraged to exercise as possible and receive vaccinations. Anticoagulants are generally not given to PoPH patients as they have coagulopathy, thrombocytopenia, and varices.

Patients with PoPH should receive treatment for portal hypertension. β blockers and TIPS are not indicated in these patients (management modality of portal hypertension). β blockers should be avoided as they can worsen right heart failure due to reduction in right ventricular output and increase in PVR [47]. TIPS can increase preload to right ventricle and worsen heart failure. In moderate PoPH, TIPS should be avoided.

Esophageal varices should be managed with banding. Balloon-occluded retrograde transvenous obliteration (BRTO) is a newer therapy in the management of acute bleeding from gastric varices.

12.18 Specific Therapy

12.18.1 PAH-Specific Therapy Includes

1. Prostacyclin pathway agonist—Epoprostenol, Iloprost, Treprostinil, and Beraprost are used for pretransplant management of PoPH. Epoprostenol is a potent vasodilator and is given as continuous intravenous infusion (short half-life 3–5 min). Some common side effects of epoprostenol are diarrhea, nausea, flushing, headache, jaw ache, and leg pain. The infusion should not be stopped abruptly as it may cause sudden rebound vasoconstriction and elevation of PAP. Treprostinil can be given intravenously or by subcutaneous route. Iloprost can be given intravenously, orally, or by inhalation route. **Selexipag**, an, oral prostacyclin agonist used in the treatment of pulmonary hypertension has not been tested in patients with PoPH.
2. Endothelin receptor antagonist—Bosentan, Macitentan, and Ambrisentan target endothelin-1 pathway. Bosentan has been shown to be effective in the management of PoPH [48]. However, it can cause liver injury, so monthly liver function tests are mandatory. Ambrisentan and Macitentan do not require frequent monitoring but baseline liver function tests must be done.
3. Phosphodiesterase—5 inhibitors—the drugs in this group act through cAMP and nitric oxide pathway and cause vasodilatation. Sildenafil, Tadalafil, and Vardenafil are some of the agents. Sildenafil is a selective lung tissue phosphodiesterase-5 inhibitor and is effective in reducing PAP in liver transplant patients. Combination therapy with two or three drugs may be given in severe PoPH.
4. Guanylate cyclase stimulant—Riociguat is a guanylate cyclase stimulant.
5. Calcium channel blockers—they are used in idiopathic PAH but avoided in PoPH. Calcium channel blockers may cause hypotension and splanchnic vasodilatation resulting in an increase in hepatic venous pressure gradient.

In the past, liver transplant was considered a contraindication for patients with PoPH but now transplant has been done successfully in patients with mild to moderate PoPH. Although liver transplant is not a treatment for PoPH, but it can be done in these patients provided their PAH is treatment responsive. In some studies, improvements in pulmonary dynamics have been reported after liver transplant in patients with treated PoPH [49].

In patients with mPAP > 50 mmHg, liver transplant is absolutely contraindicated. Guidelines [2] recommend treatment of PoPH with PAH-specific therapy in patients with mPAP > 35 mmHg with the aim to reduce mPAP < 35 mmHg, PVR to <2 Wood units, and improve right ventricular function.

MELD SCORE: As with HPS, patients with PoPH also receive MELD exception score of 22. Every 3 months, they undergo right heart catheterization and get their score upgraded by 10% while they are on liver transplant wait list.

12.19 Hepatic Hydrothorax

Management of hepatic hydrothorax is similar to ascites. Diuretics and salt restriction are the first line of management. The aim of management is to relieve symptoms and to prevent infection and complications. Therapeutic thoracocentesis and paracentesis are done in symptomatic patients and may be required before liver transplant surgery. Refractory hydrothorax refers to persistent pleural effusion despite salt restriction <2 g/day and high-dose diuretic therapy and repeated thoracocentesis [26]. In these cases, transjugular intrahepatic portosystemic shunt (TIPS) may be considered to control pleural effusion.

Chest tube should not be inserted for HH only because it can result in massive protein and electrolyte depletion, infection, renal failure, and bleeding [50]. Once inserted, it is very difficult to remove chest tube in these patients and also it has been associated with increased mortality and longer hospital stay [51]. Chest tube insertion is done in patients with SBE.

Pleurodesis is challenging in these HH, although it has been tried in patients with refractory HH. It is difficult to keep the two surfaces of pleura apposed for long time for inflammation to occur, as there is rapid filling of fluid in pleural cavity. Moreover this technique is associated with multiple complications [52].

Thoracoscopic mesh repair of diaphragmatic defects may be done for refractory HH [53].

12.20 Summary

In patients undergoing liver transplantation, pulmonary diseases are common and invariably affect prognosis. A thorough preoperative evaluation and management of pulmonary issues is mandatory in these patients to improve outcome.

Key Points
- A careful pulmonary evaluation and optimization of liver transplant patients improve the outcome.
- Hepatopulmonary syndrome is a clinical trial of abnormal arterial oxygenation caused by intrapulmonary vasodilatation in the setting of liver disease.
- Portopulmonary hypertension is pulmonary hypertension (>25 mmHg) associated with portal hypertension and the gold standard for diagnosing portopulmonary hypertension is right heart catheterization.
- Hepatic hydrothorax is collection of fluid (>500 mL) in patients with chronic liver disease in the absence of cardiac, pulmonary, or pleural disease.
- Patients with HPS have severe hypoxia and improve with liver transplant, whereas patients with portopulmonary hypertension have mild hypoxia and have variable outcome after liver transplant.

References

1. Lee KN, Lee HJ, Shin WW, Webb WR. Hypoxemia and liver cirrhosis (hepatopulmonary syndrome) in eight patients: comparison of the central and peripheral pulmonary vasculature. Radiology. 1999;211(2):549–53.
2. Krowka MJ, Fallon MB, Kawut SM, Fuhrmann V, Heimbach JK, Ramsay MA, Sitbon O, Sokol RJ. International liver transplant society practice guidelines: diagnosis and management of hepatopulmonary syndrome and portopulmonary hypertension. Transplantation. 2016;100(7):1440–52.
3. Fallon MB, Krowka MJ, Brown RS, Trotter JF, Zacks S, Roberts KE, Shah VH, Kaplowitz N, Forman L, Wille K, Kawut SM. Pulmonary Vascular Complications of Liver Disease Study Group. Impact of hepatopulmonary syndrome on quality of life and survival in liver transplant candidates. Gastroenterology. 2008;135(4):1168–75.
4. Roberts KE, Kawut SM, Krowka MJ, Brown RS Jr, Trotter JF, Shah V, Peter I, Tighiouart H, Mitra N, Handorf E, Knowles JA, Zacks S, Fallon MB. Pulmonary Vascular Complications of Liver Disease Study Group. Genetic risk factors for hepatopulmonary syndrome in patients with advanced liver disease. Gastroenterology. 2010;139(1):130–9.
5. Rolla G, Brussino L, Colagrande P, Dutto L, Polizzi S, Scappaticci E, Bergerone S, Morello M, Marzano A, Martinasso G, Salizzoni M, Bucca C. Exhaled nitric oxide and oxygenation abnormalities in hepatic cirrhosis. Hepatology. 1997;26(4):842–7.
6. Krowka MJ, Cortese DA. Hepatopulmonary syndrome: an evolving perspective in the era of liver transplantation. Hepatology. 1990;11(1):138–42.
7. Rodríguez-Roisin R, Krowka MJ, Hervé P, Fallon MB. ERS Task Force Pulmonary-Hepatic Vascular Disorders (PHD) Scientific Committee. Pulmonary-hepatic vascular disorders (PHD). Eur Respir J. 2004;24(5):861–80.
8. DuBrock HM, Krowka MJ. Pulmonary evaluation of liver transplant candidates. In: Bezinover D, Saner F, editors. Pulmonary evaluation of liver transplant candidate. New York, NY: Springer; 2019. p. 25–45.

9. Yoshida EM, Erb SR, Ostrow DN, Ricci DR, Scudamore CH, Fradet G. Pulmonary hypertension associated with primary biliary cirrhosis in the absence of portal hypertension: a case report. Gut. 1994;35(2):280–2.

10. Hervé P, Lebrec D, Brenot F, Simonneau G, Humbert M, Sitbon O, Duroux P. Pulmonary vascular disorders in portal hypertension. Eur Respir J. 1998;11(5):1153–66.

11. Savale L, Sattler C, Coilly A, Conti F, Renard S, Francoz C, Bouvaist H, Feray C, Borentain P, Jaïs X, Montani D, Parent F, O'Connell C, Hervé P, Humbert M, Simonneau G, Samuel D, Calmus Y, Duvoux C, Durand F, Duclos-Vallée JC, Sitbon O. Long-term outcome in liver transplantation candidates with portopulmonary hypertension. Hepatology. 2017;65(5):1683–92.

12. Krowka MJ, Swanson KL, Frantz RP, McGoon MD, Wiesner RH. Portopulmonary hypertension: results from a 10-year screening algorithm. Hepatology. 2006;44(6):1502–10.

13. Kawut SM, Krowka MJ, Trotter JF, Roberts KE, Benza RL, Badesch DB, Taichman DB, Horn EM, Zacks S, Kaplowitz N, Brown RS Jr, Fallon MB. Pulmonary Vascular Complications of Liver Disease Study Group. Clinical risk factors for portopulmonary hypertension. Hepatology. 2008;48(1):196–203.

14. Roberts KE, Fallon MB, Krowka MJ, Brown RS, Trotter JF, Peter I, Tighiouart H, Knowles JA, Rabinowitz D, Benza RL, Badesch DB, Taichman DB, Horn EM, Zacks S, Kaplowitz N, Kawut SM. Pulmonary Vascular Complications of Liver Disease Study Group. Genetic risk factors for portopulmonary hypertension in patients with advanced liver disease. Am J Respir Crit Care Med. 2009;179(9):835–42.

15. Mandell MS, Groves BM. Pulmonary hypertension in chronic liver disease. Clin Chest Med. 1996;17(1):17–33.

16. Edwards BS, Weir EK, Edwards WD, Ludwig J, Dykoski RK, Edwards JE. Coexistent pulmonary and portal hypertension: morphologic and clinical features. J Am Coll Cardiol. 1987;10(6):1233–8.

17. Hoeper MM, Krowka MJ, Strassburg CP. Portopulmonary hypertension and hepatopulmonary syndrome. Lancet. 2004;363(9419):1461–8.

18. Mandell MS, Groves BM. Pulmonary hypertension in chronic liver disease. Clin Chest Med. 1996;7:17–33.

19. Tilg H, Wilmer A, Vogel W, Herold M, Nölchen B, Judmaier G, Huber C. Serum levels of cytokines in chronic liver diseases. Gastroenterology. 1992;103(1):264–74.

20. Swanson KL, Johnson CM, Prakash UB, McKusick MA, Andrews JC, Stanson AW. Bronchial artery embolization: experience with 54 patients. Chest. 2002;121(3):789–95.

21. Alberts WM, Salem AJ, Solomon DA, Boyce G. Hepatic hydrothorax. Cause and management. Arch Intern Med. 1991;151(12):2383–8.

22. Abba AA, Laajam MA, Zargar SA. Spontaneous neutrocytic hepatic hydrothorax without ascites. Respir Med. 1996;90(10):631–4.

23. Serrat J, Roza JJ, Planella T. Hepatic hydrothorax in the absence of ascites: respiratory failure in a cirrhotic patient. Anesth Analg. 2004;99(6):1803–4.

24. Rubinstein D, McInnes IE, Dudley FJ. Hepatic hydrothorax in the absence of clinical ascites: diagnosis and management. Gastroenterology. 1985;88(1 Pt 1):188–91.

25. Serena A, Aliaga L, Richter JA, Calderon R, Sanchez L, Charvet MA. Scintigraphic demonstration of a diaphragmatic defect as the cause of massive hydrothorax in cirrhosis. Eur J Nucl Med. 1985;11(1):46–8.

26. Krowka MJ, Wiesner RH, Heimbach JK. Pulmonary contraindications, indications and MELD exceptions for liver transplantation: a contemporary view and look forward. J Hepatol. 2013;59(2):367–74.

27. Rybak D, Fallon MB, Krowka MJ, Brown RS Jr, Reinen J, Stadheim L, Faulk D, Nielsen C, Al-Naamani N, Roberts K, Zacks S, Perry T, Trotter J, Kawut SM. Pulmonary Vascular Complications of Liver Disease Study Group. Risk factors and impact of chronic obstructive pulmonary disease in candidates for liver transplantation. Liver Transpl. 2008;14(9):1357–65.

28. van der Heide F, Dijkstra G, Porte RJ, Kleibeuker JH, Haagsma EB. Smoking behavior in liver transplant recipients. Liver Transpl. 2009;15(6):648–55.

29. Mesarwi OA, Loomba R, Malhotra A. Obstructive sleep apnea, hypoxia, and nonalcoholic fatty liver disease. Am J Respir Crit Care Med. 2019;199(7):830–41.

30. Carey EJ, Iyer VN, Nelson DR, Nguyen JH, Krowka MJ. Outcomes for recipients of liver transplantation for alpha-1-antitrypsin deficiency–related cirrhosis. Liver Transpl. 2013;19(12):1370–6.

31. Lomas DA, Evans DL, Finch JT, Carrell RW. The mechanism of Z alpha 1-antitrypsin accumulation in the liver. Nature. 1992;357(6379):605–7.

32. Stoller JK, Aboussouan LS. A review of α1-antitrypsin deficiency. Am J Respir Crit Care Med. 2012;185(3):246–59.

33. Dupuis-Girod S, Ginon I, Saurin JC, Marion D, Guillot E, Decullier E, Roux A, Carette MF, Gilbert-Dussardier B, Hatron PY, Lacombe P, Lorcerie B, Rivière S, Corre R, Giraud S, Bailly S, Paintaud G, Ternant D, Valette PJ, Plauchu H, Faure F. Bevacizumab in patients with hereditary hemorrhagic telangiectasia and severe hepatic vascular malformations and high cardiac output. JAMA. 2012;307(9):948–55.

34. Chung F, Abdullah HR, Liao P. STOP-bang questionnaire: a practical approach to screen for obstructive sleep apnea. Chest. 2016;149(3):631–8.

35. Netzer N, Eliasson AH, Netzer C, Kristo DA. Overnight pulse oximetry for sleep-disordered breathing in adults: a review. Chest. 2001;120(2):625–33.

36. Machicao VI, Balakrishnan M, Fallon MB. Pulmonary complications in chronic liver disease. Hepatology. 2014;59(4):1627–37.

37. Benza RL, Miller DP, Gomberg-Maitland M, Frantz RP, Foreman AJ, Coffey CS, Frost A, Barst RJ, Badesch DB, Elliott CG, Liou TG, McGoon MD. Predicting survival in pulmonary arterial hypertension: insights from the Registry to Evaluate Early and Long-Term Pulmonary Arterial Hypertension Disease Management (REVEAL). Circulation. 2010;122(2):164–72.

38. Martin P, DiMartini A, Feng S, Brown R Jr, Fallon M. Evaluation for liver transplantation in adults: 2013 practice guideline by the American Association for the Study of Liver Diseases and the American Society of Transplantation. Hepatology. 2014;59(3): 1144–65.

39. Raevens S, Colle I, Reyntjens K, Geerts A, Berrevoet F, Rogiers X, Troisi RI, Van Vlierberghe H, De Pauw M. Echocardiography for the detection of portopulmonary hypertension in liver transplant candidates: an analysis of cutoff values. Liver Transpl. 2013;19(6):602–10.

40. Rodríguez-Roisin R, Krowka MJ. Hepatopulmonary syndrome--a liver-induced lung vascular disorder. N Engl J Med. 2008;358(22):2378–87.

41. Porter TR, Mulvagh SL, Abdelmoneim SS, Becher H, Belcik JT, Bierig M, Choy J, Gaibazzi N, Gillam LD, Janardhanan R, Kutty S, Leong-Poi H, Lindner JR, Main ML, Mathias W Jr, Park MM, Senior R, Villanueva F. Clinical applications of ultrasonic enhancing agents in echocardiography: 2018 American Society of Echocardiography guidelines update. J Am Soc Echocardiogr. 2018;31(3):241–74.

42. Krowka MJ. Management of pulmonary complications in pretransplant patients. Clin Liver Dis. 2011;15(4):765–77.

43. Enright PL. The six-minute walk test. Respir Care. 2003;48(8):783–5.

44. Carey EJ, Steidley DE, Aqel BA, Byrne TJ, Mekeel KL, Rakela J, Vargas HE, Douglas DD. Six-minute walk distance predicts mortality in liver transplant candidates. Liver Transpl. 2010;16(12):1373–8.

45. Taillé C, Cadranel J, Bellocq A, Thabut G, Soubrane O, Durand F, Ichaï P, Duvoux C, Belghiti J, Calmus Y, Mal H. Liver transplantation for hepatopulmonary syndrome: a ten-year experience in Paris, France. Transplantation. 2003;75(9):1482–9.

46. Arguedas MR, Abrams GA, Krowka MJ, Fallon MB. Prospective evaluation of outcomes and predictors of mortality in patients with hepatopulmonary syndrome undergoing liver transplantation. Hepatology. 2003;37(1):192–7.

47. Provencher S, Herve P, Jais X, Lebrec D, Humbert M, Simonneau G, Sitbon O. Deleterious effects of beta-blockers on exercise capacity and hemodynamics in patients with portopulmonary hypertension. Gastroenterology. 2006;130(1):120–6.

48. Hoeper MM, Halank M, Marx C, Hoeffken G, Seyfarth HJ, Schauer J, Niedermeyer J, Winkler J. Bosentan therapy for portopulmonary hypertension. Eur Respir J. 2005;25(3):502–8.

49. Kett DH, Acosta RC, Campos MA, Rodriguez MJ, Quartin AA, Schein RM. Recurrent portopulmonary hypertension after liver transplantation: management with epoprostenol and resolution after retransplantation. Liver Transpl. 2001;7(7):645–8.

50. Borchardt J, Smirnov A, Metchnik L, Malnick S. Treating hepatic hydrothorax. BMJ. 2003;326(7392):751–2.

51. Ridha A, Al-Abboodi Y, Fasullo M. The outcome of thoracentesis versus chest tube placement for hepatic hydrothorax in patients with cirrhosis: a nationwide analysis of the national inpatient sample. Gastroentero Research. Practice. 2017;2017:5872068.

52. Hou F, Qi X, Guo X. Effectiveness and safety of pleurodesis for hepatic hydrothorax: a systematic review and meta-analysis. Dig Dis Sci. 2016;61(11):3321–34.

53. Huang PM, Kuo SW, Chen JS, Lee JM. Thoracoscopic mesh repair of diaphragmatic defects in hepatic hydrothorax: a 10-year experience. Ann Thorac Surg. 2016;101(5):1921–7.

Coagulation in Liver Disease

13

Vijay Vohra

13.1 Introduction

The liver plays an important role in coagulation pathways which is involved in primary and secondary tertiary haemostasis. It is the site of production for most of the coagulation factors except for von Willebrand factor (vWf) which is synthetised by the vascular endothelium. The liver also produces anticoagulant factors—Anti-thrombin III, Protein C and Protein S. Patients with advanced liver disease are associated with impairment of coagulation. Normally there is a balance between procoagulant and anticoagulant system which can be disturbed during progression of liver disease. As the liver disease advances multiple changes occur in the haemostatic system, thereby leading to reduced level of both procoagulative and anticoagulative factors—which were being synthetised by the hepatocytes and sinusoidal cells. In addition to this there could be deficiency of vitamin K which leads to abnormal clotting factor production as this vitamin (vitamin K) is required for gamma carboxylation. So the coagulation factors produced by the liver, which is already damaged, produce clotting factors which may be abnormal in nature. In End Stage Liver Disease (ESLD) there is also reduced capacity to clear the activated clotting factors and their inhibitor complexes from the circulation. So the overall effect of the liver disease is quite complex and can lead to bleeding as well as thrombotic complications. As the disease progresses it leads to development of portal hypertension which results in splenomegaly and thrombocytopenia. Thrombocytopenia can further be accentuated due to decreased synthesis of thrombopoietin in the failing liver.

13.2 Haemostasis in Health

Haemostasis is a physiological process whereby coagulation is initiated when there is a breach in the integrity of the vessel wall leading to clot formation and minimizing bleeding. This is followed by appropriately timed lysis of this clot and restoring normal circulation. The coagulation and clot dissolution are inter-linked and are regulated in a precise manner with their own inhibitors being activated in the process. The outcome of this finally balanced process may result in bleeding or thrombosis.

The haemostatic balance is dependent on a very complex interaction between pro- and anti-coagulants as well as the effect of fibrinolytic proteins. The process of coagulation starts when tissue factor is exposed on sustaining injury to the vessel wall. This leads to activation of Factor VIIa which further activates Factor X–Xa.

V. Vohra (✉)
Liver Transplant, GI Anesthesia & Intensive Care,
Medanta the Medicity, Gurgaon, India
e-mail: vijay.vohra@medanta.org

Thrombin is generated by the effect of Factor Xa on prothrombin (Factor II). Protein C, S and antithrombin have an inhibitory effect on thrombin generation (Fig. 13.1).

Thrombomodulin also plays an important part in haemostasis. This glycoprotein is present on the endothelial surface and acts as an anticoagulant by activating protein C. Activated protein C has an inhibitory effect on thrombin [1].

There are complex enzymatic reactions taking place simultaneously through the tissue factor pathway (extrinsic pathway) as well as intrinsic pathway (contact activation pathway). Besides other factors involved, fibrinogen and platelets are two very important ingredients required to repair the damage to the injured vessel wall.

Standard laboratory tests of coagulation—Prothrombin Time (PT) or International Normalized Ratio (INR) and Activated Partial Thromboplastin Time (APTT)—guide the management of patients with deranged coagulation. There are many limitations to these tests includ-

ing a long turnaround time when prompt treatment of bleeding is required. A ratio of 1.5 times the normal of PT/APTT is considered abnormal and may warrant correction depending on the clinical status. PT primarily gives information about intrinsic pathway whereas APTT is influenced by the processes involved in the intrinsic pathway (Fig. 13.2).

Information received from PT or APTT is generally used for assessing bleeding risk or when an invasive procedure/surgery is to be performed. It should be kept in mind that PT and APTT are plasma-based coagulation tests and they were initially designed to monitor treatment with vitamin K antagonists and heparin therapy. These tests therefore have limited value in assessing peri-operative bleeding risk. Another whole blood coagulation test Viscoelastic Test probably would give better information on management of bleeding patients and guiding therapy on the basis of abnormalities seen on thromboelastography (TEG).

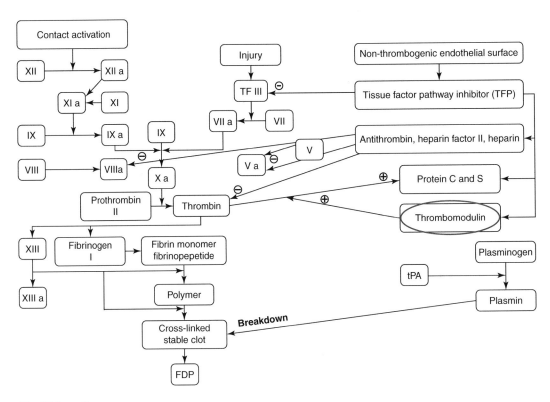

Fig. 13.1 pathways

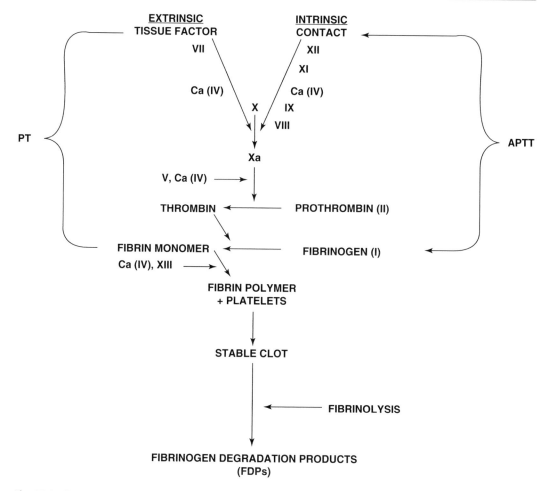

Fig. 13.2 Coagulation and conventional testing. PT—extrinsic pathway primarily, APTT—intrinsic pathway mainly

13.3 Coagulation in Chronic Liver Disease

The haemostatic system in liver disease patients affects the initial clot formation, secondary clot formation as well as tertiary haemostasis. All three phases of coagulation are altered in liver disease patients to a varying degree, disease aetiology playing an important role.

In primary haemostasis, the vessel wall injury results in exposure of platelet adhesion protein to the platelets which results in the formation of a platelet plug. Release of tissue factor leads to activation of coagulation cascade in the plasma and quickly results in the formation of a fibrin mesh. In chronic liver disease there is thrombocytopenia due to various reasons which can alter

the primary haemostasis—platelet plug formation. To counter this there is high level of vWf. The elevated levels of vWf are as a result of endothelial activation. Activity of vWf is enhanced further because of reduced clearance by the cirrhotic liver as well as increased synthesis in the liver.

As the coagulation cascade gets activated during secondary haemostasis, complex reactions involving both pro- and anti-haemostatic proteins come into play (Fig. 13.1) [2].

The coagulation factors II, V, VII, IX and XI are reduced in patients with chronic liver disease but on the other hand factor VIII levels are often elevated [3]. This is due to increased synthesis from extrahepatic sites such as spleen, kidney and lung [4]. Factor VIII activity is further enhanced due to increased level of vWf which is the carrier protein for factor VIII. The clearance of activated factor VIII is also reduced in the failing liver. Counting the decreased production of procoagulant factors, there is decreased production of anticoagulants like protein C, protein S, anti-thrombin and heparin co-factor II—all being produced in the liver. As a result there is a fine balance of pro- and anticoagulant proteins which are very much lower than the levels seen in healthy individual.

After the bleeding which stops on formation of a fibrin clot, there is dissolution of this fibrin clot—fibrinolysis (Fig. 13.2). The fibrinolytic system is again balanced by pro- and anti-fibrinolytic proteins. There are low levels of plasminogen and high levels of Plasminogen Activator Inhibitor 1 (PAI-1) which prevent fibrinolysis whereas high levels of Tissue Plasminogen Activator (t-PA) and low levels of factor XIII facilitate fibrinolysis. Exaggerated hyperfibrinolysis is quite often seen during liver transplantation during anhepatic phase as the clearance of t-PA is hampered.

Coagulation disorders produced in chronic liver disease may require correction if there is a gross deterioration in prothrombin time or before doing any invasive procedures. Non-bleeder with abnormal clotting studies may not require any correction during the normal course of management. The standard screening tests for assessing clotting status may not depict any abnormality till the procoagulant levels are reduced by 60–70% of the normal values [5]. There is no utility of measuring individual clotting factor concentrations in the normal course of the disease except in acute liver failure where factor V levels less than 20%/30% indicate need for liver transplantation (Clichy Criteria). This is relevant only if you have a practice to list your patients for transplantation on the basis of Clichy Criteria instead of the more universally used King's College Hospital (KCH) criteria.

13.4 Coagulation in Acute Liver Failure

In candidates for transplantation in Acute Liver Failure (ALF), there is gross derangement of prothrombin time but this is not replicated in the viscoelastic tests—TEG in up to 35% patients shows a hypercoagulable graph. This can be explained by the reduction in both procoagulant and anticoagulant factors along with increase in vWF and factor VIII in circulation (Fig. 13.3) [6].

In acute liver failure there is no evidence of prophylactic use of blood products to correct the abnormal coagulation profile though PT can be grossly deranged.

Thrombin generation in ALF is near normal after initial thrombin formation with activation of factor VIII, IX and XI. The rapid production of thrombin is facilitated by the availability of increased level of factor VIII. This process is further enhanced by reduced thrombin inactivation due to activated protein C resistance.

The platelet size in ALF is increased which is evident by the increase in the mean platelet volume, although the platelet count may even be reduced. This viewpoint is supported by the fact that in majority of the patients with ALF, TEG shows a hypercoagulable pattern. Platelet and fibrinogen contribute equally to the clot strength in healthy individuals whereas in ALF platelets can contribute up to 75% of clot strength [6, 7]. This shows there could be disproportionate functional hypofibrinogenemia.

The belief that increasing bleeding tendency in ALF as shown by traditional clotting test is not borne out by the assessment of clot using TEG and thrombin generation test.

% CHANGE IN FACTORS IN ALF

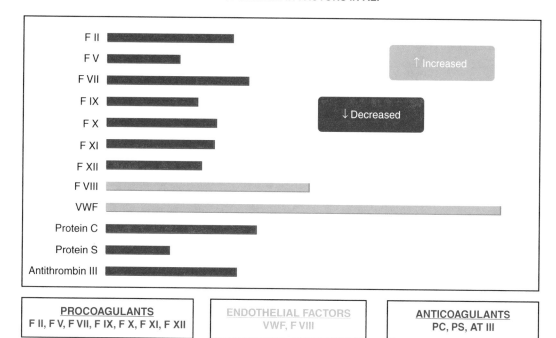

PROCOAGULANTS
F II, F V, F VII, F IX, F X, F XI, F XII

ENDOTHELIAL FACTORS
VWF, F VIII

ANTICOAGULANTS
PC, PS, AT III

Adapted from Reference No. 6

Fig. 13.3 Percentage change in factors in ALF. (Adapted from Agarwal B, Wright G, Gatt A, Riddell A, Vemala V and Mallett S et al. Evaluation of coagulation abnormalities in acute liver failure. Journal of Hepatology 2012;57(4):780–786)

13.5 Procoagulant Factors

The liver is the site of production of majority of the procoagulant factors—Factors II, V, VII, VIII, IX, X, XI, XII and XIII besides producing anticoagulant factors as well. As the synthetic function of the liver deteriorates, there is marked decline in the production of coagulation factors. However one procoagulant factor which is increased is factor VIII—This is produced mainly by the sinusoidal cells of the liver with minor contribution from the spleen, endothelial cells and the lung (Table 13.1).

Majority of the procoagulant factors are vitamin K dependant, which is deficient in chronic liver disease. Vitamin K deficiency could be because of reduction in the dietary intake, inadequate absorption due to bile acids, diminished storage and decreased production in the intestines. Treatment with antibiotics can also destroy the intestinal bacteria that syntheses vitamin K [8]. There are instances in end-stage liver disease when there are high levels of clotting factors in the presence of near-normal vitamin K—primary biliary cirrhosis and primary sclerosing cholangitis are examples of such states. This can even result in hypercoagulable states as seen in viscoelastic testing with decreased reaction time (r time), increased alpha angle and maximum Amplitude (mA) on TEG.

Table 13.1 Sites of synthesis of clotting factors

Factors	Synthesis	Half-life (h)
Factor I or fibrinogen	Liver, extrahepatic sites	72–120
Factor II or prothrombin	Liver	72
Factor V (labile)	Liver, endothelium, platelets	36
Factor VII (stable)	Liver	3–6
Factor VIII (AHF-A)	Liver, extrahepatic sites	12
Factor IX (Christmas, AHF-B)	Liver	24
Factor X (Stuart-Prower)	Liver	40
Factor XI	Liver	80
Factor XII (Hageman)	Liver	50
Factor XIII	Liver, extrahepatic sites	120–200
vWf	Endothelium	10–24

Adapted from Bolliger D, Gorlinger K, Tanaka KA and Warner DS. Pathophysiology and treatment of coagulopathy in massive haemorrhage and hemodilution. Anesthesiology 2010;113(5):1205–1219
AHF-A anti-haemophilic factor A, *AHF-B* anti-haemophilic factor B

13.6   Fibrinogen

This acute phase reactant protein is produced in the hepatocytes and consists of six polypeptide chains. High levels of fibrinogen concentration are seen in cholestatic jaundice and hepatocellular carcinoma whereas low fibrinogen concentration is seen as the patient progresses towards end-stage disease [9, 10]. In advanced liver failure, there is reduced level of fibrinogen as well as there is qualitative abnormality leading to dysfibrinogenemia which is functionally abnormal. There is abnormal alpha chain with raised sialic acid content in fibrinogen.

The normal level of fibrinogen in the blood is 2–4 g/L, which makes it the most abundant coagulation factor found in the plasma. A large amount of fibrinogen is engulfed in the formation of stable thrombus. Fibrinogen above 3 g/L is generally considered as adequate for producing

haemostasis whereas plasma levels below 1 g/L are considered inadequate. Looking at the influence of fibrinogen correction on transfusion requirement in liver transplant recipients, Roullet et al. found that there was no decrease in blood transfusion related to fibrinogen level in the blood [11]. Fibrinogen given pre-emptively to liver transplant recipients does produce change in the thromboelastographic parameters leading to increase in the maximum amplitude (mA) but these improvements did not translate into a reduction in blood transfusions. In both acute and chronic liver disease, there is qualitative change seen in the fibrinogen with quantitative effect seen only during end-stage liver failure.

13.7   von Willebrand Factor (vWf)

vWf is a high molecular weight protein multimer and an important partner in supporting haemostasis. The importance of vWf lies in the fact that this protein has a high affinity for collagen present on the vessel wall as well as glycoprotein 1b which is present on the platelet surfaces. This factor acts as a combining medium between platelets and the vessel wall where the clot formation takes place. High levels of vWf are seen in patients with chronic liver disease and cirrhosis. The mechanisms responsible for the elevated levels of vWf are possibly due to inflammation or infection and the other reason being reduced clearance of this factor by the liver. vWf levels are substantially increased in acute liver failure where there is other evidence of systemic inflammatory response (SIRS) as well. In chronic liver disease there is formation of nitric oxide due to the underlying portal hypertension. The nitric oxide acts as a stimulus for liberation of vWf from the endothelium. In essence there are increased plasma level of vWf in both acute and chronic liver disease.

The activity of vWf is controlled to an extent by ADAMTS13. In chronic liver disease ADAMTS13 levels are reduced in the plasma thereby promoting procoagulant effect of vWf [12].

13.8 Platelets

Thrombocytopenia is seen in 49–60% of the patients with end-stage liver disease. Generally the platelet count is not below 30,000/cmm and spontaneous bleeding is not seen because of low platelet count. The main cause of thrombocytopenia is due to portal hypertension leading to enlargement of the spleen causing sequestration platelets. Besides there is impaired production of platelets, increased platelet destruction due to immunological reasons. Other causes such as alcohol, disseminated intravascular coagulation, sepsis, folate deficiency and drugs may be responsible for platelet deficiency. A markedly enlarged spleen can sequestrate up to 90% of the total platelet mass [13, 14].

A normal platelet count of 150,000/cmm to 450,000/cmm offers a huge functional reserve which is also observed in the various other biological parameters like haemoglobin, WBC, etc.

Thrombocytopenia of chronic liver disease is partly because of lack of thrombopoietin (TPO) and treatment with TPO agonists leads to increase in platelet count and reduced platelet transfusion and bleeding. This also led to increased incidence of portal vein thrombosis and termination of the clinical study [15, 16].

Platelets play a very important role in clot formation; it helps in clot formation in two stages:

1. **Primary Haemostatic Plug**—Platelets through an interaction with vWf adhere to the damaged vessel wall, thereby leading to aggregation of platelets and formation of primary haemostatic plug. Platelets in the presence of exposed collagen and vWf leads to alteration in the shape of platelets and release of adenosine diphosphate and thromboxane A2, both of which cause the platelets to aggregate.

2. **Thrombin Generation**—In the presence of activated clotting factors platelets support the formation of thrombin leading to stable clot formation. Platelets count up to 60,000/cmm are usually enough to generate this response [17].

In liver disease ADAMTS13 levels are decreased in the plasma. ADAMTS13 normally makes a cleavage in the platelet vWF and thereby promotes clot formation (Fig. 13.4) [12, 18].

Myelosuppression can also contribute to the low platelet count, and this can be seen in hepatitis C virus (HCV infection), other acute viral infections, folic deficiency and chronic alcohol use [19, 20].

A large amount of platelets—up to 90%—are sequestrated in the spleen but splenectomy is generally not indicated in these patients with chronic liver disease. Splenectomy is associated with a risk of secondary portal vein thrombosis which can lead to bleeding from oesophageal varices and a difficult subsequent liver transplant [21]. There are reports of splenic artery embolization with reduction in the splenic blood flow leading to improvement in platelet count [22].

Intrinsic defects in the platelets as well as abnormalities in other plasma factors also add to the hand in cholestatic liver disease there can be hyperactive platelet functioning which can be abnormal functioning of platelets. This can be detected either by platelet function assay (PFA-100) or on the other hand by thromboelastography (TEG) [23]. Thromboelastography is a test of whole blood clotting and measures platelet function which is detected by maximum amplitude (mA) on the graph [24].

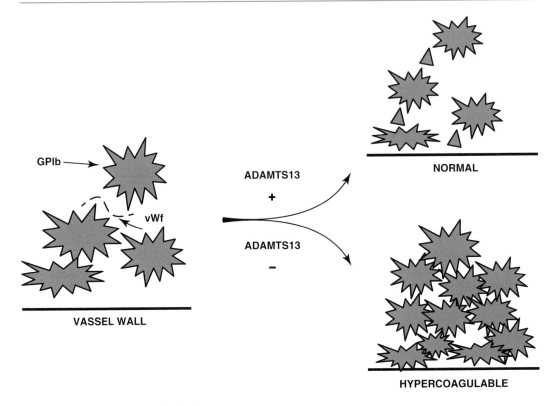

Fig. 13.4 Role of ADAMTS13 in clot formation

13.9 Anticoagulant Factors

1. **Anti-Thrombin III:** This is a glycoprotein which is synthesized by the liver and endothelium and does not require vitamin K for its activation. Anti-thrombin III levels are reduced in liver disease as the synthetic function are affected with the progression of the disease. The levels are also decreased due to its consumption during the process of fibrinolysis seen in end-stage liver disease. There are no preparations of anti-thrombin III available and its replacement is generally not indicated (Table 13.2).

2. **Protein C and Protein S:** These are also glycoproteins which are synthesized mainly by the hepatocytes and are dependent on vitamin K. Disease progression in the liver leads to decline in both protein C and protein S but their levels rarely fall below 20% of the normal (Table 13.2).

Table 13.2 Sites of synthesis of anticoagulant factors

Factors	Synthesis	Half-life (h)
Anti-thrombin II	Liver, extrahepatic sites	48–72
Protein C	Liver, endothelium	10
Protein S	Liver, endothelium	42

Adapted from Bolliger D, Gorlinger K, Tanaka KA and Warner DS. Pathophysiology and treatment of coagulopathy in massive haemorrhage and hemodilution. Anesthesiology 2010;113(5):1205–1219

13.10 Fibrinolytic and Antifibrinolytic System

In advanced liver disease, it is not uncommon to find evidence of fibrinolysis. The laboratory tests revealed elevated level of fibrinogen degradation products, raised level of plasma D-Dimer and shortened whole blood Euglobulin clot lysis time. There are high levels of circulating plasminogen activators due to their decreased clearance in the liver. The increase in tissue plasminogen activator (tPA) is also accompanied with normal or even elevated levels of tPA inhibitor. Hyperfibrinolysis is not seen in patients with acute liver disease but is seen in up to 31% of patients with compensated cirrhosis [25]. Hyperfibrinolysis is almost universal in patients with uncontrolled ascites. Agarwal S et al. reported an incidence of hyperfibrinolysis in 93% of the patients with ascites [26]. On analysing the ascitic fluid of patients with severe liver disease there was evidence of low fibrinogen, and increased levels of FDPs and D-Dimer. This is evidence of hyperfibrinolytic activity which could be because of absorption of ascitic fluid into the systemic circulation. Hyperfibrinolysis can contribute to increased incidence of bleeding from mucus membranes.

13.11 Disseminated Intravascular Coagulation (DIC)

As the liver disease progresses and reaches the end stage, there is evidence of low-grade disseminated intravascular coagulation (DIC). This coagulation concept involves formation of fibrin deposits and their partial breakdown. There is increase in fibrin degradation products (FDPs) as well as reduction in serum fibrinogen levels. DIC in end-stage liver disease is typically accompanied with prolongation of PT and PT, APTT as well as reduction in the platelet count. As the disease progresses, there is tendency to increase in severity of DIC [27, 28]. The suspicion of DIC in cirrhotic patient is based on worsening of coagulation test results and disproportionate reduction in platelet count. There is generally a triggering clinical event like bleeding or infection. In the presence of DIC there is also reduction of factor VIII as well as factor V.

Central to the development of DIC is activation of thrombin due to high level of tissue factor and consequently activation of extensive coagulation pathway [29]. There is fibrin deposition in small vessels leading to venous and arterial thrombosis which finally affects various organs and may even lead to multi-organ failure. On consumption of various clotting factors as well as

activation of DIC there is wide spread bleeding manifestation. Accelerated intravascular coagulation and fibrinolysis (AICF) has been reported in about 30% of the patients with cirrhosis and this is dependent on the severity of the liver disease. This phenomenon is seen more in the portal venous system compared to the arterial system [30]. The trigger for AICF could be endotoxaemia which is evident in the portal circulation, leading to the release of IL6 and TNFα which stimulate intravascular coagulation [31].

13.12 Hypercoagulability

This refers to the propensity of developing an appropriate clot in a patient although bleeding is the more recognized complication of chronic liver disease. Portal vein thrombosis has been reported in up to 26% of patients with cirrhosis [32] and a variable number of patients also develop deep vein thrombosis or pulmonary emboli. The risk of portal vein thrombosis increases with the severity of liver disease and increased mortality in those who undergo orthotopic liver transplant (OLT) [33].

There is an increase in vWf in chronic liver disease and this remains elevated for up to 10 days after OLT. The activity of vWf is further enhanced due to a lack of ADAMTS13 which results in the stability of platelets in circulation.

Hypercoagulability can lead to Hepatic Artery Thrombosis (HAT) post-operatively in OLT. There is an increased risk of HAT in patients who have familial amyloidotic polyneuropathy and acute intermittent porphyria. Similarly cytomegalovirus (CMV) is also known to increase the risk of developing HAT [34]. The risk of HAT is significantly reduced in these patients by treatment with aspirin.

The incidence of deep vein thrombosis can be minimized by use of Low Molecular Weight Heparin (LMWH) but this has to be weighed against the risk of bleeding post-operatively. The monitoring of LMWH is difficult as anti-Xa testing in the laboratory is not freely available. This therapy works both for DVT prophylaxis and for preventing HAT.

13.13 Assessment and Correction of Coagulation Status Before Invasive Procedures

1. **Paracentesis:** There may not be any signs of bleeding in advanced liver disease if there is not intervention. Minor intervention can trigger the bleeding process in patients with end-stage liver disease and may have serious or even life-threatening consequences. Ascites is a common manifestation in ESLD which may or may not respond to conservative management of diet and diuretic. Such refractory ascites requires paracentesis. Some patients may end up having serial therapeutic paracentesis requiring drainage every 2 weeks. Haemoperitoneum and damage to the intestine during needle insertion are potential serious complication of paracentesis. Up to 3% of patients undergoing paracentesis may develop excessive bleeding to haemoperitoneum and some of them even require transfusion. Severe coagulation defects (INR > 1.5 and Platelets <50,000/cmm) may require transfusion of FFP and platelets respectively. In presence of portal hypertension there are multiple porto-systemic shunts, some of which could be seen in the anterior abdominal wall. Ultrasound-guided paracentesis can minimize these complications in most of the patients with refractory ascites. Large volume paracentesis normally requires supplementation of albumin—8 g/L or fluid removed to maintain the haemodynamic stability [35]. Paracentesis normally would not require any support of coagulation unless the platelet count is <30,000/cmm or INR is >2.5. Carefully selected needle placement for paracentesis, avoiding inferior epigastric artery and the porto-systemic shunt, enables a safe therapeutic intervention (Fig. 13.5). To support this, there is a large study of 11,000 patients where no haemorrhagic complication was seen in patients with platelet counts as low as 19,000/cmm and INR upto 8.7 [36].

2. **Liver Biopsy:** It is not uncommon to do a liver biopsy to establish the diagnosis of advancing liver disease. There is always a

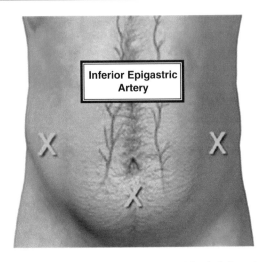

Fig. 13.5 Safe sites of paracentesis avoiding inferior epigastric artery

hazard of developing intra-peritoneal bleeding in the process of doing liver biopsy. Earlier bleeding time was used as a reference to know the suitability to do this procedure but has become an obsolete investigation. Platelet count is a value which is relied upon and a value above 60,000–80,000/cmm is considered safe [37]. Another parameter used to assess the coagulation status is prothrombin time (PT). Prolonged PT > 4–6 s is considered abnormal with likelihood of bleeding after the procedure. One study coated International Normalize Ratio (INR) > 1.5 as a risk factor for post-procedure bleeding [38]. There are other options to minimize the risk of bleeding following liver biopsy. A transjugular biopsy or a plugged biopsy can be used to minimize the risk of bleeding [39]. Most centres have their own cut-off values for performing a liver biopsy, one of the UK guidelines requires platelet count above 80,000/cmm and a survey from Mayo Clinic suggested a count of >50,000/cmm [40].

3. **Central Venous Access:** Accessing the central vein has a potential of forming haematoma or even intrathoracic collection of blood—haemothorax. The preferred site to avoid these complications would be access through internal jugular vein. In this era of ultrasound central vascular access has become

less traumatic with minimal bleeding complication (Fig. 13.6). Reported major bleeding complications in patients with end-stage liver disease are in the range 0–0.2%. It is therefore not necessary to administer blood products before obtaining central venous access, especially if it is done under the ultrasound guidance [41, 42].

4. **Coronary Angiography:** Up to 28% of patients over the age of 50 years may have coronary artery disease in patients with CLD [43, 44]. Patients with risk factors for CAD, aetiology of NASH and those with noncoronary artery disease may need to undergo coronary artery angiography before liver transplantation. Performing coronary angiography can lead to haematoma formation, pseudoaneurysm as well as increased bleeding from the puncture site in a coagulopathic liver transplant recipient. Bleeding issue can be minimized for this investigative procedure of coronary angiography by using radial artery route instead of the traditional femoral artery (Fig. 13.7). One drawback of this procedure is also because of the use of contrast used in angiography. Renal function can be compromised and may lead to overt renal failure in susceptible individuals. The measures taken

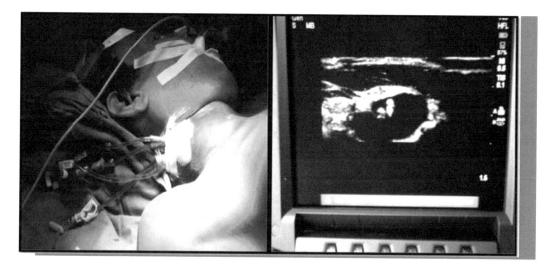

Fig. 13.6 Ultrasound-guided central venous access

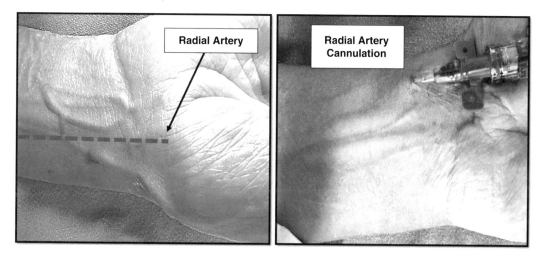

Fig. 13.7 Percutaneous radial artery cannulation

to offset development of renal compromise can be in the form of adequate hydration as well as use of free radical scavenger *N*-acetylcysteine given prophylactically.

13.14 Coagulation and Infection

Infection has been reported in cirrhotic patients which can lead to complication of bleeding. Sepsis is known to result in bleeding from oesophageal varices resultant from portal hypertension. Infection produced by the bacteria leads to production of endotoxin which produces tissue factors expression on macrophages and activation of clotting and fibrinolytic mechanism. Infection in advanced liver disease leads to production of cytokines—interleukin-1 (IL1), IL6 and tumour necrosis factor (TNF). These cytokines are precursor to fibrinolysis and can also activate clotting by stimulating the extrinsic coagulation pathway [45]. Generally a hypocoagulable state evolves in cirrhotic patients with sepsis which can manifest as bleeding from oesophageal varices [46].

13.15 Portal Hypertension and Bleeding

The risk of bleeding in end-stage liver disease is either because of a procedure being carried out or this can happen spontaneously due to the presence of portal hypertension. The patients with cirrhosis are not spontaneously anticoagulated but are in a state of rebalanced haemostasis. In a patient with oesophageal varices, reduction of portal pressures leads to control of bleeding. Institution of Transjugular Intrahepatic Portosystemic Shunt (TIPS) in patients with high HVPG gradient results in control of active bleeding. In the presence of high portal pressure there is no evidence to control bleeding with fresh frozen plasma or platelet transfusion. These interventions have the potential of increasing the risk of acute lung injury as well as further increasing the portal pressures. Other methods to control bleeding is use of non-selective beta-blockers, endoscopic ligation of varices, prophylactic des-

mopressin, anti-fibrinolytic agents or recombinant factor VIIa [47, 48].

13.16 Conclusion

Chronic and acute liver disease is frequently accompanied with changes in the coagulation parameters which can cause concern. There is an imbalance of haemostatic factors—pro- and anti-haemostatic—with a rebalance created at a different level which makes them prone to bleeding as well as hypercoagulable state. Conventional routine laboratory tests are not able to identify patients at risk. Point of care testing like TEG has the potential to identify the coagulation abnormalities. Still a lot of work needs to be done to validate the results of viscoelastic test in predicting bleeding or thrombosis. Prophylactic transfusion of blood product before any procedure needs to be guided by viscoelastic test. There is a strong recognition of thrombotic complications in patients with liver disease and the need to use necessary anti-thrombotic therapy.

Key Points
- Liver disease can result in both bleeding and thrombotic complications.
- Conventional tests of coagulation—PT/APTT—do not predict risk of thrombosis or bleeding.
- There is a delicate balance between pro- and anticoagulant in liver disease.
- Portal hypertension is more of a culprit in bleeding patients.
- Liver disease patients do not always require correction of coagulation parameters.
- Diagnostic/therapeutic procedures like paracentesis and coronary angiography do not always require correction of coagulation.
- Surgical intervention can upset the rebalanced haemostasis.
- Acute liver failure may exhibit hypercoagulable state in spite of normal PT.

References

1. Conway EM. Thrombomodulin and its role in inflammation. Semin Immunopathol. 2012;34(1):107–25.
2. Karlekar A. Understanding hemostasis: the knowns and the unknowns. Jaypee Brothers Yearb Anesthesiol. 2018;7:16–35.
3. Hollestelle MJ, Geertzen HGM, Straatsburg IH, Gulik TM, Mourik JA. Facotr VIII expression in liver disease. Thromb Haemost. 2004;91(2):267–75.
4. Hollestelle MJ, Poyck PP, Hollestelle JM, Marsman HA, Van Mouri JA, Van Gulik TM. Extra-hepatic factor VIII expression in porcine fulminant hepatic failure. J Thromb Haemost. 2005;3(10):2274–80.
5. Duchemin J, Pan-Petesch B, Arnaud B, Blouch MT, Abgrall JF. Influence of coagulation factors and tissue factor concentration on the thrombin generation test in plasma. Thromb Haemost. 2008;99(4):767–73.
6. Agarwal B, Wright G, Gatt A, Riddell A, Vemala V, Mallett S, et al. Evaluation of coagulation abnormalities in acute liver failure. J Hepatol. 2012;57(4):780–6.
7. Gottumukkala VN, Sharma SK, Philip J. Assessing platelet and fibrinogen contribution to clot strength using modified thromboelastography in pregnant women. Anesth Analg. 1999;89:1453–5.
8. Sherlock S. Nutritional complications of biliary cirrhosis. Chronic cholestasis. Am J Clin Nutr. 1970;23(5):640–4.
9. Lisman T, Ariens R. Alterations in fibrin structure in patients with liver diseases. Semin Thromb Hemost. 2016;42(4):389–96.
10. Lisman T, Porte R. Value of preoperative hemostasis testing in patients with liver disease for perioperative hemostatic management. Anesthesiology. 2017;126(2):338–44.
11. Roullet S, Freyburger G, Cruc M, Quinart A, Stecken L, Audy M, et al. Management of bleeding and transfusion during liver transplantation before and after the introduction of a rotational thromboelastometry based algorithm. Liver Transpl. 2015;21(2):169–79.
12. Lisman T, Bongers TN, Adelmeijer J, Janssen HLA, de Maat MPM, de Groot PG, et al. Elevated levels of von Willebrand Factor in cirrhosis support platelet adhesion despite reduced functional capacity. Hepatology. 2006;44(1):53–61.
13. Aster RH. Pooling of platelets in the spleen: role in the pathogenesis of "hypersplenic" thrombocytopenia. J Clin Invest. 1966;45(5):645–57.
14. Stein SF, Harker LA. Kinetic and functional studies of platelets, fibrinogen, and plasminogen in patients with hepatic cirrhosis. J Lab Clin Med. 1982;99(2):217–30.
15. Afdhal N, Duggal A, Ochiai T, Motomiya T, Kano T, Nagata T, et al. Platelet response to lusutrombopag, a thrombopoietin receptor agonist, in patients with chronic liver disease and thrombocytopenia undergoing non-emergency invasive procedures: results form a phase 3 randomized, double-blind, placebo controlled study. Blood. 2017;130(Suppl 1):291.
16. Terrault N, Chen Y-C, Izumi N, Kayali Z, Mitrut P, Young W, et al. Avatrombopag before procedures reduces need for platelet transfusion in patients with chronic liver disease and thrombocytopenia. Gastroenterology. 2018;155:705–18.
17. Tripodi A, Primignani M, Chantarangkul V, Clerici M, Dell'Era A, Fabris F, et al. Thrombin generation in patients with cirrhosis: the role of platelets. Hepatology. 2006;44(2):440–5.
18. Uemura M, Fujimura Y, Ko S, Matsumoto M, Nakajima Y, Fukui H. Pivotal role of ADAMTS13 function in liver diseases. Int J Hematol. 2010;91(1):20–9.
19. Nagamine T, Ohtuka T, Takehara K, Arai T, Takagi H, Mori M. Thrombocytopenia associated with hepatitis C viral infection. J Hepatol. 1996;24(2):135–40.
20. Peck-Radosavljevic M. Thrombocytopenia in liver disease. Can J Gastroenterol. 2000;14(Suppl D):60D–6D. https://doi.org/10.1155/2000/617428. PMID: 11110614.
21. Bolognesi M, Merkel C, Sacerdoti D, Nava V, Gatta A. Role of spleen enlargement in cirrhosis with portal hypertension. Dig Liver Dis. 2002;34(2):144–50.
22. N'Kontchou G, Seror O, Bourcier V, Mohand D, Ajavon Y, Castera L, et al. Partial splenic embolization in patients with cirrhosis: efficacy, tolerance and long-term outcome in 32 patients. Eur J Gastroenterol Hepatol. 2005;17(2):179–84.
23. Pihusch R, Rank A, Gohring P, Pihusch M, Hiller E, Beuers U. Platelet cirrhosis rather than plasmatic coagulation explains hypercoagulable state in cholestatic liver disease. J Hepatol. 2002;37(5):548–55.
24. Ben-Ari Z, Panagou M, Patch D, Bates S, Osman E, Pasi J, et al. Hypercoagulability in patients with primary biliary cirrhosis and primary sclerosing cholangitis evaluated by thromboelastography. J Hepatol. 1997;26(3):554–9.
25. Hu K-Q, Yu AS, Tiyyagura L, Redeker AG, Reynolds TB. Hyperfibrinolytic activity in hospitalisation cirrhotic patients in a referral liver unit. Am J Gastroenterol. 2001;96(5):1581–6.
26. Agarwal S, Joyner KA, Swaim MW. Ascites as a possible origin for hyperfibrinolysis in advanced liver disease. Am J Gastroenterol. 2000;95(11):3218–24.
27. Violi F, Ferro D, Basili S, Cimminiello C, Saliola M, Vezza E, et al. Prognostic value of clotting and fibrinolytic systems in a follow-up of 165 liver cirrhotic patients. CALC group. Hepatology. 1995;22(1):96–100.
28. Kemkes-Matthes B, Bleyi H, Matthes KJ. Coagulation activation in liver diseases. Thromb Res. 1991;64(2):253–61.
29. Levi M, ten Cate H. Disseminated intravascular coagulation. N Engl J Med. 1999;341(8):586–92.
30. Ben-Ari Z, Osman E, Hutton RA, Burroughs AK. Disseminated intravascular coagulation in liver cirrhosis: fact or fiction? Am J Gastroenterol. 1999;94(10):2977–82.
31. Basili S, Ferro D, Violi F. Endotoxaemia, hyperfibrinolysis, and bleeding in cirrhosis. Lancet. 1999;353(9158):1102.

32. Hodge A, Crispin P. Coagulopathy in liver disease: the whole is greater than the sum of its parts. J Gastroenterol Hepatol. 2010;25(1):1–2.

33. Duffy JP, Hong JC, Farmer DG, Ghobrial RM, Yersiz H, Hiatt JR, et al. Vascular complications of orthotopic liver transplantation: experience in more than 4200 patients. J Am Coll Surg. 2009;208(5):896–903.

34. Madalosso C, de Souza N, Ilstrup D, Wiesner R, Krom R. Cytomegalovirus and its association with hepatic artery thrombosis after liver transplantation. Transplantation. 1998;66(3):294–7.

35. Tito L, Gines P, Arroyo V, Planas R, Panes J, Rimola A, et al. Total paracentesis associated with intravenous albumin management of patients with cirrhosis and ascites. Gastroenterology. 1990;98:146–51.

36. Grabau CM, Crago SF, Hoff LK, Simon JA, Melton CA, Ott BJ, Kamath PS. Performance standards for therapeutic abdominal paracentesis. Hepatology. 2004;40:484–8.

37. Piccinino F, Sagnelli E, Pasquale G, Giusti G, Battocchia A, Bernardi M, et al. Complications following percutaneous liver biopsy. J Hepatol. 1986;2(2):165–73.

38. Gilmore IT, Burroughs A, Murray-Lyon IM, Williams R, Jenkins D, Hopkins A. Indications, methods, and outcomes of percutaneous liver biopsy in England and Wales: an audit by the British Society of Gastroenterology and Royal College of Physicians of London. Gut. 1995;36(3):437–41.

39. Papatheodoridis GV, Patch D, Watkinson A, Tibballs J, Burroughs AK. Transjugular liver biopsy in the 1990s: a 2 year audit. Aliment Pharmacol Ther. 1999;13(5):603–8.

40. MacGill DB, Rakela J, Zinsmeister AR, Ott BJ. A 21 year experience with major haemorrhage after percutaneous liver biopsy. Gastroenterology. 1990;99(5):1396–400.

41. DeLoughery TG, Liebler JM, Simonds V, Goodnight SH. Invasive line placement in critically ill patients: do hemostatic defects matter? Transfusion. 1996;36(9):827–31.

42. Fisher NC, Mutimer DJ. Central venous cannulation in patients with liver disease and coagulopathy – a prospective audit. Intensive Care Med. 1999;25(5):481–5.

43. Donovan CL, Marcovitz P, Punch J, Bach D, Brown KA, Lucey MR, et al. Two-dimensional and dobutamine stress echocardiography in the preoperative assessment of patients with end stage liver disease prior to orthotopic liver transplantation. Transplantation. 1996;61(8):1180–8.

44. Plotkin JS, Benitez RM, Kuo PC, Njoku MJ, Ridge LA, Lim JW, et al. Dobutamine stress echocardiography for preoperative cardiac risk stratification in patients undergoing orthotopic liver transplantation. Liver Transpl Surg. 1998;4(4):253–7.

45. Grignani G, Maiolo A. Cytokines and hemostasis. Haematologica. 2000;85(9):967–72.

46. Papatheodoridis GV, Patch D, Webster GJ, Brooker J, Barnes E, Burroughs AK. Infection and hemostasis is decompensated cirrhosis: a prospective study using thromboelastography. Hepatology. 1999;29(4):1085–90.

47. Franchini M. The use of desmopressin as a hemostatic agent: a concise review. Am J Hematol. 2007;82(8):731–5.

48. Marti-Carvajal AJ, Karakitsiou DE, Salanti G. Human recombinant activated factor VII for upper gastrointestinal bleeding in patients with liver disease. Cochrane Database Syst Rev. 2012;3:CD004887.

Nutrition in Chronic Liver Disease

14

Amey Sonavane and Narendra S. Choudhary

14.1 Introduction

The liver is the principal site of metabolism in the body. Patients with cirrhosis remain at a higher risk of malnutrition due to several reasons. Malnutrition is defined as deficiencies, excesses or imbalances in a person's intake of energy and/ or nutrients. Malnutrition includes both under-nutrition and over-nutrition (overweight, obesity and related complications), but is generally used as a synonym to under-nutrition. Under-nutrition and sarcopenia (muscle depletion) in patients with cirrhosis are associated with higher risk of morbidity and mortality. Even in obese cirrhosis patients, there can be muscle mass depletion (sarcopenic obesity) that may be clinically overlooked. In addition, morbid obesity adds to morbidity and mortality in patients with cirrhosis. We further discuss assessment and management of nutritional status in patients with cirrhosis.

14.2 Prevalence and Causes of Malnutrition in Cirrhosis

As stated earlier, most of data on malnutrition in cirrhosis is available on under-nutrition. The implications of under-nutrition and results of interventions are better known/discussed than over-nutrition in patients with cirrhosis. We have used the term malnutrition for under-nutrition for the purpose of current review, and obesity in cirrhosis has been discussed separately. Malnutrition is one of the most common complications associated with cirrhosis and is reported in majority of patients, particularly in presence of decompensated cirrhosis [1, 2].

Patients with advanced liver failure (Child's C class) have high prevalence of under-nutrition. Table 14.1 shows various factors contributing to under-nutrition in patients with cirrhosis. Broadly, inadequate intake, poor absorption and catabolic state all contribute to under-nutrition of cirrhosis [1, 3]. Indian studies assessing nutritional status in patients with cirrhosis are shown in Table 14.2 [4–6]. The prevalence of malnutrition ranged from 60% to 86% in these studies. Malnutrition was more common in advanced cirrhosis (Child's C) and in patients with alcohol-related cirrhosis. Approximately one-third of patients had severe malnutrition in two studies. Patients with malnutrition had more hospitalisations and mortality before or after liver transplantation [6].

A. Sonavane
Institute of Liver Transplantation, Apollo Hospitals, Navi Mumbai, India

N. S. Choudhary (✉)
Institute of Liver Transplantation and Regenerative Medicine, Medanta the Medicity, Delhi, India

© The Author(s), under exclusive license to Springer Nature Singapore Pte Ltd. 2023
V. Vohra et al. (eds.), *Peri-operative Anesthetic Management in Liver Transplantation*,
https://doi.org/10.1007/978-981-19-6045-1_14

Table 14.1 Causes of malnutrition in patients with cirrhosis

Category	Causes
Inadequate calorie/protein intake	Anorexia due to disease, socioeconomic factors, abnormal taste, decreased oral intake (frequent hepatic encephalopathy, early satiety due to abdominal distension by ascites and splenomegaly), slow gastric emptying, sodium restriction due to ascites, keep fasting for tests and procedures, unnecessary protein restrictions for hepatic encephalopathy management
Digestion and absorption	Decreased luminal bile salt availability leading to decreased micelle formation (particularly in cholestatic liver diseases), portal hypertensive enteropathy pancreatic insufficiency due to chronic pancreatitis in alcoholics, laxatives impairing absorption
Altered metabolism	Protein catabolism, insulin resistance, impaired glycogen synthesis, increased lipolysis
Hypermetabolism	Increased beta-adrenergic activity partly responsible

Table 14.2 Indian studies regarding malnutrition in cirrhosis

Author (reference)	N	Results	Comments
Sasidharan [4]	73, 6 months follow-up, used RFH-SGA	28.8% mild to moderate and 39.7% were severely malnourished	Multivariate analysis: increased Child's grade, increased creatinine, lower sodium levels and longer prothrombin time predictive of malnutrition
Maharshi [5]	247, 12 months follow-up	59.5% malnourished according to traditional model, 66.8% by body composition analysis and 71.4% by handgrip.	Worse in alcoholics
		44.5%, 73.3% and 94.4% in CTP A, B and C	Hospitalisation (71.3% versus 38.2%; 0.002) and mortality (41.1% versus 18.2%; $p = 0.001$) more in malnourished
Yadav [6]	117, Used subjective global assessment	Mild to moderate malnutrition 51.3%	Poor nutrition in Child's C, alcoholics, more risk of post-transplantation infections and mortality
		Severe malnutrition 35%	

14.3 Causes of Under-Nutrition

The pathogenesis of malnutrition is complex and multifactorial in patients with cirrhosis. The causes of malnutrition in cirrhosis include inadequate intake (due to anorexia of disease, abnormal taste secondary to zinc deficiency, dietary restrictions advised by physicians, socioeconomic factors, alcohol intake, chronic encephalopathy, to keep fasting for investigations, co-existent pancreatitis in alcoholics, ascites and splenomegaly leading to early satiety), poor absorption (decreased bile salt pool, intestinal congestion secondary to portal hypertension, pancreatic insufficiency, bacterial overgrowth) and raised energy expenditure. In addition, impaired nutrient intake/metabolism due to liver disease may also contribute to under-nutrition.

14.4 Screening for Malnutrition in Patients with Chronic Liver Disease

The purpose of assessment of nutrition is to identify protein-energy malnutrition and other macro- and micro-nutrient deficiencies that are not easily identified on regular outpatient visits. A comprehensive nutritional assessment requires good history, physical examination, evaluation of anthropometrics and laboratory evaluation. As no single parameter is sensitive or specific enough to assess protein-energy malnutrition, a combination of tools is more effective during assessment [1, 7].

14.4.1 History

Unintentional weight loss is a practical predictor of clinically significant degree of protein-energy malnutrition. However, it can be confounded by changes in hydration status and extracellular fluid accumulation or diuresis. Any change in the habitual diet pattern should be carefully looked into. The treating physician should actively look for symptoms consistent with malabsorption and nutritional deficiencies. The functional (ability to prepare meals if staying alone) and financial status (financial interruption to purchase wholesome nutritious food) of the patient should also be factored in during assessment.

14.4.2 Physical Examination

Patients should be evaluated for signs of dehydration, excess body fluid and sarcopenia. There are various manifestations of micronutrient deficiencies that can be clinically diagnosed with careful physical examination.

14.4.3 Anthropometry, Biochemical Measures and Rapid Screening Tests for Nutritional Status

Various screening tools are available to quantify the nutritional status of patients with cirrhosis. These tools include anthropometric measurements, handgrip strength using a hand-held dynamometer, laboratory tests, evaluation of subjective global assessment (SGA), physical frailty (evaluated by the Fried frailty index), short physical performance battery, whole body dual-energy X-ray absorptiometry (DEXA), tetrapolar bioelectrical impedance analysis (BIA) and royal free hospital subjective global assessment (RFH-SGA) [1, 7–9]. The advantages and pitfalls of each of these modalities are discussed in Table 14.3. SGA is generally used to assess malnutrition in cirrhosis. It should be noted that agreement of SGA with other modalities of nutritional status (total lymphocyte count, mid-arm muscle circumference, mid-arm muscular area, subscapular skinfold thickness, body mass index (BMI) and handgrip measurement) is low. Also, SGA underestimates the prevalence of sarcopenia in liver disease patients. As BMI will remain falsely higher in patients with fluid overload

Table 14.3 Various modalities to assess malnutrition (modified from reference [8])

Screening tool	Components	Advantages	Pitfalls
Anthropometry	Body mass index (BMI); triceps skinfold (TSF); mid-arm muscle circumference (MAMC); corrected arm muscle area; mid-arm muscular area (MAMA); adductor pollicis muscle thickness; waist circumference	Low cost	Initial training required
		Rapid	Influenced by ascites and oedema
		Non-invasive	Underestimates malnutrition
		MAMC and TSF have a prognostic value for mortality	Established cut-off values not well defined in cirrhosis
		Objective	
		Good intra- and inter-observer agreement	
		Correlates with Child's score	

(continued)

Table 14.3 (continued)

Screening tool	Components	Advantages	Pitfalls
Handgrip strength	Grip strength measured by a hand-held dynamometer	Simple	Values differ with sex and age of the patient
		Bedside tool	Inability to identify muscle wasting
		Inexpensive	
		Correlates with severity of cirrhosis	
		Not influenced by water retention	
		Accurately indicates impaired muscle function	
Subjective Global Assessment (SGA)	Components include: weight, dietary intake, physical examination, functional impairment	Simple bedside tool	Subjective method
		Good inter-observer reproducibility	Poor agreement with other methods of nutritional status assessment (total lymphocyte count, MAMC, MAMA, TSF, subscapular skinfold thickness, BMI and handgrip measurement)
		Predicts outcomes in cirrhosis	Requires patient comprehension and collaboration
		Recommended by ESPEN for nutritional assessment	Underestimates muscle loss
Frailty	Fried frailty index. Components include: unintentional weight loss, self-reported exhaustion, weakness (grip strength), slow walking speed and low physical activity	Bedside tool	Required patient comprehension and co-ordination
		Predicts waitlist mortality, even after adjusting for MELD score	
Short Physical Performance Battery (SPPB)	SPPB consists of timed repeated chair stands, balance testing, and a timed 13-ft walk and takes 2–3 min to complete	Bedside tool	Needs validation
		Inexpensive	Does not correlate with CT-based muscle mass in both men and women
		Predicts transplant waitlist mortality	
Quantitative laboratory investigation	Albumin; Transthyretin (prealbumin); retinol combined protein; ferritin; transferrin; vitamin levels; resting energy expenditure; creatinine height index	Blood tests	Laboratory value can be abnormal due to underlying liver disease rather than malnutrition
		Simple to perform	Affected by pregnancy, kidney diseases, acute catabolic states, hyperthyroidism
Muscle assessment	USG, CT, MRI	Highly accurate skeletal muscle mass estimation	Trained manpower required
		Estimation can be performed during imaging done for other reasons	Cost factor
			Logistical issues
			Affected by fluid status
			Ionising radiation (CT)

Table 14.3 (continued)

Screening tool	Components	Advantages	Pitfalls
Whole body dual-energy X-ray absorptiometry	DEXA	Detailed assessment of bone mineral density	High cost
		Measures fat mass and fat-free mass	Logistical issues
		Muscle depletion measured accurately	Affected by ascites
		Good reproducibility	Low dose of ionising radiation exposure
Tetrapolar Bioelectrical Impedance Analysis (BIA)	Two-compartment model. Principle: electrical current is conducted faster in water and fat-free tissues and slower in fat tissue. Based on the measured electrical current transmitted through tissues, one can estimate the proportion of fat-free mass and fat mass	Safe	Validity questionable in patients with fluid retention
		Easy to perform	Results influenced by physical activity and eating or drinking before the examination, diuretics
		Portable equipment	Underestimates malnutrition
		Segmental BIA allows limb non-fat mass quantification	
		Correlates with outcomes in cirrhotic patients	
Royal Free Hospital-Nutritional Prioritizing Tool (RFH-NPT)	Modified SGA	Reproducible	Need external validation
		Incorporates both subjective and objective parameters	Cumbersome
		Correlates with other measures of body composition	Needs trained personnel
		Predicts survival and post-transplant complications	

(ascites or oedema), following has been suggested to remove the effect of fluid overload: post-paracentesis body weight, weight recorded before fluid retention (if known), or by subtracting a % of weight based on the severity of ascites (5% for mild; 10% for moderate and 15% for severe ascites), with an additional 5% subtraction for bilateral pedal oedema (if present) [1].

14.5 Assessment and Implications of Sarcopenia

Sarcopenia is defined as a generalised reduction in muscle mass and function due to ageing (primary sarcopenia), or due to acute or chronic illness (secondary sarcopenia) including chronic liver disease [10]. Sarcopenia is an important component of malnutrition. Computed tomographic assessment at the L3 vertebra helps to quantify muscle loss. Psoas muscle and the paraspinal muscles are rarely affected by fluid status but are consistently altered by metabolic fluctuations in cirrhosis [11]. Muscle mass estimation can be performed during usual CT screening done for hepatocellular carcinoma, portal vein patency and pre-transplant assessment. Recently the cut-off values for patients with cirrhosis have been suggested as 50 cm^2/m^2 for men and 39 cm^2/m^2 for women [12]. However, these values need validation.

Various mechanisms leading to sarcopenia include decreased protein and calorie intake

(Table 14.1), alterations in amino acid profiles, endotoxaemia, decreased mobility of patients and hyperammonaemia. Increased muscle ammonia may cause sarcopenia by multiple mechanisms [13]. Sarcopenia adds to poor prognosis of a patient with cirrhosis independent of portal hypertension and model for end-stage liver disease (MELD) score. Sarcopenia has been shown to decrease survival and is associated with increased post liver transplantation infections, ventilator requirement and higher ICU stay. Some of studies have shown that muscle function (and not muscle mass) predicts mortality.

Various strategies that have been tried for sarcopenia in patients with cirrhosis include supplemental nutrition, exercise and physical activity and anabolic steroids [14]. Although ammonia lowering therapies hold promise to treat or slow sarcopenia development, data is lacking. A combination of resistance and endurance exercise has potential to improve muscle mass and functional capacity but such studies have not been performed in cirrhosis. Studies have shown improvement in short-term outcomes in response to exercise in cirrhotics [15]. In a systemic review of 24 studies, 60% of studies on the nutritional intervention, two studies on testosterone replacement in hypogonadal men and studies on transjugular intrahepatic portosystemic shunt showed improvement of sarcopenia in patients with cirrhosis [14].

14.6 Recommendations

A rapid nutritional screen should be performed for all patients with cirrhosis. A detailed assessment is needed for patients at risk of malnutrition, CTP-C state or with BMI < 18.5 kg/m² [1, 7]. Sarcopenia and muscle function should be assessed with nutritional assessment. Dietary intake should be assessed including quality and quantity of food and supplements, fluids, sodium in diet, number and timing of meals during the day and barriers to eating. Ideally, a dietician working as part of a team with the hepatologist should perform the assessment. It is important to remember that frequent meals are better to avoid

prolonged periods of fasting. A late evening or mid-night snack has been shown to improve survival. Guo et al. performed a meta-analysis of 14 trials including 478 patients [16]. The authors found that both carbohydrate and fat oxidation improved significantly with late-evening snack. The levels of serum albumin also improved significantly, without change of serum bilirubin values.

Tolerance to vegetable and dairy proteins may be better in patients with hepatic encephalopathy (HE). Decreasing protein intake in fear of hepatic encephalopathy is not advisable as it contributes to sarcopenia [1]. Enteral feeding can be used in patients with decreased oral intake. Although some studies have shown better outcomes with enteral feeding, studies have not shown consistent benefits [17, 18]. Supplemental nutrition has been shown to improve quality of life and reduce risk of minimal hepatic encephalopathy and HE [19].

Increased physical activity and exercise are anabolic stimuli that can improve muscle mass and function. Patients should be encouraged to increase physical activity to prevent and/or ameliorate sarcopenia. The daily energy intake should not be lower than recommended 35 kcal/kg of actual body weight/day (in non-obese individuals) and optimal daily protein intake should not be lower than 1.2–1.5 g/kg actual body weight/day [1, 7]. The late-evening oral nutritional supplementation and breakfast should be included in the dietary regimen of malnourished cirrhotic patients. Branched-chain amino acids (BCAA) supplements and leucine-enriched amino acid supplements can be considered if adequate protein intake is not achieved by oral diet. Enteral nutrition is recommended for patients with inadequate intake. A moderately hypocaloric (−500 to −800 kcal less than required/day) diet with adequate protein intake (>1.5 g proteins/kg of ideal body weight/day) can be given to achieve weight loss in patients with BMI > 30 kg/m² (corrected for water retention). Micronutrients and vitamins should be used to treat confirmed or clinically suspected deficiency. Most of patients with cirrhosis remain vitamin D deficient; vitamin D levels should be checked and supplementation should be provided. BCAA supplementation may be considered in patients with hepatic encephalopathy. Simple advice on nutritional management that can be suggested bedside or on outpatient basis to patients with cirrhosis is given below.

- One should try to consume a variety of healthy foodstuff.
- To avoid tobacco chewing and alcohol consumption.
- To avoid unsafe food and drinking water.
- One should attempt to split the daily food intake into three main meals (breakfast, lunch and dinner) and three snacks (mid-morning, mid-afternoon, late evening). The late-evening/pre-bed snack is of paramount importance as it covers the long interval between dinner and breakfast.
- Patients with ascites should have less salt (not more than 2 g added salt a day).
- Decreasing water intake is not advisable unless asked by a doctor for gross fluid overload or hyponatraemia.

14.7 Effect of Obesity on Cirrhosis

Morbid obesity affects a patient with cirrhosis in multiple ways. These patients have higher risk of hepatocellular carcinoma and hepatic decompensation. Also, non-alcoholic steatohepatitis (NASH) is a common diagnosis in these patients, which may be associated with comorbidities like diabetes, hypertension, chronic kidney disease and cardiovascular disease. In fact, patients with NASH have higher risk of perioperative (liver transplantation) and post-operative risk of cardiovascular events. The presence of obesity also makes liver transplantation difficult and increases the risk of complications and mortality. The living donor liver transplantation is the predominant form of liver transplantation in Asia. There may be a difficulty in finding a suitable live donor for morbidly obese patients due to risk of low graft to recipient ratio (GRWR) and subsequent risk of poor graft function and higher mortality in the post-operative period. The presence of morbid

obesity is shown to be associated with poor outcomes (graft loss, blood transfusion requirements, sepsis, multiorgan failure, wound complications, biliary complications, deep venous thrombosis and incisional hernia) after liver transplantation [20].

Weight loss by bariatric surgery or lifestyle modification is often not possible in patients with decompensated cirrhosis. Bariatric surgery is associated with higher risk (than patients without cirrhosis) of complications and not advisable in patients with decompensated cirrhosis. Although intragastric balloon is minimally invasive, there is not much data. We published a series of endoscopic intragastric balloon placement in eight prospective liver transplantation recipients, aged 46 ± 5 years [21]. The mean BMI before balloon placement was 43.5 ± 6.9 kg/m^2. The mean Child score was 8.5 ± 1.6; only one patient had Child's C cirrhosis. Five of them had successful liver transplantation later (three deceased and two living donor liver transplantation) after weight loss. All these five patients had uneventful post-transplant course. The volume of balloon was decreased in one patient due to persistent vomiting; all but one patient achieved weight loss. One patient with diabetes had meaningful improvement of HBA1c also [21]. A later study by Watt et al. also showed efficacy of endoscopic intragastric balloon placement in weight loss without loss of lean mass [22]. These findings should be validated by other centres or in a large study.

14.8 Summary

Malnutrition is a common problem in patients with end-stage liver disease. Both under-nutrition and obesity are associated with worse outcomes; most of data is available on under-nutrition. Sarcopenia is increasingly being recognised in patients with cirrhosis and affects prognosis adversely. Various methods of nutritional status screening and treatment have been discussed. Improved nutrition and sarcopenia management lead to better survival and quality of life in patients with end-stage liver disease.

Acknowledgements None.

Funding None.

Conflict of Interest None.

References

1. Puri P, Dhiman RK, Taneja S, Tandon P, Merli M, Anand AC, et al. Nutrition in chronic liver disease: consensus statement of the Indian National Association for Study of the Liver. J Clin Exp Hepatol. 2021;11:97–143.

2. Nutritional Status in Cirrhosis. Italian multicenter cooperative project on nutrition in liver cirrhosis. J Hepatol. 1994;21:317–25.

3. Saunders J, Brian A, Wright M, Stroud M. Malnutrition and nutrition support in patients with liver disease. Frontline Gastroenterol. 2010;1:105–11.

4. Sasidharan M, Nistala S, Narendhran RT, Murugesh M, Bhatia SJ, Rathi PM. Nutritional status and prognosis in cirrhotic patients. Trop Gastroenterol. 2012;33:257–64.

5. Maharshi S, Sharma BC, Srivastava S. Malnutrition in cirrhosis increases morbidity and mortality. J Gastroenterol Hepatol. 2015;30:1507–1.

6. Yadav SK, Choudhary NS, Saraf N, Saigal S, Goja S, Rastogi A, et al. Nutritional status using subjective global assessment independently predicts outcome of patients waiting for living donor liver transplant. Indian J Gastroenterol. 2017;36:275–81.

7. European Association for the Study of the Liver. European Association for the Study of the Liver. EASL Clinical practice guidelines on nutrition in chronic liver disease. J Hepatol. 2019;70:172–93.

8. Tandon P, Raman M, Mourtzakis M, Merli M. A practical approach to nutritional screening and assessment in cirrhosis. Hepatology. 2017;65:1044–57.

9. Borhofen SM, Gerner C, Lehmann J, Fimmers R, Gortzen J, Hey B, et al. The royal free hospital-nutritional prioritizing tool is an independent predictor of deterioration of liver function and survival in cirrhosis. Dig Dis Sci. 2016;61:1735–43.

10. Cruz-Jentoft AJ, Baeyens JP, Bauer JM, Boirie Y, Cederholm T, Landi F, et al. Sarcopenia: European consensus on definition and diagnosis: report of the European Working Group on sarcopenia in older people. Age Ageing. 2010;39:412–23.

11. Giusto M, Lattanzi B, Albanese C, Galtieri A, Farcomeni A, Giannelli V, et al. Sarcopenia in liver cirrhosis: the role of computed tomography scan for the assessment of muscle mass compared with dual-energy Xray absorptiometry and anthropometry. Eur J Gastroenterol Hepatol. 2015;27:328–34.

12. Carey EJ, Lai JC, Wang CW, Dasarathy S, Lobach I, Montano-Loza AJ, et al. A multicenter study to define sarcopenia in patients with end-stage liver disease. Liver Transpl. 2017;23:625–33.

13. Dasarathy S, Merli M. Sarcopenia from mechanism to diagnosis and treatment in liver disease. J Hepatol. 2016;65:1232–44.

14. Naseer M, Turse EP, Syed A, Dailey FE, Zatreh M, Tahan V. Interventions to improve sarcopenia in cirrhosis: a systematic review. World J Clin Cases. 2019;7:156–70.

15. Jones JC, Coombes JS, Macdonald GA. Exercise capacity and muscle strength in patients with cirrhosis. Liver Transpl. 2012;18:146–51.

16. Guo Y-J, Tian Z-b, Jiang N, Ding X-L, Mao T, Jing X. Effects of late evening snack on cirrhotic patients: a systematic review and meta-analysis. Gastroenterol Res Pract. 2018;2018:9189062.

17. Koretz RL, Avenell A, Lipman TO. Nutritional support for liver disease. Cochrane Database Syst Rev. 2012;(5):CD008344.

18. Ney M, Vandermeer B, van Zanten SJ, Ma MM, Gramlich L, Tandon P. Meta-analysis: oral or enteral nutritional supplementation in cirrhosis. Aliment Pharmacol Ther. 2013;37:672–9.

19. Maharshi S, Sharma BC, Sachdeva S, Srivastava S, Sharma P. Efficacy of nutritional therapy for patients with cirrhosis and minimal hepatic encephalopathy in a randomized trial. Clin Gastroenterol Hepatol. 2016;14:454–60.

20. Kumar N, Choudhary NS. Treating morbid obesity in cirrhosis: a quest of holy grail. World J Hepatol. 2015;7:2819–28.

21. Choudhary NS, Puri R, Saraf N, Saigal S, Kumar N, Rai R, et al. Intragastric balloon as a novel modality for weight loss in patients with cirrhosis and morbid obesity awaiting liver transplantation. Indian J Gastroenterol. 2016;35:113–6.

22. Watt KD, Heimbach JK, Rizk M, Jaruvongvanich P, Sanchez W, Port J, Venkatesh SK, et al. Efficacy and safety of endoscopic balloon placement for weight loss in patients with cirrhosis awaiting liver transplantation. Liver Transpl. 2021;27:1239–47.

Part III

Intra-operative Course and Management

Intra-operative Management of Transplant Recipient: An Overview

15

Lakshmi Kumar

15.1 Introduction

Liver transplant has emerged as an option for survival amongst patients with end-stage liver disease (ESLD) and fulminant failure. While deceased donation might be the most acceptable alternative as it does not pose any donor risk, constraints on organ availability due to prevailing beliefs and social conditions limit this option [1]. Optimal management of the recipient contributes to outcomes after surgery. With evolution of concepts on patient management, an anaesthesiologist has changed and improvised practices from over a decade and refined it to its current state.

In this chapter, we bring to the anaesthetists' attention newer areas of understanding in the current management of the recipient.

15.2 Preoperative Preparation

When does an anaesthetist have concerns on the management and outcomes of transplant?

The MELD (model for end-stage liver disease) scores are currently used to assess severity of liver disease and to prognosticate risk for non-transplant surgery. In the presence of MELD scores 28 or higher, age, more than 70 years is are

associated with poorer post-transplant outcomes. Development of pre-transplant diabetes and need for mechanical ventilation preoperatively also could imply poor post-transplant outcomes [2].

Extremes of weight may affect transplant oiutcomes. An analysis of the UNOS database has shown that in comparison with a high body mass index (BMI) and higher MELD scores, lower BMI (<18 kg.m^{-2}) is associated with poorer post-transplant and graft outcomes even with low MELD scores [3].

Sarcopenia is defined as a loss of muscle mass and is evaluated by a measurement of the psoas muscle mass at the level of the fourth lumbar vertebra on a computerised tomography scan. Extreme sarcopenia is seen in 40–70% of cirrhotic patients and is a concern for transplant selection. An increase in skeletal muscle mass area by 1000 mm^2 following transplant surgery appears to provide 73% reduction in mortality [4].

Acute on chronic liver failure (ACLF) is a syndrome distinct from CLD that is characterised by multi-organ decompensation in the background of diagnosed or undiagnosed cirrhosis. The 28-day mortality in ACLF grade 2 and grade 3 is 32% and 78% respectively [5]. In any patient in ACLF grade 3, transplant is associated with poor outcomes. In ACLF 2, consideration of co-morbidities, age, pre-operative status, multi-systemic supports will have to considered before undertaking the decision to proceed with transplantation.

L. Kumar (✉)
Amrita Institute of Medical Sciences,
Kochi, Kerala, India

A BMI > 35 is associated with poor outcomes in one study and a retrospective analysis of 3937 patients with 45% amongst them identified with multiple co-morbidities, cardiovascular disease was associated with increase in post-transplant morbidity while diabetes, renal or pulmonary disease did not have an influence on outcomes [6].

Preoperative hyponatraemia (Na < 120 mEq/L) poses a challenge to the anaesthetist as it confounds encephalopathic assessment. The surges in sodium during surgery can impact outcomes and central pontine myelinolysis following correction during transplant can occur. The aim should be to keep sodium levels within 5 mEq/L of the baseline value during surgery. Surprisingly, literature does not suggest associations between hyponatraemia and poorer outcomes but hypernatraemia is associated with higher postoperative mortality [7].

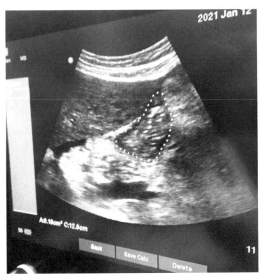

Dotted lines show the contour of the stomach shape. Cross sectional area (A=9.18 cm²)

Fig. 15.1 Posterolateral view of the gastric antrum in a liver recipient

15.3 Preoperative Fasting Guidelines and Preparation

ESLD patients have delayed gastric emptying times and are predisposed to aspiration during induction. In the presence of tense ascites, intra-abdominal pressure could increase the possibility of regurgitation particularly in the background of autonomic system dysfunction. The delay in gastric emptying appears to be related to the MELD scoring, associated thrombocytopenia, coexistent diabetes and an age less than 60 years [8]. Standard fasting instructions would include solids 8 h prior to surgery. Limited amounts of clear liquid about 200 ml or less can be given until 3 h prior to surgery to avoid dehydration and thirst. Diabetics will need blood sugar monitoring during the fasting period.

An ultrasound assessment of gastric size and residual volume in cirrhotics shows an increase in both size and residual volume in comparison to non-cirrhotic patients. Although the gastric residue shows more fluid and air, it does not result in significant Ryle's tube aspirate after intubation (Fig. 15.1) leaving us still without a clear answer on the need to perform a rapid sequence induction (RSI) in these patients. RSI can therefore be reserved for patients with tense ascites, upper GI bleed, encephalopathy, impaired airway reflexes and anticipated difficult airway amongst these patients.

Anxiolytics are avoided as premedication in view of underlying encephalopathy and aspiration risk. Preoperative medications may include beta blockers (propranolol or carvedilol) and diuretics (spironolactone/furosemide). Even diuretics can be continued in usual doses till day of surgery to avoid interference in the fluid balance. Electrolytes are monitored on the morning of surgery.

Some patients with refractory hyponatraemia and ascites are started on treatment with tolvaptan. Tolvaptan in a V2 receptor antagonist that acts at the aquaretic receptors in the distal collecting tubules of the kidney and helps in selective diuresis with retention of the sodium ion. A small study of the use of tolvaptan in cirrhotics has been encouraging in the control of sodium levels and outcomes [9], while a case report cautions on postoperative hypernatraemia in patients with renal dysfunction [10].

The coagulation in a liver recipient has a dynamic profile and can vary rapidly. Coagulation tests are ordered on the morning of surgery. Thrombocytopenia is a common accompaniment in ESLD. This does not always require a correction as there is an intrinsically rebalanced coagulation. Although platelet counts appear to be low, increased synthesis of vWF (von Willebrand factor) and decreased hepatic synthesis of ADAMTS13 (metalloprotease enzyme that cleaves vWF) compensate for the derangement in platelets and bleeding is not directly related to the extent of coagulopathy reflected by the prtohrombin time.

Platelets can be transfused prior to intubation and invasive lining can be safely performed with platelet counts more than 20–30,000/mm³. During the surgery transfusion can be guided by the ongoing bleeding in the surgical field and dynamic tests of coagulation. Transfusion of fresh frozen plasma prior to surgery can be based upon the INR. Levels more than 2.5–3 may merit transfusion at the time of invasive lines. However excessive volume related to transfusions may increase portal pressures and increase bleeding during the dissection phase.

15.4   Conduct of Anaesthesia

A preoperative checklist of the morning laboratory parameters and blood cultures close to the date of surgery are important and need to be reviewed prior to the transplant surgery.

The operating room will need to be prepared in readiness for the conduct of the surgery. A peripheral large bore venous cannula and a radial arterial cannula are placed under local anaesthesia while the patient is still on room air. A sample drawn will provide baseline oxygenation and base excess that will help in postoperative management.

Pre-transplant hypoxemia could reflect hepatopulmonary syndrome (HPS), [11] evolving chest infection or cardiogenic/non cardiogenic pulmonary oedema. Hypoxemia of new onset at the time of transplant surgery that was not present earlier may cause concern and the cause needs to be treated and evaluated prior to surgery. In case of uncertainty in diagnosis, a combined decision to postpone the transplant should be undertaken until the patient recovers and a correct diagnosis of the cause is established.

A femoral arterial catheter is often placed in addition to the radial arterial cannula to monitor pressures. Traditionally the systolic in the femoral artery is believed to be 20–30 mm Hg higher than the radial and monitoring femoral pressures allows a clearer correlate to central pressures. This is of particular value at the time of reperfusion when the radial pressures are significantly dampened. However studies have consistently shown that although the systolic variability exists the mean arterial pressures measured by both routes are comparable even at the time of reperfusion [12–14] (Fig. 15.2).

Central venous cannulation is performed after intubation and a triple or quadruple lumen catheter is used. A sheath may also be inserted for the possible need for a pulmonary artery catheter in select patients. The availability of ultrasound has improved the safety of central venous cannulations in patients with liver disease and incidence of bleeding complications is reportedly low [15, 16]. Subclavian vein cannulations are avoided due to risk of arterial puncture and uncontrolled bleeding. When more than one central venous access is planned, the same side is to be used and the catheters inserted after insertion of both guide wires in the lumen to avoid damage to the first catheter by the needle during insertion of the second central line.

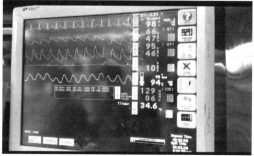

Radial artery trace, Femoral artery trace

Fig. 15.2 Radial and femoral arterial pressures at reperfusion

15.5 Haemodynamic Monitoring

15.5.1 Central Venous Pressure (CVP) Monitors

An increase in the extracellular volume and increased circulatory volume leads to an increase in the CVP. Tricuspid regurgitation often is seen in a transthoracic echocardiogram consequent to which the mean CVP is elevated. While a low to normal CVP is advised during hepatectomy, the same cannot be practised during recipient hepatectomy. The splanchnic circulation is vasodilated and is unable to contract in response to volume losses and the kidney in a patient with liver disease is sensitive to hypovolemia and acute kidney injury. Although there are reports that a reduction in the CVP to less than 6 mm Hg in the pre-anhepatic phase can reduce transfusions, decrease duration of mechanical ventilation and pulmonary complications [17], most transplant anaesthesiologists would look at indices of fluid responsiveness and not the CVP for fluid management.

15.5.2 Cardiac Output Monitors (Table 15.1)

There is no clear consensus on the optimal haemodynamic monitoring during surgery. The pulmonary artery catheter (PAC) is gradually being phased out from the operating rooms as it is known to induce arrhythmias during introduction and complications with its use [18]. There are select indications for the use of the PAC in transplant surgery. In today's scenario, mild to moderate pulmonary artery hypertension and cardiac abnormalities in a patient with large oesophageal varices contraindicating use of a transoesophageal echocardiographic probe remain as indications for its use.

Intermittent thermodilution PAC has been criticised in its accuracy for assessing cardiac output as it is dependent on volume, temperature and speed of injectate and timing of the respiratory cycle during its administration. In order to avoid this confounding effect, the continuous cardiac output (CCO) monitoring PAC was introduced. The CCO has a thermal filament located

Table 15.1 Comparison of currently available cardiac output monitors in adults

	FloTrac Vigileo	PiCCO	PAC	TEE
Device	FloTrac sensor with cable	PiCCO thermodilution with femoral artery sensor	Swan Ganz—PA catheter	TEE probe and echo machine
Principle for function	Arterial pulse contour derived cardiac output	Transpulmonary thermodilution with thermistor in femoral artery	Thermodilution derived CO	Direct estimation of cardiac output
Requirements	Radial arterial line	Central line for thermodilution and a femoral arterial line with thermistor	PAC catheter floated into the pulmonary artery	Probe placed in the oesophagus or stomach
Advantages	Simple to use, needs no calibration	Accurate measurement of cardiac output Additional parameters of GEF, EVLW available	Gold standard in CO measurement PA pressures measured	Direct estimate of cardiac function Volume replacement LVOTO, intracardiac thrombus identified
Limitations	MV at 10 ml/kg b.wt No spontaneous breath No arrhythmias Accuracy uncertain in vasoplegic states	Needs calibration Femoral arterial line in a coagulopathic patient Cost is a limitation	Invasive, ventricular arrhythmias Morbidity associated	Invasive, risk of bleeding with varices Expertise in interpretation, availability of machine and probe

PiCCO pulse contour derived cardiac output, *PAC* pulmonary artery catheter, *GEF* global ejection fraction, *EVLW* extravascular lung water, *LVOTO* left ventricular outflow tract obstruction

25 cm proximal to the tip that emits pseudo-energy random signals producing heat every 20–30 s. The change in temperature is detected at the thermistor located distally and this is used in the calculation of cardiac output. A comparison between the PAC and transpulmonary thermodilution catheter CCO appears to suggest that the values obtained by both methods are comparable but there is a poor correlate of cardiac output (CO) at reperfusion and at cross clamping [19].

15.5.2.1 Can We Derive Fluid Responsiveness?

The cardio-respiratory interactions and variations in arterial and pulse pressure are used to determine the fluid responsiveness. Reverse pulsus paradoxus is the phenomenon of increase in blood pressure during inspiration and fall in expiration in a patient on mechanical ventilation. These systems are derived from arterial pulse contour analysis. The technology varies between different monitors, uncalibrated devices using patient demographics such as the FloTrac-Vigileo (Edward Lifesciences) appear user friendly and its simplicity allows a wider use amongst non-cardiac anaesthetists.

Fluid responsiveness is measured by the variations in stroke volume across the phases of respiration. A stroke volume variation (SVV) value <10% is considered indicative of adequate filling during surgery. The pulse pressure variation (PPV) is easier in that it does not require a specialised cable but can be read off the screen of compatible monitors. Values above 14% correlate with volume responsiveness. Minimally invasive monitors however require that the person is on mechanical ventilation at 8–10 ml/kg tidal volume, in sinus rhythm without tachycardia and minimal PEEP and without an open thorax.

Newer non-invasive monitors: Clear sight (Edwards Life Sciences) can measure CO, blood pressure, PPV and systemic vascular resistance (SVR) by a digital sensor and wrist cuff. CNAP (Lid CO): Continuous non-invasive arterial pressure works on the principle of detecting blood volume changes in the finger transforming plethysmographic signals into continuous blood pressure information. The components of CNAP include an infrared light source, finger pressure cuff that inflates and deflates to maintain normal volume and an absolute brachial pressure cuff. For cardiac output monitoring, the continuous, non-invasive blood pressure waveform is analysed by the validated Pulse CO™ algorithm. Arterial lines will be mandatorily placed for transplant surgery; hence these non-invasive monitors may have a role as a supplementary monitor in the future.

PICCO/Volume view appears the most sensitive amongst current monitors as it combines transpulmonary thermodilution with arterial contour derived cardiac output. Thermodilution assessment of cardiac output is derived by a change in temperature of ice-cold saline that is detected in the thermistor located in the femoral artery. In addition it can determine global end diastolic volume and extravascular lung water that can predict early volume overload. The advantages with the use of these advanced monitors are that it allows an assessment of the systemic vascular resistance and fluid responsiveness and allows titration of vasopressors during surgery. A comparison of the EV 1000 (Volume view) with the PAC has shown that although the limits of agreement was acceptable, trending was unreliable between both techniques [20].

The TEE has emerged as a potentially useful tool that can give an ongoing feedback of the volume status, both right and left ventricular contractility, development of outflow tract obstruction and diagnosis of rarer embolic and thrombotic cardiac events during reperfusion [21].

A recent analysis of 318 patients who underwent transplant with either or both PAC and TEE concluded that outcomes and LOHS were lower in patients who had dual monitoring [22]. Concerns on the safety of TEE in the presence of oesophageal varices were evaluated in 232 patients. The incidence of variceal rupture and haemorrhagic complications was 0.4%. Guidelines for the safe use of TEE in liver transplant suggest use of the probe at mid-oesophageal level, avoidance of advancement in the flexed position, refraining from excessive manipulation in difficult advancement and to keep the probe in freeze position when not in use [23] (Table 15.1).

15.5.2.2 Induction Agents

Anaesthesia induction is performed with an anxiolytic, lorazepam 1–2 mg, along with fentanyl 2 μg/kg and propofol titrated to a loss of verbal response. Lorazepam has a high hepatic extraction ratio and is predominantly metabolised by conjugation in the liver. Its duration of action is not altered in cirrhotics. Benzodiazepines can cause hepatic encephalopathy after 2–3 days of administration but in the setting of transplant is unlikely to cause residual effects. Lignocaine 1 mg/kg can obtund the intubation responses and is given prior to thge administration of propofol.

Among induction agents, propofol appears to be the safest in patients with CLD. Thiopentone and etomidate can decrease hepatic blood flow by an increase in hepatic vascular resistance and decrease in cardiac output. Propofol can increase total hepatic blood flow by increasing the portal and hepatic arterial blood flow component. Propofol, etomidate and ketamine are lipid soluble with a high hepatic extraction ratio. Their duration of action is not prolonged and elimination half-lives are similar to normal adults. Ketamine and etomidate can be used when the blood pressures are low when the use of propofol can decrease the blood pressures. Dexmedetomidine has a decreased half-life and prolonged clearance in patients with hepatic dysfunction part of which could be due to altered protein binding [24].

Although fentanyl is lipid soluble with a short half-life, redistribution to storage sites occurs and prolonged administration results in cumulative effects. Remifentanil is metabolised by tissue esterases that hydrolyse the ester linkage and its elimination is independent of liver function and is the safest opioid for use in patients with liver diseases.

Volatile anaesthetics: The hepatic blood flow is determined by dual flow through the portal vein and hepatic artery, the two having a semi-reciprocal relationship called the hepatic arterial buffer response (HABR). This implies that a fall in portal vein flow is compensated by an increase in hepatic arterial flow through the release of adenosine which is a vasodilator but the converse cannot occur. A fall in blood pressure can reduce the liver blood flow and this can be corrected by drugs that increase the mean arterial pressure (MAP).

The role of inhalational gents in patients with liver disease is thought provoking. The only agents consistently known to decrease hepatic blood flow are halothane and enflurane that are not used today. Sevoflurane prevents hepatic arterial vasoconstriction and is equivalent or superior to isoflurane in preservation of hepatic arterial blood flow. Sevoflurane preserves hepatic oxygen delivery and oxygen consumption delivery ratio as measured by hepatic venous oxygen saturation. Compound A that is produced with prolonged anaesthesia with sevoflurane is devoid of side effects on the liver. All inhalational anaesthetics can produce a mild transaminitis that is clinically not relevant. Desflurane, sevoflurane and isoflurane are safe for use in CLD patients undergoing transplant.

Ischaemic preconditioning with sevoflurane has provoked interest in hepatic surgery. Animal studies have shown that sevoflurane preconditioning reduces hepatocellular injury and reduces acidosis in liver ischaemia. Postconditioning with sevoflurane promoted superior haemodynamic recovery with a decrease in inflammatory responses [25]. Currently it is perhaps the most widely used inhalational anaesthetic during liver transplantation surgery.

15.5.3 How Do I Intubate a Patient with CLD for Transplant? Is RSI Mandatory?

There is evidence of delayed gastric emptying in patients with ESLD. Gastric volumes and contents are higher with more advanced liver disease (Child C), concurrent opiate usage and co-existent diabetes [26] (Fig. 15.2). Need for RSI is at the discretion and experience of the anaesthesiologist. In any ESLD patient, large tense ascites, bleeding esophageal varices and a history of esophageal reflux may mandate RSI while lower MELD scores and controlled ascites can allow intubation by conventional techniques.

The use of succinylcholine in RSI should be with the knowledge of a possible prolonged duration of action due to decreases in the enzyme pseudocholinesterase produced by the liver. In the presence of contraindications for the use of suxamethonium, rocuronium can be used to facilitate an RSI in a reduced dose 0.9 mg/kg. Sugammadex is not freely available as yet in many institutions hence the use of rocuronium should be limited in patients in whom airway control can be established with reasonable safety.

Atracurium and cis atracurium have non-end organ-dependent routes of elimination and are preferred over vecuronium or pancuronium for maintenance of neuromuscular blockade. Atracurium at a dose of 0.5 mg/kg for intubation followed by 0.3–0.6 mg/kg/h and cis atracurium at 0.15 mg/kg for intubation and 2 mcg/kg/min as infusion can be used.

15.6 Depth of Anaesthesia Monitoring During Liver Transplant Surgery

The Bispectral Index (BIS) monitor is useful to monitor the depth of anaesthesia during transplant surgery. The BIS is a weighted sum of several EEG parameters that is summated as a number ranging from 0 (EEG silence) to 100. A value between 40 and 60 correlates with an adequate depth of anaesthesia. In a study looking at end tidal (ET) concentrations of isoflurane in healthy liver donors, patients with HCC and cirrhotis revealed lowest values of ET isoflurane in cirrhotics emphasising the need for a depth of anaesthesia monitoring in patients with impairment of liver function [27]. The requirement of desflurane guided by the BIS is significantly reduced in the anhepatic and neohepatic phases of orthotopic liver transplant surgery [28].

NIRS (near infrared spectroscopy) is a non-invasive measurement of cerebral oxygenation. Studies evaluating this have shown absence of cerebral blood flow autoregulation during liver transplantation [29]. A decrease in cerebral oximetry was seen preceding onset of vascular complications during orthotopic liver transplantation surgery [30].

15.7 Fluid Management in Liver Surgery

Balanced salt solutions are emerging as replacement solutions of choice as they contain a base of lactate or acetate. Normal saline administration raises concerns regarding hyperchloremia and dilutional acidosis. Hyperchloremia could increase renal dysfunction by activation of the rennin angiotensin aldosterone axis and by renal arteriolar vasoconstriction. In the context of hepatic hypoperfusion or dysfunction, lactate administered extraneously is inadequately broken down in the liver and lactic acidosis could ensue. Acetate solutions do not interfere with lactate metabolism by the liver as they have an extrahepatic metabolism. Additionally they do not increase gluconeogenesis in the liver, release bicarbonate faster than lactate containing solutions and may be superior in diabetics and in situations where lactate measurements are followed as markers of tissue perfusion.

The SOLAR trial that evaluated Ringer's lactate versus normal saline in elective colorectal and orthopaedic surgery concluded that the overall outcomes and renal injury were similar between both groups [31].

However, the SALT-ED trial and the SMART study showed that the use of balanced salt solutions versus normal saline significantly reduced the incidence of AKI. The SMART trial showed an improved postoperative outcome in the balanced salt groups [32, 33].

It appears intuitive that administration of colloid can reduce the volume of transfusion; however amongst synthetic colloids, starches have fallen in disrepute after several studies have shown a higher incidence of renal dysfunction in sepsis. A retrospective analysis of 174 liver transplants at a single centre showed that the risk of AKI was threefold in patients who received HES 130/0.5 in comparison to patients who had received albumin [34].

Gelatins are possible alternatives although concerns regarding anaphylaxis and coagulation remain. Albumin is the colloid of choice in liver dysfunction but at a high cost; availability and potential disease transmission remain as concerns.

15.8 Coagulation Monitoring and Guidelines for Product Transfusion

It is now well understood that the coagulation in liver disease is "rebalanced". This implies that despite a platelet count that is lower or a pro-thrombin time that is prolonged, patients may be predisposed to thrombosis and that this delicate balance can be pushed to either hyper- or hypo-coagulability.

Transfusions during liver transplantation are associated with higher rates for re-exploration, length of hospital stay and mortality. An increased use of products also has a negative impact on 1-year and 5-year graft survival [35]. Transfusion of FFP besides increasing the concentration of deficient clotting factors can also increase levels of factor VIII and vWF and precipitate thrombosis [36].

Static tests such as the prothrombin time and activated partial thromboplastin time cannot reliably predict coagulation within the body as they only measure the availability of clotting factors and do not measure the absence of naturally occurring anticoagulant substances. In liver disease, along with the decrease in clotting factors, there is a decrease in the circulating anticoagulants, protein C and protein S. Also the decrease in thrombomodulin found on the endothelial surface that activates the protein C cannot be measured by static tests.

Studies have shown that viscoelastic tests of coagulation are normal in stable cirrhotics even when static tests are deranged [37].

Viscoelastic coagulation monitoring or point of care tests (POCT) involve graphs derived from viscoelastic strength of clot from a sample of blood that is agitated after the addition of a clot initiator. The two currently popular tests include thromboelastography TEG (Haemonetics Corporation, Braintree, MA) and rotational thromboelastometry ROTEM (TEM International GmbH, Munich, Germany) [38]. ROTEM appears to be more refined in its technique for automatic sampling and reagent wise grouping of coagulation defects and thereby directed transfusion of specific products. The FLEV in TEG is a modification that allows an estimate of fibrinogen levels at the time of measurement and is used similar to the FIBTEM in ROTEM assays (Figs. 15.3 and 15.4). A combination of EXTEM and FIBTEM has been found to be useful in the coagulation management of transplant (Fig. 15.5). The indications for fibrinogen correction are laboratory values less than 100 mg/dL or between 100 and 200 mg/dL in the presence of bleeding. The 10-minute amplitude on the FIBTEM A_{10} below 5–8 mm is also considered an indication for fibrinogen transfusion [39]. It is prudent to base all transfusions based upon a clinical assessment of bleeding in combination with the POCT.

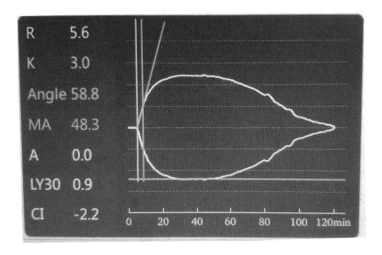

Fig. 15.3 TEG with kaolin showing delayed lysis

Fig. 15.4 TEG functional fibrinogen (FF/FLEV) showing fibrinolysis

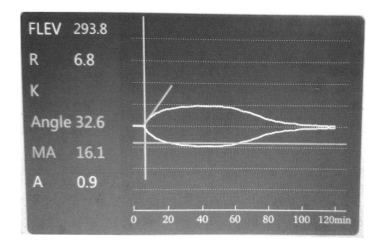

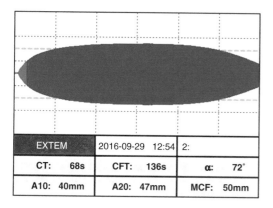

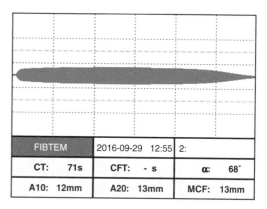

Fig. 15.5 EXTEM and FIBTEM assays of ROTEM viscoelastic testing

Prothrombin complex concentrates (PCC) are prepared from the supernatant of pooled cryoprecipitate by ion exchange chromatography. A three factor PCC contains factors II, IX and X and four factor PCC additional factor VII alongwith endogenous inhibitor proteins C and S. A vial reconstituted to 20 ml provides 25 IU/ml standardised to the factor IX level. A retrospective study in 120 patients undergoing transplant has shown that the use of PCC as a primary modality for coagulation correction reduced transfusion of red cells and did not increase incidence of thromboembolic complications [40].

15.8.1 Fast Tracking in Liver Transplant

In a country constrained by financial and hospital resources fast tracking appears as an option that can be considered. A retrospective study on fifteen patients at an Indian centre has suggested the option of fast tracking in a select group of patients with stable haemodynamics, minimal transfusion and optimal vascular anastomosis and good-sized graft [41]. This may become an accepted management in this select group with time.

15.9 Conclusion

The advances in surgery and anaesthesia care are evolving and the anaesthetist needs to update with ongoing practices. Appropriate preoperative assessment and optimal haemodynamic monitoring and meticulous attention to the finest detail are crucial for the best outcomes after surgery. Ultrasonography is becoming irreplaceable for safe insertion of invasive lines in these patients. Transoesophageal echocardiography despite being rated as the best is slow to appear in the transplant scene, probably due to bleeding concerns and costs. Viscoelastic testing of coagulation and availability of clotting factor concentrates have avoided fluid overloading in patients and improved outcomes. Improved experience in management has introduced fast tracking as part of management strategies. With growing awareness of the risk profiles an optimal management directed postoperatively can improve outcomes.

Key Points
- Optimal preoperative preparation improves patient outcome after LT.
- High-risk patients are those with higher MELD score, low BMI, hyponatraemia, extreme sarcopenia and those on mechanical ventilation.
- Preoperative monitoring of laboratory parameters and blood cultures close to surgery are important.
- Ultrasonography is becoming irreplaceable for safe insertion of invasive line.
- CVP monitoring is still essential although its role in fluid management is debated.
- Newer non-invasive cardiac output monitor measuring CO, PPV and SVR is a good guide in patient management intra-operatively.
- TEE is a useful tool for giving information on volume status, right and left ventricular contractility and to detect thromboembolic issue during reperfusion.
- Balanced salt solutions are the fluids of choice.
- Viscoelastic test guides blood and product transfusion.

References

1. Navin S, Suriyamoorthi S. Current state of acceptance of brain stem death and organ donation in India. Amrita J Med. 2020;16:87–94.
2. Sharpton SR, Feng S, Hameed B, Yao F, Lai JC. Combined effects of recipient age and model for end-stage liver disease score on liver transplantation outcomes. Transplantation. 2014;98:557–62.
3. Bambha KM, Dodge JL, Gralla J, Sprague D, Biggins SW. Low, rather than high, body mass index confers increased risk for post-liver transplant death and graft loss: risk modulated by model for end-stage liver disease. Liver Transpl. 2015;21:1286–94.
4. Lai JC. Defining the threshold for too sick for transplant. Curr Opin Organ Transplant. 2016;21:127–32.
5. Arroyo V, Moreau R, Kamath PS, Jalan R, Ginès P, Nevens F, et al. Acute-on-chronic liver failure in cirrhosis. Nat Rev Dis Primers. 2016;2:16041.
6. Tovikkai C, Charman SC, Praseedom RK, Gimson AE, van der Meulen J. Time-varying impact of comorbidities on mortality after liver transplantation: a national cohort study using linked clinical and administrative data. BMJ Open. 2015;5:e006971.
7. Leise MD, Yun BC, Larson JJ, Benson JT, Yang JD, Therneau TM, et al. Effect of the pretransplant serum sodium concentration on outcomes following liver transplantation. Liver Transpl. 2014;20:687–97.
8. Snell DB, Cohen-Mekelburg S, Weg R, Ghosh G, Buckholz AP, Mehta A, Ma X, Christos PJ, Jesudian AB. Gastric food retention at endoscopy is associated with severity of liver cirrhosis. World J Hepatol. 2019;11:725–34.
9. Jia J-D, Xie W, Ding HG, Mao H, Guo H, Li Y, et al. Utility and safety of tolvaptan in cirrhotic patients with hyponatremia: a prospective cohort study. Ann Hepatol. 2017;16:123–32.
10. Iida H, MaehiraH MH, Maekawa T, Tani T. Post-hepatectomy tolvaptan-induced hypernatremia in a hepatocellular carcinoma patient with cirrhosis: a case report. Surg Case Rep. 2020;61:6.
11. Grilo I, Pascasio JM, López-Pardo FJ, Ortega-Ruiz F, Tirado JL, Sousa JM, Rodríguez-Puras MJ, Ferrer MT, Gómez-Bravo MA, Grilo A. Hepato pulmonary syndrome: which blood gas analysis criteria and position should we use for diagnosis? Rev Esp Enferm Dig. 2017;109:843–9.
12. Arnal D, Garutti I, Perez-Peña J, Olmedilla L, Tzenkov IG. Radial to femoral arterial blood pressure differences during liver transplantation. Anaesthesia. 2005;60:766–71.
13. Shin BS, Kim GS, Ko JS, Gwak MS, Yang M, Kim CS, et al. Comparison of femoral arterial blood pressure with radial arterial blood pressure and non-invasive upper arm blood pressure in the reperfusion period during liver transplantation. Transplant Proc. 2007;39:1326–8.
14. Thomas M, Kumar L, Jain P, Sarma C, Paul S, Surendran S. Correlation between radial and femoral arterial blood pressure during reperfusion in liv-

ing donor liver transplantation. Indian J Anaesth. 2021;65:302–8.

15. Sanei B, Shahabi S, Malek-Hosseini SA, Nikeghbalian S, Shamsaeifar A, Kakaei F, et al. Central venous catheterization in patients with liver disease and coagulopathy. Indian J Transplant. 2017;11:123–6.

16. Singh AS, Sharma S, Singh A, Singh AK, Sharma U, Bhadoria AS. The safety of ultrasound guided central venous cannulation in patients with liver disease. Saudi J Anaesth. 2015;2:155–60.

17. Kim JH. Should low central venous pressure be maintained during liver transplantation? Open Anesthesiol J. 2017;11:17–28.

18. Schechter MC, Prezzi EDV, Cabral G, Fernandes ESM, Vianna AOA. Pulmonary artery rupture with a Swan-Ganz catheter. Revista Brasileira de Terapia Intensiva. 2009. https://doi.org/10.1590/S0103-507X2009000200017.

19. Rudnick MR, De Marchi L, Plotkin JS. Hemodynamic monitoring during liver transplantation: a state of the art review. World J Hepatol. 2015;7:1302–11.

20. Vetrugno L, Bignami E, Barbariol F, Langiano N, De Lorenzo F, et al. Cardiac output measurement in liver transplantation patients using pulmonary and transpulmonary thermodilution: a comparative study. J Clin Monit Comput. 2019;33:223–31.

21. Robertson AC, Eagle SS. Trans esophageal echocardiography during orthotopic liver transplantation: maximizing information without the distraction. J Cardiothorac Vasc Anesth. 2014;28:141–54.

22. Hofer RE, Vogt MNP, Taner T, Findlay JY. Influence of intraoperative trans esophageal echocardiography and pulmonary artery catheter monitoring on outcomes in liver transplantation. Transplant Direct. 2020;6:e525.

23. Pai SL, Aniskevich S, Feinglass NG, Ladlie BL, CrawfoPeiris P, et al. Complications related to intraoperative trans esophageal echocardiography in liver transplantation. SpringerPlus. 2015;4:480.

24. Rothenberg DM, O'Connor CJ, Tuman KJ. Chapter 73, Anaesthesia and the hepatobiliary system. In: Miller RD, editor. Miller's anaesthesia. 8th ed. Philadelphia: Elsevier Saunders; 2014. p. 2244–61.

25. Figueira ERR, Rocha-Filho JA, Lanchotte C, Coelho AMM, Nakatani M, Tatebe ER, et al. Sevoflurane preconditioning plus postconditioning decreases inflammatory response with hemodynamic recovery in experimental liver ischemia reperfusion. Gastroenterol Res Pract. 2019;2019:5758984.

26. Snell DB, Cohen Mekelburg S, Weg R, Ghosh G, Buckholz AP, Mehta A, et al. Gastric food retention at endoscopy is associated with severity of liver cirrhosis. World J Hepatol. 2019;11:725–34.

27. Wang CH, Chen CL, Cheng KW, Huang CJ, Chen KH, Wang CC, et al. Bispectral index monitoring in healthy, cirrhotic, and end-stage liver disease patients undergoing hepatic operation. Transplant Proc. 2008;40:2489–91.

28. Kumar G, Sethi N, Pant D, Sood J, Singh A, Pandey S, et al. Comparison of bispectral index targeted end-tidal concentration of desflurane during three phases

of orthotopic liver transplantation. Indian J Anaesth. 2019;63:225–30.

29. Nissen P, Pacino H, Frederiksen HJ, Novovic S, Secher NH. Near-infrared spectroscopy for evaluation of cerebral autoregulation during orthotopic liver transplantation. Neurocrit Care. 2009;11:235. https://doi.org/10.1007/s12028-009-9226-8.

30. Ghidini F, Benetti E, Zucchetta P, Amigoni A, Gamba P, Castagnetti M. Transcutaneous near-infrared spectroscopy (NIRS) for monitoring kidney and liver allograft perfusion. Int J Clin Pract. 2021;75:e14034. https://doi.org/10.1111/ijcp.14034.

31. Maheshwari K, Turan A, Makarova N, Ma C, Esa WAS, Ruetzler K, et al. Saline versus lactated Ringer's solution: the saline or lactated Ringer's (SOLAR) trial. Anesthesiology. 2020;132:614–24.

32. Self WH, Semler MW, Wanderer JP, Wang L, Byrne DW, Collins SP, et al. SALT-ED Investigators. Balanced crystalloids versus saline in noncritically ill adults. N Engl J Med. 2018;378:819–28.

33. Brown RM, Wang L, Coston TD, Krishnan NI, Casey JD, Wanderer JP, Ehrenfeld JM, Byrne DW, Stollings JL, Siew ED, Bernard GR, Self WH, Rice TW, Semler MW. Balanced crystalloids versus saline in sepsis. A secondary analysis of the SMART clinical trial. Am J Respir Crit Care Med. 2019;200:1487–95.

34. Hand WR, Whiteley JR, Epperson TI, Tam L, Crego H, Wolf B, et al. Hydroxyethyl starch and acute kidney injury in orthotopic liver transplantation. Anesth Analg. 2015;120:619–26.

35. Clevenger B, Mallett SV. Transfusion and coagulation management in liver transplantation. World J Gastroenterol. 2014;20:6146–58.

36. Saner FH, Gieseler RK, Akız H, Canbay A, Görlinger K. Delicate balance of bleeding and thrombosis in end-stage liver disease and liver transplantation. Digestion. 2013;88:135–44.

37. Mallett SV. Clinical utility of viscoelastic tests of coagulation (TEG/ROTEM) in patients with liver disease and during liver transplantation. Semin Thromb Hemost. 2015;41:527–37.

38. Whiting D, DiNardo JA. TEG and ROTEM: technology and clinical applications. Am J Hematol. 2014;89:228–32.

39. Chow JH, Lee K, Abuelkasem E, Udekwu OR, Tanaka KA. Coagulation management during liver transplantation: use of fibrinogen concentrate, recombinant activated factor VII, prothrombin complex concentrate, and antifibrinolytics. Semin Cardiothorac Vasc Anaesth. 2018;22:164–73.

40. Srivastava P, Agarwal A, Jha A, Rodricks S, Malik T, Makki K, Singhal A, Vij V. Utility of prothrombin complex concentrate as first-line treatment modality of coagulopathy in patients undergoing liver transplantation: a propensity score-matched study. Clin Transpl. 2018;32:e13435.

41. Bhangui P, Bhangui P, Gupta N, Jolly AS, Bhalotra S, Sharma N, et al. Fast tracking in adult living donor liver transplantation: a case series of 15 patients. Indian J Anaesth. 2018;62:127–30.

Ischemia–Reperfusion Injury

16

Chandra Kant Pandey ⓘ, S. S. Nath ⓘ,
and Manish Tandon ⓘ

Abbreviations

ALT	Alanine aminotransferase
AST	Aspartate aminotransferase
ATP	Adenosine triphosphate
cAMP	Cyclic adenosine monophosphate
DNA	Deoxyribonucleic acid
ER	Endoplasmic reticulum
GM-CSF	Granulocyte-macrophage colony-stimulating factor
HO-1	Hemeoxygenase-1
HSP-70	Heat shock protein 70
IL	Interleukin
IPC	Ischemic preconditioning
IPostC	Ischemic postconditioning
IR	Ischemia reperfusion
IRI	Ischemia–reperfusion injury
KC	Kupffer cells
LDH	Lactate dehydrogenase
LT	Leukotriene
MDA	Malondialdehyde
NO	Nitric oxide
PKA	Protein kinase A
RAS	Renin angiotensin system
ROS	Reactive oxygen species
SIRT	Sirtuin
TNF	Tumor necrotizing factor

C. K. Pandey (✉)
Anesthesiology, Medanta Hospital, Lucknow, India

S. S. Nath
Anesthesiology and Critical Care Medicine, Dr.
RMILS, Lucknow, India

M. Tandon
Department of Anesthesia, Dharamshila Narayana
Superspeciality Hospital, New Delhi, India

16.1 Introduction

Ischemia has always been associated with immediate as well as delayed adverse consequences. Restoration of perfusion to ischemic tissues can also have adverse consequences. Reperfusion being invariably associated with ischemia and consequences of reperfusion are clubbed with those of ischemia and are together referred to as ischemia–reperfusion injury (IR).

Ischemia–reperfusion injury is referred in the context of solid organ transplantation, but has implications for varied vascular intervention like for peripheral vascular diseases, cardiac coronary interventions, and for vascular composite free myo-cutaneous flap surgery. The clinical manifestations of ischemia–reperfusion injury include myocardial hibernation, reperfusion arrhythmias, renal dysfunction, and multiple organ dysfunction syndrome. The pathophysiology underlying IR injury is same, yet subtle differences exist depending upon the organ and tissue bed affected. Therapeutic approaches therefore differ according to the injured organ, and it is important to manage immediate consequences of reperfusion following ischemia and subsequent impact on outcome of surgical intervention and implications for patient mortality and morbidity.

The pathophysiology of ischemia–reperfusion injury and pharmacological and non-pharmacological interventions to curtail the ischemia–reperfusion injury and recent advances in this context are discussed in this chapter.

16.2 Pathophysiology

There are two components of ischemia–reperfusion injury:

1. Ischemia
2. Reperfusion

16.2.1 Ischemia

Ischemia/reperfusion injury (IRI) is tissue damage induced by blood deprivation (ischemia) followed by reperfusion, during which a large number of various mediators are released that can lead to cellular and, eventually, organ dysfunction. The injury process is more extensive during the reperfusion period than the period of ischemia [1]. Ischemia deprives the tissue of metabolic supplies and oxygen leading to accumulation of metabolic wastes. Absence of oxygen supply causes depletion of energy reserves, Adenosine triphosphate (ATP) and glycogen in the ischemic tissue. Sodium-Potassium (Na-K) pumps that maintain the electrolytes gradient across the cell membrane being energy dependent, depleted energy reserves following ischemia, and shut down these NA-K pumps. Ion gradients across the cellular membrane are therefore not maintained [1]. Sodium ions move down the concentration gradient from extracellular space into the cells, whereas potassium ions move from intracellular space to extracellular milieu. The metabolic activity in the tissue switches from aerobic to anaerobic pathways causing lactate accumulation and intracellular acidosis. A vicious cycle is created with progressive decrease in efficacy of the energy apparatus of the cells. Reduced intracellular pH further inhibits glycolysis that cur-

tails the safe ischemia period and glycogen reserves remain underutilized [2].

Reduced intracellular pH with increased hydrogen ion concentration activates the Sodium/Hydrogen antiporter pumps to cause rise in intracellular sodium concentration. Increased intracellular sodium concentration causes secondary rise in intracellular calcium concentration. Sodium-calcium antiporter exchange pumps are inhibited with resultant accumulation of calcium in the cytosol [1, 2]. Calcium is also released from mitochondria via the mitochondrial Na^+-H^+/Ca^{2+} exchange pumps following rise in sodium and hydrogen ion concentration in cytosol. The raised intracellular calcium ion concentration binds and activates the regulatory protein calmodulin, which then activates Ca^{2+}-calmodulin-dependent protein kinases, phospholipase A_2, and proteases and causes degranulation from vesicles thereby releasing proinflammatory chemokines and cytokines like interleukin-8, Von-Willebrand factor, p-selectin, etc. [2].

Intracellular acidosis disrupts the hydrogen ion gradient across the mitochondrial membrane and thus ATP generation comes to a halt. Increases in reactive oxygen species (ROS) in the mitochondria, in the setting of increased intracellular Ca^{2+} and elevation of inorganic phosphate (Pi) levels due to accelerated ATP breakdown, prime the Mitochondrial-membrane Permeability Transition Pore (MPTP). But during the ischemic phase the low intracellular pH inhibits the MPTP opening [1, 2]. Thus, the duration of ischemia that a tissue may tolerate is decided by the extent of metabolic activity of the tissue and the tissue reserves for metabolic supplies. Brain with very high metabolic activity with no or very minimal metabolic reserves is highly susceptible to ischemia whereas muscles with reasonable glycogen reserves can tolerate ischemia for a considerable period of time before irreversible injury may happen.

16.2.2 Reperfusion

The reperfusion of ischemic tissue triggers a series of local and systemic pathophysiologic pathways which culminate in cell death by necrosis, apoptosis (programmed death), and autophagy. Necrosis is an uncontrolled phenomenon and is associated with the state of inflammation whereas apoptosis is a regulated and programmed cell death without inflammation. Apotosis is a form of programmed cell death that is achieved by intracellular changes associated with reperfusion following ischemia and includes increased ROS production and sequestration of intracellular Ca^{2+} into mitochondria via the Na^+-Ca^{2+} antiporter upon return to normal intracellular pH. Oxygen free radicals generated during ischemia and upon reperfusion are key for opening of MPTP. During the ischemic phase, MPTP which was kept from opening by low intracellular pH, correction of acidosis upon reperfusion, allows opening of MPTP and drives necrotic cell death by mitoptosis. MPTP pore opening results in increased permeability of the outer mitochondrial membrane and the release of proapoptotic proteins (such as cytochrome C). Loss of cytochrome C from the mitochondrial membrane initiates the vicious cycle of decreased aerobic cellular respiration and increased ROS and consequently increased apoptosis activity [1, 2]. During normal physiological conditions also, there is a continuous, low magnitude leak of electrons from the electron transport chain resulting in the formation of ROS. But during IR, this electron leak is amplified and ROS formation is enhanced. Mitochondria contain Mn-superoxide dismutase (MnSOD), glutathione and glutathione peroxidase, thioredoxin-2, and glutaredoxin, which neutralize the ROS and help repair the cell but these are overwhelmed during ischemia and reperfusion [1, 2].

ROS generated during IR activate proapoptotic proteins, e.g., B cell lymphoma-2 gene (Bcl-2) homology (BH) domains coded BH_3-only proteins. These ROS are produced from enzymatic sources as well as from non-enzymatic sources [2]. Enzymatic sources include the xanthine oxidase system, NADPH oxidase system, mitochondrial electron transport chain, and uncoupled nitric oxide synthase (NOS) system. Non-enzymatic sources include hemoglobin and myoglobin [2]. Xanthine oxidase system,

NADPH oxidase system, and mitochondrial electron transport chain are implicated in oxidative stress induced dysfunction in the intestine, lung, heart, brain, muscle, liver, pancreas, stomach, and kidney, whereas the NOS is considered to play a role in the liver, heart, and aortic endothelial cells dysfunction [2]. These enzymatic systems are the targets of virtually all the therapeutic interventions aimed at managing the ischemia–reperfusion injury.

Neo-antigens are expressed in ischemic tissue. Innate and adaptive immune systems of body mount autoimmune response subsequently upon reperfusion against these neo-antigens with consequent activation of the complement system and inflammatory pathways [2]. Leukocytes, neutrophils, and platelets are activated which then propagate the systemic ill effects of reperfusion following ischemia [2]. Tumor necrosis factor-α (TNF-α) is released from activated macrophages and is an important proapoptotic agent through the induction of multiple cellular pathways, including non-canonical Nuclear Factor-kappa B (NF-κB). The activation of NF-kB regulates cell survival, apoptosis, and inflammation, via effectors such as MnSOD, Bcl-2, TNF-α, ICAM, and P-selectin [2].

The liver is one of the most frequently affected organs. Liver transplantation-associated IRI plays an important role in the induction of graft injury. Prolonged cold ischemia time remains a risk factor for poor liver graft outcome, especially when steatosis is present. Steatotic liver exhibits endoplasmic reticulum (ER) stress, which occurs in response to cold IRI. Also, there is defective liver autophagy which correlates with liver damage [3]. IR (ischemia–reperfusion) associated with hepatic resections and liver transplantation remain a serious complication in clinical practice. The redox balance, which is pivotal for normal function and integrity of tissues, is dysregulated during IR, leading to an accumulation of reactive oxygen species (ROS). ROS are normally generated during the mitochondrial energy metabolism via oxidative phosphorylation in the respiratory chain. The redox balance is well maintained because of the presence of antioxidant systems. During IR the production of

ROS is increased manyfold and so this delicate balance is disturbed. This increased ROS consumes the endogenous antioxidants and induces the expression of antioxidant enzymes in order to maintain the redox balance. When the IR is severe, inadequacy of the compensatory responses becomes evident. This gives rise to oxidant stress leading to inflammatory responses and hepatic damage [4].

The destructive effects of IR result from the acute generation of ROS subsequent to oxygenation. These ROS inflict tissue damage and initiate a cascade of deleterious cellular responses leading to inflammation, cell death, and organ failure. This is the reason why formation of ROS and oxidative stress are the mechanisms of IR that are most commonly debated upon. During IR-induced donor hepatic damage, oxidant stress depends on the donor conditions (steatotic, small for size, and aged livers). These marginal livers suffer more pronounced oxidant stress from exposure to IR compared to histologically normal livers [4].

The hepatic IR injury can be divided into initial and late phases. The initial phase which occurs within 2 h of reperfusion wherein the excessive ROS cause tissue damage and cell death by binding and altering cellular macromolecules (including DNA, proteins, and lipids), thus affecting their function. There is also activation of macrophages which are the primary source of extracellular ROS. This, in turn, leads to endothelial injury and further release of proinflammatory cytokines [5, 6]. There is also activation of Kupffer cells (KC), which is further amplified by CD4+ T lymphocytes via Granulocyte-Macrophage Colony-Stimulating Factor (GM-CSF) and interferon gamma. Xanthine dehydrogenase is metabolized to xanthine oxidase during hypoxia, and upon reperfusion, it reacts with oxygen to produce ROS. Oxidant stress is a potent trigger of mitochondria permeability and transition pore opening in hepatocytes. As a result, the mitochondrial membrane potential collapses leading to failure

of ATP production and finally cell death [7]. In the late phase of injury, which occurs between 6 and 24 h after reperfusion, an evolving inflammatory process occurs that is mediated by oxidants of extrahepatic cellular origin [8]. This late phase of IR injury is caused by neutrophil activation, ROS, TNF-alpha, and IL-1beta, and it results in more substantial injury. There is also upregulation of and expression of inducible nitric oxide synthase, creating large quantities of NO that results in further creation of ROS and oxidative stress in marginal livers undergoing IR [9].

1. **Steatotic liver:** Fatty hepatocytes have an increased sensitivity to the injurious effects of ROS and thus they tolerate poorly the onslaught of IR. These livers are more susceptible than nonsteatotic livers to lipid peroxidation because of either lower antioxidant defense or their greater production of ROS or both [10].

2. **Aged liver:** Age had been postulated to influence the sensitivity of the liver to oxidative stress. All the information had been derived from animal studies. During warm ischemia, mature adult mice had increased neutrophil function, increased intracellular oxidant, and decreased mitochondrial function compared with young adult mice. A vicious cycle has been proposed, in which damaged mitochondria produce progressively greater amounts of ROS, leading to progressively greater damage to mitochondrial, cytosolic and nuclear components, and finally resulting in dysfunctional mitochondria. Also, mature mice liver had much lower hepatic expression of a cytoprotective protein, heat shock protein 70 (HSP70), than did young adult mice [4].

3. **Small-for-size liver graft**: Small-for-size liver grafts are more vulnerable to IR injury after transplantation than are standard-size liver grafts [11]. ROS originating after reperfusion are known to induce DNA damage and inhibit cell division after hepatectomy [12].

16.3 Global Effects of Hepatic Ischemia–Reperfusion Injury

Deleterious effects of hepatic ischemia–reperfusion injury are not limited to the liver alone but also involve several distant organs like kidneys, myocardium, lungs, pancreas, intestine, and adrenals leading to their dysfunction and injury. Thus, it represents an event with global consequences. This involvement of multiple organs leads to multiple organ dysfunction syndrome. Remote organ injury seems to be, in part, the result of the oxidative burst and the inflammatory response following reperfusion [13].

1. **Injury to the Kidneys:** The mechanism of renal injury following hepatic IRI is multifactorial. The trigger for renal injury seems to be portal hypertension, which occurs due to portal vein occlusion, which is an important step in the vascular control of the liver during hepatic surgery. This leads to splanchnic vasodilation with subsequent infrarenal vasoconstriction. Splanchnic vasodilation leads to hypotension which in turn leads to activation of renin angiotensin system (RAS). Upregulation of RAS can cause severe reduction of glomerular filtration rate, urinary sodium excretion, and free water excretion. It has been proposed that intense infrarenal ischemia subsequent to RAS activation leads to renal tubular necrosis and renal dysfunction [13]. Other mechanisms have also been proposed including systemic inflammatory response following hepatic IRI leading to renal injury [14].

2. **Myocardial Injury:** A porcine model of liver IR showed a relatively subtle yet consistent injury to the myocardium early after liver ischemia/reperfusion, manifested mainly by increase in cardiac troponin I blood levels and confirmed histologically by myocardiocyte necrosis [15].

3. **Lung Injury:** Lung injury and acute respiratory distress syndrome can severely complicate the postoperative course following liver transplantation. Lung injury occurs following extensive hepatectomies and reperfusion of

donor liver during transplantation. The mechanism is again multifactorial. One of the proposed mechanisms is the release of TNF-α from reperfused Kupffer cells, which interacts with pulmonary capillaries and elicits the expression of adhesion molecules, such as E-selectin, leading to migration of neutrophils and subsequent lung injury [16]. In combination with TNF-α, a variety of proinflammatory molecules are released from the reperfused liver and have been found to mediate lung injury after hepatic IR. Another important mechanism is the translocation of endotoxin to the systemic circulation and spill over into the pulmonary circulation because of insufficiency of Kupffer cells. Bacterial translocation is evident after liver resection under vascular control even after the creation of a portosystemic shunt. Oxidative stress during hepatic IR has been consistently shown to play a crucial role in the development of lung injury.

4. **Gut Injury**: Gut barrier failure in the form of bacterial and/or endotoxin translocation as well as other forms of intestinal dysfunction including motility, transit time, and absorption function changes has been reported following liver IR [17]. Multiple causes have been proposed, but the exact pathophysiology is unclear. Experimental data suggest that intestinal mucosa oxidative injury results from the effect of liver-produced ROS, which are "spilled" in the systemic circulation. The proposed mechanism of oxidative injury to the gut mucosa from liver derived ROS is damage of the tight junctions between enterocytes, which results in increased permeability and gut barrier failure. Another suggested mechanism is congestion of the portal venous system because of the Pringle maneuver. Apoptosis is also implicated in gut mucosal injury following liver ischemia and reperfusion, since it is already known that extracellular free radicals can induce cell apoptosis [17].

5. **Pancreatic Injury:** Pancreatic dysfunction and rarely acute pancreatitis have been reported following hepatectomies. Although

the reason is unclear, the key factor of post-hepatectomy pancreatitis is thought to be the production of ROS, resulting in remote organ injury. The measured MDA (malonaldehyde) content of portal blood and pancreatic tissue samples, which suggested lipid peroxidation and oxidative damage, increased during liver reperfusion. In addition, there was increased amylase and c-peptide levels during reperfusion and histological evidence of pancreatic necrosis [18]. These data support the hypothesis that ROS and oxidative stress, as assessed by lipid peroxidation and tissue necrosis, play a crucial role in pancreatitis following liver ischemia/reperfusion combined with hepatectomy [18].

6. **Adrenal Injury:** Relative adrenal dysfunction following liver ischemia/reperfusion has been reported to have an incidence of 92% [19]. Moreover, there are reports of macroscopic injury to the adrenals following hepatectomy under vascular control and orthotopic liver transplantation. A possible proposed mechanism is the decreased levels of high-density lipoprotein (HDL) after liver transplantation and thus decreased cortisol synthesis. HDL levels have been shown to be a predictor of posttransplant relative adrenal insufficiency [20]. During the anhepatic phase, the liver does not produce apoA-1 (which is essential for the formation of HDL) for a number of hours. In addition, the transplanted liver suffers IRI that is responsible for postoperative liver dysfunction. ApoA-1 has a relatively short half-life and, therefore, the HDL levels are decreased after transplantation. Liver IR has been shown to increase the levels of endotoxin, as well as various cytokines, which have been shown to inhibit steroidogenesis. These cytokines have been shown to decrease synthesis and secretion of apoA-1 [21]. Endotoxin has been reported to bind to the HDL receptor, neutralizing it [20]. Also, TNF-α has been demonstrated to directly inhibit steroidogenesis and increase resistance to cortisol [20].

16.4 Measures to Ameliorate Hepatic Ischemia–Reperfusion Injury

16.4.1 Pharmacological Measures

1. **Melatonin:** Melatonin is a powerful antioxidant produced by the pineal gland. Melatonin and its metabolites have potent antioxidant/anti-inflammatory properties and have been proved to be highly effective in a variety of disorders linked to inflammation and oxidative stress. Melatonin not only neutralizes reactive nitrogen species (RNS) and reactive oxygen species (ROS) but also stimulates several antioxidant enzymes, such as SOD, GRed, and GPx thereby stabilizing cell membranes [21]. The combined protective effects of melatonin and trimetazidine as additives to the Institute George Lopez 1 (IGL-1) solution improved steatotic liver graft preservation. It achieves this through activation of adenosine monophosphate activated protein kinase (AMPK) which in turn reduces ER stress and promotes autophagy after cold IR [22]. Since melatonin is endogenously produced and has a low toxicity profile, and upto 5 miligrams per kilograms of melatonin is well tolerated. Beyond 5 mg/kg, melatonin has been reported to cause elevation of liver enzymes, plasma creatinine, and LDH levels [22]. Thus, although melatonin shows promise in reducing damage and molecular changes associated with IRI, the biological functions of melatonin remain only partially characterized and further human studies are needed [21].

2. **Role of Anesthetic Inhalational Agents:** The prognosis of IRI can be improved by inhibiting the expression of endogenous cytokines. Also, sevoflurane pretreatment group had significantly lower TNF-alpha, IL-8, and IL-6 concentration. There was much increased IL-10 level. Also, MDA (malondialdehyde) and nitric oxide (NO) were lower and SOD concentrations were significantly higher in this group compared with the group not

treated with sevoflurane. Sevoflurane had been reported to significantly reduce IRI by a variety of physiological processes like reducing oxygen free radicals, inhibiting inflammatory reactions, reducing intracellular calcium overload as well as improving the energy metabolism of liver cells [23, 24]. Isoflurane, another inhalation agent, which is more commonly used, also can protect against ischemia–reperfusion injury at clinically relevant levels [25].

3. **Sirtuins:** To date, seven sirtuins have been described in mammals. Sirtuin 1 (SIRT1) plays an important role in several processes ranging from cell cycle regulation to energy homeostasis. They have emerged as critical modulators of various processes including those that contribute to pathogenesis of IRI. SIRT1 has been shown to exert its beneficial effect against oxidative stress and hypoxic injury or inflammation associated with IRI. Also, studies have demonstrated key roles for SIRT1 and SIRT3 in brain, heart, and kidney IRI. However, the protective effects of these sirtuins against IRI in the liver have not been demonstrated [26]. SIRT1 had been shown to have protective effects of hyperbaric oxygen preconditioning against apoptosis in the rat brain. However, its possible implication in IPC-related mechanisms in other organs, including the liver or kidney, remains to be elucidated [26].

4. **Octreotide:** Octreotide is a synthetic octapeptide. It resembles somatostatin in physiological activities, reduces portal hypertension, retards gastrointestinal tumor growth, and also inhibits the release of growth hormone. Inhibition of autophagy after IR can lead to increased hepatocyte death. Induction of autophagy can protect animals from hepatic IR injury. In a rat IR model, it was shown that single dose of octreotide conferred hepatoprotective effects [27]. It was speculated that the protective effects of octreotide was by induction of heme-oxygenate 1 enzyme (HO-1). HO-1 is a stress inducible enzyme that has anti-inflammatory, antiapoptotic, and antioxi-

dant properties. During hepatic IR, HO-1 has been shown to confer its protection by modulating oxidative stress and inflammation [27].

5. **Montelukast:** Montelukast is a selective reversible cys LT-1 receptor antagonist which was used in asthma and reduced eosinophilic inflammation. In a rat model, rats were pretreated with 7 mg/kg of montelukast 30 min prior to ischemia. Compared to control group, those pretreated with montelukast had markedly attenuated liver tissue injury and liver damage as evidenced by reduced serum AST, ALT, LDH, TNF-alpha, IL-1B, MDA (malondialdehyde), and myeloperoxidase (MPO) levels after hepatic ischemia of 45 min. In the control group, hepatic IRI induced marked increase in cysL TR1, Caspase-8 and caspase-9 protein expression in the liver [28]. Thus, it was concluded that montelukast reduces IR-induced neutrophil accumulation, oxidative stress, and liver dysfunction. The therapeutic effects of montelukast on IRI can be attributed to its ability to inhibit neutrophil infiltration and regulate generation of inflammatory mediators. Thus, it could have a future role in the treatment of liver failure due to IRI [28].

6. **Milrinone:** Some agents like milrinone had been postulated to demonstrate effects akin to mechanical postconditioning, so-called pharmacological inducers of postconditioning. Milrinone, a phosphodiesterase-3 inhibitor, is an inotropic agent, acting through elevation of intracellular cyclic adenosine monophosphate (cAMP) and protein kinase A (PKA) activation. It has been shown that it also has preconditioning properties against hepatic IR injury, exerted via the same pathway (cAMP/PKA activation) [29]. In a liver warm ischemia model of 1-h duration followed by 5 h of reperfusion showed that milrinone administered as an intravenous bolus immediately after reperfusion effectively attenuated liver injury, as demonstrated by reduced AST, ALT, and LDH serum levels and reduced histologic damage and apoptotic scores in milrinone-treated animals, as compared to controls [30].

16.4.2 Surgical

1. **Ischemic Preconditioning (IPC):** IPC is the method by which the target organ is conditioned with a brief ischemic period followed by reperfusion prior to the subsequent prolonged ischemic insult in order to attenuate the extent of injury [31]. IPC has been adopted in liver surgery and tested in several experimental and clinical contexts, proving to be an effective intervention, since it seems to increase the ability of the liver to withstand the subsequent prolonged period of ischemia [32]. Adenosine and NO seem to play a significant role in the IPC effect and favorable responses such as decreased hepatocellular injury, inhibition of apoptosis, improved liver microcirculation, and enhanced energy metabolism have been documented through the application of IPC [33]. Regarding the clinical setting, in spite of favorable effects of enzyme markers of liver injury, recent meta-analyses failed to reveal a sustained clinical benefit of IPC, in terms of duration of hospital stay, perioperative morbidity, or mortality [34, 35]. The main limitation of IPC techniques in the clinical context is that they must be initiated before the ischemic insult, which is not always predictable [31].

2. **Ischemic Postconditioning (IPostC):** IPostC consisted of several brief pre-reperfusions, consecutively, each separated by short occlusion time, followed by the sustained reperfusion. The beneficial effects of IPostC have been documented in several experimental studies in different organs and confirmed in human clinical studies in the heart [31]. In adult cadaveric liver transplantation, grafts subjected to postconditioning presented less severe histopathological lesions of IR injury and increased activation of autophagy in periportal areas [36]. Unlike donor preconditioning, which is not always feasible, graft postconditioning in the recipient seems to be more attractive since it can be applied selectively in settings prone to greater risks for IR injury due to donor, procurement, or recipient-related factors and can prove useful in complex cases requiring long periods of ischemia or with marginal grafts [36]. IPostC may also be incorporated in non-transplant complex cases needing long periods of ischemia, in cases of unexpected ischemia, where there is limited clinical applicability for IPC, and during major hepatectomies, with marginal liver remnants. By applying IPostC, a 30% reduction of liver cell necrosis was demonstrated which could be crucial for compromised livers [37]. Such resections can be complicated by bleeding, which is often unpredictable, and bleeding has to be controlled by clamping. In this context, IPC is not a feasible option and IPostC is the technique of choice because it can be applied after clamping to ensure the survival of as much liver parenchyma as possible. Further. IpostC has demonstrated favorable effect on liver regeneration as well as the requirement for less operative time, in contrast to preconditioning techniques making IPostC clinically more attractive to implement [38].

16.5 Summary

Hypoxia and ischemia induce anaerobic metabolism and dysfunction of the electron transport chain in mitochondria. Decreased ATP production that occurs causes dysfunction of ion-exchange channels, leading to retention of sodium, hydrogen, and calcium, which results in cell swelling and impaired enzyme activity in the cytoplasm.

The outcome of ischemia is thus dependent on the duration of ischemia. Prolonged ischemia and reperfusion lead to apoptosis, autophagy, necrosis, and necroptosis whereas moderate duration of ischemia followed by reperfusion induces ischemia–reperfusion injury and activates recovery systems and damage control mechanisms. A shorter duration of ischemia followed by reperfusion is considered to activate cell survival programs to control ROS generation and cell damage. Strategies are being explored in lab and in clinical setting using pharmacological and mechanical means to confer protection against ischemia and reperfusion injury. Application of the available modalities in combination like combining ischemic pre- and postconditioning, pharmacological with mechanical pre- and post-ischemic preconditioning is being tried until such time that a standard ischemic conditioning organ-specific protocol evolves which would require better understanding of the molecular mechanisms involved.

References

1. Kalogeris T, Baines CP, Krenz M, Korthuis RJ. Cell biology of ischemia/reperfusion injury. Int Rev Cell Mol Biol. 2012;298:229–317.
2. Fukazawa K, Lang JD. Role of nitric oxide in liver transplantation: should it be routinely used? World J Hepatol. 2016;8:1489–96.
3. Murry CE, Jennings RB, Reimer KA. Preconditioning with ischemia: a delay of lethal cell injury in ischemic myocardium. Circulation. 1986;74:1124–36.
4. Elias Miro M, Jimenez Castro MB, Rotes J, Peralta C. Current knowledge on oxidative stress in hepatic ischemia/reperfusion. Free Radic Res. 2013;47:555–68.
5. Tapuria N, Kumar Y, Habib MM, Abu Amara M, Seifalian AM, Davidson BR. Remote ischemic preconditioning: a novel protective method from ischemia reperfusion injury. J Surg Res. 2008;150:304–30.
6. Cutrin JC, Perrelli MG, Cavalieri B, Peralta C, Rosell Catafau J, Poli G. Microvascular dysfunction induced by reperfusion injury and protective effect of ischemic preconditioning. Free Radic Biol. 2002;33:1200–8.
7. Casillas-Ramirez A, Mosbah IB, Ramalho F, Rosello-Catafau J, Peralta C. Past and future approaches to ischemia reperfusion lesion associated with liver transplantation. Life Sci. 2006;79:1881–94.
8. Fernandez L, Heredia N, Grande L, Gomez G, Rimola A, Marco A, et al. Preconditioning protects liver and lung damage in rat liver transplantation: role of xanthine/xanthine oxidase. Hepatology. 2002;36:562–73.
9. Jaeschke H. Xanthine oxidase-induced oxidant stress during hepatic ischemia-reperfusion: are we coming full circle after 20 years? Hepatology. 2002;36:761–3.
10. Massip-Salcedo M, Rosello-Catafau J, Prieto J, Avila MA, Peralta C. The response of hepatocyte to ischemia. Liver Int. 2007;27:6–16.
11. Theodoraki K, Arkadopoulos N, Nastos C, Vassilios I, Karmaniolou I, Smyrniotis V. Small liver remnants are more vulnerable to ischemia/reperfusion injury after extended hepatectomies: a case control study. World J Surg. 2012;36:2895–900.
12. Franco-Gou R, Rosello-Catafau J, Casillas-Ramirez A, Massip-Salcedo M, Rimola A, Calvo N, et al. How ischemic preconditioning protects small liver grafts. J Pathol. 2006;208:62–73.
13. Nastos C, Kalimeris K, Papoutsidakis N, et al. Global consequences of liver ischemia/reperfusion injury. Oxidative Med Cell Longev. 2014;2014:906965. https://doi.org/10.1155/2014/906965.
14. Davis CL, Gonwa TA, Wilkinson AH. Pathophysiology of renal disease associated with liver disorders: implications for liver transplantation. Part I. Liver Transpl. 2002;8:91–102.
15. Papoutsidakis N, Arkadopoulos N, Smyrniotis V, et al. Early myocardial injury is an integral component of experimental acute liver failure—a study in two porcine models. Arch Med Sci. 2011;l7:217–23.
16. Colletti LM, Cortis A, Lukacs N, Kunkel SL, Green M, Strieter RM. Tumor necrosis factor up-regulates intercellular adhesion molecule 1, which is important in the neutrophil-dependent lung and liver injury associated with hepatic ischemia and reperfusion in the rat. Shock. 1998;10:182–91.
17. Zheyu C, Lunan Y. Early changes of small intestine function in rats after liver transplantation. Transplant Proc. 2006;38:1564–8.
18. Arkadopoulos N, Nastos C, Defterevos G, et al. Pancreatic injury after major hepatectomy: a study in a porcine model. Surg Today. 2012;42:368–75.
19. Iwasak I, Tominaga M, Fukumoto T, et al. Relative adrenal insufficiency manifested with multiple organ dysfunction in a liver transplant patient. Liver Transpl. 2006;12:1896–9.
20. Marik PE, Gayowski T, Starzl TE. The hepatoadrenal syndrome: a common yet unrecognized clinical condition. Crit Care Med. 2005;33:1254–9.
21. Li Y, Yang Y, Feng Y, et al. A review of melatonin in hectic ischemia/reperfusion injury and clinical liver disease. Ann Med. 2014;46:503–11.
22. Zaouli MA, Boncompagni E, Reiter RJ, et al. AMPK involvement in endoplasmic reticulum stress and autophagy modulation. after fatty liver graft preservation: a role for melatonin and trimetazidine cocktail. J Pineal Res. 2013;55:65–78.
23. Lucchinetti E, Wang L, Ko KWS, et al. Enhanced glucose uptake via GLUT4 fuels recovery from calcium overload after ischemia reperfusion injury in sevoflurane but not propofol treated hearts. Br J Anesth. 2011;106:792–800.
24. Li J, Yuang T, Zhao X, et al. Protective effects of sevoflurane in hepatic ischemia reperfusion injury. Int J Immunopathol Pharmacol. 2016;29:300–7.
25. Lv X, Yang L, Tao K, et al. Isoflurane preconditioning at clinically relevant doses induce protective effects of heme oxygenase-1 on hepatic ischemia reperfusion in rats. BMC Gastroenterol. 2011;11:31.
26. Yan W, Fang Z, Yang Q, Dong H, Lu Y, Lei C, Xiong L. SirT1 mediates hyperbaric oxygen preconditioning-induced ischemic tolerance in rat brain. J Cereb Blood Flow Metab. 2013;33:396–406.
27. Zou S, Sun H, Candiotti KA, et al. Octreotide protects against hepatic ischemia/reperfusion injury via HO-1 mediated autophagy. Acta Biochem Biophys Sin. 2018;50:316–8.

28. Lee JC. Therapeutic effects of montelukast in hepatic ischemia reperfusion injury in rats. Our J Anat. 2018;22:201–12.

29. Satoh K, Kume M, Abe Y, et al. Implication of protein kinase A for a hepato-protective mechanism of milrinone pretreatment. J Surg Res. 2009;155:32–9.

30. Toyoda T, Tosaka S, Tosaka R, et al. Milrinone-induced postconditioning reduces hepatic ischemia-reperfusion injury in rats: the roles of phosphatidylinositol 3-kinase and nitric oxide. J Surg Res. 2014;186:446–51.

31. Theodoraki K, Karmaniolou I, Tympa A, Tasoulis MK, Nastos C, Vassiliou I, Arkadopoulos N, Smyrniotis V. Beyond preconditioning: postconditioning as an alternative technique in the prevention of liver ischemia-reperfusion injury. Oxidative Med Cell Longev. 2016;2016:8235921. https://doi.org/10.1155/2016/8235921.

32. Suzuki S, Inaba K, Konno H. Ischemic preconditioning in hepatic ischemia and reperfusion. Curr Opin Organ Transplant. 2008;13:142–7.

33. Alchera E, Dal Ponte C, Imarisio C, Albano E, Carini R. Molecular mechanisms of liver preconditioning. World J Gastroenterol. 2010;16:6058–67.

34. Gurusamy KS, Kumar Y, Pamecha V, Sharma D, Davidson BR. Ischemic pre-conditioning for elective liver resections performed under vascular occlusion. Cochrane Database Syst Rev. 2009;(1):CD007629.

35. O'Neill S, Leuschner S, McNally SJ, Garden OJ, Wigmore SJ, Harrison EM. Meta-analysis of ischemic preconditioning for liver resections. Br J Surg. 2013;100:1689–700.

36. Ricca L, Lemoine A, Cauchy F, Hamelin J, Sebagh M, Esposti DD, Salloum C, Vibert E, Balducci G, Azoulay D. Ischemic postconditioning of the liver graft in adult liver transplantation. Transplantation. 2015;99:1633–43.

37. Knudsen AR, Kannerup AS, Grønbæk H, Dutoit SH, Nyengaard JR, Funch-Jensen P, Mortensen FV. Quantitative histological assessment of hepatic ischemia-reperfusion injuries following ischemic pre- and post-conditioning in the rat liver. J Surg Res. 2013;180:e11–20.

38. Young SB, Pires ARC, Boaventura GT, Ferreira AMR, Martinho JMSG, Galhardo MA. Effect of ischemic preconditioning and postconditioning on liver regeneration in prepubertal rats. Transplant Proc. 2014;46:1867–71.

C. Patrick Henson and Ann Walia

Over the last five decades, Liver Transplantation (LT) surgical technique, anesthetic management and graft, and patient survival have undergone significant improvement. Despite these improvements, the intraoperative management of the patient undergoing LT remains challenging and is often accompanied by hemodynamic instability [1]. The pathophysiology of cirrhotic liver disease results in systemic vasodilation, altered circulating and total body volume status, and may be complicated by other organ system dysfunction [2]. This level of hemodynamic instability requires the use of a variety of hemodynamic monitors.

Liver transplant itself can be divided into three distinct phases: the pre-anhepatic phase, the anhepatic phase, and the neohepatic phase. Each phase has its own distinctive hemodynamic challenges [3, 4].

The pre-anhepatic phase is the dissection phase and is marked by significant changes in preload from large volume ascites drainage and acute and occasionally large volume blood loss, in addition to procedurally necessary manipulation of the liver and the vena cava.

During the anhepatic phase, the portal vein and inferior vena cava (IVC) are clamped and may result in decreased cardiac output (CO) by up to 50% under total venous occlusion (TVO) technique. This decrease is less dramatic under "piggyback" technique when the IVC is only partially occluded. Other forms of liver isolation which decrease blood loss include portocaval shunt and venovenous bypass. The technique for liver isolation is center dependent and patient specific [1, 5].

The neohepatic stage is when the newly implanted liver is reperfused and connected to the systemic circulation. This phase is marked by hemodynamic changes due to rapid return of blood from a previously obstructed portal system and the returned blood tends to be cold, acidotic, hyperkalemic, and contains a variety of inflammatory and vasoactive mediators [3, 5].

This results in transient but often significant decrease in myocardial contractility, systemic vascular resistance (SVR), chronotropy, and possible rise in pulmonary pressure.

C. P. Henson
Clinical Anesthesiology, Division of Critical Care, Vanderbilt University Medical Center, Nashville, TN, USA
e-mail: Patrick.henson@vumc.org

A. Walia (✉)
Chair, Anesthesiology, Perioperative, Pain Management and Critical Care, Tennessee Valley Healthcare System, Nashville, TN, USA

Professor of Anesthesiology, Vanderbilt University Medical Center, Nashville, TN, USA
e-mail: Ann.walia@vumc.org, ann.walia@va.gov

17.1 Blood Pressure

Given the potential for rapid changes in hemodynamics, invasive blood pressure (BP) monitoring is the standard for patients undergoing LT [1, 6]. The number and location of these lines vary by individual preference and center protocols. Cannulation of the radial artery provides safe and reliable blood pressure monitoring in nearly all patients. However, monitoring at a distal site, while convenient, does come with limitations. In certain situations, such as when high-dose vasopressors are being administered or when patients are in circulatory shock, the systolic pressures measured at the radial site are less reliable, and measurement of central arterial pressure via the femoral artery may provide more consistent pressure monitoring. However, even with this discrepancy, the mean arterial pressure tends to be consistent between the two sites [6, 7].

Risks of arterial cannulation for blood pressure monitoring include arterial or venous injury, bleeding, and nerve damage. While these risks are not theoretically different between femoral and peripheral sites, the femoral site cannot be visualized or easily evaluated during the procedure, and problems such as vascular bleeding may not be readily apparent. Specific situations may require more central cannulation despite the slightly higher risks of cannulating the femoral artery in select patients. Cannulation of the axillary or brachial artery can be considered, as well. Historically, there has been concern that the risk of nerve injury and ischemic injury may be higher with more proximal upper extremity cannulation, although recent data suggests that both are safe alternatives [8, 9]. Our observation over the past three decades has shown consistent discrepancies in radial and central pressures (systolic, diastolic, and mean) especially right after reperfusion and with the use of high-dose vasopressors. Extreme vasodilatory state which decreases distal pressure disproportionately to central pressure may be the cause of the variance post-reperfusion although none of the studies have consistently demonstrated this [10, 11]. Interestingly, one study showed that noninvasive BP measurement in the upper extremity more closely reflected central pressures than the radial invasive pressure, presumably due to the proximal location of the cuff [12].

In addition to the hemodynamic monitoring provided by arterial lines, the ability to measure arterial blood for gas exchange and metabolic demand is absolutely necessary for the safe performance of liver transplantation, given the potential risk of profound acid-base and electrolyte derangement.

17.2 Central Venous Pressure

Central venous access and measurement of central volume status via a catheter placed in the superior vena cava is standard practice during LT, although its utility in predicting such is often called into question.

The ideal use of CVP appears to be as a practical measure of volume status, where high values suggest volume adequacy or overload, and low values hypovolemia or underfilling. Unfortunately, in nearly all clinical scenarios, CVP as a variable only poorly reflects stroke volume and cardiac output, which are the clinically significant variables of concern. In cirrhotic patients with hyperdynamic circulations, some degree of portopulmonary hypertension, and concomitant ventricular hypertrophy and cardiomyopathy, the reliability of CVP is even more questionable. Additionally, studies of the impact of CVP in non-cirrhotic patients should not necessarily be expected to accurately reflect the altered physiology that occurs during LT.

Increased CVP has been implicated as a risk factor for complications during liver resection [13]. Maintenance of lower CVP during liver resection surgery has been associated with reduced blood loss, transfusion, risk of postoperative fluid overload, and secondary complications, such as pulmonary and gastrointestinal edema [13–15]. Reduced CVP/right atrial pressure allows for passive reduction in IVC pressure, which helps drainage of the hepatic venous system, reduced tension on the liver and associated venous structures. This may directly impact surgical bleeding during dissection and postoperatively, but also may increase the risk of air embolism and hypotension as a result of low stroke volume.

In patients with significant portal hypertension, the portomesenteric vasculature is already under pressure, and maintaining low CVP will theoretically help reduce this.

However, studies and expert opinion are mixed with regard to the actual benefit of low CVP in the LT patient, as most studies have excluded these patients in favor of those undergoing liver resection. In addition, use of artificial means to lower this number, such as systemic vasodilators and phlebotomy, may increase other risks of end-organ hypoperfusion. Thus, the accuracy and utility of the actual number remains unclear, and, ultimately, trends in CVP during the surgical procedure may be of most value [16, 17].

17.3 Invasive Cardiac Output Monitoring

In addition to the ability to measure CVP and administer vasopressors and accomplish large volume resuscitation, the presence of a central venous catheter of adequate size (typically at least eight French) may provide a conduit for pulmonary artery catheterization. Data from a pulmonary artery catheter (PAC) can provide information on intracardiac filling pressures, pulmonary hypertension, or alterations in cardiac output (CO), which all may be useful, especially in the patient with preexisting cardiac dysfunction (Fig. 17.1). Hemodynamic derangements are to be expected during all phases of LT, and monitoring of CO using PAC may provide valuable

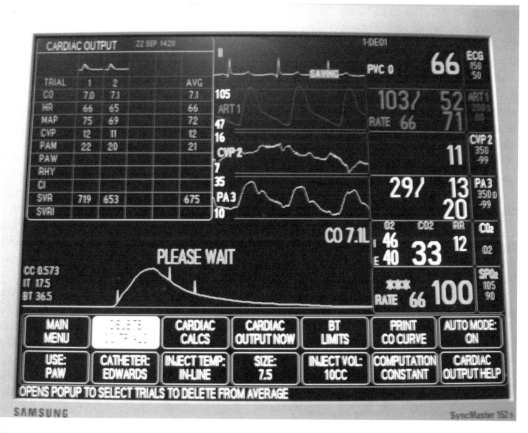

Fig. 17.1 Invasive hemodynamic monitor

real-time data to guide management in appropriate patients [4].

The PAC can deliver data on right-sided filling pressures directly, left-sided filling pressures indirectly, SVR, and CO, through either thermodilution or oximetric approaches. These data, when taken together, can provide numerical evidence of the cardiac function and quantify the degree of pulmonary hypertension, should any exist. In addition, changes in the measured pressures and calculated variables, such as end-diastolic volumes, can suggest altered central volume status. As referenced previously, there may be benefit in maintaining a normal or slightly reduced central volume status in LT patients, when appropriate, and PAC data can help with this guidance.

CO data can be assessed intermittently or continuously, depending on the choice of device. Typically, thermodilution CO is checked at intervals, while oximetric catheters report CO continuously through optical assessment of mixed venous oxygen, after an initial calibration.

The accuracy of the continuous cardiac output (CCO) monitors may decrease with time from calibration, while the use of intermittent monitors requires action on the part of the provider, which may not be feasible in times of high stress. Otherwise, these may be considered reasonably equitable approaches to measuring CO [18].

The presence of cirrhosis is typically associated with high CO states due to alterations in SVR and circulating volume status [19]. Altered systemic perfusion as measured by BP, acidosis, and urine output may not necessarily correlate with numerical changes in CO, especially if the absolute numbers remain above normal. Thus, the trend of CO and filling pressures may provide more useful data in many circumstances. In addition, cardiac contractility may be abnormal in cirrhotic patients even in the setting of normal or elevated CO.

The presence of cirrhotic cardiomyopathy may add complexity to the intraoperative management, as heart rate, CO, and BP can all be adversely impacted. Hypertrophic obstructive cardiomyopathy (HOCM) is also evident in some patients with cirrhotic liver disease, and manage-

ment of these patients can present challenges during LT [20].

The PAC can provide many data points, which may help guide hemodynamic management of the LT patient. However, use of this monitor has become less common in LT over the years due to a slight increase in risk of the procedure, unclear benefit of the data provided, and desire for reduced resource utilization [21]. Of particular importance, CO data from PAC monitoring may be less precise in patients with hyperdynamic cardiac function, such as those with cirrhotic liver disease.

The PAC remains an important monitor in certain ESLD diagnoses such as portopulmonary hypertension and HOCM. The emergence of arterial pressure waveform analysis and increased use of transesophageal echocardiography have provided alternative monitoring strategies to conventional PAC [18].

17.4 Minimally Invasive Cardiac Output Monitoring

Arterial pressure-based CO calculations interpret the pulse pressure waveform presented by an arterial line. These have been validated to provide data comparable to that of the PAC, especially in prediction of CO response to fluid administration [22, 23]. Variations in pulse pressure, stroke volume, and systolic pressure are commonly used hemodynamic variables in the evaluation of CO in critically ill patients, although some difficulty exists when extrapolating these data to operative patients (Fig. 17.2).

Cardiac stroke volume can be interpreted from the arterial line waveform, which can be used to calculate CO. The fidelity of these devices is dependent on a properly functioning arterial line, and changes in patient positioning, manipulation of the abdominal structures, and altered vascular tone may all reduce the accuracy of the information gathered in this manner.

As referenced previously, peripheral arterial line hemodynamic measurements, such as those from radial arterial lines, may be impaired in

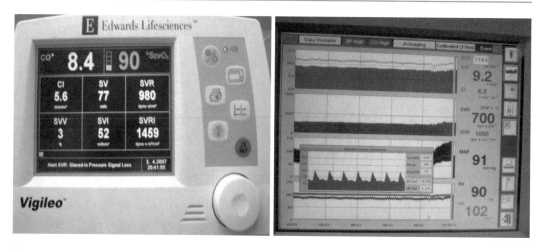

Fig. 17.2 Minimally invasive cardiac output monitor - VIgileo/ FloTrac and LiDCO

patients with high vasopressor requirement or those in shock, and in situations such as this, stroke volume calculations are likely to be less accurate.

Ultimately, the CO data generated from these devices are not as accurate as thermodilution methods using PAC, and in cases where CO monitoring is imperative, these devices should not be used as a substitute [23–25]. Direct measurement via thermodilution through a PAC remains the gold standard for measurement of CO.

17.5 Transesophageal Echocardiography

Transesophageal echocardiography (TEE) is able to provide real-time, dynamic, information about right and left heart systolic and diastolic function, volume status, regional wall motion as well as valvular function [26–28]. Intraoperative TEE has also been valuable in detecting conditions like cirrhotic or Takotsubo cardiomyopathy, HOCM, pulmonary hypertension, intracardiac air or thromboembolic events, and pericardial tamponade.

Use of TEE during LT is increasing, as it is seen as both more accurate and less invasive than other monitors of cardiac function, such as the PAC [29].

In a multicenter study of 244 patients undergoing LT, stroke volume index determined by TEE more strongly corelated with right ventricular end-diastolic volume index than CVP or PAOP [30]. CVP is also an unreliable indicator of stroke volume and intravascular volume [30].

Coronary artery disease (CAD) is not uncommon in patients undergoing LT. TEE has been shown to be more sensitive in detecting ischemia based on regional wall motion abnormalities as compared to other monitors including PAC [31].

Intracardiac thromboemboli may arise in association with caval manipulation, coagulopathy, and resuscitation, and TEE may provide evidence prior to catastrophic complication. The presence of thromboemboli is likely underappreciated, as one prospective study discovered 44% of patients with microemboli and 27% with larger emboli [32]. While smaller emboli are typically handled well by the pulmonary circulation, right ventricular dysfunction, failure and cardiovascular collapse can occur with larger ones. TEE provides real-time monitoring of the intracardiac status and is very useful in visualizing intracardiac thrombi, as well as "pre-thrombotic" characteristics such as microemboli and "smoke," suggestive of lower-flow states.

Paradoxical air embolus is a concern in liver transplant surgery. Patent foramen ovale (PFO), which predisposes to right-to-left intracardiac shunting, should be diagnosed by preoperative echocardiography, but these can be missed, or may not be evident with normal right-sided pressures. In addition, patients with cirrhosis often have a high degree of intrapulmonary shunting. This commonly exacerbates hypoxemia in these patients, but in rare cases, entrained venous air and microdebris can cross into the systemic circulation, with subsequent embolization to the brain, other organs, and extremities [33, 34]. Use of TEE in LT can alert the anesthesiologist to the presence of this air or debris in the cardiac chambers, even without hemodynamic changes, where standard monitoring is likely to miss this until manifested as hemodynamics change.

Placement and manipulation of a TEE probe is relatively simple in skilled hands, but patients with cirrhotic liver disease are at increased risk of esophageal pathology such as varices and stricture, and the presence and severity of these should be assessed prior to probe placement. Active bleeding and known esophageal pathology are two of the more common absolute contraindications to TEE. Risk of complication, such as major bleeding, is low [35] when used in liver transplant patients, even those with high MELD [36]. We recommend that the ability to rapidly tamponade a rupture gastric or esophageal varix be available for these patients, especially if TEE is used. Risks and benefits should be weighed prior to planned TEE placement, and it is perhaps reasonable to consider TEE as a focused therapy for a specific condition, rather than a monitor to be used in all liver transplant patients [37].

Key Points

- Proper hemodynamic monitoring is imperative in the management of the liver transplant recipient.
- Arterial blood pressure should be measured directly. The site chosen should balance the need for the reliability of proximal measurement and the complication risk of the site chosen.
- Central venous pressure monitoring is recommended, and following trends of this value may provide evidence of shifts in circulating volume status.
- In cases where precise cardiac output measurement is desired, use of the pulmonary artery catheter is recommended. In some circumstances, less invasive devices (LidCO, PicCO, etc.) may provide similar information based upon arterial waveform analysis.
- Transesophageal echocardiography is recommended as a tool for assessment of dynamic cardiac function, especially during complicated liver transplant cases. Placement and interpretation should only be undertaken by experienced providers.

References

1. Schumann R, Mandell MS, Mercaldo N, Michaels D, Robertson A, Banerjee A, Pai R, Klinck J, Pandharipande P, Walia A. Anesthesia for liver transplantation in United States academic centers: intraoperative practice. J Clin Anesth. 2013;25(7):542–50. https://doi.org/10.1016/j.jclinane.2013.04.017. Epub 2013 Aug 30. PMID: 23994704.
2. Schuppan D, Afdhal NH. Liver cirrhosis. Lancet. 2008;371:838–51.
3. Ozier Y, Klinck JR. Anesthetic management of hepatic transplantation. Curr Opin Anaesthesiol. 2008;21:391–400. https://doi.org/10.1097/ACO.0b013e3282ff85f4.
4. Hori T, et al. Systemic hemodynamics in advanced cirrhosis: concerns during perioperative period of liver transplantation. World J Hepatol. 2016;8:1047–60.
5. Walia A, Schumann R. Intraoperative resource utilization in anesthesia for liver transplantation in the United States: a survey. Anesth Analg. 2003;97:21–8, table of contents [PMID: 12818937]. https://doi.org/10.1213/01.ANE.0000068483.91464.2B.
6. Rudnick MR, Marchi LD, Plotkin JS. Hemodynamic monitoring during liver transplantation: a state of the art review. World J Hepatol. 2015;7:1302–11.
7. Arnal D, Garutti I, Perez-Peña J, Olmedilla L, Tzenkov IG. Radial to femoral arterial blood pressure differences during liver transplantation. Anaesthesia. 2005;60:766–71.
8. Nuttall G, et al. Surgical and patient risk factors for severe arterial line complications in adults. Anesthesiology. 2016;124:590–7.

9. Singh A, et al. Brachial arterial pressure monitoring during cardiac surgery rarely causes complications. Anesthesiology. 2017;126:1065–76.

10. Krenn CG, De Wolf AM. Current approach to intraoperative monitoring in liver transplantation. Curr Opin Organ Transplant. 2008;13:285–90. https://doi.org/10.1097/MOT.0b013e3283005832. PMID: 18685319.

11. De Wolf AM. Perioperative assessment of the cardiovascular system in ESLD and transplantation. Int Anesthesiol Clin. 2006;44:59–78. https://doi.org/10.1097/01.aia.0000210818.85287.de. PMID: 17033479.

12. Shin BS, Kim GS, Ko JS, Gwak MS, Yang M, Kim CS, Hahm TS, Lee SK. Comparison of femoral arterial blood pressure with radial arterial blood pressure and noninvasive upper arm blood pressure in the reperfusion period during liver transplantation. Transplant Proc. 2007;39:1326–8. https://doi.org/10.1016/j.transproceed.2007.02.075. PMID: 17580132.

13. Melendez JA, et al. Perioperative outcomes of major hepatic resections under low central venous pressure anesthesia: blood loss, blood transfusion, and the risk of postoperative renal dysfunction. J Am Coll Surgeons. 1998;187:620–5.

14. Wang B, He H, Cheng B, Wei K, Min S. Effect of low central venous pressure on postoperative pulmonary complications in patients undergoing liver transplantation. Surg Today. 2013;43:777–81.

15. Feng Z-Y, Xu X, Zhu S-M, Bein B, Zheng S-S. Effects of low central venous pressure during preanhepatic phase on blood loss and liver and renal function in liver transplantation. World J Surg. 2010;34:1864–73.

16. Kang Y, Elia E. Contemporary liver transplantation, the successful liver transplant program. Berlin: Springer; 2017. p. 143–87. https://doi.org/10.1007/978-3-319-07209-8_9.

17. Hughes MJ, Ventham NT, Harrison EM, Wigmore SJ. Central venous pressure and liver resection: a systematic review and meta-analysis. HPB. 2015;17:863–71.

18. Kobe J, et al. Cardiac output monitoring: technology and choice. Ann Cardiac Anaesth. 2019;22:6.

19. Milani A, Zaccaria R, Bombardieri G, Gasbarrini A, Pola P. Cirrhotic cardiomyopathy. Digest Liver Dis. 2007;39:507–15.

20. Robertson A. Intraoperative management of liver transplantation in patients with hypertrophic cardiomyopathy: a review. Transplant Proc. 2010;42:1721–3.

21. Costa MG, et al. Uncalibrated continuous cardiac output measurement in liver transplant patients: LiDCOrapid™ system versus pulmonary artery catheter. J Cardiothor Vasc Anesth. 2014;28:540–6.

22. Esper SA, Pinsky MR. Arterial waveform analysis. Best Pract Res Clin Anaesthesiol. 2014;28:363–80.

23. Su BC, et al. Cardiac output derived from arterial pressure waveform analysis in patients undergoing liver transplantation: validity of a third-generation device. Transplant Proc. 2012;44:424–8.

24. Krejci V, Vannucci A, Abbas A, Chapman W, Kangrga IM. Comparison of calibrated and uncalibrated arterial pressure–based cardiac output monitors during orthotopic liver transplantation. Liver Transplant. 2010;16:773–82.

25. Wang D-J, et al. Non-invasive cardiac output measurement with electrical velocimetry in patients undergoing liver transplantation: comparison of an invasive method with pulmonary thermodilution. BMC Anesthesiol. 2018;18:138.

26. Suriani RJ. Transesophageal echocardiography during organ transplantation. J Cardiothorac Vasc Anesth. 1998;12:686–94. https://doi.org/10.1016/S1053-0770(98)90245-2. PMID: 9854670.

27. Plotkin JS, Johnson LB, Kuo PC. Intracardiac thrombus formation during orthotopic liver transplantation: a new entity or an old enemy? Transplantation. 1996;61:1131. https://doi.org/10.1097/00007890-199604150-00033. PMID: 8623204.

28. Fahy BG, Hasnain JU, Flowers JL, Plotkin JS, Odonkor P, Ferguson MK. Transesophageal echocardiographic detection of gas embolism and cardiac valvular dysfunction during laparoscopic nephrectomy. Anesth Analg. 1999;88:500–4. [PMID: 10071994].

29. Vetrugno L, et al. Transesophageal echocardiography in orthotopic liver transplantation: a comprehensive intraoperative monitoring tool. Crit Ultrasound J. 2017;9:15.

30. Rocca GD, Costa MG, Feltracco P, Biancofiore G, Begliomini B, Taddei S, Coccia C, Pompei L, Di Marco P, Pietropaoli P. Continuous right ventricular end diastolic volume and right ventricular ejection fraction during liver transplantation: a multicenter study. Liver Transpl. 2008;14:327–32. https://doi.org/10.1002/lt.21288. PMID: 18306366.

31. De Marchi L, Wang CJ, Skubas NJ, Kothari R, Zerillo J, Subramaniam K, Efune GE, Braunfeld MY, Mandel S. Safety and benefit of transesophageal echocardiography in liver transplant surgery: a position paper from the Society for the advancement of transplant anesthesia (SATA). Liver Transpl. 2020;26:1019–29. https://doi.org/10.1002/lt.25800.

32. Shillcutt SK, et al. Liver transplantation: intraoperative transesophageal echocardiography findings and relationship to major postoperative adverse cardiac events. J Cardiothor Vasc Anesth. 2016;30:107–14.

33. Velthuis S, et al. Clinical implications of pulmonary shunting on saline contrast echocardiography. J Am Soc Echocardiogr. 2015;28:255–63.

34. Badenoch A, Srinivas C, Al-Adra D, Selzner M, Wsowicz M. A case report of paradoxical air embolism caused by intrapulmonary shunting during liver transplantation. Transplant Direct. 2017;3:e134.

35. Markin NW, Sharma A, Grant W, Shillcutt SK. The safety of transesophageal echocardiography in patients undergoing orthotopic liver transplantation. J Cardiothor Vasc Anesth. 2015;29:588–93.

36. Bui CCM, et al. Gastroesophageal and hemorrhagic complications associated with intraoperative transesophageal echocardiography in patients with model for end-stage liver disease score 25 or higher. J Cardiothor Vasc Anesth. 2015;29:594–7.

37. Cywinski JB, Maheshwari K. Con: transesophageal echocardiography is not recommended as a routine monitor for patients undergoing liver transplantation. J Cardiothor Vasc Anesth. 2017;31:2287–9.

Intraoperative Coagulation Monitoring in Liver Transplant Surgery

18

Jayanti Shankar and Vijay Vohra

Abbreviations

ACT	Activated clotting time
DIC	Disseminated intravascular coagulation
DVT	Deep-vein thrombosis
ECMO	Extra-corporeal membrane oxygenation
ESLD	End-stage liver disease
FDPs	Fibrinogen degradation products
PAI-1	Plasminogen activator inhibitor-1
POC	Point-of-care
ROTEM	Rotational thromboelastometry
TEG	Thromboelastography
t-PA	Tissue plasminogen activator

18.1 Introduction

Coagulation occurs in three phases such as primary haemostasis, coagulation and fibrinolysis, and liver dysfunction affects all three functions [1]. The liver is responsible for the synthesis of all clotting factors (except von Willebrand factor—vWf), all anticoagulants, as well as production of fibrinolytic proteins [2], and therefore haemostasis abnormality in liver disease is multifactorial—Box 18.1.

Box 18.1 Haemostatic abnormalities in liver disease are due to [2]
- Thrombocytopenia and qualitative dysfunction
  - Hypersplenism contributing to sequestration of platelets
  - Decreased thrombopoietin production
  - Immune-mediated platelet destruction
  - Renal impairment and uraemia accompanying liver failure [3]
- Impaired humoral coagulation
  - Inadequate coagulation factor production
  - Increased coagulation factor consumption
  - Vitamin K deficiency (due to which abnormal clotting factors are produced as there is lack of gamma carboxylation)
- Excessive fibrinolysis
- Disseminated intravascular coagulation

J. Shankar
Transplant Anaesthesia, Sakra World Hospital, Bangalore, India

V. Vohra (✉)
Liver Transplant, GI Anesthesia & Intensive Care, Medanta The Medicity, Gurgaon, India
e-mail: vijay.vohra@medanta.org

The historical assumption that haemostasis in liver disease depicts a bleeding tendency is now replaced with the concept of a 'rebalanced' haemostasis between procoagulant, anticoagulant and fibrinolytic system due to a parallel deficiency of requisite factors. The tendency towards bleeding or thrombosis will depend on the circumstantial risk factors such as volume status, infections, alcohol, medications and renal function [4, 5]. Coagulopathy is also an essential component of acute liver failure, the other component being hepatic encephalopathy. Plasma concentration of coagulation factors is drastically reduced due to high cytokine concentration. High levels of acute phase reactant PAI-1 (plasminogen activator inhibitor-1) found in acute liver failure predispose these patients towards hypofibrinolysis [1].

Liver transplantation is the only treatment which can restore normal haemostasis in patients with end-stage liver disease or acute liver failure. It is an intricate procedure during which coagulopathy may precipitate into a catastrophe at a dramatic pace, hence requiring rapid diagnosis and management. The complex nature of haemorrhage increases the likelihood of a therapeutic misadventure, if a targeted approach is not followed [6]. Transfusion is associated with increased morbidity and mortality and may contribute to the alloantibody load and increase the risk of allograft rejection [3]. Moreover, an adverse association of red cell (RBC) transfusion on survival rates following liver transplant has been demonstrated; therefore, there is a constant endeavour to reduce transfusion [7]. Advancements in modalities for diagnosing and managing coagulopathy have been a major contributing factor in improving the 5-year survival rate from 72% in 1998 to 90% in 2010 in the United States [3].

Transfusion and coagulation management algorithms based on the point-of-care tests can be useful adjuncts to reduce transfusion requirement and thereby affect morbidity and mortality.

18.2 Intraoperative Changes in Each Phase

Management of coagulopathy in patients undergoing liver transplant poses a unique challenge due to the low haemostatic reserve in these

Table 18.1 Summary of coagulation abnormalities—phase wise

Dissection	Surgical bleeding, slight worsening of coagulopathy
Anhepatic	Loss of coagulation factors, fibrinolysis
Reperfusion/ neohepatic	Initially—hyperfibrinolysis, entrapment of platelet and release of heparin
	Followed by resolution of hyperfibrinolysis

patients, prolonged duration of surgery and phase-specific requirements during each phase of the procedure, described as below [Table 18.1]:

18.2.1 Dissection Phase

This phase involves dissection of adhesions, transection of collaterals and manipulation of major structures to facilitate mobilization of the liver, contributing to major blood loss. There is a slight deterioration of the pre-existing coagulopathy due to surgical stress; however, surgical bleeding is the hallmark of this phase.

Aetiology of the liver disease is also a factor which influences intraoperative requirement of blood products in this phase. For example, patients with hepatocellular carcinoma are usually hyper-coagulopathic. Similarly, patients with primary biliary cirrhosis and primary sclerosing cholangitis are likely to have a hyper-coagulopathic state with reduced fibrinolytic activity [8]. Enhanced fibrinolysis contributes to blood loss in only 10–20% of the cases [1].

18.2.2 Anhepatic Phase

This phase extends from occlusion of the hepatic vasculature till reperfusion of the new liver into the recipient's circulation. Major vessels have already been clamped during the dissection phase which limits the surgical bleed. However, since the liver is out of circulation, the characteristic feature of this phase is loss of synthesis and clearance of coagulation factors.

There is an increased level of t-PA (tissue plasminogen activator), due to release from endothelial cells and decreased clearance in absence of the liver, which contributes to hyperfibrinolysis seen in this phase [1]. This later continues into the reperfusion phase [9].

18.2.3 Post-reperfusion/Neohepatic Phase

This phase begins with the reperfusion of the new liver into the recipient's circulation often resulting in uncontrollable bleeding during the first few minutes, thus warranting immediate management and control [1].

During the reperfusion of the new liver, further t-PA from the endothelium of the replaced organ is released and hyperfibrinolysis is at its peak [9]. This period is further characterized by abnormalities related to thrombocytopenia and heparin-like effect of donor liver. There is a gradient of platelet count of up to 50% between the arterial and venous circulation representing the profound entrapment of platelets in the donor sinusoids. The ischemic donor liver endothelium releases heparinoids, which adds to the heparin load following heparinization of donor liver prior to harvesting [10]. This initial hyperfibrinolysis gradually resolves with clearance of t-PA and increased production of PAI-1.

18.3 Monitoring Coagulation During Liver Transplant Surgery

Bleeding during liver transplantation, as mentioned above, occurs due to several reasons [8]:

- Surgical factors—previous abdominal surgery, portal hypertension, portal vein thrombosis
- Donor-related factors—length of ICU stay, duration of cold ischaemia time
- Recipient-related factors—severity of disease, age, renal dysfunction and comorbidities
- Factors arising from operative milieu—acid-base balance, hypocalcaemia, hypothermia
- Inherent coagulopathy of the patient

Due to disparity between the increasing demand for organs and limited supply of donors, there is an increasing trend of marginal and high-risk donors being accepted. The recipients who receive organs from these donors are at an increased risk of perioperative coagulopathy resulting from delayed graft function or slow-graft function commonly seen with these donor grafts [3].

Coagulation monitoring and management for major surgical procedures is challenging and is usually based on standard laboratory tests. However, these tests, in the setting of ESLD (end-stage liver disease), are less reliable especially in the background of bleeding during liver transplant, where diagnosis has to be precise and treatment prompt. The standard laboratory tests are briefly described.

18.3.1 Standard Laboratory Tests

The clotting process can be divided into four phases [11] (Fig. 18.1):

- Primary haemostasis
- Thrombin generation
- Clot formation
- Clot breakdown/lysis

Conventional or standard laboratory tests at best reflect the thrombin generation phase.
These tests include:

- Prothrombin time (PT)
- Activated partial thromboplastin time (aPTT)
- Platelet count
- Fibrinogen levels

18.3.2 Prothrombin Time (PT)

Also called tissue factor-induced coagulation time, the prothrombin time test was developed in 1935 to titrate coumarin doses [12]. It is sensitive to factors I, II, V, VII and X and is performed by incubating plasma at 37° with tissue thromboplastin (tissue factor plus phospholipid) and cal-

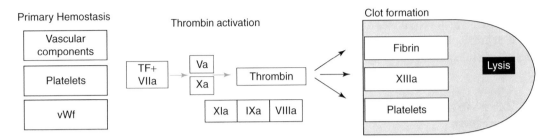

Fig. 18.1 This is the arbitrary subdivision of the coagulation system which is an interaction between vascular, cellular and humoral components

cium at standard pH. It detects the time needed for platelet-poor plasma to clot and reflects the integrity of the extrinsic and common coagulation pathway [13]. Detection of fibrin strands using either a photo-optical or electromechanical device is the end point of the test [10]. It is reported in seconds and normal value is 0.9–0.12 s [13].

18.3.3 International Normalized Ratio (INR)

Standardization is based on the responsiveness to a singular type of thromboplastin which is then measured by International Sensitivity Index and converted to the INR (international normalized ratio) value mainly to account for inter-device variations in PT measurements. INR was introduced in 1983 to harmonize results of PT across laboratories. It is defined as (patient PT/control PT)^{ISI} [12, 14].

18.3.4 Activated Partial Thromboplastin Time (aPTT)

It was developed in 1953 and then modified in 1961. It is performed to monitor heparin therapy during thrombolysis. This test is sensitive to coagulation factors I, II, V, VIII, IX, XI and XII, heparin, fibrinogen degradation products, hypothermia and hypofibrinogenaemia. The term 'partial thromboplastin' indicates that the reagent contains phospholipids (as a substitute for the platelet membrane) but no tissue factor,

distinguishing it from the PT [10]. Platelet-poor plasma is incubated with partial thromboplastins, calcium and an activator (e.g. celite, kaolin, silica) at 37° and standard pH [13]. It reflects the integrity of the intrinsic and common coagulation pathway and the normal range is between 25 and 35 s [13]. Factor deficiency must be reduced to almost 30% before the test is able to demonstrate abnormality.

18.3.5 Thrombin Time [13]

The ability of thrombin to convert fibrinogen to fibrin (fibrin polymerization) in the final stage of haemostasis is measured with this test. A standard concentration of human thrombin is added to citrated, platelet-poor plasma and time to clot formation is measured. Clot formation requires the presence of fibrinogen and the absence of thrombin inhibitors [10]. Its normal value is 15–19 s. It helps in establishing conditions such as hypofibrinogenaemia, dysfibrinogenaemia, presence of direct thrombin inhibitors, fibrinogen and FDPs (fibrinogen degradation products) since it bypasses all the preceding reactions before the conversion of fibrinogen. It is also used to monitor fibrinolytic therapy and to detect heparin resistance.

18.3.6 Platelet Count

Platelet count is routinely measured by automated machines [6]. Formation of a satisfactory platelet plug may be impaired if the platelet count is low, if platelets are functionally inert or if the patient is on antiplatelet drugs. However, the platelet count reflects the quantity of platelets in numbers and does not provide information regarding their function [13]. The normal range is between 150,000 and 440,000 cu mm and counts less than 150,000 cu mm reflect thrombocytopenia. Platelet clumping and sample haemodilution are common causes for low platelet count. Platelet count plays an important role in demonstration of HITS (heparin-induced thrombocytopenia).

18.3.7 Fibrinogen

Measures the amount of fibrinogen in the system. The two most frequently used tests in routine clinical practice are the Clauss assay and the PT-derived fibrinogen level. Fibrinogen values range between 160 and 350 mg/dL [13]. Reduced levels may be due to impaired production (such as liver disease) or increased consumption (such as disseminated intravascular coagulation (DIC) and fibrinolysis). Fibrinogen levels may also be falsely elevated in the presence of synthetic colloids such as hydroxyethyl starch often used for fluid resuscitation [6].

18.3.8 Fibrinogen Degradation Products (FDPs) and D-Dimer (Tests of Fibrinolysis)

This assay detects degeneration products of fibrin (either cross-linked or uncross-linked). The D-Dimer is specific for degraded products of cross-linked fibrin. These may be elevated in advanced liver disease, exogenous thrombolysis and fibrinolysis following cardiopulmonary bypass and DIC. Elevated levels cannot differentiate primary and secondary fibrinolysis. Elevated D-dimer is non specific and is the result widespread lysis of cross-linked fibrin of established thrombi, as seen in deep-vein thrombosis (DVT) and pulmonary embolism.

18.3.9 Limitations of Conventional Tests

Though commonly done in cirrhotic patients, these tests do not reflect the exact picture of coagulation. The levels of naturally occurring anticoagulants as protein C and antithrombin are also reduced as are procoagulants and the full anticoagulant activity cannot be expressed. These tests have a direct relationship to the degree of decompensation in cirrhosis and may be useful in predicting prognosis but not for predicting bleeding or thrombosis in these patients [15]. The coagulation system in these patients seems to be more 'balanced' than suggested by traditional tests. PT and aPTT can assess the speed of fibrin strand formation; they do not assess the mechanical and functional properties of the clot over time. INR monitoring will at best be an indicator of synthetic function rather than to assess the actual probabilty to bleed [16, 17]. The current concepts in coagulation advocate the cell-based model which emphasizes on the interaction between platelets, vascular endothelium and fibrinolytic factors in the haemostatic mechanism. Standard laboratory tests which are performed in plasma do not demonstrate these interactions and therefore cannot guide therapy [8, 18].

Fibrinogen levels coupled with platelet count would be more meaningful than INR as a measure of risk of bleeding and target values have been ascertained as 120–150 mg/dL; however, these values are with reference to trauma settings [4]. Platelets contribute to thrombin formation and therefore a theoretical possibility of reduced thrombin generation exists in cirrhosis. However, this has not been clinically demonstrated in stable cirrhotic patients with platelet count $>60 \times 10^9$. Under physiological condition of flow, platelets from these patients are able to interact normally with collagen and fibrinogen. Platelet count is purely quantitative and cannot detect platelet dysfunction. A school of thought suggests the thrombin generation test is likely to provide a better clinical picture in cirrhotic patients for the prediction of bleeding or guided decision making [12].

None of the conventional coagulation tests detect or identify the fibrinolytic process; they can only detect products of degeneration which is highly non-specific [16]. Coagulation results can be affected adversely by poor sampling technique such as underfilling the tube may prolong clotting times artefactually due to over-anticoagulation. Reduced haematocrit may reduce plasma volume and prolong clotting times in the sample [10].

18.4 Point-of-Care Coagulation Testing

Preoperative treatment of infection, optimization of renal status, surgical management of active bleeding, striving to preserve normothermia, maintaining low central venous pressure, normocalcaemia and pH levels within physiological limits during the intraoperative period contribute towards reducing bleeding during liver transplant surgery. However, despite all these measures, the delicate surgical milieu may be disrupted due to the inherent coagulation imbalances resulting in a 'dynamic haemostatic profile' [19].

Apart from a longer turnaround time, standard laboratory tests may fail to predict the risk of bleeding as they are not affected by profibrinolytic susceptibility, anticoagulant protein C, antithrombin and tissue factor pathway inhibitor, and endothelium-derived haemostatic process thus making them unsuitable for managing coagulation during liver transplant surgery. The risk of thrombotic events in these patients is substantial and mortality associated with these events is manifold. These events can be prevented by judicious administration or avoiding inadvertent transfusions of products [17]. This is where intraoperative point-of-care coagulation monitoring can aid in ensuring transfusion of blood products in a targeted manner, thus preventing unwarranted transfusion and its deleterious effect. Therefore, point-of-care devices provide immediate, accurate, real-time and comprehensive picture of the patient's coagulation status (Box 18.2).

> **Box 18.2 Advantages of point of care testing [20]**
> - Small volume of blood is needed (<1 to 5 mL).
> - Rapid availability of results; therefore decisions can be made faster.
> - Transporting time is saved.
> - Pre-analytical steps (centrifuging, etc.) can be avoided.
> - Persons without training in medical technology may perform the test.
> - Tests are easy to learn.

A point-of-care test is defined as a rapid bedside diagnostic test to aid the clinician in directing therapeutic intervention. The aim of perioperative coagulation testing is the detection of deranged haemostasis and to initiate treatment rapidly; therefore point-of-care tests would be the way forward to improve clinical efficiency. Applicable devices in the perioperative setting are classified into four broad categories [13]:

(a) Functional assay of monitoring heparin anticoagulation
(b) Platelet function monitors
(c) Near-patient clotting factor tests
(d) Viscoelastic measures of coagulation

Despite the fact that some of the classical criteria for designation of a test to be point-of-care test (includes easy measurement, easy interpretation and no handling of reagent) may not be met by some of these tests, they have still been classified as point-of-care coagulation tests [20].

18.4.1 Functional Assay of Monitoring Heparin Anticoagulation [13]

18.4.1.1 Activated Clotting Time (ACT)

This test is widely used to monitor systemic heparin therapy in cardiac surgery, haemo-filtration,

ECMO (extra-corporeal membrane oxygenation) therapy, cardiac catheterization and interventional radiology [20].

First described in 1966, it utilizes the activation of coagulation through the intrinsic pathway when fresh whole blood is incubated with glass beads, kaolin or celite at 37°. Two millilitres of whole blood is added to a test tube containing celite and a ferro-magnetic bar. The tube is gently rotated within the test well. As coagulation occurs, the bar also begins to rotate with the tube and the rotation is detected by a magnetic sensor. The time to formation is recorded by a timer; the normal value is 90–150 s. ACT is a popular test due to its low cost, simplicity and linear response at high heparin concentration [10]. The test is not sensitive at low heparin concentrations, hypothermia, coagulation factor deficiency, IIb/IIIa inhibitors, warfarin therapy, lupus antibodies and haemodilution.

There is a variant of ACT called heparin management test (HMT) which is capable of measuring prothrombin time and activated partial thromboplastin time [21].

18.4.2 Platelet Function Monitoring

Factors such as congenital and acquired defects affecting the surface receptors participating in aggregation or adhesion, storage granules or other mechanisms can contribute to platelet dysfunction. Point-of-care platelet function monitors are now available to aid the clinician to monitor platelet function. Some monitors have specific activators to detect P2Y12 antagonists such as thienopyridines (clopidogrel, prasugrel), cyclooxygenase inhibitors (aspirin) and glycoprotein IIb/IIIa antagonists (abciximab, tirofiban).

18.4.2.1 Platelet Function Analyser-100

The PFA-100 monitors measure platelet adhesion and aggregation by incorporating high-shear conditions to stimulate small vessel injury. A total of 800 µL of citrated whole blood is drawn through a 150 µm hole in a collagen-coated membrane bonded with either epinephrine or ADP. The shear stress of whole blood being drawn through a vacuum leads to platelet activation and promotes platelet adherence and aggregation and proceeds to form a primary plug which seals the hole [21]. This is sensed by a pressure transducer and usually occurs in 81–166 s with epinephrine and 54–109 s with ADP [10].

The response to epinephrine detects aspirin-induced platelet dysfunction. Both channels detect dysfunction in patients with von Willebrand's disease and uraemia [21].

The drawback is the analysis has to be performed 30–120 min after venepuncture. Haemodilution and interference by thrombocytopenia are some of the limitations.

18.4.3 Near-Patient Clotting Factor Test

Point-of-care coagulation tests are also available for the evaluation of PT, aPTT and INR.

Hemochron Jr. signature is a hand-held device used to derive ACT, aAPTT and PT. Test-specific cuvettes are pre-warmed to 37 °C, onto which 50 µL of fresh or citrated whole blood is placed and then mixed with the test-specific reagent. As coagulation occurs, optical sensors detect the impeded movement.

CoaguChek is another near-patient test that uses reflectance photometry to derive INR.

These point-of-care tests (of PT and APTT) can be affected to a variable extent in patients with liver disease, septicaemia, trauma, etc. Hence, these point-of-care tests for PT and APTT are approved only for monitoring anticoagulation therapy and their value in other clinical situations is limited.

18.4.4 Viscoelastic Measures of Coagulation

Standard laboratory tests (other than platelet count), being plasma-based tests, only reflect the initial stages of the coagulation. Viscoelastic, point-of-care coagulation tests use whole blood and can provide insight into all components such as coagulation initiation to fibrinolysis, the strength and stability of the clot.

The point-of-care viscoelastic tests validated for liver transplant include:
1. Thromboelastography (TEG)
2. Rotational thromboelastometry (ROTEM)
3. Sonoclot

18.4.4.1 TEG/ROTEM: Introduction

Invented in 1948 by Hartert, they assess the viscoelastic properties of whole blood under low shear conditions and provide valuable information about all stages of haemostasis until resolution of the clot [22]. Use in liver transplant was first described in 1985 by Kang et al. and later in cardiac surgery in 1995 [9].

In contrast to many other coagulation tests where the time to first fibrin formation is used as an end point [13], these tests are based on the clinical principle that

- The end result of haemostasis is formation of clot and
- The physical properties of this clot (rate of formation, strength and stability) are a reflection of the patients' in vivo haemostasis status [22, 23].

Specific activators have been used to improve standardization and practicability [11]. Formation of the clot is a result of interaction between the cellular components of blood and coagulation proteins. The interaction between fibrinogen, platelets and clotting factors are therefore assessed with a single test [10]. The physical properties of the clot are measured and translated into electrical signals which are used to create graphic and numerical output which are interpreted in terms of hypocoagulable, normal or hypercoagulable state, with or without lysis.

Of course, the importance of periodic assessment of surgical field and communication with surgical teams cannot be underestimated. Surgical attempts to control visible source of bleeding, temperature monitoring, acid base and electrolyte monitoring contribute to monitoring coagulopathy during the transplant procedure [6].

18.4.4.2 Thromboelastography (TEG)

The term thromboelastograph is used to describe the trace produced during the test. The term thromboelastography and TEG have been used to describe the technique (Fig. 18.2). In 1996, TEG® became the registered trademark of the Haemoscope Corporation [9].

TEG gives a graphic representation of clot formation and subsequent lysis; 340-360 μL of whole blood sampled from the patient is incubated in a heated cup at 37°. Care should be taken not to underfill the cups as this will result in prolongation of the coagulation time. A pin connected to a detector system (a torsion wire) is suspended in the cup. The cup oscillates through an arc of 4°45′ in either direction, each rotation

Fig. 18.2 Components of thromboelastography (TEG) instrument

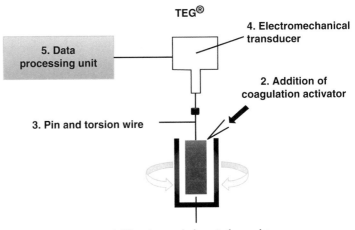

lasting 10 s, aiming to reproduce sluggish venous flow. These mimic low shear conditions similar to those present in the vena cava and well below those seen in venules, small veins and arterial system [19]. Initially the pin remains stationary generating a straight line on the tracing. As the clot begins to form, the pin gets embroiled within the clot and the torque of the cup is transmitted across the pin and the torsion wire to a mechano-electrical transducer [13]. The electric signal thus generated gets converted into a graphic display demonstrating the shear-elastic characteristic of clot (Y axis) against time (X axis).

The shape provides a rapid assessment of different coagulation states (hypo, normal, hyper) and also provides information regarding specific abnormalities in clot formation and fibrinolysis. A strong clot causes the pin to move directly in phase with the cup creating a broad TEG, whereas a weak clot stretches and delays the arc movement of the pin creating a narrow TEG. As the clot retracts or lyses, the bonds between the cup and pin are broken and the motion is again diminished and eventually stops, depicted by diminishing amplitude followed by a straight line [24].

Various variants of the TEG assay are available to give assessment of tissue factor, effect of heparin, assessment of function fibrinogen as well as platelet functioning (Table 18.2) (Box 18.3).

Table 18.2 Variants of the TEG assay [19, 24]

Kaolin	Contact activation. The standard test is performed with kaolin activator and gives an assessment of overall coagulation
Rapid TEG	Tissue factor and contact activation. Roughly analogous to ACT
HTEG	Kaolin plus Heparinase is used to specifically detect presence of heparin as the enzyme Heparinase will inactivate heparin
Functional fibrinogen	Contains TF (tissue factor) and abciximab that blocks platelet contribution to clot formation and therefore assesses fibrinogen contribution to clot strength
Platelet mapping	TEG platelet mapping assay measures platelet inhibition in comparison with the patient's baseline profile [18]

Box 18.3 Platelet Mapping: Adenosine Diphosphate (ADP) and Arachidonic acid (AA) are used to monitor antiplatelet therapy [18, 24]

A baseline kaolin-activated TEG is done to measure the thrombin-induced clot strength ($MA_{thrombin}$).

After this, a heparinized blood sample to which Reptilase and Factor XIIIa are added to inhibit all effects of thrombin, thus generating a cross-linked fibrin clot demonstrating clot strength coming from fibrin (MA_{fibrin}).

The third and fourth cup require heparinized sample with Reptilase and factor XIIIa (to block thrombin) and activate platelet at the ADP-activated receptor (that thienopyridines or GPIIb/IIIa drugs inhibit) or thromboxane A2 receptor (that aspirin affects) and therefore demonstrate the clot strength which platelets are activated though those specific receptors (MA_{AA} or MA_{ADP}).

Percentage platelet aggregation is calculated by the formula

$$\left[(MA_{AA} - MA_{fibrin}) / (MA_{thrombin} - MA_{fibrin}) \right] \times 100.$$

Platelet mapping assay measures clot strength at maximum amplitude and therefore quantifies platelet function. It also measures contribution of ADP and thromboxane A2 receptors to clot formation [16].

Nomenclature of measured values [10, 19].

Quantitative analysis of the TEG is performed by assessment of five main parameters; four related to clot formation and one to clot lysis (Figs. 18.3 and 18.4, Table 18.3).

Reaction (R) time—time in minutes taken to reach an amplitude of 2 mm. This corresponds to initial fibrin formation and is related to plasma clotting and inhibitor factor activity.

- Normal range: whole blood: 4–8 min, Kaolin: 3–8 min

Fig. 18.3 TEG. *R*—reaction time, *K*—amplitude progression from 2 to 20 mm, α—rate of clot formation, MA—maximum amplitude, LY30—clot lysis at 30 min after achieving maximum amplitude

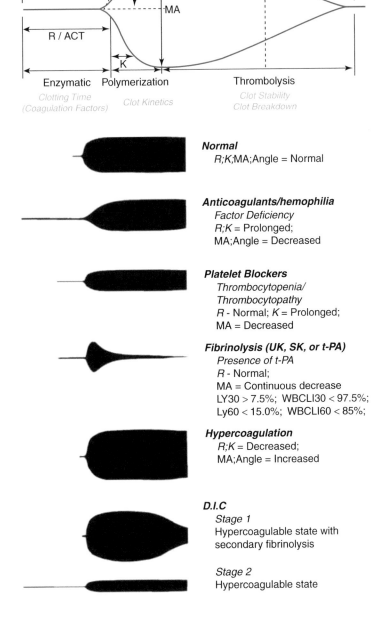

Fig. 18.4 TEG graphs in common conditions

Normal
  R;*K*;MA;Angle = Normal

Anticoagulants/hemophilia
  Factor Deficiency
  R;*K* = Prolonged;
  MA;Angle = Decreased

Platelet Blockers
  Thrombocytopenia/
  Thrombocytopathy
  R - Normal; *K* = Prolonged;
  MA = Decreased

Fibrinolysis (UK, SK, or t-PA)
  Presence of t-PA
  R - Normal;
  MA = Continuous decrease
  LY30 > 7.5%; WBCLI30 < 97.5%;
  Ly60 < 15.0%; WBCLI60 < 85%;

Hypercoagulation
  R;*K* = Decreased;
  MA;Angle = Increased

D.I.C
  Stage 1
  Hypercoagulable state with
  secondary fibrinolysis

  Stage 2
  Hypercoagulable state

Table 18.3 Derived parameters [19]

CI—clotting index	Global estimation of clot formation using a combination of variables R, K, MA and α angle, calculated continuously
G (shear modulus strength)	Clot strength in TEG represented by computer generated G value. G = (5000 × amplitude)/(100 − amplitude), normal 5.3–12.4 dynes/cm² (TEG 11)
E	Elasticity constant—normalized value of G
TPI	Thrombodynamic potential index-E obtained at maximum amplitude divided by K EMA/K
CL₃₀, CL₆₀—clot lysis index 30, 60	Measure of lysis calculated as the relationship of amplitudes at 30 and 60 to maximum amplitude
EPL— estimated percent lysis	It is the degree of lysis 30 min after MA is reached, computed 30 s after MA is reached and continuously updated till 30 min after MA is reached [22]

- Prolonged by anticoagulants, factor deficiencies and severe hypofibrinogenaemia
- Reduced by hypercoagulable conditions

Kinetics (K) time—time necessary for the clot to reach an amplitude of 20 mm from 2 mm. The *K*-time is a measure of clot formation kinetics.

- Normal range: whole blood: 1–4 min, Kaolin: 1–3 min
- Prolonged by anticoagulants, hypofibrinogenaemia, thrombocytopenia
- Shortened by increased fibrinogen level, increased platelet function

α **angle**—determined by creating a tangent line from the point of clot initiation (*R*) to the slope of the developing curve. It represents the speed at which solid clot forms and reflects the fibrinogen activity [25].

- Normal range: whole blood: 47–74°, Kaolin: 55–78°
- Increased by increased fibrinogen level, increased platelet function
- Decreased by anticoagulants, hypofibrinogenaemia, thrombocytopenia

MA (maximum amplitude)—is the peak amplitude of the clot. This is the maximum width, in millimetres, reached on the trace and is representative of the maximum strength of the haemostatic plug. It is directly related to the quality of fibrin and platelet interaction. MA is significantly altered by changes in platelet number or function.

- Normal range: whole blood: 50–73 mm, Kaolin: 51–69 mm
- Increased by hypercoagulable states, thrombocytosis
- Decreased by thrombocytopenia, platelet blockers, fibrinolysis, factor deficiencies (lesser extent)

18.4.4.3 Decrease in Amplitude Measurement A30 and A60
[22]

A30—amplitude of the trace 30 min after MA is reached.

A60—amplitude of the trace 60 min after MA is reached.

LY30 and LY 60—percentage reduction in area under TEG curve at 30 and 60 min. LY30 reflects fibrinolysis and measures percent lysis 30 min after MA is reached.

Normal range: 7.5%.

There is another variant of thromboelastography (TEG) available in the name of BIOTEM (Fig. 18.5).

18.4.4.4 Clot Pro

Another viscoelastic analyser is now available in Europe with few modifications to the currently

Fig. 18.5 BIOTEM—4 chambers instrument

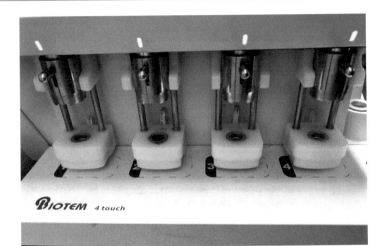

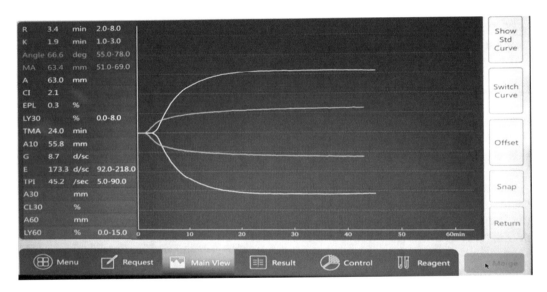

Fig. 18.6 Clot Pro Graph

available analysers. In this analyser they have removed the need to pipette liquid reagents, and these reagents are present in dried form in the pipette itself. When the blood is drawn in through the pipette, the dried reagent present in the sponge of the pipette activates the blood sample (Figs. 18.6 and 18.7). The basic principle of the CLOTPRO is similar to Thromboelastography (TEG), wherein the cup rotates and the pin is static. This design significantly mitigates the potential for error and eliminates reagent handling, which, combined with its ease of use, provides more flexibility and increased throughput in lab-based and clinical settings. ClotPro enables the detection and assessment of factor deficiencies,

low fibrinogen, platelet contribution (to whole blood coagulation), heparin and DOAC effects, fibrinolysis and antifibrinolytic drugs [26].

18.4.5 Rotational Thromboelastometry (ROTEM)

Similar to thromboelastography, rotational thromboelastometry (ROTEM) is a viscoelastic whole blood test which analyses the clotting process under low shear conditions and reflects the kinetics of all stages in thrombus formation, clot stability and strength as well as fibrinolysis [16].

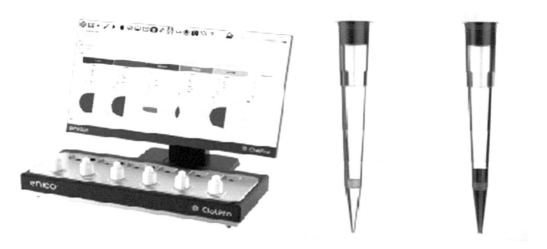

Fig. 18.7 Clot Pro

Fig. 18.8 Components
of ROTEM instrument

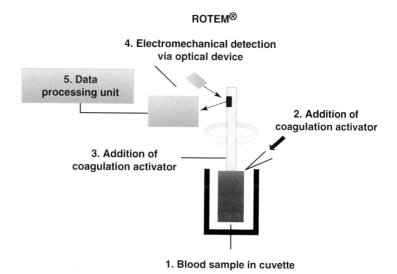

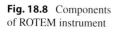

ROTEM is considered to be an improvement of the TEG as there is less vibrational interference. Also, it permits differential diagnosis of underlying patho-mechanism by implementing test modifications. Transfusion requirements after implementation of ROTEM were statistically significantly lower than without, making it a valuable guide in management algorithms (Fig. 18.8).

The ROTEM device uses 300 μL of whole blood with activators incubated at 37° in a heated holder which remains fixed. Activators used are tissue factor in the EXTEM cuvette and contact activator in INTEM cuvette [13, 18, 19]. Care should be taken not to underfill the tubes which may contribute to erroneous values [9,

18]. The difference in the working principle is that the cup is immobile and rotational movement arises from the pin suspended on a ball-bearing mechanism oscillating at 4°75′ every 6 s with a constant force. An optical sensor is attached to the pin (as compared to the torsion wire in the TEG). As fibrin begins to form and the viscoelastic strength of the clot increases, the movement of the pin is impeded, which is detected by an optical system consisting of a light-emitting diode, a mirror on the steel axis and an electronic camera. This is translated into a characteristic trace from which the parameters are assessed.

Nomenclature used in ROTEM [8, 11, 19].

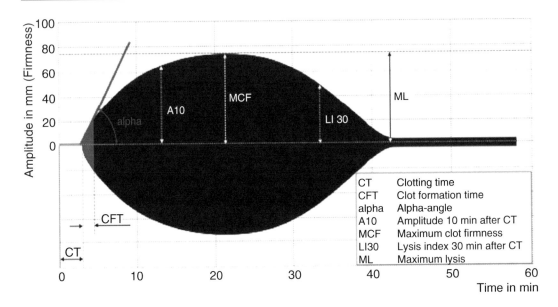

Fig. 18.9 ROTEM graph

Clotting time (CT)—time in minutes taken to reach an amplitude of 2 mm. It is the time to initial fibrin formation and signifies soluble clotting factors in plasma (Fig. 18.9).

- Normal—INTEM: 130–246 s, EXTEM: 42–74 s
- Prolonged by anticoagulants, factor deficiencies and severe hypofibrinogenaemia
- Reduced by hypercoagulable conditions

Clot formation time (CFT)—time necessary for the clot to reach an amplitude of 20 mm from 2 mm. It measures the kinetics of clot formation.

- Normal—INTEM: 40–100 s, EXTEM: 46–148 s
- Prolonged by anticoagulants, hypofibrinogenaemia, thrombocytopenia
- Shortened by increased fibrinogen level, increased platelet function

α angle—angle between tangent to a tracing at 2 mm amplitude and horizontal line. Relates to rapidity of fibrin cross-polymerization

- Normal—INTEM: 71–82°, EXTEM: 63–83°
- Increased by increased fibrinogen level, increased platelet function

- Decreased by anticoagulants, hypofibrinogenaemia, thrombocytopenia

Maximum clot firmness (MCF)—Greatest vertical height of tracing or the peak amplitude. Depicts stability and strength of the clot and platelet number and function.

EXTEM is a baseline test which supports rapid generation of a clot. The MCF$_{extem}$ gives information on clot strength and stability which depends on platelet and fibrinogen level. The FIBTEM test used a platelet inhibitor and therefore MCF$_{fibtem}$ gives an insight to the fibrinogen contribution to the clot. Therefore, comparing these two values can help differentiate platelet-related issues from hypofibrinogenaemia. A low MCF$_{fibtem}$ is indicative of fibrinogen transfusion and a normal MCF$_{fibtem}$ in presence of a low MCF$_{extem}$ would be indicative of need of platelets.

- Normal—INTEM: 52–72 mm, EXTEM: 49–71 mm
- Increased by hypercoagulable states, thrombocytosis
- Decreased by thrombocytopenia, platelet blockers, fibrinolysis, factor deficiencies (lesser extent)

Lysis Index 30 (LI30) is the percent reduction in MCF that exists whose amplitude is measured

30 min after CT is detected. Depicts clot stability and fibrinolysis (Box 18.4).

Box 18.4 ROTEM ASSAYS [19, 24]

INTEM—Contact activation. Reagent containing phospholipid and ellagic acid as activators. This provides information similar to the aPTT (intrinsic pathway).

Assessment of clot formation and fibrin polymerization

EXTEM—Tissue factor activation. Reagent contains tissue factor and provides information similar to PT (extrinsic pathway).

Fast assessment of clot formation and fibrinolysis

HEPTEM—Contains lyophilized heparinase for neutralizing unfractionated heparin, basically a modified INTEM by adding heparinase to inactivate present heparin.

To analyse heparin effect

APTEM—Contains aprotinin in addition to tissue factor. Used together with EXTEM.

Fast detection of fibrinolysis

FIBTEM—Uses cytochalasin D which blocks platelet contribution to the clot formation. When compared to the EXTEM analysis, it allows qualitative assay of fibrinogen contribution to clot strength.

Measure of functional fibrinogen levels

NATEM—Native whole blood sample—impractical and not used due to long CFT time.

The TEG is capable of analysing two samples at a time whereas ROTEM can analyse four samples simultaneously.

The traces of TEG and ROTEM appear similar; however, it is important to remember that terminologies and reference ranges are unique to each device and not interchangeable (Table 18.4). The differences may be explained due to different cups and pins used in both systems—ROTEM cups are composed of plastic with greater surface charge which may result in greater contact activation. There is also a variability in the activators and reagents used contributing to the significant difference in their results.

Table 18.4 Operating characteristics of TEG and ROTEM [19]

Characteristics	TEG	ROTEM
Pipetting	Manual	Automated
Cup motion	Moving	Fixed
Pin motion	Fixed	Moving
Angle of rotation	4°45′/5 s	4°75′/6 s
Detection	Pin transduction	Impedance of rotation
Temperature control	24–40	30–40
Cup interior	Smooth	Ridged (thickness 0.6–0.9 mm)
Cup material	Cryolite (acrylic polymer)	Polymethylmethacrylate

18.4.5.1 Diagnostic Power of TEG/ROTEM [11]

1. *Heparin effect/factor deficiency*

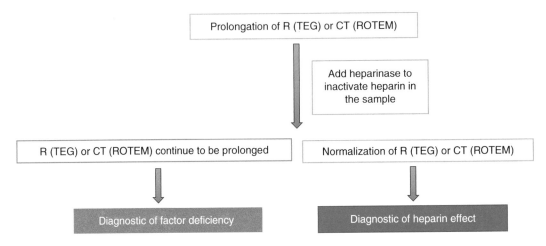

2. *Clot firmness*

    Strength of clot is determined by

    (a) Fibrinogen
    (b) Platelets
    (c) Factor XIII (by assay)

    ROTEM can be efficiently used to differentiate the cause of bleeding.

    FIBTEM and EXTEM are performed simultaneously [11, 27] (Fig. 18.10).

    The MCFextem gives information on clot strength and stability which depend on platelet and fibrinogen level.

    MCFfibtem gives an insight to the fibrinogen contribution to the clot.

    Therefore, comparing these two values can help differentiate platelet-related issues from hypofibrinogenaemia. A low MCFfibtem is indicative of fibrinogen transfusion and a normal MCFfibtem in presence of a low MCFextem would be indicative of need of platelets.

    In TEG

    Decreased α and prolonged K will signify fibrinogen deficiency and decreased MA will signify platelet deficiency.

3. *Hyperfibrinolysis*

    TEG and ROTEM are considered the gold standard for diagnosis of hyperfibrinolysis by measuring lysis.

    Example: in a case of severe hyperfibrinolysis, there may be no clot formation with the EXTEM. Addition of aprotinin and performing APTEM will trigger clotting by inhibiting the fibrinolytic component, thus demonstrating the presence of fibrinolysis. If the MCF of APTEM is reduced, thrombocytopenia may also coexist with hyperfibrinolysis.

18.4.6 The Sonoclot

The sonoclot analyser was introduced by von Kaulla et al. in 1975 as a modality of measuring viscoelastic changes in whole blood [28, 29]. The entire haemostatic process is measured and depicted in the form of a graph known as Sonoclot signature (Fig. 18.11a, b).

Fig. 18.10 ROTEM in use—FIBTEM

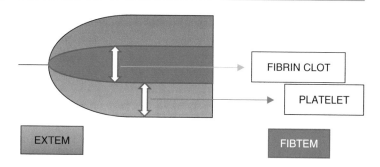

a

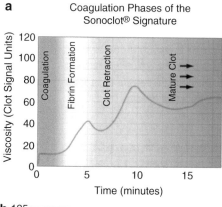

Coagulation Phases of the Sonoclot® Signature

b

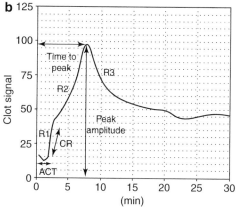

Fig. 18.11 (**a**) Sonoclot. (**b**) Sonoclot showing different components—ACT, R1, R2, R3 and Peak amplitude

18.4.6.1 Principle

The analyser consists of a hollow open-ended disposable probe, vibrating vertically at a distance of 1 μm at a frequency of 200 Hz, mounted on an ultrasonic transducer. This is immersed to a depth in a cuvette containing 0.4 mL of whole blood which exerts a viscous drag on probe, impeding its free vibration. As fibrin strands begin to form and the sample begins to clot, the drag on the probe increases further, effectively increasing the mass of the probe. This increase in impedance is sensed by the electronic circuit and converted to an output signal on a paper in the form of a curve describing the whole process from the start of fibrin formation, through polymerization of the fibrin monomer, platelet interaction and eventually clot and lysis. Usually a plain cuvette is used, without an activator, to derive sonoclot signature [13]. However, two other types of cuvettes, both containing celite activator, are better suited for intraoperative monitoring (the red cap tube contains low concentration and white cap tube contains high concentration of the activator).

The graph is plotted on a 100 mm wide recorder chart with X axis in minutes and Y axis as clot signal.

Measurements obtained [28]:

Sonoclot activated clotting time (SONACT)—time taken for upward deflection of 1 mm. It represents time (in seconds) for fibrin formation. It corresponds to ACT. Range 85–145 s without heparin.

Clot rate (CR)—rate (units/minute) of fibrin formation (from fibrinogen) depicted by the gradient of primary slope R1. The rate can also be expressed as a percentage of the peak amplitude per unit time—15–45% being normal.

An inflection point can be seen between R1 and R2 representing the start of contraction of fibrin strands by the action of platelets.

Secondary slope R2—represents further fibrinogenesis, fibrin polymerization and platelet-fibrin interaction.

R2 peak (PEAK)—indicates completion of fibrin formation. It has two variables:

- Time to peak (in minutes)—index rate of conversion of fibrinogen to fibrin (<30 min)
- Peak amplitude (in units)—index of fibrinogen concentration

Downward slope R3—represents platelets induced contraction of completed clot after which the clot mass decreases as the serum is squeezed out of clot matrix. Low platelets and/or poor function produce a shallow R3. Decreased signal of R3 will represent fibrinolysis.

Platelet function (PF)—the slope gradient of R3 represents the number of platelets and level of platelet function and is recorded as PF by the analyser.

The signal decreases further as fibrinolysis takes place and eventually returns to pre-immersion values which is seen only in patients with accelerated fibrinolysis. Therefore, the decrease in signal after R3 slope is the measure of fibrinolysis (Box 18.5).

Box 18.5 Variations of Sonoclot [8]

SonACT with celite activator for rapid assessment

k-ACT with kaolin activator for heparin management

gb-ACT + glass beads—overall coagulation and platelet function assessment

gb-ACT + glass beads + heparinase—assessment in presence of heparin

The results are influenced by age, sex and platelet count and have shown poor reproducibility. However, some studies have demonstrated the sonoclot analyser's precision to be quite comparable to that of thromboelastography [16].

18.4.7 Use of Standard/Conventional Tests in Liver Transplant

Routine coagulation tests have not been found to be accurate to predict bleeding events in patients with cirrhosis. PT/INR and aPTT are sensitive to procoagulant factors and do not account for anticoagulant factors. Moreover, they are performed in plasma and do not reflect the interaction of cellular components, vascular endothelium and fibrinolytic systems [8].

The standard laboratory tests have a long turnaround time which may not be appropriate for timely intervention often warranted during liver transplant surgery. They do not offer a differential diagnosis of impaired haemostasis and therefore may be inadequate to specify which component therapy is indicated.

Due to these shortcomings, standard laboratory tests have made way for the use of point-of-care viscoelastic coagulation monitoring devices during liver transplant.

18.4.8 Use of Point-of-Care (POC) Devices in Liver Transplant

Intraoperative red cell transfusion (>10 units) was found to be an independent risk factor for in-hospital mortality after liver transplant in a multivariate analysis by Li et al. [8]. Transfusion of ≥ 3 units PRBC (packet red blood cell) and ≥ 3 units FFP (fresh frozen plasma) was independently associated with poor graft survival at 1 and 5 years [30]. Platelet transfusion causing acute lung injury which ultimately contributes to mortality has also been mentioned in the literature.

There is evidence that point-of-care guided factor replacement aids in reducing red cell as well as volume of plasma transfusion during liver transplantation [2]. In fact, the reduction of FFP has been found to be >90% and there have been reports of significant reduction in incidence of massive transfusion. This surely translates into benefit with respect to both risk-benefit ratio and cost-effectiveness [8].

Data also suggests that these devices are reflective of the rebalanced haemostasis which has been described in cirrhotic patients and evidence, albeit limited, suggests that patients with compensated cirrhosis often maintain normal global haemostasis. There are no prospective studies validating the accuracy of TEG or

ROTEM for predicting procedural bleeding in cirrhotic patients.

Transfusion of blood during liver transplant has been thought to be inevitable. TEG-guided component therapy was described in 1985 for the first time and has been a topic of interest thereafter given the fact that minimizing transfusion will always have beneficial effect on outcome. Using parameters such as an increased R-time which reflects time to fibrin formation, as an indicator for fresh frozen plasma transfusion, decreased angle denotes a requirement of cryoprecipitate as it indicates speed of clot formation, decreased MA which denotes the clot strength is indicative of platelet transfusion—a reduction of transfusion was demonstrated [9].

18.4.8.1 Pre-transplant Liver Failure Patients

TEG values and standard laboratory tests in the preoperative period do not corelate on a consistent basis. These patients had deranged PT, INR and aPTT which was not consistent with the finding on TEG which corelated with the clinical picture [31]. Studies found that TEG-based algorithms are superior to conventional lab tests such as INR, fibrinogen and platelet count to guide transfusion [23]. There have been descriptions of patients with high INRs and MELD score with haemostatic profile ranging from normal to hypercoagulable [32]. MA of less than 47 mm was found to have 90% sensitivity and 72% specificity to predict the need for massive transfusion [3, 33].

18.4.8.2 Intraoperative Use of TEG During Liver Transplant

Studies have demonstrated a significant reduction in transfusion volume compared to a cohort of patients transplanted prior to development of the protocol. Kang and many authors have dem-

onstrated that viscoelastic testing can offer valuable insight and potentially guide transfusions [34]. Patients who underwent liver transplant with a stringent transfusion protocol received fewer plasma transfusions than patients who underwent transfusion based on less extreme TEG values [35]. Patients who underwent POC testing and were managed by algorithms based on these received significantly lower platelet concentrate transfusion rate as well as less packed red cell transfusions [20, 36] (Table 18.5). POC group had fewer thrombotic complications. There was no significant difference in perioperative mortality and no beneficial effect on mortality could be demonstrated either [17].

TEG has also been useful in detecting hyperfibrinolysis and therefore guiding antifibrinolytic therapy during liver transplant thus limiting empirical use of these drugs and thereby reducing incidence of thrombotic episodes.

Another study comparing ROTEM-based protocols demonstrated that there were reduced red blood cell transfusion and decreased complication rates with these patients. ROTEM was also efficient in picking up hyperfibrinolysis during reperfusion phase. While TEG and sonoclot provide a global picture of haemostasis, ROTEM offers a number of test variants which facilitate differential diagnosis.

Use of a TEG-based transfusion algorithm intraoperatively during liver transplant had no adverse effect on survival at 30 days and 6 months after liver transplant [37] (Fig. 18.12). Perioperative TEG values also have potential value at predicting outcomes from liver transplants. TEG values obtained preoperatively could be valuable in predicting early hepatic artery thrombosis following liver transplant [38].

An example of how POC viscoelastic tests can be used to manage transfusion.

Table 18.5 Transfusion triggers generally used in liver transplant [8]

	Trigger for FFP	Trigger for platelet	Trigger for fibrinogen
TEG	$R > 14$ min	MA < 45 mm	
ROTEM	$CT_{intem} > 4$ min	$MCF_{intem} < 45$ mm	$MCF_{fibtem} < 8$ mm
		With $MCF_{fibtem} > 8$ mm	
		Or $MCF_{intem} < 25$ mm	
Conventional tests	INR > 1.5	Platelet <50 × 10^9/dL	Fibrinogen <1 g/dL

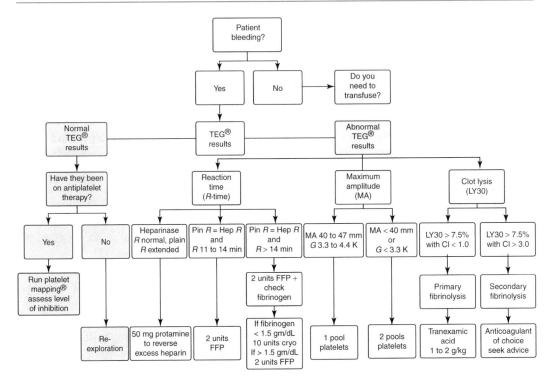

Fig. 18.12 Algorithm using viscoelastic test for transfusion management

18.4.8.3 Sonoclot in Liver Transplant

Though the literation is not extensive, Sonoclot has been used in liver transplant surgery and diagnosis of platelet dysfunction or clotting factor deficiency correlated well with clinical scenario. It has been shown to be sensitive compared to laboratory tests in detecting platelet dysfunction and fibrinolysis as well [16, 29].

18.4.8.4 Application of Platelet Function Testing in Liver Transplant [8]

In patients with hypercoagulable states (such as Budd-Chiari syndrome) coming for transplant, prevention of postoperative thrombotic events is crucial for which antiplatelet therapy has to be instituted at the earliest. Thromboelastography has been reported to be less accurate in detecting hypercoagulable states as compared to hypocoagulable states. Therefore, platelet mapping may be synergistic in managing perioperative coagulopathy in hypercoagulable cirrhosis patients during liver transplant.

18.4.9 Limitations [23]

TEG requires daily calibration (two or three times a day calibration of the machine is recommended).

Point-of-care machines do not undergo same quality testing and evaluation processes like those of conventional tests.

It is imperative that some kind of training be given for anyone performing the test. Standard technique with adherence to time guidelines must be complied with.

Though meaningful information can be obtained in 10 min of initiating the test, the whole test takes 30–60 min to complete.

Reagent sensitivity may differ between manufacturers.

Equipment, activators and other test modifications alter the specificity of the test and make inter-laboratory standardization a distant possibility, therefore limiting comparison of results [16].

Another limitation of TEG was inability to detect platelet impairment due to antiplatelet drugs which was later overcome by platelet mapping.

Bacterial infections in cirrhotics may trigger release of heparin-like substances which may be demonstrated as a prolonged R-time in the TEG. This would require antibiotic therapy rather than product administration [2].

The coagulation profile in cirrhotic patients is a dynamic process rather than a static one; therefore, TEG/ROTEM done at the baseline may not reflect and predict the risk of bleeding or thrombosis over a longer period of time [17]. Having said that, it would not be reasonable to perform repeated assessments during the entire hospitalization as the cost associated with this may not be justified.

There is a plethora of literature indicating the lack of utility of traditional laboratory tests; however, studies and evidence available to ascertain utility and efficiency of point-of-care monitoring are still not substantial. Prospective, randomized studies are required to strengthen the evidence of its use [17].

Viscoelastic tests do not detect the effects of hypothermia as the sample is measured at 37°. Neither do they test the effect of hypocalcaemia on clot strength and platelet function [30].

Nuances of the tests, such as use of reagents and stimulators and analysis of the traces obtained, are still not well-defined and standardized and have subjective variability [4].

No beneficial effect of POC-based coagulation has been demonstrated on postoperative mortality [16].

Results of the sonoclot are influenced by factors such as age, sex and platelet count, and it has been criticized for the same. The sonoclot analyser's role may be limited in acutely bleeding patients, and its application may be limited to goal-directed management algorithms [16] (Box 18.6).

Box 18.6 Summary

Pathophysiologically speaking, coagulation can be broken down into [20]:

- Primary hemostasis
- Thrombin generation
- Clot formation/stabilization
- Fibrinolysis

Most standard laboratory tests reflect only time to fibrin formation while others are only quantitative and therefore do not reflect the entire clotting process [39].

Viscoelastic tests are useful in measuring time until clot formation, dynamics of clot formation and stability and integrity of the clot over time.

These tests have been used in liver transplantations and there is evidence to show that transfusion protocols based on point-of-care tests have reduced red cell and plasma transfusion and therefore contributed to reduction in complications due to transfusion.

There is evidence that point-of-care monitoring also reduces the incidence of postoperative thrombotic complications, and this is especially of importance in cirrhotic patients undergoing transplant.

Literature does not indicate effect of POC testing on perioperative mortality [16].

While TEG and sonoclot describe the global picture of hemostasis, ROTEM has a repertoire of test variations which enable a differential diagnosis [16].

Some studies correlating POC devices with standard laboratory tests found that MA correlates with both platelet count and fibrinogen concentration in hypercoagulable patients, a significant correlation between PTT and R-time and euglobulin clot lysis time and lysis time, while other studies demonstrated poor correlation between these [9, 23].

More evidence, in the form of randomized trials, regarding key issues such as standardization, algorithms, outcomes and economic viability, is required.

The motto of management of coagulation in a bleeding patient is to replace what is missing in a timely efficient manner and in transplant recipients; this is best achieved by using point-of-care monitoring devices.

18.5 Conclusion

Bleeding in liver failure patients is a unique and multifactorial phenomenon, and it is important to understand the rebalanced haemostasis occurring in these patients. Conventional testing may be inappropriate in these patients and the use of point-of-care coagulation testing has emerged as a valuable adjunct in establishing goal-directed transfusion of blood products. Transfusion of blood and blood products has been significantly reduced, and this has a major impact on postoperative complications and morbidity following liver transplant. These techniques should be advocated more routinely as there is evidence to suggest that there is a scope for increasing their implementation.

References

1. Senzolo M, Burra P, Cholongitas E, Burroughs AK. New insights into the coagulopathy of liver disease and liver transplantation. World J Gastroenterol. 2006;12(48):7725–36.
2. Kujovich JL. Coagulopathy in liver disease: a balancing act. Hematology Am Soc Hematol Educ Program. 2015;2015:243–9.
3. Hawkins RB, Raymond SL, Hartjes T, Efron PA, Larson SD, et al. Review: the perioperative use of thromboelastography for liver transplant patients. Transplant Proc. 2018;50(10):3552–8.
4. O'Leary JG, Greenberg CS, Patton HM, Caldwell SH. AGA clinical practice update: coagulation in cirrhosis. Gastroenterology. 2019;157(1):34–43.
5. Monroe DM, Hoffman M. The coagulation cascade in cirrhosis. Clin Liver Dis. 2009;13(1):1–9.
6. Kozek-Langenecker SA. Perioperative coagulation monitoring. Best Pract Res Clin Anaesthesiol. 2010;24(1):27–40.
7. Dalmau A, Sabaté A, Aparicio I. Hemostasis and coagulation monitoring and management during liver transplantation. Curr Opin Organ Transplant. 2009;14(3):286–90.
8. Agarwal A, Sharma N, Vij V. Point-of-care coagulation monitoring during liver transplantation. Trends Anaesth Crit Care. 2013;3:42–8.
9. Luddington RJ. Thrombelastography/thromboelastometry. Clin Lab Haematol. 2005;27(2):81–90.
10. Curry AN, Pierce JT. Conventional and near-patient tests of coagulation. Contin Educ Anaesth Crit Care Pain. 2007;7:45–50.
11. Lang T, Depka M. Possibilities and limitations of thrombelastometry/-graphy. Hamostaseologie. 2006;26:20–9.
12. Tripodi A. Tests of coagulation in liver disease. Clin Liver Dis. 2009;13(1):55–61.
13. Thiruvenkatarajan V, Pruett A, Adhikary SD. Coagulation testing in the perioperative period. Indian J Anaesth. 2014;58(5):565–72.
14. Arjal R, Trotter JF. International normalized ratio of prothrombin time in the model for end-stage liver disease score: an unreliable measure. Clin Liver Dis. 2009;13(1):67–71.
15. Intagliata NM, Argo CK, Stine JG, Lisman T, Caldwell SH, Violi F. Concepts and controversies in haemostasis and thrombosis associated with liver disease: proceedings of the 7th international coagulation in liver disease conference. Thromb Haemost. 2018;118(8):1491–506.
16. Jakoi A, Kumar N, Vaccaro A, Radcliff K. Perioperative coagulopathy monitoring. Musculoskelet Surg. 2014;98(1):1–8.
17. Harrison MF. The misunderstood coagulopathy of liver disease: a review for the acute setting. West J Emerg Med. 2018;19(5):863–71.
18. Srivastava A, Kelleher A. Point-of-care coagulation testing. BJA Educ. 2013;13(1):12–6.
19. Whiting D, DiNardo JA. TEG and ROTEM: technology and clinical applications. Am J Hematol. 2014;89(2):228–32.
20. Weber CF, Zacharowski K. Perioperative point of care coagulation testing. Dtsch Arztebl Int. 2012;109(20):369–75.
21. Enriquez LJ, Shore-Lesserson L. Point-of-care coagulation testing and transfusion algorithms. Br J Anaesth. 2009;103(1):14–22.
22. Narani KK. Thrombelastography in the perioperative period. Indian J Anaesth. 2005;49(2):89–95.
23. Luz D, Nascimento. B, Bartolomeu, Rizoli S. Thrombelastography (TEG®): practical considerations on its

clinical use in trauma resuscitation. Scand J Trauma Resusc Emerg Med. 2013;21(1):21–9.

24. Ganter MT, Hofer CK. Coagulation monitoring: current techniques and clinical use of viscoelastic point-of-care coagulation devices. Anesth Analg. 2008 May;106(5):1366–75.

25. Chen A, Teruya J. Global hemostasis testing thromboelastography: old technology, new applications. Clin Lab Med. 2009;29(2):391–407.

26. https://www.clot.pro/site/assets/files/1054/clotpro_brochure_en_rev002_enicor_web.pdf.

27. Roullet S, Pillot J, Freyburger G, Biais M, Quinart A, Rault A, Revel P, Sztark F. Rotation thromboelastometry detects thrombocytopenia and hypofibrinogenaemia during orthotopic liver transplantation. Br J Anaesth. 2010;104(4):422–8.

28. Saxena P, Bihari C, Rastogi A, Agarwal S, Anand L, Sarin SK. Sonoclot signature analysis in patients with liver disease and its correlation with conventional coagulation studies. Adv Hematol. 2013;2013:237351.

29. Hett DA, Walker D, Pilkington SN, Smith DC. Sonoclot analysis. Br J Anaesth. 1995;75(6):771–6.

30. Ho KM, Pavey W. Applying the cell-based coagulation model in the management of critical bleeding. Anaesth Intensive Care. 2017;45:166.

31. Agarwal B, Wright G, Gatt A, Riddell A, Vemala V, Mallett S, Chowdary P, Davenport A, Jalan R, Burroughs A. Evaluation of coagulation abnormalities in acute liver failure. J Hepatol. 2012;57(4):780–6.

32. Stravitz RT. Potential applications of thromboelastography in patients with acute and chronic liver disease. Gastroenterol Hepatol (N Y). 2012;8(8):513–20.

33. Lawson PJ, Moore HB, Moore EE, et al. Preoperative thrombelastography maximum amplitude predicts massive transfusion in liver transplantation. J Surg Res. 2017;220:171–5.

34. Kang YG, Martin DJ, Marquez J, Lewis JH, Bontempo FA, Shaw BW Jr, et al. Intraoperative changes in blood coagulation and thrombelastographic monitoring in liver transplantation. Anesth Analg. 1985;64(9):888–96.

35. Mallett SV. Clinical utility of viscoelastic tests of coagulation (TEG/ROTEM) in patients with liver disease and during liver transplantation. Semin Thromb Hemost. 2015;41(5):527–37.

36. https://litfl.com/thromboelastogram-teg/.

37. De Pietri L, Ragusa F, Deleuterio A, Begliomini B, Serra V. Reduced transfusion during OLT by POC coagulation management and TEG functional fibrinogen: a retrospective observational study. Transplant Direct. 2016;2:e49.

38. Zahr Eldeen F, Roll GR, Derosas C, Rao R, Khan MS, Gunson BK, et al. Preoperative thromboelastography as a sensitive tool predicting those at risk of developing early hepatic artery thrombosis after adult liver transplantation. Transplantation. 2016;100(11):2382–90.

39. Hugenholtz GGC, Porte RJ, Lisman T. The platelet and platelet function testing in liver disease. Clin Liver Dis. 2009;13(1):11–20.

Parshotam Lal Gautam

Liver transplantation (LT) is the standard surgical definite treatment for end-stage liver disease (ESLD) with different indications encompassing a wide spectrum of liver failure patients with variable clinical profile and status ranging from fulminant to chronic liver failure. It is a high-risk surgery requiring critical vascular volume assessment and fluid management; there are multiple hemodynamic drifts resulting from major blood loss, fluid shifts, and vasomotor tone. Liver transplant recipients suffer many complications, some of which are intervention or approach related. On an average, liver transplant recipients suffer more than three postoperative complications, with over half of them being severe. Perioperative acute renal failure is frequent (13–71%) and is associated with postoperative mortality [1, 2]. Several perioperative events and factors including inappropriate fluid therapy seem associated with the risk of complications ranging from insignificant insult to multiorgan dysfunction syndrome and mortality as a consequence of hypoperfusion and tissue hypoxia, often exacerbated by a microcirculatory injury and increased tissue metabolic demands [3, 4]. This insult sets in a chain of sequential molecular reactions resulting in further ischemic and hypoxic tissue injury. This may be further compounded by cytopathic hypoxic injury due to mitochondrial dysfunction [5, 6]. If not all, many of these complications are preventable, but at least can be minimized with good perioperative care. Liver transplantation is a growing and evolving specialty. Strategies to improve recipient's survival are needed. One of these strategies is restrictive fluid strategies and has been found better postoperative outcomes than liberal fluid management strategies.

Fluid management strategy is one of the important aspects of perioperative care in liver transplant surgery. In critically ill cirrhotic patients with altered pathophysiology at different levels including organ dysfunction, endocrine imbalance, and receptor response alteration, volume status evaluation is difficult leading to inappropriate fluid therapy. Fluid overload is related to several complications like pulmonary edema, ileus, cardiac failure, delayed wound healing and tissue breakdown, infections, and increased mortality. Therefore, the evaluation of volume status is crucial in the optimal management of fluid therapy. Successful fluid overload treatment depends on the precise assessment of individual volume status, understanding the pathophysiology and principles of perioperative fluid management, concerns of volume over- and underload on graft function and other organs, and clear treatment goals. Perioperative fluid therapy is not just simple fluid to supplement volume for hemodynamics but needs to be prescribed as any other drug prescription. If fluid administration is in excess, it leads to

P. L. Gautam (✉)
Critical Care Division, Dayanand Medical College & Hospital, Ludhiana, Punjab, India

tissue edema of every organ including the gut and lungs affecting adversely translocation of bacteria and oxygenation resulting in delayed recovery. It may lead to graft congestion particularly in living transplant recipients. If there is deficit and hypovolemia, it increases the risk of ischemic and thrombotic complications (Table 19.1). More importantly,

Table 19.1 Fluid overload and adverse effects

Systemic and organ effects	Adverse effects	Remarks
Systemic, organ, and tissue effects		
Body systemic effects	Increased tissue edema	Increased morbidity and mortality
	Infection	Prolonged ICU stay
	Impaired perfusion of tissues	
	Abdominal compartment syndrome	
Tissue edema	Poor wound healing	Difficult IV access
	Wound infection	
	Pressure ulceration	
Organ/tissue edema		
Cerebral edema	Impaired cognition	Patients with acute liver failure and risk of further rise in ICP
Cardiac	Conduction disturbance	Pericardial effusion can result in cardiac tamponade and is difficult to drain in coagulopathic patients
	Impaired contractility	
	Diastolic dysfunction	
	Pericardial effusion	
Pulmonary	Impaired gas exchange	Increased ventilator days, VAP and ICU stay
	Reduced compliance	
	Increased work of breathing	
	Pleural effusion	
Renal	Interstitial edema	Patients with previous renal injury or HRS are at great risk of further AKI
	Reduced RBF	
	Increased interstitial pressure	
	Reduced GFR	
	Uremia	
	Salt and water retention	

Table 19.1 (continued)

Systemic and organ effects	Adverse effects	Remarks
Liver and gut edema	Impaired synthetic function	Graft dysfunction
	Cholestasis	Increased abdominal drain output
	Malabsorption	Translocation of bacteria
	Ileus	

a recent multicenter clinical trial showed an increased incidence of acute renal failure when a fixed restrictive perioperative fluid strategy was compared to a liberal one during a major abdominal surgery [7]. There is substantial data against the use of starch-based solutions in septic patients where endothelial capillary leak fails to retain fluid intravascularly and detrimental effects on the kidney and immune system.

Current fluid therapy-related practice issues. There is wide variation in practice. The choice of fluids is largely based on traditional beliefs, context of practice, location, and cost. It seems that there is more of personnel choices rather than scientific approach. Most of transplant anesthesiologists are quite experienced and skillful. Despite the knowledge and skills there is ample evidence that practices are not uniform and there is wide deviation in choice of goals and parameter targets, monitoring, and type of fluids and management strategy. Secondly as outcome is dependent on many factors so this makes difficult to design evidence-based fixed fluid therapy protocols. All choices and preferences are not having equivalent outcome. However, everyone justifies his/her own approach being an expert and experienced senior. Thus, there is a need to find the best strategy. The Liver Transplant Anesthesia Consortium (LTrAC) did a series of four comprehensive, web-based surveys in the United States and internationally. There was a very interesting finding that there were geographical differences in practice pattern. Clinicians from the UK, China, and Australia relied primarily on colloid therapy (55–75% of time), whereas only 13% of clinicians in the United States used colloid for treating hypovolemia. In the United

States, normal saline was a frequent choice, followed by a pH-adjusted crystalloid in 74%. Albumin was a common colloid for volume expansion (85%; 95% CI, 70–93%). The synthetic colloids HES in saline (Hespan) or HES in balanced electrolyte solution (Hextend) had been used nearly in half of programs at that time prior to restriction by many international agencies on starch fluids [8].

Understanding altered pathophysiology and perioperative fluid management. It is well established that fluid balance has an impact on outcome in liver transplant surgery or any other major abdominal surgery, particularly in high-risk candidates. It is important to understand that it is not only the type of fluid or over-jealous fluid therapy consequences but also happens because of capillary leak which may occur due to sepsis or reperfusion or altered membrane function resulting from other perioperative insults. This happens secondary to the release of host responses in the form of complement factors, cytokines and prostaglandin products, and altered organ microcirculation [9–11]. In presence of increased capillary permeability to proteins and increased trans-capillary hydrostatic pressure, hypervolemia secondary to inappropriate fluid administration to maintain pressures results in excessive leak [12]. There is neurohumoral alteration in body homeostasis with marked activation of sympathetic and renin-angiotensin-aldosterone systems in these patients resulting in sodium retention with very low urinary excretion of sodium. The "splanchnic steal" and leaky endothelium in cirrhotic make fluid management difficult. There is an inability of body to mobilize ascites despite adherence to the dietary salt restriction. There is rapid reaccumulation of fluid after therapeutic paracentesis despite adherence to a sodium-restricted diet. These changes put cirrhotic patients at risk of renal and another organ failure in the perioperative period, and a challenging situation for the treating physician [13]. The amount of fluid that leaks into the interstitium correlates with infused fluid volume and that remained intravascular varies with the type of fluid and it's terminal half life [14]. There is a paradigm shift in membrane function conceptualization. Traditionally it was thought that fluid transfer across endothelial membrane is based on oncotic and hydrostatic pressure balance, i.e., Starling principle. Current concept is "Double-barrier concept" or endothelial Glycocalyx layer. The endothelial glycocalyx layer is a web of membrane-bound glycoproteins and proteoglycans. Sub-glycocalyx intercellular spaces are almost protein-free. Capillaries filter fluid to ISF throughout their length. Absorption through venous capillaries/venules does not occur. Most filtered fluid returns to circulation via lymph. Oxidative stress, attenuation of leucocyte, and platelet adhesion lead to damage of endothelial glycocalyx layer, thus resulting in capillary leak. The integrity or leakiness of this layer and hence potential to develop interstitial edema varies substantially among organ systems, particularly under reperfusion and other inflammatory conditions like sepsis, SIRS of surgery, trauma, and overfluid resuscitation [15].

19.1 Vascular Component Approach for Guiding Fluid Therapy: A Novel and Critical Way of Volume Status Assessment [16]

The blood volume and the portion of the volume containing red blood cells represent the vital elements of the **Vascular content** (vC). If the patient has a decreased vC irrespective of the reason, it equals "hypovolemia." Here, it is important to understand that the vC may be low relatively secondary to vasodilator drugs, in response to anesthesia or redistribution of volume. The classical scenario is that of vasoplegia. The definite therapy will be to restore the vascular tone to normal range but at times may be difficult. Clinically, an important feature of any clinical assessment is "the patient's volume status." However, for better management, we need to look at all components tone, integrity, and hemodynamics rather than volume status only resulting in inappropriate therapy. The separate evaluation of these different components allows better assessment and management of the patient. These four main components are

1. Blood flow (BF)
2. Vascular content (vC)
3. Vascular barrier (vB)
4. Vascular tone (vT)

An obvious limitation to assess each component reliably bedside is not easy with routine monitoring tools. This concept needs translation in clinical practice to avoid unnecessary fluids in volume responsive patient where vasopressors may prove to be a better option.

19.2 Restrictive vs. Liberal Strategy

The impact of perioperative fluid balance and fluid therapy has been studied on postoperative complications in last decades in complex surgical populations and septic patients including cardiac, liver transplant and liver resections, with many different combinations of fluid management protocols, strategies, and hemodynamic goals. It is difficult to find the ideal or optimal protocol. ERAS guidelines emphasize on restrictive fluid strategy for enhanced recovery in major abdominal surgery. Perioperative fluid imbalance, defined as too little or too much fluid, had been associated with a greater than 60% increase in postoperative complications after major abdominal surgery [17, 18].

Even in restrictive strategy, there is a need to define target if zero balance or negative balance or minimal positive balance or to which side we can err while moving in gray shades. To implement a strategy, there is a need to know the best monitoring tool to guide fluid therapy. All devices and related parameters to guide fluid management protocol have some caveats and limitations. If the physician is unaware of these pitfalls, one can make mistakes not only in therapy but in research analysis leading to biased results. There are many restrictive fluid strategies such as early

goal-directed protocols, weight-based protocols, low-CVP protocols, SVV or cardiac output or PAP-based protocols. Recent systematic reviews done on major surgeries particularly abdominal suggest that cardiac output-guided fluid administration, compared to either fixed restrictive or fixed liberal strategies, reduces postoperative complications by 20–30% in patients undergoing major surgery highlighting and signifying preference to restrictive fluid strategy in these subgroups of these patients [19–21].

Thus, current evidence favors to a specific target using restrictive strategy. Sometimes when the patient is too leaky to hold fluid into the vascular compartment, edema sets in despite keeping low vascular volume. Fluid overload is not only a consequence of fluid therapy but also occurs because of altered capillary endothelial function and high hydrostatic pressure from volume overload resulting in leak during severe sepsis secondary to the release of complement factors, cytokines and prostaglandin products, and altered organ microcirculation. Edema in a vicious cycle results in impaired oxygen and metabolite diffusion, distorted tissue architecture, obstruction of capillary blood flow and lymphatic drainage, and disturbed cell to cell interactions that may then contribute to progressive organ dysfunction. Encapsulated organs suffer these insults greater than other organs and tissues [22, 23].

19.3 Composition of Fluids and Its Impact on Outcome

The right choice of fluid replacement has been a matter of debate. We have three types of fluids broadly: crystalloids, colloids, and albumin. Further we have balanced and non-balanced crystalloid fluids with different electrolyte composition. Colloids include starch-based, gelofusine-based, and albumin with different strengths. Colloids have an edge over crystalloids in expanding the plasma volume and stays longer in the intravascular compartment. The volume administered is less thereby lower incidence of pulmonary, and other organ edema. There is substantial evidence that supports its benefits on microcirculation, blood rheology, and inflammatory mediators. However, starch-based fluids are almost out particularly in septic patients and other critically ill patients because of their adverse effects and ban by various regulatory agencies. Some of the adverse effects are acute and chronic toxicity, coagulopathy, and hypersensitivity reactions in addition to its cost [24, 25]. Most of these studies are from intensive care settings where most of these patients are septic with altered endothelial function. There are few studies from cardiac surgeries debating for the safety of these HES fluids. These studies underlined the difficulties in establishing hardcore outcome data, even in large cohort studies. Although the findings seemed to diminish the magnitude of risk using HES, it cannot nullifies the results of metanalysis and systemic reviews [26–29]. There is data from animal studies suggesting that 6% HES 130/0.4 exerts protective effects on glycocalyx integrity and attenuates the increase of vascular permeability during systemic inflammation [30]. However, with current literature the safety of starch-based colloids is questionable in critically ill patients.

Human serum albumin has been widely used for many decades in clinical settings with variable reputation as choice over time, but a frequent choice in cirrhotic patients. Albumin is the most abundant protein in the human body, accounting for ~55% of the total protein content in plasma, with many physiologic functions including binding and transporting a large number of drugs and both endogenous and exogenous substances. It plays an important role as defensive quality by trapping the toxic matter. Moreover, it has antioxidant, free radical scavenger, antithrombotic, and anticoagulant effects and seems to limit increased capillary permeability during inflammation [31, 32]. Albumin as a perioperative fluid therapy is not the first choice as it is costly. However, it is often used whenever there is large ascites and fluid requirement is large. Currently it is recommended in spontaneous bacterial peritonitis with ascites, refractory ascites not responsive to diuretics, large-volume paracentesis,

post-paracentesis syndrome, and the treatment of hepatorenal syndrome as an adjunct to vasoconstrictors. New indications for albumin therapy include the antioxidant activity and its effects on capillary integrity. In recent years, large-pore hemofiltration and albumin exchange have emerged as promising liver support therapies for liver failure and other toxic syndromes. They are designed to remove a broad range of blood-borne toxins and to restore normal functions of the circulating albumin by replacing defective forms of albumin and albumin molecules saturated with toxins with normal albumin [32]. In recent years, the use of albumin has been questioned in many studies by the growing concern about the cost-effectiveness of medical treatments. Many of the metanalysis comparing saline and albumin has not shown discernible benefit of albumin [33–38]. In a recent study in cardiac surgical intensive care, albumin infusion decreased the need for fresh frozen plasma transfusion, reduced mortality, and lowered serum lactate level but increased financial burden for patients, compared to normal saline group [39]. However, currently careful patient assessment is necessary before administering albumin to see appropriateness as there are a number of contraindications and growing concern of cost-effectiveness [34–36, 40]. The adverse effects of albumin have been reported such as interstitial pulmonary edema, multiorgan failure in capillary leak syndrome, or antihemostatic and antiplatelet properties that may worsen blood loss, particularly in post-surgical or trauma patients. In view of high cost and some other associated concerns, appropriateness of prescription is paramount.

In a recent review by Zhou et al. comparing the efficacy and safety of normal saline (NS) for fluid therapy in critically ill with other fluids and colloids, there is no significant different in mortality and incidence of AKI when compared with 10% HES, albumin, and buffered crystalloid solution [41]. A good understanding of individual fluid with its advantage and disadvantage and its interaction in liver recipient with altered homeostasis and neurohumoral response when compared with other fluids prescribed for critically ill patients is conducive to make good clinical decision. There is substantial evidence and experience to support the use of albumin as a part of fluid therapy in liver transplant recipients but its use should be restricted and prescribed judiciously to make liver transplant economical.

19.4 Monitoring of Volume Status and Perioperative Fluid Management

Intravenous fluid therapy plays a key role in the perioperative management of transplant, and many authors believe that it should be like drug prescription where drug, dose, time, and route matter. Considering the type, dose-effect relationship, and side effects of fluids, fluid therapy should be regarded similar to other drug therapy with specific indications and tailored recommendations. By emphasizing the necessity to individualize fluid therapy, we hope to reduce the risk to our patients and improve their outcome. Weight gain greater than 10% is considered a risk factor for increased pulmonary complications in major abdominal surgeries. Observational studies in nontransplant critically ill patients who required continuous renal replacement therapy (CRRT) have shown an association between fluid overload and mortality [42, 43].

The clinical determination of the intravascular volume can be extremely difficult in critically ill and surgical patients who have altered vascular tone and volume due to anesthesia and major surgery. This is problematic as fluid loading is considered the first step in the resuscitation of hemodynamically unstable patients. However, recent data suggest that only about 50% of hemodynamically unstable patients in the ICU and operating room respond to a fluid challenge [44–46]. Traditionally used CVP and other cardiac filling pressures over the last many decades are unable to predict fluid responsiveness. Over the last decade a number of studies have been reported where heart–lung interactions have been used to assess fluid responsiveness in mechanically ventilated patients. Particularly, the pulse pressure variation derived from analysis of the arterial waveform and the stroke volume variation derived from pulse contour analysis have been found to be highly predictive of fluid responsiveness and a better tool to guide fluid therapy. In difficult situations and particularly transplant surgery, transesophageal echocardiography is a more accurate measure of preload than either the central venous pressure or pulmonary artery occlusion pressure using left ventricular end-diastolic area as TEE not only predicts fluid responsiveness but provides functional status of the heart as well as the dynamic indices. There are always controversial results as study design and bias factors change. However, with less expertise and cost issues, TEE in many centers is underutilized.

Although there is current trend in using SVV calibrated and uncalibrated both in liver transplant recipients despite controversial literature, many centers use uncalibrated SVV along with derived cardiac index and SVRI as a routine tool. There are many studies where authors have documented poor performance with uncalibrated SVV. A couple of studies using pulse pressure variations and protocolized fluid therapy based on pulse pressure variation and cardiac index in the setting of brain death donors to guide fluid therapy failed to demonstrate any discernible benefit [47].

In transplant recipients, in order to maintain perfusion of graft and vital organs, restore cardiac output, systemic blood pressure, and renal perfusion an adequate fluid resuscitation is essential. Overload is detrimental to gut function and overall recovery delay. Low perfusion state carries the risky of hepatic artery thrombosis. Achieving an appropriate level of volume management requires knowledge of the underlying pathophysiology, evaluation of volume status, and selection of appropriate monitoring device or making good judgment from corroborative multiple data, appropriate solution for volume repletion, and maintenance and modulation of the tissue perfusion [48–51].

Fluid overload recognition and assessment requires an accurate documentation of all intakes and outputs, yet there is a wide variation in practice: how it is evaluated, reviewed, and utilized.

But in a nutshell it is equally important to look at assessing the intravascular status and cumulative balance. Accurate volume status evaluation is essential for appropriate therapy since errors of volume evaluation can result in either lack of essential treatment or unnecessary fluid administration, and both scenarios are associated with increased mortality. It is important to discuss fluid therapy in the team meeting - whether to adopt restrictive or liberal fluid regime. There are several methods to evaluate the fluid status; however, most of the tests currently used are fairly inaccurate. Diuretics, especially loop diuretics, remain a valid therapeutic alternative in posttransplant period to optimize the balance. Fluid overload refractory to medical therapy requires the application of extracorporeal therapies [52].

19.5 Fluid Assessment in ICU

It is challenging at times to evaluate a critically ill or transplant recipient in the perioperative period with altered vascular tone particularly if there is an element of sepsis. Fluid evaluation requires a critical review of intake and output chart to monitor with advance gadgets in collaboration considering the limitations of each device. Accurate volume status evaluation is essential and critical for appropriate fluid prescription. Volume status assessment errors can result in over- or under-fluid treatment, both associated with increased dysfunction of different organs leading to morbidity and mortality. There are several clinical and device tools to evaluate the fluid status; however, most of the tests currently used are fairly inaccurate at times. We need to understand and know the limitation of the device and pitfalls in the monitoring technique. Each method has gray areas where the performance is equivocal. We should try to consider other data streams and interpret in collaboration.

1. **Nursing documentation calculations**
   (a) **Daily fluid balance**: daily difference in all intakes and all outputs including drains, CRRT fluid removal if applied

which frequently does not include insensible losses.
   (b) **Cumulative fluid balance**: sum of each day fluid balance over a period of time including intraoperative balance.
   (c) **Weight gain**: Percentage of fluid overload adjusted for bodyweight: cumulative fluid balance that is expressed as a percent.

Fluid overload or weight gain
$$= \frac{\text{Total fluid in} - \text{total fluid out}\%}{\text{Admission body weight}} \times 100$$

   (d) **Clinical signs of fluid overload:** usually implies a degree of pulmonary edema (PaO_2/FiO_2 ratios) or peripheral edema (chemosis).

2. **Radiological Imaging**
   (a) **Chest X-ray** Chest X-ray has been one of the most used tests to evaluate for hypervolemia. Radiographic sings of volume overload include dilated upper lobe vessels, cardiomegaly, interstitial edema, enlarged pulmonary artery, pleural effusion, alveolar edema, prominent superior vena cava, and Kerley lines. However, a reliable single tool is not available to comment on fluid overload or cardiac dysfunction may not be good tool as may miss subtle changes.
   (b) **Ultrasonographic assessment of IVC, lung ultrasound and jugular veins.** Blue protocol and Sonographic artifacts known as B-lines that suggest thickened interstitial or fluid-filled alveoli can be detected using thoracic ultrasound. PCWP and fluid accumulation in lungs have been correlated with the presence of B-lines ("comet-tail images") in patients with congestive heart failure and volume overload. Agricola et al. found significant correlations between comet-tail images score and extravascular lung water determined by the PiCCO System, between comet score and PCWP, and between comet-tail images score and radiologic sings of fluid overload in the lungs [34]. The measurement of the inferior vena

cava (IVC) diameter can also be used to assess volume status. Normal diameter of IVC is 1.5–2.5 cm (measured 3 cm from the right atrium); volume depletion is considered with an IVC diameter <1.5 cm while an IVC diameter >2.5 cm suggests volume overload. Other IVC signs are collapsibility and distensibility in spontaneously breathing patients and in mechanically ventilated patients respectively. In an observational study Lyon et al. found significant differences between the inferior vena cava diameter during inspiration (IVCdi) and during expiration (IVCde), before and after blood donation of 450 mL [35]. There are other studies supporting the use of IVC diameter. We also use ultrasonography quite a lot in the perioperative period to evaluate the fluid and cardiac status. We try eyeballing different parameters of ultrasonography such as lung ultrasound, IJV and IVC diameters and collapsibility along with cardiac chamber sizes. In patients treated for hypovolemia, Zengin et al. evaluated the IVC and right ventricle (RVd) diameters and diameter changes with the diameters and diameter changes of healthy volunteers. The IVCd was measured ultrasonographically by M-mode in the subxiphoid area and the RVd was measured in the third and fourth intercostal spaces before and after fluid resuscitation. As compared with healthy volunteers, average diameters in hypovolemic patients of the IVC during inspiration and expiration, and right ventricle diameter were significantly lower. After fluid resuscitation, there was a significant increase in mean IVC diameters during inspiration and expiration as well as in the right ventricle diameter [36]. Bedside inferior vena cava diameter and right ventricle diameter evaluation could be a practical noninvasive instrument for fluid status estimation and for evaluating the response to fluid therapy in critically ill patients.

3. **Biochemistry: BNP levels** High levels of BNP can be found with diastolic dysfunction and volume overload commonly; however, some conditions like myocardial infraction and pulmonary embolism can cause elevated levels of BNP. Other conditions that have to be taken into account when evaluating BNP levels are renal failure, which is associated with high BNP levels and obesity where there is lower BNP levels. The greatest utility of BNP levels is in the absence of elevation, since low BNP levels have a high negative predictive value for excluding heart failure diagnosis [53–55].

Medical history, record review, clinical signs along with routine diagnostic studies (chest radiograph, electrocardiogram, and serum B-type natriuretic peptide (BNP)) helps in overload assessment as well as to differentiate heart failure from other causes.

4. **Bioimpedance analysis**

It is a noninvasive and inexpensive versatile test that transforms electrical properties of tissues into clinical information. Bioimpedance vector analysis (BIVA) measures whole body water. This technology is evolving to evaluate hydration status in the postoperative period particularly in patients who are on dialysis [56]. Its role may get more explored in the perioperative period to assess the excess water gain.

19.6   Special Considerations

19.6.1 LDLT vs. Cadaveric

Brain-dead donors currently remain the primary source of grafts for solid organ transplantation in the western world except in southeast Asian countries where live donor program is the backbone. In this context, appropriate management of organ donors from the diagnosis of brain death to the end of the organ procurement (OP) procedure is of paramount importance to optimize the function of potential grafts. As there is altered patho-physiology in brain-dead donors, there is dying endocrine function leading to diabetes insipidus and hemodynamic instability requiring special attention to maintain organ function of individual organ. Thus, it is of utmost importance to maintain strict balance as per the organ retrieval. However, data is limited to make an evidence-based recommendation. The current practice is of restrictive strategy using fluids with chloride restriction and starch free balanced salt solutions in this subset of patients. A French survey done by Champigneulle et al. in collaboration with SFAR research network also found similar practices and concerns by the respondents [57].

Hormonal substitution should be used to maintain hemodynamics for organ procurement particularly where retrieval is delayed in days.

As most of LDLT cases are performed electively, living donor recipients may have better compensated liver disease at the time of surgery than cadaver donor recipients. A study by Niemann et al. found that while intraoperative fluid and transfusion requirements are similar in LDLT and cadaveric recipients, the impact of transplantation on pulmonary gas exchange and reperfusion syndromes is more pronounced in patients receiving organs from cadaveric donors. Intraoperative transfusion and fluid requirements were also not significantly different in recipients from living donors versus cadaveric donors with regard to red blood cells, fresh frozen plasma, platelets, and cryoprecipitate. Authors thought that this difference probably arose from longer cold ischemia times present in the cadaveric donor group [58].

References

1. Parikh A, Washburn KW, Matsuoka L, Pandit U, Kim JE, Almeda J, et al. A multicenter study of 30 days complications after deceased donor liver transplantation in the model for end-stage liver disease score era. Liver Transpl. 2015;21:1160–8.
2. Pereira AA, Bhattacharya R, Carithers R, Reyes J, Perkins J. Clinical factors predicting readmission after orthotopic liver transplantation. Liver Transpl. 2012;18:1037–45.
3. Ince C, Sinaasappel M. Microcirculatory oxygenation and shunting in sepsis and shock. Crit Care Med. 1999;27:1369–77.
4. Beal AL, Cerra FB. Multiple organ failure syndrome in the 1990's: systemic inflammatory response and organ dysfunction. JAMA. 1994;271:226–33.
5. Fink MP. Bench-to-bedside review: cytopathic hypoxia. Crit Care. 2002;6:491–9.
6. Fink MP, Cytopathic hypoxia. Is oxygen use impaired in sepsis as a result of an acquired intrinsic derangement in cellular respiration? Crit Care Clin. 2002;18:165–75.
7. Myles PS, Bellomo R, Corcoran T, Forbes A, Peyton P, Story D, et al. Restrictive versus liberal fluid therapy for major abdominal surgery. N Engl J Med. 2018;378(24):2263–74.
8. LTrAC survey report: US choice of resuscitation fluid in OLT. Transpl Proc. 2013;45:2258–62.
9. Andreucci M, Federico S, Andreucci VE. Edema and acute renal failure. Semin Nephrol. 2001;21(3):251–6.
10. Schrier RW, Wang W. Acute renal failure and sepsis. N Engl J Med. 2004;351(2):159–69.
11. Murphy CV, Schramm GE, Doherty JA, Reichley RM, Gajic O, Afessa B, et al. The importance of fluid management in acute lung injury secondary to septic shock. Chest. 2009;136(1):102–9.
12. Bouchard J, Mehta RL. Fluid balance issues in the critically ill patient. Contrib Nephrol. 2010;164:69–78.
13. McAvoy NC, et al. Alimentary pharmacology & therapeutics, vol. 43. Hoboken: Wiley; 2016. p. 947–54.
14. Hahn RG, Lyons G. The half-life of infusion fluids. Eur J Anaesthiol. Jul 2016;3(7):75–482.
15. Myburgh JA. Resuscitation fluids. N Engl J Med. 2013;369:1243–51.
16. Chawla LS, Ince C, Chappell D, Gan TJ, Kellum JA, Mythen M, Shaw AD. Vascular content, tone, integrity, and haemodynamics for guiding fluid therapy: a conceptual approach. Br J Anaesth. 2014;113(5):748–55.
17. Wilms H, Mittal A, Haydock MD, van den Heever M, Devaud M, Windsor JA. A systematic review of goal directed fluid therapy: rating of evidence for goals and monitoring methods. J Crit Care. 2014;29:204–9.
18. Varadhan KK, Lobo DN. A meta-analysis of randomised controlled trials of intravenous fluid therapy in major elective open abdominal surgery: getting the balance right. Proc Nutr Soc. 2010;69:488–98.
19. Corcoran T, Emma Joy Rhodes J, Clarke S, Myles PS, Ho KM. Perioperative fluid management strategies in major surgery. Anesth Analg. 2012;114:640–51.
20. Pearse RM, Harrison DA, MacDonald N, Gillies MA, Blunt M, Ackland G, et al. Effect of a perioperative, cardiac output–guided hemodynamic therapy algorithm on outcomes following major gastrointestinal surgery. JAMA. 2014;311:2181.
21. Boland MR, Noorani A, Varty K, Coffey JC, Agha R, Walsh SR. Perioperative fluid restriction in major abdominal surgery: systematic review and meta-analysis of randomized clinical trials. World J Surg. 2013;37:1193–202.

22. Schumann R, Mandell S, Mercaldo N, Michaels D, Robertson A, Banerjee A, et al. Anesthesia for liver transplantation in United States academic centers: intraoperative practice. J Clin Anesth. 2013;25:542–50.

23. Gurusamy KS, Pissanou T, Pikhart H, Vaughan J, Burroughs AK, Davidson BR. Methods to decrease blood loss and transfusion requirements for liver transplantation. In: Gurusamy KS, editor. Cochrane database of systematic reviews, vol. 63. Chichester: Wiley; 2011. p. CD009052.

24. Wiedermann CJ, Joannidis M. Accumulation of hydroxyethyl starch in human and animal tissues: a systematic review. Intensive Care Med. 2014;40(2):160–70.

25. Serpa Neto A, Veelo DP, Peireira VG, de Assunção MS, Manetta JA, Espósito DC, Schultz MJ. Fluid resuscitation with hydroxyethyl starches in patients with sepsis is associated with an increased incidence of acute kidney injury and use of renal replacement therapy: a systematic review and meta-analysis of the literature. J Crit Care. 2014;29(1):185.

26. Van der Linden P, Dumoulin M, Van Lerberghe C, Torres CS, Willems A, Faraoni D. Efficacy and safety of 6% hydroxyethyl starch 130/0.4 (Voluven) for peri-operative volume replacement in children undergoing cardiac surgery: a propensity-matched analysis. Crit Care. 2015;19(1):87.

27. Ryhammer PK, Tang M, Hoffmann-Petersen J, Leonaviciute D, Greisen J, Storebjerg Gissel M, Jakobsen CJ. Colloids in cardiac surgery-friend or foe? J Cardiothorac Vasc Anesth. 2017;31(5):1639–48.

28. Raiman M, Mitchell CG, Biccard BM, Rodseth RN. Comparison of hydroxyethyl starch colloids with crystalloids for surgical patients: a systematic review and meta-analysis. Eur J Anaesthesiol. 2016;33(1):42–8.

29. He B, Xu B, Xu X, Li L, Ren R, Chen Z, Xiao J, Wang Y, Xu B. Hydroxyethyl starch versus other fluids for non-septic patients in the intensive care unit: a meta-analysis of randomized controlled trials. Crit Care. 2015;19:92.

30. Margraf A, Herter JM, Kühne K, Stadtmann A, Ermert T, Wenk M, Meersch M, Van Aken H, Zarbock A, Rossaint J. 6% hydroxyethyl starch (HES 130/0.4) diminishes glycocalyx degradation and decreases vascular permeability during systemic and pulmonary inflammation in mice. Crit Care. 2018;22(1):11.

31. Quinlan GJ, Martin GS, Evans TW. Albumin: biochemical properties and therapeutic potential. Hepatology. 2005;41:1211–9.

32. Farrugia A. Albumin usage in clinical medicine: tradition or therapeutic? Transfus Med Rev. 2010;24:53–63.

33. Rozga J, Piątek T, Małkowski P. Human albumin: old, new, and emerging applications. Ann Transplant. 2013;18:205–17.

34. Vanek VW. The use of serum albumin as a prognostic or nutrition marker and the pros and cons of IV albumin therapy. Nutr Clin Pract. 1998;3:110–22.

35. Yim JM, Vermeulen LC, Erstad BL, et al. Albumin and nonprotein colloid solution use in US academic health centers. Arch Intern Med. 1995;155:2450–5.

36. Tarín Remohí MJ, Sánchez Arcos A, Santos Ramos B, et al. Costs related to inappropriate use of albumin in Spain. Ann Pharmacother. 2000;34:1198–205.

37. Schierhout G, Roberts I. Fluid resuscitation with colloid or crystalloid solutions in critically ill patients: a systematic review of randomized trials. BMJ. 1998;316:961–4.

38. Casuccio A, Nalbone E, Immordino P, Laseta C, Sanfilippo P, Tuttolomondo A, Vitale F. Appropriateness of requests for human serum albumin at the University Hospital of Palermo, Italy: a prospective study. Int J Qual Health Care. 2015;27(2):154–60.

39. Zhang Z, Dai X, Qi J, Ao Y, Yang C, Li Y. Effect of albumin administration on post-operation mortality, duration on ventilator, and hospital stay on patients in cardiac intensive care: an observational study. Trop J Pharm Res. 2019;18(6):1339–45.

40. Boldt J, Knothe C, Zickmann B, et al. Influence of different intravascular volume therapies on platelet function in patients undergoing cardiopulmonary bypass. Anesth Analg. 1993;76:1185–90.

41. Zhou FH, Liu C, Mao Z, Ma PL. Normal saline for intravenous fluid therapy in critically ill patients (Review Article). Chin J Traumatol. 2018;21:11–5.

42. Bouchard J, Soroko SB, Chertow GM, Himmelfarb J, Ikizler TA, Paganini EP, et al. Fluid accumulation, survival and recovery of kidney function in critically ill patients with acute kidney injury. Kidney Int. 2009;76(4):422–7.

43. Hoste EA, Maitland K, Brudney CS, Mehta R, Vincent JL, Yates D, Kellum JA, Mythen MG, Shaw AD, ADQI XII Investigators Group. Four phases of intravenous fluid therapy: a conceptual model. Br J Anaesth. 2014;113(5):740–7.

44. Marik PE. Hemodynamic parameters to guide fluid therapy. Transfus Alter Transfus Med. 2010;11(3):102–12.

45. Marik PE, Cavallazzi R, Vasu T, et al. Dynamic changes in arterial waveform derived variables and fluid responsiveness in mechanically ventilated patients. A systematic review of the literature. Crit Care Med. 2009;37:2642–7.

46. Michard F, Teboul JL. Predicting fluid responsiveness in ICU patients: a critical analysis of the evidence. Chest. 2002;121:2000–8.

47. Cinotti R, Roquilly A, Mahé P-J, Feuillet F, Yehia A, Belliard G, et al. Pulse pressure variations to guide fluid therapy in donors: a multicentric echocardiographic observational study. J Crit Care. 2014;29:489–94.

48. Al-Khafaji A, Elder M, Lebovitz DJ, Murugan R, Souter M, Stuart S, et al. Protocolized fluid therapy in brain-dead donors: the multicenter randomized MOnIToR trial. Intensive Care Med. 2015;41:418–26.

49. Prowle JR, Echeverri JE, Ligabo EV, Ronco C, Bellomo R. Fluid balance and acute kidney injury. Nat Rev Nephrol. 2010;6(2):107–15.

50. Levy MM, Artigas A, Phillips GS, Rhodes A, Beale R, Osborn T, et al. Outcomes of the Surviving Sepsis Campaign in intensive care units in the USA and Europe: a prospective cohort study. Lancet Infect Dis. 2012;12(12):919–24.

51. Kellum JA, Lameire N, Kidney Disease Improving Global Outcomes (KDIGO) Working Group. Section 3: prevention and treatment of AKI. Kidney Int Suppl (2011). 2012;2(1):37–68.

52. Mehta RL, Bouchard J. Controversies in acute kidney injury: effects of fluid overload on outcome. Contrib Nephrol. 2011;174:200–11.

53. Granado RC-D, Mehta RL. Fluid overload in the ICU: evaluation and management. BMC Nephrol. 2016;17:109.

54. Peacock WF, Soto KM. Current techniques of fluid status assessment. Contrib Nephrol. 2010;164:128–42.

55. Bagshaw SM, Cruz DN. Fluid overload as a biomarker of heart failure and acute kidney injury. Contrib Nephrol. 2010;164:54–68.

56. Lukaski HC, Diaz NV, Talluri A, Nescolarde L. Classification of hydration in clinical conditions: indirect and direct approaches using bioimpedance. Nutrients. 2019;11:809.

57. Champigneulle B, Arthur Neuschwander A, Bronchard R, Favé G, Josserand J, Lebas B, Bastien O, Pirracchio R, SFAR Research Network. Intraoperative management of brain-dead organ donors by anesthesiologists during an organ procurement procedure: results from a French survey. BMC Anesthesiol. 2019;19:108.

58. Carrier FM, Chassé M, Wang HT, Aslanian P, Bilodeau M, Turgeon AF. Effects of perioperative fluid management on postoperative outcomes in liver transplantation: a systematic review protocol. Syst Rev. 2018;7:180.

Role of Vasopressors in Liver Transplant Surgery

20

Sonali Saraf

20.1 Introduction

Liver transplant is the only treatment for patients with end-stage liver disease (ESLD), regardless of the aetiology of liver failure. Patients with ESLD typically have hyperdynamic circulation with increased cardiac output (CO), heart rate (HR) and decreased systemic vascular resistance (SVR) [1, 2], resembling patients with sepsis. During liver transplant (LT) surgery, these haemodynamic responses are further exacerbated after induction of general anaesthesia (GA), increased blood loss during surgery, massive fluid shifts intra-operatively and post-reperfusion of the new graft. Strategies to maintain haemodynamics include maintaining adequate intravascular volume, managing coagulopathy with the use of blood products and combating vasodilatation due to impaired vascular tone with the use of vasopressors. Vasopressors are agents that induce vasoconstriction, thereby elevating MAP [3, 4]. Some vasopressors also have inotropic effects. This chapter outlines the different vasopressors used in LT surgery.

20.2 Aetiopathogenesis

The patients with ESLD typically have a high CO, cardiac index (CI) with normal-to-low mean blood pressure (MBP), variable central venous pressure (CVP) along with decreased SVR secondary to portal hypertension [1, 2]. They may have underlying cirrhotic cardiomyopathy, underlying coronary artery disease (CAD), and porto-pulmonary hypertension which need to be evaluated in the pre-anaesthesia check-up. Mediator-induced vasodilation in splanchnic and peripheral circulation reduces the effective circulatory blood volume, resulting in a compensatory increase in HR and CO. Decreased perfusion pressure can also lead to diminished renal blood flow in cirrhotic patients which in turn stimulates the renal angiotensin aldosterone system (RAAS) and antidiuretic hormone (ADH) production. This results in renal artery vasoconstriction, sodium retention and volume expansion [1, 2].

It is recognized that type 1 HRS is reversible following treatment with intravenous albumin and vasoconstrictors in 60–75% of patients, as serum creatinine levels drop to below 1.5 mg/dL, resulting in improved survival. However, both therapeutic components are necessary (i.e. albumin and vasoconstrictor), as a single-agent treatment did not revert HRS.

Numerous vasodilatory mediators have been recognized in circulation in ESLD patients, most important of which is nitric oxide (NO).

S. Saraf (✉)
Jupiter Hospital, Pune, Maharashtra, India

Cytokines, especially TNF α, are considered to be NO inducers. Endothelial NO synthase is the main source of NO production. In ESLD patient's sensitivity of β-adrenoreceptors is relatively decreased causing attenuated cardiovascular response to endogenic catecholamines [1, 2].

20.3 Haemodynamic Changes During LT Surgery

20.3.1 Anaesthesia-Related Factors

All general anaesthesia techniques reduced the hepatic blood flow (HBF) by about 30% secondary to the fall in the systemic arterial blood pressure in a dose-dependent manner. Use of isoflurane and sevoflurane for anaesthesia maintenance may cause only minimal reduction in HBF and does not have any significant influence on oxygen transport and extraction ratio in the liver [1, 2, 5]. Short-acting opioids, especially fentanyl, has no effect on HBF. Initiation of mechanical ventilation, positive end-expiratory pressure (PEEP), systemic hypotension, hypoxemia, hypocapnia and alkalosis reduce HBF. Hence it is important to maintain mean arterial pressure (MAP) around 75–85 mmHg, HR below 100/min, SVR more than 500 dynes/s/cm^{-5} with normal central venous pressure (CVP) and CO of more than 4 L/min.

20.3.2 Surgery-Related Factors [1, 2]

LT surgery is accomplished in four stages.

First stage—Preanhepatic or dissection phase where the diseased liver is prepared for removal. Portal vein clamping followed by hepatic artery and hepatic veins clamping denotes the start of anhepatic phase.

Second stage—Anhepatic phase where the diseased liver is removed from the body and vascular anastomoses are being performed on the donor organ.

Third stage—Reperfusion and post-reperfusion phase where the vascular venous clamps are

released and organ is reperfused. This is the shortest phase with most significant haemodynamic impact.

Fourth stage—Post-reperfusion phase includes hepatic artery and bile duct reconstruction.

Phase 1: Dissection phase (preanhepatic)—during this phase massive fluid shifts are common due to ascites evacuation causing a drop in intra-abdominal pressure with increase in splanchnic volume. Blood loss may be substantial due to abundance of venous collaterals secondary to portal hypertension and presence of infection. Adhesions due to previous surgeries results in blood loss and metabolic acidosis which further contributes to decrease in CO, CI and MBP. Transfusion is recommended for haemorrhage; however, overtransfusion should be avoided. Colloid (e.g. 5% albumin) infusion can also be considered to preserve intravascular volume, with additional vasopressor infusion also in consideration.

Phase 2: Anhepatic phase—during this phase portal cross clamp can reduce the venous return but is generally well tolerated in cases of well-developed porto-systemic collaterals (secondary to portal hypertension). Inferior vena cava (IVC) complete cross clamp leads to a more substantial and poorly tolerated (approximately 50%) decrease of venous return. Partial IVC clamp reduces venous return by 25–50% and may be well tolerated. ESLD patients have a very limited capacity to compensate for this rapid decrease in venous return. Veno-venous bypass (VVV) should be a standby in operation theatres (OT) if severe haemodynamic instability presents during test clamping.

Phase 3: During graft reperfusion major haemodynamic changes are seen that may result in end organ injuries. This is the ischaemia reperfusion syndrome (IRS) which may result in tachy/brady arrythmias, direct myocardial depression, profound vasoplegia (rapid drop of SVR), hypotension, cardiac arrest, acute interstitial pulmonary oedema leading to right ventricular overload, rise in CVP and pulmonary artery pressure (PAP). Blood loss, hypovolaemia, hypothermia and lactic acidosis all contribute to decreased sensitivity to catecholamines and efficiency of vasopressors.

Ischaemia reperfusion syndrome is defined as more than 30% decrease in MBP from that in anhepatic phase, lasting longer than 1 min during the first 5 min after reperfusion of liver graft. During the periods of ischaemia and reperfusion of the liver, there is a microcirculatory failure, activation of Kupffer cells and production of reactive oxygen species, inflammatory responses and apoptosis of the hepatocytes.

Ischaemia reperfusion injury (IRI) is associated with primary graft dysfunction and delayed graft function. Strategies of prevention of IRI include ischaemic preconditioning (IP) and pharmacological management.

Ionotrope infusion of choice in many centres is norepinephrine alone. Other agents may be added to this during the most critical anhepatic phase maintenance during reperfusion. Epinephrine may be added, with the purpose of using its β-stimulation activity. Some centres use "pretreatment" with epinephrine and phenylephrine combination for post-reperfusion syndrome prevention.

Vasopressin in small boluses, 1–2 U, may be highly efficient in opposing the significant and rapid decrease of SVR, and calcium chloride, up to 100 mg, may enhance inotropic effects of epinephrine. Methylene Blue, 2 mg/kg, has been reported as very efficient and "last resort" drug for prolonged and profound hypotension, refractory to treatment with other vasoactive drugs. The presence of significant metabolic, mainly lactic, acidosis is a well-known cause of decreased vasoactive agent's efficiency. To overcome hyporesponsiveness to vasopressors, sodium bicarbonate infusion may be necessary.

Phase 4: In post-reperfusion phase (Neohepatic phase) the major factors contributing to haemodynamic instability include ongoing blood loss, deficiency of coagulation factors by the liver graft, hypocalcaemia secondary to blood transfusions and lactic acidosis. While combating the loses, close communication with the surgeons and the surgical field is important to avoid over-

zealous correction of volume. Graft congestion causes substantial perfusion and oxygen delivery impairment in the newly transplanted liver that delays normal function restoration, specifically restart of coagulation components synthesis, which, in turn, exacerbates and prolongs the coagulation deficit. Maintenance of low central venous pressure to decrease graft congestion is important at this stage.

Continued use of vasopressors in low doses may help prevent this. Some centres advocate a background infusion of Nitroglycerin (NTG) to prevent this complication [5]. NTG has proved to be an effective agent for treatment of pulmonary hypertension. It has been shown that nitroglycerin infusion resulted in pulmonary vascular resistance decrease by 43% and mean pulmonary artery pressure decrease by 19%. Boluses of diuretics, e.g. furosemide, may be required as well.

Due to rapid ongoing fluid shifts in LT surgery these patients need invasive advanced haemodynamic monitoring for continuous pressure monitoring, meticulous fluid balance, blood gas analysis and determining haemodynamic response to vasopressors. The pulse contour analysis is useful for monitoring cardiac output, for e.g. the PiCCO system, the Flowtrach, the LiDCO and Transoesophageal echocardiography (TEE).

Many studies have shown that the use of an adjuvant vasopressor, together with controlled fluid administration, to maintain a stable haemodynamic status during GA reduced the need for endotracheal reintubation and its associated morbidities in the postoperative period [4, 6].

20.4 Vasoactive Agents Used During Orthotopic Liver Transplant (OLT) [3, 4, 6]

Vasopressors are indicated in liver transplant when the BP falls more than 30 mmHg from the baseline systolic pressure, or a MAP less than 60 mmHg, when there is a risk of end organ dysfunction due to hypoperfusion. Hypovolaemia needs to be corrected prior to the institution of vasopressor therapy as vasopressors will be ineffective or only partially effective in a settling of coexisting hypovolaemia [3–7].

Adrenergic Agents Adrenergic agents, such as norepinephrine, epinephrine, phenylephrine, dopamine and dobutamine, are the most commonly used vasopressor and inotropic drugs in ESLD patients undergoing LT [3–6].

20.4.1 Norepinephrine

Norepinephrine acts on both alpha-1 and beta-1 adrenergic receptors (α1 >β1). Norepinephrine-induced β1 adrenergic stimulation would cause tachycardia; however elevated MAP from its α adrenergic receptor-induced vasoconstriction results in a reflex decrease in the heart rate, so the net result is a stable or slightly reduced heart rate when the drug is used. It should be given in an infusion, preferably through a central line, in a dose of 0.01–3.0 mcg/kg/min. It is an agent of choice used in most centres for combating hypotension during liver transplant.

20.4.2 Phenylephrine

Phenylephrine has purely alpha-adrenergic agonist activity and therefore results in vasoconstriction with minimal cardiac inotropy or chronotropy. The drug is useful in the setting of hypotension with an SVR <700 dynes × s/cm^5 (e.g. hyperdynamic sepsis, neurologic disorders, anaesthesia-induced hypotension).

SVR elevation increases cardiac afterload, which is tolerated among patients without pre-existing cardiac dysfunction. The drug is contraindicated if the SVR is >1200 dynes × s/cm^5 and those having previous cardiac dysfunction.

Due to phenylephrine's almost purely α-mimetic activity, its use actually addresses the low SVR problem, a main culprit for low MABP in majority of cases, provided that volume status correction and maintenance is being performed properly. Hence it is used in some centres in infu-

sion during the preanhepatic phase and along with other agents like norepinephrine or vasopressin during the reperfusion phase. Some centres give phenylephrine as intermittent boluses of 10–100 mcgs during the reperfusion phase.

20.4.3 Epinephrine

Epinephrine has potent beta-1 adrenergic receptor activity and moderate beta-2 and alpha-1 adrenergic receptor effects. Clinically, low doses of epinephrine increase CO because of the beta-1 adrenergic receptor inotropic and chronotropic effects, while the alpha-adrenergic receptor-induced vasoconstriction is often offset by the beta-2 adrenergic receptor vasodilation. The result is an increased CO, with decreased SVR and variable effects on the MAP. However, at higher epinephrine doses the alpha-adrenergic receptor effect predominates, producing increased SVR in addition to an increased CO.

Other disadvantages of epinephrine include dysrhythmias (due to beta-1 adrenergic receptor stimulation) and splanchnic vasoconstriction. Epinephrine and norepinephrine decrease liver and kidney tissue perfusion, thereby reducing lactate clearance, promote lactic acidosis and cause temporary alterations of hepatic macro- and microcirculation (return to baseline 2 h after onset of infusion). Dose-dependent progressive decline of hepatic macro- (33–75% reduction) and microcirculation (39–58% reduction) was found in transplanted livers. Norepinephrine has a direct constrictor effect on liver sinusoids, thereby reducing hepatic blood volume/flow and aggravating portal hypertension [5].

It is recommended to be given as an infusion via a central line, in a dose of 0.01–2.0 mcg/kg/min.

Its use is restricted to second-line vasopressor in case of hypotension unresponsive to noradrenaline infusion during reperfusion phase with myocardial depression. In some centres, pretreatment with epinephrine with phenylephrine is used prior to reperfusion. Bolus doses of 10 mcgs may be reserved for use during the reperfusion phase.

However, in paediatric age group, hypotension is largely dependent on heart rate rather than the SVR. In these patients, epinephrine is mainly the first choice of ionotrope.

20.4.4 Ephedrine

Similar to epinephrine, ephedrine acts primarily on beta 1 adrenergic receptors, but with less potency. It also has an effect by leading to release of endogenous norepinephrine. Since tachycardiac is not desired, it is rarely used except in the setting of post-anaesthesia-induced hypotension.

20.4.5 Dopamine

Dopamine has a variety of effects depending upon the dose range administered. It is most often used as a second-line alternative to norepinephrine in patients with absolute or relative bradycardia and a low risk of tachyarrhythmias.

- At doses of 1 to 2 mcg/kg/min, dopamine acts predominantly on dopamine-1 (D1) receptors in the renal, mesenteric, cerebral and coronary beds, resulting in selective vasodilation. Some reports suggest that dopamine increases urine output by augmenting renal blood flow and glomerular filtration rate and natriuresis by inhibiting aldosterone and renal tubular sodium transport.
- At 5 to 10 mcg/kg/min, dopamine also stimulates beta-1 adrenergic receptors and increases cardiac output, predominantly by increasing stroke volume with variable effects on heart rate.
- At doses >10 mcg/kg/min, the predominant effect of dopamine is to stimulate alpha-adrenergic receptors and produce vasoconstriction with an increased SVR. However, the overall alpha-adrenergic receptor effect of dopamine is weaker than that of norepinephrine and the beta-1 adrenergic receptor stimulation of dopamine at doses >2 mcg/kg/min can result in dose-limiting dysrhythmias.

Intraoperative use of dopamine, 3 mcg/kg/min in OLT, is intended to preserve and protect the adequate renal function, especially in cases of hepatorenal syndrome. Higher rates of dopamine infusion, 5–10 to 20 mcg/kg/min, increase cardiac output and SVR. However, gaining CO/CI increase at the expense of tachycardia and, potentially, some rhythm disturbances makes dopamine a less desirable agent during liver transplant surgery.

20.4.6 Dobutamine

Dobutamine is not a vasopressor but rather is an inotrope that causes vasodilation. Dobutamine causes predominant beta-1 adrenergic receptor effect which increases inotropy and chronotropy and reduces left ventricular filling pressure. In patients with heart failure this results in a reduction in cardiac sympathetic activity. The net effect is increased CO, with decreased SVR with or without a small reduction in blood pressure.

Dobutamine is most frequently used in severe, medically refractory heart failure and cardiogenic shock. Given as an infusion in the dose of 2.5–10.0 mcg/kg/min. It is of use in cardiac evaluation of patients undergoing transplant surgery, the Dobutamine stress echocardiography. It is reserved in treatment during liver transplant when the patient develops cardiac failure refractory to other treatment.

20.4.7 Isoproterenol

Isoprenaline acts upon beta-1 adrenergic receptors and, unlike dobutamine, has a prominent chronotropic effect. It also acts on beta 2 adrenergic receptor causing vasodilation and a decreasing MAP. Therefore, its utility in hypotensive patients is limited to situations in which hypotension results from bradycardia.

20.4.8 Vasopressin and Analogues

Vasopressin (antidiuretic hormone ADH) is used in the management of diabetes insipidus and oesophageal variceal bleeding. It is primarily used as a second-line agent in refractory vasodilatory shock, particularly septic shock or anaphylaxis that is unresponsive to epinephrine [7].

Terlipressin, a vasopressin analogue, has been used successfully in the treatment of hepatorenal syndrome (HRS) and variceal bleeding [8–10]. Terlipressin is a pro-hormone of Triglycyl-Lysine-Vasopressin. Following intravenous administration, the glycyl residues are cleaved from the pro-hormone by endothelial peptidases, allowing prolonged release of lysine-vasopressin. It can be given in divided doses or as an infusion. Terlipressin has affinity for both V1 and V2 receptors and selectively causes splanchnic and extra-renal vasoconstriction by V1 vascular smooth muscle receptor stimulation. It thereby reduces the splanchnic blood flow and portal pressure, diverting the volume to systemic circulation, thereby improving the effective circulatory volume and renal perfusion pressure. There is an increase in MAP and SVR while the HR, CO, hepatic venous pressure gradient and portal venous blood flow decrease. V2 receptor stimulation by Terlipressin increases water resorption by collecting ducts and can result in hyponatraemia in some patients [8–10].

Peri-operative use of Terlipressin during liver transplantation has been shown to improve the SVR and BP with reduced need for catecholamine support and with less renal dysfunction in LDLT in numerous studies. Normalizing low SVR in cirrhotic patients with portal hypertension helps to return the hepatosplanchnic blood to the central compartment and improves perfusion into major organs. The peak portal blood flow is reduced with terlipressin without hepatic artery vasoconstriction or signs of splanchnic hypoperfusion. Reducing portal vein pressure is postulated to decrease the amount of bleeding and transfusion requirements. Hepatic artery buffer response (HABR) is preserved during the use of terlipressin to maintain total hepatic blood flow (when portal vein blood flow reduces, hepatic artery blood flow increases) [8]. Given as an infusion in the dose of 1–4 mcg/kg/h.

20.5 Nonadrenergic Agents

A number of agents produce vasoconstriction or inotropy through nonadrenergic mechanisms, including phosphodiesterase inhibitors and nitric oxide synthase inhibitors, calcium sensitizers or angiotensin II. Their uses are extensively studied in septic shock, but data in cirrhotic patients is very limited.

PDE Inhibitors Phosphodiesterase (PDE) inhibitors, such as inamrinone (formerly known as amrinone) and milrinone, are nonadrenergic drugs with inotropic and vasodilatory actions. They have a lower risk of dysrhythmias than Dobutamine. PDE inhibitors most often are used to treat patients with impaired cardiac function and medically refractory heart failure, but their vasodilatory properties limit their use in hypotensive patients.

NOS Inhibitors Nitric oxide overproduction appears to play a major role in vasodilation induced by sepsis. Only sepsis is not good enough for liver patients.

Studies of nitric oxide synthase (NOS) inhibitors such as N-monomethyl-L-arginine (L-NMMA) in sepsis demonstrate a dose-dependent increase in systemic vascular resistance (SVR). However, cardiac index (CI) and heart rate (HR) decrease, even when patients are treated concomitantly with norepinephrine or epinephrine. The increase in SVR tends to be offset by the drop in CI, such that mean arterial pressure (MAP) is only minimally augmented. The clinical utility of this class of drugs remains unproven.

Calcium sensitizers—Several agents increase myocardial contractility (e.g. pimobendan, levosimendan) but conclusive evidence of improved outcomes with their use is lacking.

Angiotensin II—Preliminary trials have reported an adequate vasopressor effect when synthetic angiotensin II is exogenously administered for vasodilatory shock (e.g. septic shock).

Methylene Blue Dye (MB) Though not a conventional vasopressor drug, it has been used as a vasopressor in sepsis and acute liver failure where conventional vasopressors do not produce the desired response [11]. The IRS observed during liver transplant surgery may manifest a state of vasoplegia where occasionally the conventional treatment (e.g. Norepinephrine, epinephrine and vasopressin) is not sufficient to restore adequate SVR and BP. Like in sepsis, these changes are associated with excess nitric oxide (NO). MB has properties to stop NO production by inhibition of guanylate cyclase. MB also acts as an antioxidant; pro-oxidant inhibiting the synthesis of prostacyclin and accelerates reductive processes in the cell. Dose of MB is 2 mg/kg loading dose over 30 min followed by an infusion of 0.5 mg/kg/h over 6 h.

20.6 Complications of Vasopressor Use

Vasopressors and inotropic agents have the potential to cause a number of significant complications, including hypoperfusion, dysrhythmias, myocardial ischaemia, local effect and hyperglycaemia. In addition, a number of drug interactions exist [3–6].

Hypoperfusion—Excessive vasoconstriction in response to hypotension and vasopressors can produce inadequate perfusion of the extremities, mesenteric organs or kidneys. Excessive vasoconstriction with inadequate perfusion, usually with a systemic vascular resistance (SVR) >1300 dynes × s/cm^5, commonly occurs in the setting of inadequate cardiac output or inadequate volume resuscitation.

The initial findings are dusky skin changes at the tips of the fingers and/or toes, which may progress to frank necrosis with autoamputation of the digits. Compromise of the renal vascular bed may produce renal insufficiency and oliguria, while patients with underlying peripheral artery disease may develop acute limb ischaemia.

Inadequate mesenteric perfusion increases the risk of gastritis, shock liver, intestinal ischaemia, or translocation of gut flora with resultant bacteraemia. Despite these concerns, maintenance of MAP with vasopressors appears more effective in maintaining renal and mesenteric blood flow than allowing the MAP to drop, and maintenance of MAP with vasopressors may be lifesaving despite evidence of localized hypoperfusion.

Dysrhythmias—Many vasopressors and inotropes exert powerful chronotropic effects via stimulation of beta-1 adrenergic receptors. This increases the risk of sinus tachycardia (most common), atrial fibrillation (potentially with increased atrioventricular nodal [A-V] conduction and therefore an increased ventricular response), re-entrant atrioventricular node tachycardia or ventricular tachyarrhythmias.

Adequate volume loading may minimize the frequency or severity of dysrhythmias. Despite this, dysrhythmias often limit the dose and necessitate switching to another agent with less prominent beta-1 effects.

Myocardial ischaemia—The chronotropic and inotropic effects of beta-adrenergic receptor stimulation can increase myocardial oxygen consumption. While there is usually coronary vasodilation in response to vasopressors, perfusion may still be inadequate to accommodate the increased myocardial oxygen demand. Daily electrocardiograms on patients treated with vasopressors or inotropes may screen for occult ischaemia, and excessive tachycardia should be avoided because of impaired diastolic filling of the coronary arteries.

Local effects—Peripheral extravasation of vasopressors into the surrounding connective tissue can lead to excessive local vasoconstriction with subsequent skin necrosis. To avoid this complication, vasopressors should be administered via a central vein whenever possible. If infiltration occurs, local treatment with phentolamine (5–10 mg in 10 mL of normal saline) injected subcutaneously can minimize local vasoconstriction.

Hyperglycaemia—Hyperglycaemia may occur due to the inhibition of insulin secretion. The magnitude of hyperglycaemia generally is minor and is more pronounced with norepinephrine and epinephrine than dopamine. Monitoring of blood glucose while on vasopressors can prevent complications of untreated hyperglycaemia.

20.7 Conclusion

LT surgery poses a challenge to anaesthetists. The ongoing fluid losses, coagulopathy and haemodynamic instability need to be meticulously balanced with the use of advanced haemodynamic monitoring. Optimum fluid replacement and judicious use of vasopressors optimize the cardiac output and adequate tissue oxygen delivery to improve surgical outcomes.

References

1. Kim MY, Baik SK, Lee SS. Hemodynamic alterations in cirrhosis and portal hypertension. Korean J Hepatol. 2010;16:347–52. https://doi.org/10.3350/kjhep.2010.16.4.347.
2. Hori T, Ogura Y, Onishi Y, Kamei H, Kurata N, Kainuma M, Takahashi H, Suzuki S, Ichikawa T, Mizuno S, Aoyama T, Ishida Y, Hirai T, Hayashi T, Hasegawa K, Takeichi H, Ota A, Kodera Y, Sugimoto H, Iida T, Yagi S, Taniguchi K, Uemoto S. Systemic hemodynamics in advanced cirrhosis: concerns during perioperative period of liver transplantation. World J Hepatol. 2016;8(25):1047–60.
3. Zhang LP, Li M, Yang L. Effects of different vasopressors on hemodynamics in patients undergoing orthotopic liver transplantation. Chin Med J. 2005;118:1952–8.
4. Manaker S. Use of vasopressors and inotropes. Literature Review Current Through. 2020.
5. Vitin AA, Tomescu D, Azamfirei L. Hemodynamic optimization strategies in anesthesia care for liver transplantation. 2017. https://doi.org/10.5772/intechopen.68416.
6. Ponnudurai RN, Koneru B, Akhtar SA, Wachsberg RH, Fisher A, Wilson DJ, de la Torre AN. Vasopressor administration during liver transplant surgery and its effect on endotracheal reintubation rate in the postoperative period: a prospective, randomized, double-blind, placebo-controlled trial. Clin Ther. 2005;27(2):192–8.
7. Moreau R, Liberec D. The use of vasoconstrictors in patients with cirrhosis: type 1 HRS and beyond. Hepatology. 2006;43(3):385–94.
8. Wagener G, Gubitosa G, Renz J, Kinkhabwala M, Brentjens T, Guarrera JV, Emond J. H. Thomas Lee and Donald Landry. Vasopressin decreases portal vein pressure and flow in the native liver during liver transplantation. Liver Transpl. 2000;14:1664–70.
9. Ibrahim N, Hasanin A, Allah SA, Sayed E, Afifi M, Yassen K, Saber W, Khalil M. The haemodynamic effects of the perioperative terlipressin infusion in living donor liver transplantation: a randomised controlled study. Indian J Anaesth. 2015;59(3):156–64.
10. Karaaslan P, Sevmiş Ş. Effect of terlipressin infusion therapy on recipient's hepatic and renal functions in living donor liver transplantations: experience from a tertiary hospital. Niger J Clin Pract. 2019;22(2):265–9.
11. Hong SH, Lee JM, Choi JH, Chung HS, Park JH, Park CS. Perioperative assessment of terlipressin infusion during living donor liver transplantation. J Int Med Res. 2012;40:225–36.

Minimizing Blood Loss in Recipient Surgery

21

Ravi Raya

21.1 Introduction

Interventions to reduce blood loss during Orthotopic Liver Transplant (OLT) have been surgical, anaesthesia-related and pharmacological. Intraoperative blood loss is a predictor of perioperative outcome following liver resection and transplantation and may have an effect on short-term and long-term survival. The liver plays a central role in the haemostatic system as it synthesizes the majority of coagulation factors and proteins involved in fibrinolysis. Although anticoagulant factors are decreased as well, blood loss during orthotopic liver transplantation can still be excessive in view of interplay between multiple factors. In patients with cirrhosis, the synthesis of coagulation factors can fall short, reflected by a prolonged prothrombin time. Patients undergoing orthotopic liver transplantation are at high risk of bleeding complications. Several authors have shown that thromboelastography (TEG)-based coagulation management and the administration of fibrinogen concentrate reduce the need for blood transfusion. The reduction in blood loss has also led to the successful transplantation of livers in Jehovah's witnesses. Timely prevention and identification of "triangle of death" (hypothermia, acidosis and coagulopathy) play an important role in reducing

blood loss. It is well known that blood transfusions are associated with an increased risk of postoperative complications, such as infections, pulmonary complications, protracted recovery and a higher rate of reoperations. Blood loss during orthotopic liver transplantation is currently managed by transfusion of red blood cell concentrates, platelet concentrates, fresh frozen plasma and fibrinogen concentrate. Increasing experience and improvements in surgical technique, anaesthesia care and better graft preservation methods have contributed to a steady decrease in blood transfusion requirements in most liver transplant programmes.

21.2 Why to Minimize Transfusion?

Intraoperative transfusion of at least 6 units of RBCs decreases survival rates during medium- and long-term follow-up after Liver Transplant (LT). RBCs transfusion has been independently correlated with the rate of postoperative infections in the unit-dependent manner [1]. The number of transfused RBCs units during LT is also a predictor of early surgical re-intervention, which in turn increases postoperative mortality threefold. Platelet transfusion is associated with increased postoperative mortality due to a higher prevalence of acute lung injury (ALI). FFP used for volume replacement or pre-emptive non-specific correction of coagulopathy in the dissec-

R. Raya (✉)
Department of Anaesthesiology, Asian Institute of
Gastroenterology, Axon Anaesthesia Associates,
Hyderabad, Telangana, India

tion phase of LT may exacerbate splanchnic hyperaemia and portal hypertension. A transfusion-free perioperative period was associated with improved early outcomes, fewer infections, reduced dialysis requirement, shorter hospital LOS and a reduction in mortality compared with a transfused group with similar recipient, graft and donor quality variables.

21.3 Coagulation Derangements (Preoperative and Intraoperative)

The new paradigm relies entirely on the concept of a rebalanced coagulation state, where all of the components of the system are significantly altered (both pro- and anticoagulant portions) but maintained in a precarious equilibrium (Fig. 21.1). External disruption of this balance, whether a consequence of disease progression or from intervention, can thrust the balance into bleeding or thrombosis. Liver transplantation represents one of the greatest physiological insults to this balance (Table 21.1).

Disruptions in pro- and anticoagulant factors and portal hypertension increase the risk of haemorrhage. Changes in platelet and endothelial function in liver failure also may delay clot formation. Additionally, patients with liver failure can experience hyperfibrinolysis, dysfibrinogenemia and renal failure, which may further increase the risk of prolonged bleeding.

Fig. 21.1 Rebalanced coagulation in liver disease

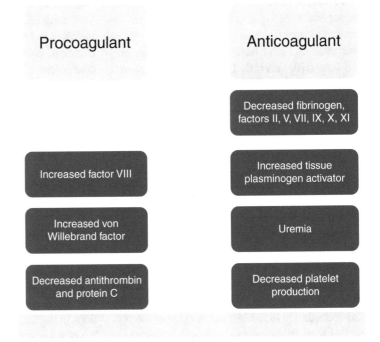

Table 21.1 Changes in haemostatic system of patients with chronic liver disease

Anticoagulant	Procoagulant
Thrombocytopenia	Elevated levels of von Willebrand factors (vWf)
Platelet dysfunction	Decreased levels of ADAMTS-13
Enhanced production of nitric oxide and prostacyclin	Increased factor VIII level
Factors II, V, VII, IX, X & XI deficiency	Decreased levels of protein C, protein S, antithrombin, α2-macroglobulin and heparin cofactor II
Lack of vitamin K	Low levels of plasminogen
Low fibrinogen	
Low levels of α2-antiplasmin, factor XIII and TAFI	
Elevated t-PA levels	

21.4 Risk Factors (Recipient, Surgery and Graft-Related Risk Factors)

Patient-related factors are pre-operative high MELD score, severe coagulopathy (platelet count <50,000 and low fibrinogen) and low haematocrit and renal dysfunction. The recipients present differing degrees of preoperative haemostasis disorders and may also present intraoperative coagulopathy. Changes in the production and clearance of coagulation proteins in the course of LT may lead to severely disturbed haemostasis, further aggravated by ischaemia of the hepatic graft and the splanchnic network [2]. Hyperfibrinolysis has been described as a major cause of non-surgical bleeding during LT. The results for many potential predictive variables (age, starting haemoglobin value, international normalized ratio [INR], platelets count, creatinine, albumin and second OLT) for intraoperative bleeding are conflicting. It has been shown that central venous pressure (CVP) and the splanchnic venous pressure are key factors in the haemostatic balance during liver surgery [3, 4], a fact that is supported by the finding that maintaining a low CVP intraoperatively significantly reduces

blood loss and the need for transfusion during liver transplantation and liver resection [3–5]. The donor's older age is associated with a higher risk of massive transfusion.

Other technical factors, such as the decreased size of the donor liver, portal vein hypoplasia and an inadequate graft-recipient body weight ratio, were associated with transfusion requirements in several studies. Prolonged cold ischaemia time and poor graft function due to decreased production of coagulation factors also significantly increase the risk of massive transfusion [6].

21.5 Prevention of Excessive Bleeding

Identifying and planning the management of patients at high risk of bleeding is the key to minimize blood loss and can be implemented as early as the preoperative assessment visit. Interestingly, several patient and operative characteristics were associated with an increased risk of receiving a transfusion of blood products. Specifically, older patients and individuals with more comorbidities were at markedly higher risk of receiving a transfusion. Patients are categorized into good risk and bad risk in terms of need for blood and blood product reserves [7]. Patients with severe liver failure have significant derangement of their clotting function due to impaired production of procoagulant and anticoagulant factors. Traditional coagulation studies are limited by the short time needed for the result and provide little information about the dynamics and strength of clot formation. According to a recent study, a parameter derived from ROTEM, the time required for the maximum clotting velocity, can identify cirrhotic patients at high risk of bleeding. VETs can be an aid in LT by limiting the transfusion of labile blood products, probably at the cost of an increase in the transfusion of fibrinogen. VETs lack sensitivity for the diagnosis of hyperfibrinolysis. It is wise not waiting for the appearance of typical hyperfibrinolysis plots to use antifibrinolytics if other clinical features are present such as diffuse or massive bleeding. Inhibition of clot lysis in

VET is another approach to promoting haemostasis. Amongst specific actions to minimize perioperative blood loss and transfusion requirements during LT, we can distinguish nonpharmacological and pharmacological interventions.

21.5.1 Nonpharmacological Interventions

Fluid management is considered a key player in haemostatic management. Avoiding excessive fluid transfusions and maintaining low CVP during dissection phase is a well-established measure to minimize intraoperative blood loss. Fluid restriction not only helps one to maintain low CVP but also prevents dilutional coagulopathy associated with excessive transfusion of crystalloids and colloids. Relative hypovolaemia due to low CVP might also increase the risk of significant tissue hypoperfusion, air embolism, as well as acute renal failure. Standard coagulation tests do not reflect the functional haemostatic status. Therefore, the use of modern viscoelastic tests such as thromboelastography (TEG) or rotational thromboelastometry (ROTEM) allows us to assess humoral and cellular components of the haemostatic system (both coagulation and fibrinolysis), helping to identify the cause of intraoperative bleeding, targeting specific problems and evaluating management. Recent guidelines of the European Society of Anaesthesiology recommend to use perioperative global coagulation tests (TEG/ROTEM) for targeted management of coagulopathy in patients undergoing LT [8].

Another important surgical measure to reduce perioperative blood product transfusions is use of intraoperative cell salvage (CS). Nowadays, a "stand by" set-up rather than routine application of CS is recommended. It must be emphasized that as salvaged washed erythrocytes do not contain clotting factors or platelets, haemostatic replacement therapy must be managed accordingly. To minimize the risk of bacterial contamination it is recommended to start collecting blood after the removal of ascitic fluid and cease it once biliary anastomosis begins.

21.5.2 Pharmacological Interventions

21.5.2.1 Antifibrinolytics

Derivatives of the amino acid lysine, 6-aminohexanoic acid (aminocaproic acid) and 4-(aminomethyl) cyclohexanecarboxylic acid (tranexamic acid), are grouped in the class of medications named antifibrinolytics. Fibrinolysis is an important process developing during anhepatic phase and progressing massively after reperfusion due to the alterations in haemostatic system (t-PA) [8] (Fig. 21.2). Hyperfibrinolysis or dysfibrinogenemia should be suspected in the presence of mucosal (gum) bleeding or late bleeding (such as hours post line placement), suggesting that clot has formed and prematurely dissolved. According to the current guidelines, consider administration of antifibrinolytic drugs when fibrinolysis is either confirmed in viscoelastic tests (TEG/ROTEM) or is clinically evident from microvascular oozing, but not as a routine practice [9].

21.5.2.2 Prothrombin Complex Concentrate (PCC)

Prothrombin complex concentrate (PCC) comprises either 3 or 4 vitamin K-dependent procoagulant factors (II, ± VII, IX, X) and the anticoagulants protein C and S, extracted from pooled plasma. PCCs can improve haemostasis where loss or dilution of prothrombotic factors is contributing to bleeding. In LT a dose of 25 iu/kg is advocated if there is severe bleeding associated with prolonged clotting time on VETs (TEG R time or EXTEM Clotting time > 80 s) after excluding a HLE. PCC may be the ideal therapy to restore thrombin generation in dilutional coagulopathy.

21.5.2.3 Fibrinogen Concentrate

Fibrinogen concentrate substitution was also found to restore MCF after in vitro haemodilution in blood from LT recipients, its potential role in the treatment of dilutional coagulopathy. Cryoprecipitate is still used as the most abundant source of fibrinogen. It is recommended that as fibrinogen concentrates contain standard doses of fibrinogen, carry lower risk of pathogen and

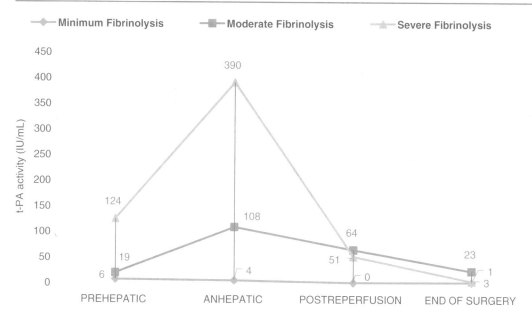

Fig. 21.2 t-PA levels in different phases of transplantation {Adapted from Dzik WH et al. Blood 1988;71(4):1090–1095 [8]}

immune-mediated complications and should be the preferred source of fibrinogen, in comparison to cryoprecipitate, for the treatment of the quantitative functional deficits of fibrinogen in bleeding patients, unless the former is unavailable. The fibrinogen dose can be calculated as follows: Fibrinogen concentrate dose (g) = [target FIBTEM MCF (mm) − actual FIBTEM MCF (mm)] × [body weight (kg)/70] × 0.5 g/mm. Dosing range is 25 mg/kg to 50 mg/kg.

21.6 Others

Piggyback hepatectomy (PGB) is a surgical technique increasingly utilized in both DDLT and LDLT (Caval preservation technique).

21.6.1 Strategies

1. Maintain adequate blood viscosity (Hb).
2. Maintenance of haemostatic conditions for clotting.
3. During the intraoperative period, local haemostasis is the most important factor in the control of bleeding; in this context, surgical technique and meticulous haemostasis are fundamental measures.
4. MAP range between 60 mmHg and 65 mmHg during dissection phase.
5. Maintenance of a low central venous pressure (CVP) and even reduction of CVP by phlebotomy is a beneficial strategy in minimizing blood loss during liver resection or liver transplantation [5].
6. Use of viscoelastic coagulation tests performed bedside (point-of-care [POC]), including rotational thromboelastometry (ROTEM) and thromboelastography (TEG).
7. Use of transfusion algorithms based on VETs can reduce perioperative bleeding and the rate of transfusion of allogeneic blood products [10–12].
8. VETs can be an aid by limiting the transfusion of labile blood products, probably at the cost of an increase in the transfusion of fibrinogen. (VETs may lack sensitivity for the diagnosis of hyperfibrinolysis.)
9. Predictive models to identify higher risk patients for bleeding and transfusions should be developed.

10. Measuring portal pressure intraoperatively and correlation with CVP.
11. Define the nature of the coagulopathy in a given patient who has liver disease at given time.
12. Recombinant factor VIIa (rFVIIa) procoagulant drug can facilitate clot formation through amplifying the thrombin burst and accentuation of platelet function.
13. Prothrombin complex concentrate (frequently) and fibrinogen concentrate use is on the rise.

All the strategies that we may use to reduce or avoid transfusions will have important benefits not only in decreasing transfusion-associated risks [13, 14] but in preserving blood stores and reducing costs as well. Recourse to transfusion may vary depending on the device used, confirming that transfusion thresholds are not well defined. Measures to reduce the filling status of the patient and to lower the CVP through volume contraction and no routine correction of laboratory coagulation test with large-volume blood products are effective and safe.

Key Points
- LT is associated with massive blood loss.
- Bleeding in LT is related to aetiology and severity of liver disease.
- Pre-operative optimisation can reduce transfusion requirement.
- Restrictive transfusion protocols are preferred.
- Viscoelastic test helps reduce transfusion requirement.

References

1. Benson AB, Burton JR, Austin GL, et al. Differential effects of plasma and red blood cell transfusions on acute lung injury and infection risk following liver transplantation. Liver Transpl. 2011;17:149–58. https://doi.org/10.1002/lt.22212.
2. Ozier Y, Steib A, Ickx B, Nathan N, Derlon A, Guay J, et al. Haemostatic disorders during liver transplantation. Eur J Anaesthesiol. 2001;18:208–18.
3. Smyrniotis V, Kostopanagiotou G, Theodoraki K, Tsantoulas D, Contis J. The role of central venous pressure and type of vascular control in blood loss during major liver resections. Am J Surg. 2004;187:398–402.
4. Jones RM, Moulton CE, Hardy KJ. Central venous pressure and its effect on blood loss during liver resection. Br J Surg. 1998;85:1058–60.
5. Massicotte L, Lenis S, Thibeault L, Sassine MP, Seal RF, Roy A. Effect of low central venous pressure and phlebotomy on blood product transfusion requirements during liver transplantations. Liver Transpl. 2006;12:117–23.
6. Feltracco P, Brezzi M, Barbieri S, et al. Blood loss, predictors of bleeding, transfusion practice and strategies of blood cell salvaging during liver transplantation. World J Hepatol. 2013;5:1–15. https://doi.org/10.4254/wjh.v5.i1.1.
7. Caldwell SH, Hoffman M, Lisman T, et al. Coagulation disorders and hemostasis in liver disease: pathophysiology and critical assessment of current management. Hepatology. 2006;44:1039e46.
8. Dzik WH, Arkin CF, Jenkins RL, Stump DC. Fibrinolysis during liver transplant in humans: role of tissue type plasminogen activator. Blood. 1988;71(4):1090–5.
9. Kozek-Langenecker SA, Afshari A, Albaladejo P, et al. Management of severe perioperative bleeding: guidelines from the European Society of Anaesthesiology. Eur J Anaesthesiol. 2013;30:270–382. Review. Erratum in: Eur J Anaesthesiol 2014; 31: 247. https://doi.org/10.1097/EJA.0b013e32835f4d5b
10. McNicol PL, Liu G, Harley ID, et al. Blood loss and transfusion requirements in liver transplantation: experience with the first 75 cases. Anaesth Intensive Care. 1994;22:666–71.
11. Perry DJ, Fitzmaurice DA, Kitchen S, et al. Point-of-care testing in haemostasis. Br J Haematol. 2010;150:501–14.
12. Kang YG, Martin DJ, Marquez J, et al. Intraoperative changes in blood coagulation and thrombelastographic monitoring in liver transplantation. Anesth Analg. 1985;64:888–96.
13. Kotze A, Carter LA, Scally JA. Effect of a patient blood management programme on preoperative anaemia, transfusion rate, and outcome after primary hip or knee arthroplasty: a quality improvement cycle. Br J Anaesth. 2012;108(6):943–52.
14. Goodnough LT, Shander A. Patient blood management. Anesthesiology. 2012;116:1367–76.

Veno-Venous Bypass in Liver Transplantation

22

Komal Ray

22.1 Introduction and Historical Background

Liver transplant is an accepted standard of care worldwide for acute liver failure and chronic liver disease. The initial surgical technique also known as conventional technique for orthotopic liver transplantation (OLT) involved resection and removal of recipient's retrohepatic inferior vena cava (IVC) along with liver, requiring cross clamping of IVC and portal vein. The physiological effects of caval cross clamping for prolonged periods can be deleterious for perfusion of many organ systems in the body (Table 22.1). Conventional technique as a result was associated with cardiovascular instability, reduced perfusion to intestines, kidneys, and excessive bleeding from venous collaterals leading to poor outcomes [1–3]. To mitigate the effect of venous clamping the concept of venous bypass was proposed. It was first described and used in animal experiments as early as 1960 by Moore [4].

The first human trial of veno-venous bypass (VVBP) was performed by Starlz during OLT using a passive shunt to bypass venous blood from IVC to superior vena cava (SVC) through internal jugular vein (IJV); however, it was associated with pulmonary embolism and high mortality [5]. Later in 1979 Calne et al. used partial

Table 22.1 Physiological effects of IVC cross clamping

Cardiovascular: ↓ venous return, ↓ cardiac output, ↑heart rate, ↓ cardiac index
Renal: ↓ perfusion pressure, renal outflow obstruction →renal venous congestion
Splanchnic circulation: ↑venous congestion/ ↓ portal venous flow → ileus, bowel oedema, bacterial translocation
Central nervous system: ↓ cerebral perfusion pressure
Respiratory: ↑ pulmonary vascular resistance, ↓ mixed venous oxygen saturation

cardiopulmonary bypass system which collected blood from IVC and femoral vein, passing through oxygenator and returning to femoral artery. Although it achieved the desired haemodynamic stability, but lead to excessive bleeding due to the use of anti-coagulation, hence limiting its usefulness [6]. Further revision of cardiac support system without heparin using a constrained vortex pump by Dixon and colleagues [7]. With this background, Griffith and team designed a closed veno-venous bypass system with heparin bonded tubings and centrifugal blood pump in 1983 and later successfully used in 1984 during OLT without systemic anti-coagulation [8, 9].

Studies from 1984 to 1985 showed that the use of VVBP offered advantages of haemodynamic stability, lesser requirement for blood transfusion, better perfusion of kidneys, intestine and allowed for longer anhepatic phase with better short term patient survival (91% in VVBP group vs. 73% in non-VVBP group) [9, 10].

K. Ray (✉)
St James's University Hospital, Leeds, UK

22.2 Indications for VVBP (Table 22.2)

22.2.1 Cardiovascular Instability

Preserving haemodynamic stability remained one of the most important indications for VVBP in the initial years (1986–1992) after its introduction. Some authors suggested the use of VVBP if there was >30% reduction in mean arterial pressure or >50% decrease in cardiac index during trial clamp period of 5 mins [11]. However, other studies during 1987–2001 failed to concur with these results and showed no increase in morbidity and mortality with or without use of VVBP [12, 13].

It was further proposed that degree of haemodynamic instability is likely to be influenced by intravascular filling status, presence of underlying cardiac condition and collaterals [14].

Also venous cross clamping in patients with normal cardiac reserve would generate compensatory response to maintain cardiac output by means of increase in heart rate and systemic vascular resistance [1].

Use of fluids or blood to maintain preload in anhepatic phase can be associated with fluid overload and pulmonary oedema specially in patients with low cardiac reserve like ischaemic heart disease, pulmonary hypertension, cardiomyopathy where use of VVBP has been advocated previously in some studies [15–17]. However, further studies emerged showing fall in cardiac output, increase in systemic vascular resistance, and minimal change in cardiac filling pressure even with VVBP use [18, 19].

Table 22.2 Indications for VVBP

Cardiovascular instability
Failed trial clamp
High risk group (ischaemic heart disease, pulmonary hypertension, cardiomyopathy)
Renal impairment
Acute liver failure
Extensive bleeding during hepatectomy
Severe portal hypertension
Surgically challenging: Complex anatomy, polycystic liver, redo-transplantation

At this point alternatives to the use of VVBP for maintaining haemodynamic stability were emerging like cautious filling and titrated use of inotropes to reduce risk of volume overload in high risk patients [20, 21] and use of rapid infusion device [17]. As of now there are no studies which support use of VVBP for the purposes of haemodynamic stability even in high risk patients.

22.2.2 Renal Impairment

Renal impairment is common after liver transplant with multifold aetiology: pre-existing renal impairment, intraoperative haemodynamic instability, and use of blood products, post-reperfusion syndrome, immunosuppressants. Whilst advantages of *VVBP* to offer haemodynamic stability and reduce venous congestion is likely to be beneficial for renal perfusion and therefore renal function. Study from Pittsburgh 1984 showed lower serum creatinine levels and reduced the rate of haemodialysis post-transplant in patients where VVBP was used [10].

But later in 1996 Grand et al. prospectively randomized and compared patients with or without VVBP, they demonstrated that patients with VVBP showed lower degree of renal impairment during anhepatic phase only with no differences during the rest of the perioperative period and also in terms of postoperative requirement for haemodialysis [18].

In patients with preoperative renal impairment there is variable opinion, some authors recommend the use of VVBP [18, 22] whilst other are not supportive as no changes found in peri and postoperative renal function when VVBP not used [23, 24].

Retrospective analysis by Cabezuelo and team showed that VVBP, postreperfusion syndrome, 20 units cryoprecipitate transfusion are independent risk factor for postoperative renal failure [25]. Also with advent of caval sparing techniques like piggyback the incidence of acute kidney injury after transplant has reduced [25].

22.2.3 Acute Liver Failure (ALF)

It is estimated that incidence of cerebral oedema is as high as 75% in patients with fulminant hepatic failure and is associated with high mortality [26, 27]. Normally cerebral blood flow is maintained independent of mean arterial pressure and $PaCO_2$. However, this autoregulation is impaired in ALF. It was believed that patients undergoing OLT are at risk of cerebral complications during anhepatic phase with caval cross clamping without VVBP related to significant haemodynamic instability [9, 10].

In addition administration large volumes of fluids to address haemodynamic instability phases can precipitate cerebral oedema. This phenomenon can be exacerbated during reperfusion by release of anaerobic metabolites leading to cerebral vasodilatation [27]. Some authors have suggested judicious use of perioperative monitoring and inotropes to help maintain cerebral blood flow and intracranial pressure in ALF patients with Grade 3/4 encephalopathy undergoing OLT without VVBP [28, 29].

22.2.4 Severe Portal Hypertension

The logic of using VVBP in portal hypertension is to reduce portal venous pressure and mesenteric venous congestion. Most patients with cirrhosis undergoing OLT generally have well established portal venous collaterals, therefore impact of portal vein clamping on haemodynamic stability should be minimal [14], however, this cannot be generalized [30]. Some authors recommend the use of VVBP in severe portal hypertension to reduce bleeding from large varices in retrohepatic areas which may lead to prolonged and complicated hepatectomy without VVBP [27].

22.2.5 Massive Bleeding During Hepatectomy and Other Indications

Over the year advancements in surgical and anaesthetic techniques, careful use coagulation monitoring, antifibrinolytic drugs have tapered transfusion requirements. However, there are many confounding factors which can contribute and worsen bleeding during OLT these are portal hypertension, intrinsic coagulopathy due to liver disease, previous surgery, redo-liver transplantation, and polycystic liver disease. VVBP during its introductory years showed a spectacular drop in transfusion requirements, 33 units vs. 18.9 in VVBP group, which was related to venous decompression [9]. However, as surgical and haemostatic techniques improved, further studies showed no difference in transfusion requirements in VVBP or no VVBP groups [23, 31].

Some studies have shown that VVBP can be associated with increase transfusion requirement related to platelet adhesion, haemolysis, and fibrinolysis caused by bypass tubing [32–34].

22.3 Contraindications

The only absolute contraindication of using VVBP is acute Budd-Chiari syndrome as often linked with poor flow rate and high incidence of thromboembolic phenomenon [9].

22.4 Insertion and Management of VVBP

When VVBP was first introduced the vascular access was obtained by insertion of outflow cannula into PV, femoral vein (FV), and inflow cannula into axillary vein by means of surgical cutdown. This was associated with higher incidence of complications (details next section). This was later replaced by percutaneous technique, first described by Oken et al. in 1994 [35].

Percutaneous approach has been described as simple, safe, and rapid with added advantages of better flow rates [36, 37]. VVBP cannula are available in sizes: 18–21 French. The inflow cannula is inserted into internal jugular vein (IJV) and outflow cannula is inserted into FV after induction of anaesthesia. In our institute we use 21Fr percutaneous bypass catheters (Femoral arterial cannula with introducing trocar set, Medtronic, MN, USA, Fig. 22.1). The catheter is 17 cm in length with a radio opaque dilator which

Fig. 22.1 21 French
Medtronic Femoral
arterial catheter and
introducing trocar set (**a**)
Needle with guide wire
(**b**) Stiff dilator (**c**) Soft
polyurethane catheter
(17 cm in length) and
dilator (60 cm) (**d**)
extension tubing for
catheter with a luer lock
aspiration port

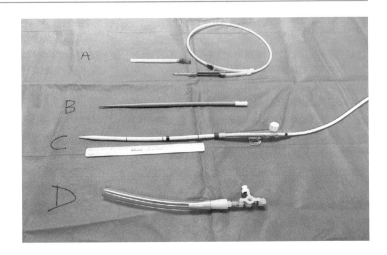

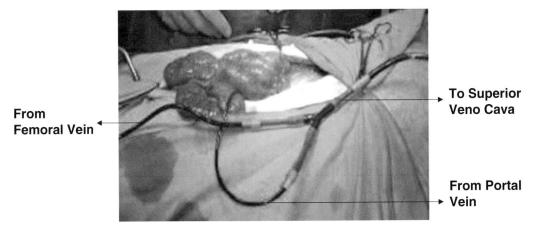

Fig. 22.2 VVBP system. Blood flows from outflow cannulas (portal vein, femoral vein) into centrifugal pump and then returned back into the body through inflow cannula (Internal Jugular vein (IJV))

is 60 cm in length. The catheter and dilator are made of polyurethane which makes it flexible and kink resistant. Cannulas are inserted under strict asepsis with ultrasound guidance using Seldinger technique. This is followed by careful incision around guidewire to allow dilatation before cannula is inserted. At this point it is important to avoid any force to advance dilator or cannula if met with resistance. The first set of dilator is stiff and can cause venous wall injury and advances should be limited to <2 cm, ensuring that guidewire is freely mobile after each advance as this may be an indicator of problem. IJV and FV cannula are connected to an extension tubing approximately 15 cm long with luer lock port for aspiration and flushing as shown in Fig. 22.1. Lines are then flushed with plenty of saline and secured with sutures. The position of

IJV cannula in superior vena cava can be verified with Trans oesophageal echocardiography (TOE) probe or by means of bubble test (immediate appearance of micro-bubbles in the right atrium after normal saline injection through the cannula) if good view not obtainable [38]. Portal vein (PV) cannula is inserted by surgeon. VVBP is commenced during dissection phase of surgery. VVBP circuit (Fig. 22.2) is established by connecting outflow cannulae (PV + FV) to heparin coated circuit primed with normal saline via centrifugal pump to inflow cannula (IJV).

When VVBP is commenced, anaesthetists using TOE monitors can look for the following: bubble in right atrium for position check, stable chamber size, and wall motion to rule out any leak into pericardium, mediastinum or thoracic cavity. Any concerns for malpositioning should be addressed using

TOE, chest X-ray or a scan as deemed appropriate. Also it is important to start at low flow rate initially to allow clamping of VVB tubing adjacent to IJV cannula to prevent any air emboli reaching IJV. Once column of blood established without issues then flow rate can be enhanced to desire rate to achieve an optimal flow of 40 mL/kg/min.

We use Bio-Medicus Perfusion system Fig. 22.3 (Bio-Pump plus centrifugal blood pump and Bio-Console 560, Medtronic, Minneapolis) which is run by dedicated operating department practitioner/perfusionist. The importance here is to ensure

adequate competency and training schedule for the VVBP practitioners, which is a growing concern as lesser numbers of OLT are performed using VVBP. Advanced nonocclusive design of centrifugal pump promotes laminar flow decreasing blood cell trauma including reduced platelet and complement activation. Pump flow ranges from 1.5 to 6 L/min and with an average duration on VVBP of 100 mins (range: 70–158 min) and is generally terminated post-reperfusion [39]. After discontinuation of VVBP the blood column from the circuit is carefully allowed to return to circulation ensuring no air is entrained in the process. IJV and FV cannulae should be removed soon after as they carry risk of disconnection leading to exsanguination. The site of insertion would require sutures and manual compression to ensure haemostasis.

22.5 Complications of VVBP (Table 22.3)

22.5.1 Vascular Access Related

When VVBP was first introduced the standard practice was to insert inflow cannula by surgical cutdown of axillary vein and FV. This was associ-

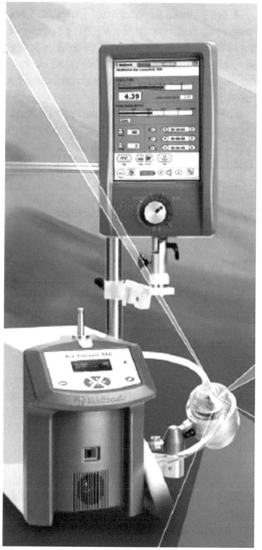

Fig. 22.3 Medtronic: Bio-medicus perfusion system, Bio-pump, Centrifugal blood pump with Bio-console 560

Table 22.3 Complications of VVBP

Insertion related
Percutaneous approach
Haemothorax
Haemomediastinum
Thrombosis
Air emboli
Malposition
Pneumothorax
Open surgical approach
Infection
Lymphorrhoea
Seroma
Nerve damage
Reduced flow rate
VVBP circuit related
Hypothermia
Bleeding: Haemolysis, fibrinolysis
Thromboembolism: Platelet adhesion
Post reperfusion syndrome (PRS): Higher incidence
Increased cost and duration of procedure
Staff training and competency

ated with high incidence of wound infection, seromas, lymphocoele and nerve injury [40–42]. Additionally there were issues around reduced flow rates and prolongation of surgical time.

Percutaneous approach is overall considered safe but it can be associated with life threatening complications and mortality. Single centre study involving 312 patients described morbidity of 1.28% related to intrathoracic haemorrhage requiring thoracotomy/sternotomy and mortality of 0.32% due to cardiovascular collapse [43]. Another study of 94 patients requiring veno-venous cannulation for extra corporal life support had 1 death related SVC perforation [44]. Hilmi and colleagues reviewed 326 patient where percutaneous approach was used, showed a failure rate of 1.8% due to technical difficulties and 2.2% of other complications including: air embolism, low flow rate, hypotension, atrial fibrillation, delayed start to verify position [38]. There has been a case report of fatal haemothorax related to superior vena cava perforation following insertion of IJV bypass cannula [45]. One catheter related death in a paediatric liver transplant patient has also been reported [46].

There is only one trial comparing open vs. percutaneous technique. Although the study showed no statistically significant difference in the incidence of complications but primary/secondary outcomes were not available to compare between the two approaches. The trial was not suitably powered and had possibility of random errors related to small numbers hence difficult to establish that any one technique better than the other [47]. As of current available evidence there are no clear advantages in using open technique which not only adds to operating time and contributes to bigger scar in addition to other risks described above.

22.5.2 Extracorporeal/Bypass Circuit Related

Extracorporeal or commonly known as bypass circuit has undergone many refinements since first introduced. Complications related to VVBP circuit include hypothermia, thrombosis, pulmonary embolism, and haemolysis.

Hypothermia is a frequent issue during liver transplant as a result of many factors (anaesthesia induced peripheral vasodilatation, cold operating theatres, loss of heat from open abdomen, large incision, prolonged operating time, and anhepatic phase) this can have deleterious effect on coagulation, cardiac function. Addition of extracorporeal circuit during liver transplantation can worsen hypothermia with heat loss of 0.75 °C/h, this can be avoided by addition of heat exchanger in the circuit [48].

A few authors have reported increased transfusion requirements in the VVBP group which could be related to haemolysis, platelet adhesion, fibrinolysis [32–34]. But other studies have shown no differences in the blood products given between the two groups [49].

There have been reports of mortality related to pulmonary embolism with origin of thrombus in bypass circuit or translocated from IVC to right atrium during low flow rates of <1 L/min [50].

22.5.3 Post-Reperfusion Syndrome (PRS)

This was described in 1987 by Aggarwal et al. as phenomenon of cardiovascular collapse related to release of vasoactive substances from reperfused liver with an incidence of 30% [51]. Later redefined by Estrin and colleagues as syndrome of bradycardia, hypotension (MAP<60 mmHg in adults or <50 mmHg in children) following liver reperfusion with incidence of 3.7% in their study which was without VVBP. They suggested that lower incidence PRS in their study is related to higher volume of fluids administered without VVBP which led to better haemodynamic stability during PRS [2].

Studies have shown that extracorporeal circulation leads to activation of inflammatory cytokines which leads to vasodilatation and hypotension [52].

22.6 Caval Preserving Options

VVBP carries morbidity risk, although it may be useful in certain situation but is not essential for liver transplant. Over the years there have been research into caval preserving techniques.

One such technique is piggyback technique (PT) suggested by Tzakis in 1989 [53]. This is useful in maintaining venous return to the heart during anhepatic phase. PT offers advantages of haemodynamic stability, preserved renal function, shorter anhepatic phase, lesser bleeding. Since introduction of PT the use of VVBP has fallen across many transplant centres [54].

PT is commonly used in paediatric live related liver transplantation and in reduced size grafts. The reluctance to use PT in some centres without a passive shunt or VVBP is due to anxiety around venous complications [55]. However studies have shown that outflow complications can be managed by surgical or radiological interventions [56, 57].

22.7 Selective Use of VVBP

Rapidly rising number of liver transplants across the world has been accompanied by advancements in surgical and anaesthesia techniques resulting in excellent outcomes.

Survey by Chiari et al. showed decline in routine use of VVBP from 91% in 1987 to 42% in 1998 [58]. This was related to increased reporting of VVBP associated complications and emerging caval sparing techniques with good outcomes. Whilst a survey in UK in 2003 revealed a variable practice centres, VVBP was used routinely in two centres, rarely used in two others and selectively used for 10–30% cases in 2 centres [27]. VVBP has been reappraised and advocated when establishing a new liver transplant programme [59].

In a review conducted by Guruswamy [60] there was no difference in the perioperative mortality, re-transplantation, renal function at 24 h or other side effects between the VVBP/No-VVBP groups although graft survival was not reported in the trials. Blood transfusion requirements were similar in the two groups. There are no trials comparing routine/selective use of VVBP. Currently, there is no evidence to support the use of VVBP and as it can be associated with complications therefore routine use is not recommended.

22.8 Conclusion

There continues to be varied practice regarding VVBP use across liver transplant centres. The use of caval preserving techniques is rapidly expanding and the indications for VVBP dwindling. In the current climate it would be difficult to design high quality multicentre trials looking at outcomes using different surgical techniques with or without VVBP. It is increasingly accepted that VVBP is not without risks and its use should be considered based on professional judgement, personal experience, and institutional practice.

References

1. Pappas G, Palmer WM, Martineau GL, et al. Hemodynamic alterations caused during orthotopic liver transplantation in humans. Surgery. 1971;70(6):872–5.
2. Estrin JA, Belani KG, Ascher NL, Lura D, Payne W, Najarian JS. Hemodynamic changes on clamping and unclamping of major vessels during liver transplantation. Transplant Proc. 1989;21(3):3500–5.
3. Kang Y. Hemodynamic changes during intraabdominal organ transplantation. Transplant Proc. 1993;25:2583–7.
4. Moore FD, Smith LL, Burnap TK, Dallenbach FD, Dammin GJ, Gruber UF, et al. One-stage homotransplantation of the liver following total hepatectomy in dogs. Transplant Bull. 1959;6(1):103–7.
5. Starzl TE, Marchioro TL, Vonkaulla KN, Hermann G, Brittain RS, Waddell WR. Homotransplantation of the liver in humans. Surg Gynecol Obstet. 1963;117:659–76.
6. Calne RY, Smith DP, McMaster P, Craddock GN, Rolles K, Farman JV, et al. Use of partial cardiopulmonary bypass during the anhepatic phase of orthotopic liver grafting. Lancet. 1979;2:612–4.
7. Dixon CM, Magovern GJ. Evaluation of the bio-pump for long-term cardiac support without heparinization. J Extra Corp Technol. 1982;14:331–6.

8. Griffith BP, Shaw BW Jr, Hardesty RL, Iwatsuki S, Bahnson HT, Starzl TE. Veno-venous bypass without systemic anticoagulation for transplantation of the human liver. Surg Gynecol Obstet. 1985;160:270–2.

9. Shaw BW Jr, Martin DJ, Marquez JM, Kang YG, Bugbee AC Jr, Iwatsuki S, et al. Venous bypass in clinical liver transplantation. Ann Surg. 1984;200:524–34.

10. Shaw BW Jr, Martin DJ, Marquez JM, Kang YG, Bugbee AC Jr, Iwatsuki S, et al. Advantages of venous bypass during orthotopic transplantation of the liver. Semin Liver Dis. 1985;5:344–8.

11. Veroli P, el Hage C, Ecoffey C. Does adult liver transplantation without venovenous bypass result in renal failure? Anesth Analg. 1992;75:489–94.

12. Schwarz B, Pomaroli A, Hoermann C, Margreiter R, Mair P. Liver transplantation without venovenous bypass: morbidity and mortality in patients with greater than 50% reduction in cardiac output after vena cava clamping. J Cardiothorac Vasc Anesth. 2001;15:460–2.

13. Wall WJ, Grant DR, Duff JH, Kutt JL, Ghent CN, Bloch MS. Liver transplantation without venous bypass. Transplantation. 1987;43:56–61.

14. Hilmi IA, Planinsic RM. Con: venovenous bypass should not be used in orthotopic liver transplantation. J Cardiothorac Vasc Anesth. 2006;20:744–7.

15. Gifford DJ. Support perfusion for liver transplantation. Perfusion. 1991;6:203–8.

16. Beltran J, Taura P, Grande L, Garcia-Valdecasas JC, Rimola A, Cugat E. Venovenous bypass and liver transplantation. Anesth Analg. 1993;77:42.

17. Stock PG, Payne WD, Ascher NL, Roberts JP, Belani K, Estrin J, et al. Rapid infusion technique as a safe alternative to veno-venous bypass in orthotopic liver transplant (TX). Transplant Proc. 1989;21(1Pt 2):2322–5.

18. Grande L, Rimola A, Cugat E, Alvarez L, Garcia-Valdecasas JC, Taura P, et al. Effect of venovenous bypass on perioperative renal function in liver transplantation: results of a randomized, controlled trial. Hepatology. 1996;23:1418–28.

19. Paulsen AW, Whitten CW, Ramsay MA, Klintmalm GB. Considerations for anesthetic management during veno-venous bypass in adult hepatic transplantation. Anesth Analg. 1989;68:489–96.

20. Wu Y, Oyos TL, Chenhsu RY, Katz DA, Brian JE, Rayhill SC. Vasopressor agents without volume expansion as a safe alternative to venovenous bypass during cavaplasty liver transplantation. Transplantation. 2003;76:1724–8.

21. Cheema SP, Hughes A, Webster NR, Bellamy MC. Cardiac function during orthotopic liver transplantation with venovenous bypass. Anaesthesia. 1995;50:776–8.

22. Kai Sun MD, Fu Hong MD, Wang Y. Venovenous bypass is associated with a lower incidence of acute kidney injury after liver transplantation in patients with compromised pretransplant renal function. Anesth Analg. 2017;125(5):1463–70.

23. Johnson MW, Powelson JA, Auchincloss H Jr, Delmonico FL, Cosimi AB. Selective use of veno-venous bypass in orthotopic liver transplantation. Clin Transpl. 1996;10:181–5.

24. Corti A, Degasperi A, Colussi S, Mazza E, Amici O, Cristalli A, et al. Evaluation of renal function during orthotopic liver transplantation. Minerva Anestesiol. 1997;63:221–8.

25. Cabezuelo JB, Ramirez P, Acosta F, Torres D, Sansano T, Pons JA, et al. Does the standard vs piggyback surgical technique affect the development of early acute renal failure after orthotopic liver transplantation? Transplant Proc. 2003;35:1913–4.

26. Lee WM. Acute liver failure. N Engl J Med. 1993;329:1862–72.

27. Reddy K, Mallett S, Peachey T. Venovenous bypass in orthotopic liver transplantation: time for a rethink? Liver Transpl. 2005;11:741–9.

28. Pere P, Hockerstedt K, Isoniemi H, Lindgren L. Cerebral blood flow and oxygenation in liver transplantation for acute or chronic hepatic disease without venovenous bypass. Liver Transpl. 2000;6:471–9.

29. Prager MC, Washington DE, Lidofsky SD, Kelley SD, White JD. Intracranial pressure monitoring during liver transplant without venovenous bypass for fulminant hepatic failure. Transplant Proc. 1993;25:1841.

30. Shaw BW Jr. Some further notes on venous bypass for orthotopic transplantation of the liver. Transplant Proc. 1987;9(Suppl 3):13–6.

31. Stegall MD, Mandell S, Karrer F, Kam I. Liver transplantation without venovenous bypass. Transplant Proc. 1995;27:1254–5.

32. Scholz T, Solberg R, Okkenhaug C, Videm V, Gallimore MJ, Mathisen O, et al. Veno-venous bypass in liver transplantation: heparin-coated perfusion circuits reduce the activation of humoral defense systems in an vitro model. Perfusion. 2001;16:285–92.

33. Eleborg L, Sallander S, Tollemar J. Minimal haemolytic effect of veno-venous bypass during liver transplantation. Transpl Int. 1991;4:157–60.

34. Van der Hulst VP, Henny CP, Moulijn AC, Engbers G, ten Cate H, Grundeman PF, et al. Veno-venous bypass without systemic heparinization using a centrifugal pump: a blind comparison of heparin bonded circuit versus a non heparin bonded circuit. J Cardiovasc Surg (Torino). 1989;30:118–23.

35. Oken AC, Frank SM, Merritt WT, Fair J, Klein A, Burdick J, et al. A new percutaneous technique for establishing venous bypass access in orthotopic liver transplantation. J Cardiothorac Vasc Anesth. 1994;8:58–60.

36. Frenette L, Cox J, Singer D, Ronderos J, Steele S, Eckhoff D, Bynon S. Five years of experience with percutaneous cannula for establishing venous bypass access in orthotopic liver transplantation. Transplant Proc. 1996;28:2974–7.

37. Scherer R, Giebler R, Erhard J, Lange R, Gunnicker M, Schmutizler M, et al. A new method of veno-venous bypass during human orthotopic liver transplantation. Anaesthesia. 1994;49:398–402.

38. Sakai T, Gligor S, Diulus J, McAffee R, Marsh JW, Planinsic RM. Insertion and management of percutaneous veno-venous bypass cannula for liver transplantation: a reference for transplant anesthesiologists. Clin Transpl. 2010;24:585–91.

39. Scherer RU, Giebler RM, Schmutzler MJ, Gunnicker FM, Kox WJ. Shunt flow and caval pressure gradient during veno-venous bypass in human orthotopic liver transplantation. Br J Anaesth. 1993;70:689–90.

40. Johnson SR, Marterre WF, Alonso MH, Hanto DW. A percutaneous technique for venovenous bypass in orthotopic cadaver liver transplantation and comparison with the open technique. Liver Transpl Surg. 1996;2:354–61.

41. Ozaki CF, Langnas AN, Bynon JS, Pillen TJ, Kangas J, Vogel JE, et al. A percutaneous method for venovenous bypass in liver transplantation. Transplantation. 1994;57:472–3.

42. Katirji MB. Brachial plexus injury following liver transplantation. Neurology. 1989;39:736–8.

43. Budd JM, Isaac JL, Bennet J, Freeman JW. Morbidity and mortality associated with large-bore percutaneous venovenous bypass cannulation for 312 orthotopic liver transplantations. Liver Transpl. 2001;7:359–62.

44. Pranikoff T, Hirschi RB, Remenapp R, et al. Venovenous extracorporeal life support via percutaneous cannulation in 94 patients. Chest. 1999;115:818–22.

45. Jankovic Z, Boon A, Prasad R. Fatal haemothorax following large-bore percutaneous cannulation before liver transplantation. Br J Anaesth. 2005;95:472–6.

46. Lovell M, Baines D. Case report: fatal complication from central venous cannulation in a paediatric liver transplant patient. Paediatr Anaesth. 2000;10:661–4.

47. Tisone G, Mercadante E, Dauri M, Colella D, Anselmo A, Romagnoli J, et al. Surgical versus percutaneous technique for veno-venous bypass during orthotopic liver transplantation: a prospective randomized study. Transplant Proc. 1999;31(8):3162–3.

48. Khoury GF, Kaufman RD, Musich JA. Hypothermia related to the use of venovenous bypass during liver trasnplantation. Eur J Anaesthiol. 1990;7:501–3.

49. Kuo PC, Alfrey EJ, Garcia G, Haddow G, Dafoe DC. Orthotopic liver transplantation with selective use of venovenous bypass. Am J Surg. 1995;170:671–5.

50. Navalgund AA, Kang Y, Sarner JB, Jahr JS, Gieraerts R. Massive pulmonary thromboembolism during liver transplantation. Anesth Analg. 1988;67:400–2.

51. Aggarwal S, Kang Y, Freeman JA, Fortunato FL, Pinsky MR. Postreperfusion syndrome: cardiovascular collapse following hepatic reperfusion during liver transplantation. Transplant Proc. 1987;19:54–5.

52. Solberg R, Scholz T, Videm V, Okkenhuag C, Aasen AO. Heparin coating reduces cell activation and mediator release in an in vitro venovenous bypass model for liver transplantation. Transpl Int. 1998;11:252–8.

53. Tzakis A, Todo S, Starzl TE. Orthotopic liver transplantation with preservation of the inferior vena cava. Ann Surg. 1989;210:649.

54. Lerut J, Ciccarelli O, Roggen F, Laterre PF, Danse E, Goffette P, et al. Cavocaval adult liver transplantation and retransplantation without venovenous bypass and without portocaval shunting: a prospective feasibility study in adult liver transplantation. Transplantation. 2003;75:1740–5.

55. Hesse UJ, Berrevoet F, Troisi R, Pattyn P, Mortier E, Decruyenaere J, et al. Hepato-venous reconstruction in orthotopic liver transplantation with preservation of the recipients' inferior vena cava and veno-venous bypass. Langenbecks Arch Surg. 2000;385:350–6.

56. Lerut J, Gertsch PH. Side-to-side cavo-cavostomy: a useful aid in "complicated" piggy-back liver transplantation. Transpl Int. 1993;6:299.

57. Merhav H, Bronsther O, Pinna A, et al. Significant stenosis of the vena cava following liver transplantation: a six years experience. Transplantation. 1993;56:1541.

58. Chari RS, Gan TJ, Robertson KM, et al. Venovenous bypass in adult orthotopic liver transplantation: routine or selective use? J Am Coll Surg. 1998;186:683–90.

59. Mossdorf A, Ulmer F, Junge K, Heidenhain C, Hein M, Temizel I, Neumann UP, Schöning W, Schmeding M. Bypass during liver transplantation: anachronism or revival? Liver transplantation using a combined venovenous/portal venous bypass-experiences with 163 liver transplants in a newly established liver transplantation program. Gastroenterol Res Pract. 2015;2015:967951.

60. Gurusamy KS, Koti R, Pamecha V, Davidson BR. Veno-venous bypass versus none for liver transplantation. Cochrane Database Syst Rev. 2011;3:CD007712.

Intraoperative Complications and Management

23

Sanjeev Aneja and Ashish Malik

Abbreviations

AKI	Acute kidney injury
CI	Cardiac index
CVP	Central venous pressure
FFP	Fresh frozen plasma
HR	Heart rate
LT	Liver transplant
MA	Maximum amplitude
MAP	Mean arterial pressure
MELD	Model for end stage liver disease
OLT	Orthotropic liver transplant
PAP	Pulmonary artery pressure
SAM	Systolic anterior motion
SVR	Systemic vascular resistance
TEE	Transesophageal echocardiography
TEG	Thromboelastography
TXA	Tranexamic acid
VET	Viscoelastic tests

Intraoperative course in liver transplant is lengthy and complications or conditions aggravating already existing one are very common and can occur at any phase. Complications can be related to equipment, patient or surgery and anaesthesia. Successful management of these complications requires sound knowledge, recognition and prompt treatment. Significant blood loss requiring massive blood transfusion is still one of the most dreaded intraoperative complications of liver transplantation despite advances in surgical techniques and risk stratification for bleeding. Widespread use of viscoelastic tests for coagulation has resulted in better understanding of coagulation mechanism in patients with end stage liver disease. TEG directed blood transfusion has decreased the incidence of massive blood transfusion, but normal values of TEG are derived from healthy volunteers and may not represent ESLD patients. ESLD results in several alterations which favour thrombosis which can be picked by viscoelastic methods better than conventional tests of coagulation. Intracardiac thrombus (ICT) and pulmonary embolism (PE) are the two most dreaded intraoperative complications because of high mortality. ICT and PE have been diagnosed in all phase of transplantation and their mechanism is poorly understood. Intraoperative hypothermia because of long duration of surgery in low ambient temperature of operating room is also frequently encountered despite aggressive warming measures. Hypothermia has an adverse effect on patient and has been linked to poor outcome. Air embolism, disseminated intravascular coagulation, life threatening arrythmias and haemodynamic collapse are other frequently encountered intraoperative complications. Use of technology and equipment is increasing during intraoperative

S. Aneja (✉) · A. Malik
Indraprastha Apollo Hospital, New Delhi, India

period. Many intraoperative complications may be related to equipment malfunctioning. Last but not the least, positioning of patient because of long duration of surgery and care of patient during application of retractors is also important.

Common complications seen are:
1. Massive Blood Transfusion.
2. Pulmonary Embolism.
3. Intracardiac Thrombus.
4. Vasoplegia.
5. Air Embolism.
6. Severe Post Reperfusion Syndrome.
7. Dynamic LVOTO.
8. Pulmonary Hypertension.
9. Arrhythmias.
10. Miscellaneous.

23.1 Massive Blood Transfusion in Liver Transplant

There is a wide variation in the management of coagulation and blood transfusion practice in liver transplantation. The use of blood products intraoperatively is declining, and transfusion free transplantations are taking place more frequently in the current scenario. The mean number of red cells transfused to a liver recipient was 12 units in the late 1990s but is now as low as 0.5 units, with some centres reporting almost 80% of patients not requiring any blood transfusion [1, 2]. Nevertheless, transfusion remains an essential part of the toolbox for transplantation.

Blood transfusion is one of the factors influencing graft and patient survival. Poor outcome of patients who received more blood transfusion might be attributed to more blood loss during transplantation, or adverse transfusion reaction, infectious contamination of blood products, or immune modulation of the transfused patient [1]. One-year survival rate is decreased in patients who received any amounts of FFP or more than four units of RBC [2].

Massive transfusion (MT) is defined in adults as

- Replacement of total blood volume within 24 h
- Replacement of 50% of total blood volume within 3 h or
- Transfusion of more than 4 units of red blood cells (RBCs) within 4 h with active major bleeding or more than 150 mL/min of blood loss [3].

The MT in children is defined as red blood cell transfusion of 50% of total blood volume (TBV) in 3 h, 100% in 24 h, or >10% of TBV per minute [4, 5].

In the liver transplant scenario, transfusion of more than 6 units of blood in 24 h is considered massive blood transfusion and is associated with poor outcome [6].

23.1.1 Preoperative Risk Factors for Massive Blood Transfusion

Various preoperative predictors have been identified to predict massive blood transfusion during liver transplantation. McCluskey et al. identified seven independent predictors of massive blood transfusion (age > 40 years, Hb concentration < 100 g/L, INR > 2.0, platelet count <70,000/cm and albumin <24 g/L; as well as repeat transplantation) [7]. By using these predictors, a risk index was developed that assigned each patient a score between 0 and 8. As all these predictors are related to disease severity and coagulation status, they are found to be associated with excessive blood loss in various studies. INR > 1.6 has been associated with excessive blood loss [6]. Massicotte L. et al. did not find any link between MELD score and the transfusion rate whereas starting haemoglobin was linked to rate of blood transfusion [8].

Preoperative low platelet count has been shown to be associated with excessive blood loss [9, 10]. Previous abdominal surgery, portal vein thrombosis and spontaneous bacterial peritonitis are also associated with increased blood loss.

A low baseline fibrinogen concentration can contribute to bleeding risk. Fibrinogen levels below 1.5 g/dL were associated with increased risk for transfusion of >6 units of RBC in living donor related transplant patients [11]. The quantity of fibrin degradation products has also been ascribed to an increased risk of transfusion. Patients with a low MA (<40 mm) on baseline are a high risk for bleeding [12]. A low MA and low baseline fibrinogen concentration increases the risk of fibrinolysis [13]. Recipient age and donor age is implicated in predicting transfusion [14].

23.1.2 Intraoperative Risk Factors for Massive Blood Transfusion

Increased technical difficulty of the operation, such as portal vein thrombosis, presence of collaterals increases the risk of bleeding. A hyperdynamic circulation and portal hypertension are significant contributors to the bleeding risk. Advancement in surgical techniques and experience have played crucial role in the reduction of blood loss. Use of veno-venous bypass has decreased over the years. Most of the surgeons are employing piggyback technique with preservation of recipient's Inferior vena cava. These techniques have significant impact on blood loss during surgery. Veno-venous bypass is an independent predictor of increased blood loss. It has been postulated that the contact of blood with the circuit triggers haemolysis, fibrinolysis and platelet activation, thus impairing haemostasis [15].

Use of piggyback technique and preservation of inferior vena cava has shown to decrease blood loss during surgery. Preservation of inferior vena cava reduces the requirement of extensive retroperitoneal dissection which is the seat of many collaterals in patients with portal hypertension. Many studies have reported reduction in blood loss and transfusion requirement in patients undergoing OLT using piggyback technique [16, 17]. However, a Cochrane data base review which included two randomized trials consisting of 106 patients did not find any beneficial effect of pig-

gyback technique on blood transfusion requirement as compared to conventional technique [18]. Authors concluded that there is no evidence to recommend or refute the piggyback method of liver transplantation [18].

Haemodilution secondary to fluid replacement with crystalloid and colloid solutions and the preservation solution from the donor liver, further reduce the plasma concentration of clotting factors.

Acidosis, hypothermia, hypocalcaemia and citrate toxicity can all contribute to the coagulopathy intraoperatively. Acute coagulopathy of trauma (ACOTS) characterized by ooze-type bleeding from mucosal regions, serosal surfaces and vascular access sites distinct from simple massive bleeding has also been postulated in liver transplantation because of pathophysiological similliarties [19]. High levels of syndecan-1, a marker of endothelial degradation is associated with coagulopathy in trauma patients. Patients with end stage liver disease have also demonstrated increased level of syndecan-1, which further increases during reperfusion [20].

Acute renal failure (ARF) is common in patients with cirrhosis and uraemia is associated with bleeding, particularly due to platelet dysfunction due to decreased platelet aggregation and adhesion.

23.2 The Role of Graft Function

Quality of liver graft plays a significant role in the amount of bleeding in the reperfusion phase. Poor quality of graft causes sustained deterioration of coagulation status with reduction of coagulation factors and increased fibrinolysis [21]. Predisposing factors for graft failure include marginal grafts, poor preservation and prolonged cold and warm ischaemic times. Extended donor criteria grafts are independent predictors of increased chance of reoperation in transplant recipients because of bleeding [22].

23.3 Management of Massive Blood Loss

Blood loss during liver transplant surgery can occur in a slow and protracted manner or can be rapid and cause severe hemodynamic instability. Management of both conditions differ. Slow and protracted bleeding can be managed with judicious use of fluid and vasopressors whereas rapid bleeding needs to be managed aggressively with blood products keeping lessons learnt from trauma management in mind.

23.3.1 Fluid Management

Susceptibility to increase bleeding during liver transplant surgery is related to portal hypertension. As portal hypertension develops portosystemic collaterals develop and splanchnic circulation is diverted to these collaterals. Increase blood flow in this circulation bed results in thinning of arterial walls and increased tendency to bleed during surgery.

Portal hypertension is related to central venous pressure and volume status, thus keeping low central venous pressure (CVP) or restricted fluid regimen is likely to decrease blood loss by decreasing portal hypertension.

Liberal volume loading in the dissection phase of liver transplant has several detrimental consequences. Acute volume loading in transplant recipient tends to pool in the splanchnic circulation instead of central circulation. Therefore, this volume loading does not improve cardiac preload or output. On the other hand, it increases bleeding in the dissection phase by increasing splanchnic blood volume [23]. Volume loading with crystalloid or colloid can cause dilution of clotting factors and interruption of clot formation.

Methods to lower CVP include volume restriction, phlebotomy, use of diuretics such as mannitol, low tidal volume ventilation and avoidance of high positive end expiratory pressure (PEEP) [24]. Massicotte et al. reported good outcome and decreased transfusion requirement when CVP was reduced by 40% in protocolised manner [25]. Schroeder et al. compared outcomes at two centres with contrasting protocols where CVP was maintained at either <5 mmHg or 7–10 mmHg. They reported less blood loss and transfusion requirement at centre which routinely maintains low CVP [26]. Although a Cochrane review did not find this strategy to be effective in decreasing blood transfusion in patients undergoing liver resection [27], but the strategy of restricted fluid and early use of appropriate vasopressor is practiced universally to decrease the blood loss. This is very effective strategy when there is slow and protracted blood loss. Early use of low dose of vasopressin is also effective in decreasing blood loss by reducing splanchnic blood flow. There is risk of hypoperfusion of organ with low CVP in these physiological vulnerable patients. Potential benefit of low CVP must be weighed against chances of renal impairment and dialysis requirement [26].

23.4 Maintenance of Homeostatic Conditions for Clotting

Maintenance of core body temperature >35 °C, pH > 7.2 and plasma calcium levels >1 mmol/L optimizes conditions for clot formation [28]. Hypothermia reduces fibrin and clotting factor synthesis and impairs platelet function. Acidosis reduces thrombin generation and increases clot lysis. Therefore, it is imperative to have patient and efficient patient and rapid fluid warming devices.

23.4.1 Vasopressors

Variety of vasopressors aimed at decreasing portal blood flow by targeting selective vasoconstriction of splanchnic circulation have been employed. Early use of vasopressors like phenylephrine, vasopressin and octreotide has been recommended in case of slow protracted bleeding. Use of low dose vasopressin (0.04 U/min) infusion during the dissection phase was associated with reduce blood loss compared with control group in a retrospective nonrandomized study [24]. Phenylephrine has been found to be useful for restoring blood pressure following phlebotomy. It has also been found more effective than dopamine and dobutamine for decreasing the blood loss and maintaining cardiovascular stability [29].

23.5 Coagulation Tests for Monitoring and Guiding Coagulation Management

Conventional laboratory assays offer limited and potentially misleading information in the context of liver disease. They have long turnaround times for results. Viscoelastic tests provide point of care coagulation monitoring. Viscoelastic tests provide information on the cellular and humoral contribution to clot formation. They also guide about the blood component therapy. The European Society of Anaesthesiology (ESA) guidelines recommend VETs in the management of severe bleeding in liver transplant (grade 1C evidence) [30].

TEG and ROTEM are two most commonly used devices for point of care coagulation monitoring. Clot dynamics of both devices are comparable, both use reagents to increase their diagnostic scope. Viscoelastic tests help in differentiating if platelets or fibrinogen is required for clot firmness. Decision to transfuse should not be entirely dependent on viscoelastic tests as these tests have low positive predictivity and risk over treatment. Good communication with the surgeon and visual assessment of surgical field is important. It should be acknowledged that VETs do not incorporate the endothelial, vascular or flow related contribution to clot formation in vivo.

23.5.1 Pharmacological Interventions

23.5.1.1 Antifibrinolytic Drugs
Fibrinolysis is an important process developing during anhepatic phase and progressing massively after reperfusion due to the alterations in haemostatic system explained above. Quite often it ceases spontaneously within the first hour after reperfusion, but may persist longer, especially in patients with poorly functioning grafts, leading to global microvascular oozing.

It is recommended to consider administration of antifibrinolytic drugs when fibrinolysis is either confirmed in viscoelastic tests (TEG/ROTEM) or is clinically evident from microvascular oozing, but not as a routine practice [31].

Tranexamic acid and epsilon-aminocaproic acid (EACA) competitively inhibit the activation of plasminogen to plasmin, preventing plasmin from degrading fibrin. Tranexamic acid has superior efficacy as compared to EACA. Tranexamic acid is usually given in dose of 25 mg/kg in 1–2 increments if there is continuous ooze with viscoelastic evidence of fibrinolysis. Aprotinin is available once again following a revoked suspension in 2012 by the European Medicines Agency. The response to antifibrinolytic agents should be monitored using TEG/ROTEM to guide further doses. There is variation in the literature regarding the relative efficacy of aprotinin and tranexamic acid. In two Cochrane reviews aprotinin appeared to have superior efficacy but with an increased risk of death [28, 31].

23.5.1.2 Fibrinogen
Fibrinogen is the first factor to reach critical levels when haemodilution or massive bleeding occurs. A concentration of <1.5–2 g/L increases haemorrhagic tendency, so this, or signs of functional fibrinogen deficit on TEG or ROTEM should be triggers for use [32]. It has been shown to reduce transfusion of RBCs, FFP and platelets was reduced by over 50%.

Fibrinogen concentrate substitution restores MCF in dilutional coagulopathy. Fibrinogen concentrates contain standard doses of fibrinogen, as well as carry lower risk of pathogen and immune mediated complications. They should be the preferred source of fibrinogen, in comparison to cryoprecipitate, for the treatment of the quantitative functional deficits of fibrinogen in bleeding patients, unless the former is unavailable. But in most of the centres cryoprecipitate is used as the most abundant source of fibrinogen. (50 mL fibrinogen concentration contains nearly 1 g fibrinogen; there is 250 mg fibrinogen in 100 mL of 1 FFP unit and 225 mg fibrinogen in 15 mL cryoprecipitate).

23.5.1.3 Prothrombin Complex Concentrate

Prothrombin Complex Concentrates (PCC) are purified coagulation concentrates from pooled plasma, after removal of antithrombin and factor XI, with approximately 25 times higher concentrations of clotting factors. PCC is used "off-label" during LT as a rescue therapy in catastrophic bleeding, when coagulopathy is evident.

They allow the correction of coagulation using small volumes. PCCs undergo viral reduction or elimination. A randomized controlled trial (the PROTON trial) studying PCCs effect on RBC transfusion requirements in OLT is currently in progress [33].

23.5.1.4 Recombinant Activated Factor VII

Recombinant factor VIIa binds with tissue factor at the site of injury to activate factor X and generate a thrombin burst. ESA guidelines advocate the use of rF VIIa as a rescue therapy at a dose of 40 μg/kg in the context of intractable bleeding following correction of coagulation factors, fibrinogen, platelets and calcium (grade 1A evidence). With the routinely use of POC monitoring there is declined in the use of rFVIIa.

Currently it is recommended against the prophylactic use of rFVIIa during LT and only suggests its potential role as a "rescue therapy" to control massive haemorrhage. There are concerns over thromboembolic risks following use of rFVIIa [34].

23.5.1.5 Factor XIII

Factor XIII (FXIII) contributes to clot stability by crosslinking the fibrin mesh and rendering fibrin chains insoluble. Levels can become depleted in the context of massive blood loss, reaching clinical significance when<60%. Mild reduction in MA or MCF may be seen on VETs that persists despite antifibrinolytic therapy or reverses with the addition of FXIII to whole blood. FXIII (e.g., Fibrogammin) can be supplemented at a dose of

15–30 mL/kg to help support clot durability. There is no data to show its use in LT.

23.5.2 Protamine and the Heparin Like Effect

A marked heparin like effect on the TEG at the time of reperfusion is common and is due to both exogenous heparins administered to the donor and the release of endogenous heparinoids from the vascular endothelium plus activated macrophages due to ischemia/reperfusion injury. It does not appear to contribute significantly to bleeding risk and is usually a temporary phenomenon unless graft function is poor. It is recommended to run a heparinase modified TEG in parallel with the native TEG during OLT. An empirical dose of 25–50 mg of protamine is often administered if the decision to treat this is made. At high doses protamine can exert a paradoxical anticoagulant effect by inhibiting Factor V activation and impairing endogenous thrombin potential [35].

23.5.3 Fractionated Products vs. Fresh Components

Fractionated products (also called blood derivatives) are highly purified protein concentrates.

There are three main advantages of using fractionated products.

1. Their purity and pharmaceutical-style batch production mean their contents and concentrations are known and consistent with few if any contaminating proteins.
2. Modern fractionation processes typically include one or more viral inactivation steps such as heat, pH, nanofiltration and solvents. This provides much greater confidence in the infectious safety of the products compared with fresh components.
3. Ease of delivery of the product. Fractionated products are usually stored refrigerated or at room temperature, making for faster dispensing than frozen plasma, and they have significantly smaller volumes than plasma so are quicker to administer.

Two main disadvantages of fractionated products.

1. Cost. Fractionated products costing two or more times that of plasma for the equivalent amount of the specific protein.
2. The purified products do not provide balanced coagulation support

Clonidine—A centrally acting alpha 2-adrenergic receptor agonist, significantly decreased transfusion and fluid requirements. It is hypothesized that excessive sympathetic stimulation occurred in patients with cirrhosis because of a spillover of excess epinephrine and norepinephrine. Clonidine acted to decrease sympathetic activity on the splanchnic circulation and, thus, decreased flow and pressure in the portal circulation. I/v administration of 4 μg/kg of clonidine has been shown to decrease blood loss as well fluid requirement during liver transplant [36].

Conjugated oestrogen—Administered just prior to surgery and just after graft reperfusion has been shown to decrease blood loss and transfusion requirements. Hypothesized mechanisms of action include an increased platelet count secondary to an increase in thromboxane B2 and beta-thromboglobulin. 100 mg of oestrogen was used to achieve this effect. Optimal dosing and morbid effect of oestrogen not well understood therefore oestrogen is not in mainsream use, nor it is standard of care (Flowchart 23.1) [37].

23.5.4 Preparation for Massive Bleeding

Massive bleeding is always a possibility in liver transplantation. Therefore, operating room should always be prepared to deal with massive blood loss.

- Large bore intravenous (IV) access: Pressure bags/The Level 1 Rapid Infuser—flow rates up to 1 L/min.
- Warming devices: active external warming/surface-contact warmers, counter-current

warmers, heated-saline admixture and in-line microwave blood warming technology.
- Continuous core temperature monitoring.
- Invasive arterial pressure monitoring.
- Colloid (gelatins), crystalloid, infusion sets and IV calcium preparations.
- Communication with blood bank.
- Adequate manpower.
- Point-of-care testing: Arterial blood gas (ABG) and thromboelastography (TEG).
- Postoperative intensive care.

23.5.5 Transfusion of Blood Components During Massive Blood Transfusion

23.5.5.1 Fixed Ratio Blood Products Vs. POC Directed Transfusion

Traditional management of massive blood loss during surgery was based on restoration of circulating blood volume with crystalloid until transfusion trigger was met after which packed red blood cells were to be given. American guidelines advised only giving FFP after the loss of approximately one blood volume and aiming for an INR < 1.5 [38]. Publication of papers regarding acute coagulopathy trauma shock (ACOTS) changed this practice.

Management of massive blood loss with fixed ratios of red cells to plasma more closely approximating whole blood transfusions came to the fore following a retrospective analysis of United States army combat patients requiring massive transfusion. Those that were treated with a high plasma to RBC ratio had a significantly improved survival [39].

Fixed ratio blood products can be used in patients with massive blood transfusion during liver transplant surgery in centres having no access to POC coagulation monitoring. Advantage of fixed ratio regimen is that there is less delay in obtaining the blood products from blood bank. Fixed ratio blood products promote the early use of plasma and platelets, which might otherwise be delayed if waiting for conventional laboratory coagulation test results to guide treat-

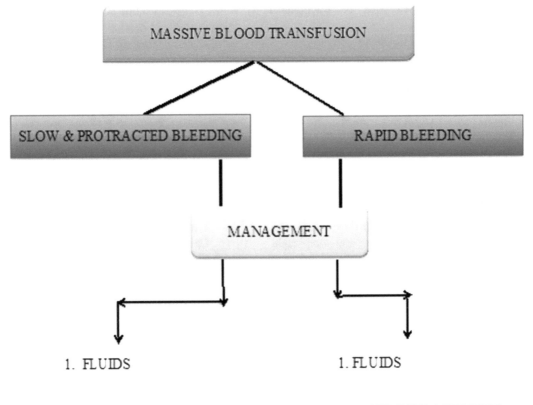

Flowchart 23.1 Management of massive blood loss

ment. Increasing availability of POC during liver transplant does not justify routine use of fixed ratio regimen. Given the lack of high-quality trials the Canadian National Advisory Committee on Blood and Blood products took the decision in 2011 that fixed ratio formula-based care could not be recommended as a standard of care [40]. Recent state of the art papers on the management of traumatic haemorrhage have viscoelastic tests integrated into fixed ratio regimen. In the presence of uncontrolled haemorrhage, fixed ratio transfusion packages are started converting to viscoelastic test guided goal-driven resuscitation once bleeding slows [41].

23.5.5.2 Targets of Resuscitation in Massive Blood Loss

- Mean arterial pressure (MAP) around 60 mmHg, systolic arterial pressure 80–100 mmHg.
- Hb 7–9 g/dL.
- INR <1.5; activated PTT <42 s.
- Fibrinogen >1.5–2 g/L.
- Platelets >50 × 109/L.
- pH 7.35–7.45,
- Core temperature > 35.0 °C.
- Base deficit <3.0 lactate <2 mEq/L.
- Fibrinogen >1.5–2 g/L.

The transfusion trigger threshold for viscoelastic tests have been described. However, the transfusion trigger thresholds described for viscoelastic tests have not been validated and large controlled clinical trials comparing strategies of coagulation management and cut-off values for transfusion of blood product components are still needed (Table 23.1).

Perioperative blood loss during LT is a complex endpoint which is affected not only by pre-existing alterations of the haemostatic system but also by surgical and anaesthetic management.

A pre-emptive and prophylactic correction of the patients' preoperative haemostatic disorders through the "watchful waiting" approach, the treatment of existing infections and the optimization of renal status minimize the transfusion-related complications in the patients undergoing liver transplantation. Besides the expert opinions the recommendations are listed for the management of perioperative bleeding for patients undergoing liver transplantation (Table 23.2).

Table 23.1 Complications related to massive blood transfusion

Complications	Reasons
Hypocalcaemia	Exhaustion of liver function for citrate clearance from circulation
Hyperkalaemia	Increased extracellular potassium in stored blood due to inactivation of the RBC membrane ATPase pump Enhanced with acidosis
Hypomagnesemia	Due to supplementation of magnesium poor fluids, along with binding of magnesium to citrates
Coagulopathy Disseminated intravascular coagulation (DIC)	Dilutional Hypothermia and acidosis may exacerbate
Hypothermia	Rapid infusion of a huge amount of inadequately warmed crystalloid solution and blood products
Immunological complications Febrile nonhemolytic transfusion reactions, refractoriness to platelet transfusions, transfusion-related lung injury (TRALI), transfusion-associated graft-vs-host disease (TAGVHD), immune suppression, allograft tolerance and development of possible autoimmune diseases	Donor leucocytes and are related to the induction of autoantibodies against, class I and class II HLA antigens which they express; T-cell activation and microchimerism Post-transfusion immunosuppression is evident in liver transplant Recent studies suggest that perioperative transfusion may increase the risk of postoperative bacterial infection reactivation of latent infection and mortality because of tolerance induction and immunosuppression

It is also important to ensure surgical management of active bleeding, achieve normothermia, keeping low CVP, calcium and pH levels within

Table 23.2 Recommendations for the management of perioperative bleeding during liver transplantation

Recommendation	Level of evidence
Antifibrinolytic therapy reduces blood loss and transfusion requirements in liver transplantation	B
Implementation of transfusion and coagulation management algorithms (based on ROTEM/TEG) can reduce transfusion-associated costs in liver transplantation	B
In acute liver failure, moderately elevated INR should not be corrected before invasive procedures, with the exception of intracranial pressure monitor insertion	1C
rFVIIa should be used only as rescue therapy for uncontrolled bleeding not for prophylaxis	1A
Point of care platelet function tests may help to stratify risk and rationalize platelet transfusion in patients taking antiplatelet drugs	C
A low central venous pressure and restrictive fluid administration reduce bleeding	

GRADE System
1A Strong Recommendation High QOE (Quality of Evidence), *1B* Strong Recommendation Mod QOE, *1C* Strong Recommendation Low QOE
2A Weak Recommendation, High QOE, *2B* Weak Recommendation Mod QOE, *2C* Weak Recommendation, Low QOE

physiological limits during the intraoperative period.

23.6 Intracardiac Thrombus (ICT) and Pulmonary Embolism (PE)

There is a state of rebalanced haemostasis in patients with end stage liver disease (ESLD) undergoing liver transplantation. This rebalanced state is less stable and may easily tip towards either bleeding or thrombosis. As a result, during intraoperative period patients are at risk of bleeding episodes as well as thrombotic complications.

Conventional coagulation panel consisting of prothrombin time (PT), International normalized ratio (INR), activated partial thromboplastin time (APTT), platelet count and fibrinogen concentra-

tion is not sensitive enough to guide transfusion in patient of ESLD undergoing liver transplantation. These tests do not reflect the interaction between platelets, vascular endothelium and fibrinolytic factors in the haemostatic mechanism. The limitations of these conventional coagulation tests during liver transplantation have shifted the focus towards viscoelastic coagulation monitoring. Routine use of viscoelastic coagulation monitoring has rationalized the use of blood products during liver transplantation. Viscoelastic coagulation monitoring can detect the tendency of blood to clot in time so that corrective measures can be taken. Despite better understanding of physiology of coagulation and routine use of viscoelastic coagulation monitoring there is significant incidence of ICT and PE in patients undergoing liver transplantation.

23.6.1 Incidence of Intraoperative Thromboembolic Events

Incidence of intracardiac thrombus and pulmonary thromboembolism depends upon the diagnostic methods utilized in the diagnosis of intracardiac pulmonary thrombo embolism. It is reported to be 1–6% if TEE is not used as routine monitor [42, 43]. With the use of TEE, incidence of pulmonary thrombo embolism defined as identification of thrombo emboli in pulmonary artery, right atrium or right ventricle with or without evidence of right ventricle dysfunction and hemodynamic instability is reported to be 26%. Intracardiac pulmonary thromboembolism are more commonly seen in reperfusion phase but have been reported in all phases [44]. ICT has also been reported before incision in a patient who had no evidence of any thrombus by trans thoracic echocardiography. Currently TEE is considered the gold standard for diagnosing intra operative pulmonary embolism. TEE has an 80% sensitivity and 100% specificity for diagnosing thrombi large enough to cause haemodynamic instability. When to start TEE monitoring in patients undergoing liver transplantation, i.e. before induction, before clamping of inferior vena cava, or before reperfusion is controversial.

Routine use of TEE before the induction may be more helpful than the practice of having TEE probe placed after hemodynamic collapse. Early placement of TEE probe can pick up small ICT which are not large enough to cause hemodynamic instability by causing complete out flow track obstruction. This also gives anaesthesiologist time to administer inotropes, anticoagulants and thrombolytics in time.

23.6.1.1 Predisposing Factors

Predisposing factors for the development of intraoperative ICT and pulmonary thromboembolism are history of preoperative venous thrombo embolism, trans jugular intrahepatic porto systemic shunt (TIPS), veno venous bypass, presence pulmonary artery and dialysis catheter and exposure to antifibrinolytic agent. Transfusion of cryoprecipitate, platelets and hepatitis immunoglobulin have also been reported as risk factors. Molly et al. in their recent article identified that patients who developed ICT had higher MELD score at the time of transplant, longer warm ischaemia time and received grafts from donors of higher BMI as compared to patients who did not.

23.6.1.2 Role of Antifibrinolytics

Antifibrinolytics comprise a group of pharmacological agents that include epsilon-aminocaproic acid (EACA), tranexamic acid (TXA) and aprotinin. Antifibrinolytics have been increasingly used in the cardiac and non-cardiac surgery to decrease the blood loss and transfusion requirement. World Health Organization has included antifibrinolytics in the list of essential medicines 2015 for decreasing the blood loss in both cardiac and non-cardiac surgery. Recently concerns have been raised over the use of antifibrinolytics in liver transplant surgery especially their association with ICT which carries very high mortality. Both lysine analogues (EACA, TXA) act to block conversion of plasminogen to plasmin whereas aprotinin inactivates free plasmin.

Antifibrinolytics have been implicated for the development of thrombotic complications in various case reports, but the association of antifibrinolytics and thrombotic complications are lacking in the large studies [45]. Most of the large studies are underpowered to detect any role of antifibrinolytics in the development of thromboembolic complications. In addition to this, subgroups at low risk of bleeding or high risk of thrombotic complications are often excluded. Selection of type and dose of antifibrinolytics is specific to institution. Adam Badenoch et al. did not detect any evidence of increased thromboembolic events in patients exposed to TXA, including patients with high risk of thromboembolic events [46]. Ramona Nicolau—Raducu et al. concluded that EACA was not associated with increased thrombotic events in liver transplantation [47].

Most of the liver transplant centres are using point of care coagulation monitoring which has improved the perioperative blood transfusion management and use of antifibrinolytics. Studies on the routine administration of antifibrinolytic after the era of POC coagulation monitoring are lacking. Large prospective studies are needed to determine the association of antifibrinolytics and thromboembolism in liver transplant patients.

23.6.1.3 Factor Concentrates

Prothrombin complex concentrates (PCC) are approved by the FDA for urgent reversal of vitamin K antagonist medications. Since PCC contains all the factors which are synthesized in the liver, their use is postulated in patients undergoing liver transplantation. Beneficial effects of PCC in liver transplantation is postulated because of less volume required to correct coagulopathy. Studies conducted to study the effect of intraoperative use of concentrates in liver transplant patients have not showed an increased risk of thromboembolic events. In addition, some PCC formulation contains protein C, protein S and antithrombin or heparin which further decrease the risk of thromboembolism (Figs. 23.1 and 23.2).

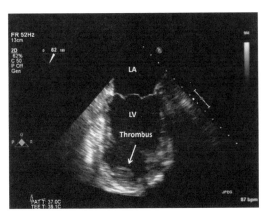

Fig. 23.1 Example of large thrombus (Th) in the right atrium (RA) shown in patient with indwelling catheter (arrow). *LA* left atrium, *SVC* superior vena cava

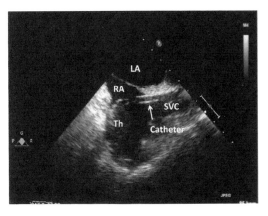

Fig. 23.2 ME commissural view of left ventricle showing apical thrombus (arrow) in a patient with apical hypokinesis. *LA* left atrium, *LV* left ventricle

23.6.2 Management of ICT

ICT presents intraoperatively as right ventricle failure. Hypoxia, hypotension, bradycardia and sudden increase or decrease of pulmonary artery pressure are hallmarks of right ventricle failure. The visualization of thrombus by using intraoperative TEE remains the gold standard [48].

Initial management consists of inotropes, fluid, chest and aortic compression as required to support the heart contractility. Calcium chloride and sodium bicarbonate are also administered to treat acidosis. Definitive treatment of ICT consists of dissolving the clot with anticoagulants. When and how to administer anticoagulants is

difficult decision which requires clear discussion with surgical team.

23.6.2.1 Anticoagulation

Various modalities have been attempted to dissolve the thrombus, i.e. administration of heparin, tissue plasminogen activator, transcatheter aspiration of thrombus and catheter directed thrombolysis. Thrombectomy on cardiopulmonary bypass remains an option. Heparin has been successfully used with good results in patients with TEE detected hemodynamic stable intra cardiac clots [49]. Heparin at the dose of 5000 units intravenously has not been found to be very helpful when ICT is accompanied with hemodynamic instability. Intravenous administration of low dose of rTPA (0.5 mg–4 mg) has been found helpful in most of the case when intracardiac thrombosis is accompanied with hemodynamic instability [50]. Low dose rTPA was successful in improving hemodynamic. It has been recommended to keep 2–4 mg of rTPA in the operating room.

23.6.2.2 Suggested Management of Intra Cardiac Thrombus

Clot <1 cm^2 AND Hemodynamic Stable ⟶ Observe.

Clot >1 cm^2 AND Haemodynamic Stable

⟶ Heparin 3000 units iv.

Clot >1 cm^2 AND Haemodynamic unstable ⟶ rTPA 0.5 to 2 mg via central line.

Repeat rTPA consider ECMO/Bypass.

23.6.3 Intraoperative Vasoplegia

Vasoplegia or distributive shock is seen in significant number of patients in the intraoperative period. This condition includes multiple aetiologies (sepsis, neurogenic, anaphylactic, etc.) and leads to profound and uncontrolled vasodilation.

In the vasoplegic state (VPS), the body is unable to maintain adequate perfusion pressure despite high cardiac output.

Vasoplegic state is different from post-reperfusion syndrome and ischemic reperfusion injury. VPS is defined as normal or high cardiac output state (cardiac index >2.2 L/m^2) with difficulty in maintaining mean arterial pressure of 60 mmHg due to low systemic vascular resistance (<800 dynes s/cm^5) despite high vasopressors (0.5 µg/kg/min of norepinephrine) in a patient without any evidence of infections. It may be difficult to differentiate VPS from ischaemic reperfusion injury or post-reperfusion syndrome. Maintenance of blood pressure with fluid and inotropes is the priority but these patients are usually not responsive to vasopressors [51].

Mortality in patients with vasoplegia because of any aetiology can be very high and can be to the extent of 50% [52]. Duration of vasoplegic syndrome is also related to outcome after transplant. Longer the vasoplegic syndrome poorer is the outcome after transplant.

Proposed mechanisms of VS in these patients include deficiency of the hormone vasopressin, massive oxidative stress triggering the release of proinflammatory mediators. With the better understanding of role of NO and other mediators' various pharmacological interventions have been suggested.

23.6.4 Methylene Blue [51]

Methylene is heterocyclic aromatic molecule with chemical formula $C_{16}H_{18}CIN_3S$. It is available as green powder which turns in to blue solution when dissolved in water. MB is metabolized to leucomethylene blue by nicotinamide adenine dinucleotide phosphate and excreted primarily in urine, turning the urine a blue green colour [53].

Methylene should be used with caution in patients who are G6PD deficient as It can cause haemolysis. The risk of serotonin syndrome

because of monoamine oxidase inhibition properties is another limitation of the use of MB. Patients at risk for serotonin syndrome with methylene blue include those on selective serotonin reuptake inhibitors (SSRIs); monoamine oxidase inhibitors; meperidine; tramadol; phenyl-piperidine narcotics (e.g., remifentanil, fentanyl, sufentanil); linezolid.

Vasoconstrictor effect of MB is seen only in case where there is upregulation of NO. MB does not cause increase in blood pressure if it is given in non vasoplegic conditions. Blue colour of the MB can also interfere with the accuracy of pulse oximetry.

MB improves vascular tone by decreasing the production of NO by directly inhibiting the enzyme NO synthase. It also competitively blocks the target enzyme of NO, thus reducing the responsiveness of vessels to cyclic GMP dependent vasodilators.

Methylene blue (MB) has been successfully used in few case reports as rescue measure for treatment of nor epinephrine resistant vasoplegia. It has been found to increase blood pressure when used in the dose of 2 mg/kg as a bolus followed by infusion of 0.5 mg/kg for 6 h [53].

Routine prophylactic use of methylene blue (MB) before reperfusion of liver cannot be recommended. Large study by Fukazawa and Pretto showed that bolus dose of MB just before reperfusion did not prevent post reperfusion syndrome or decreased the dose of vasopressors [54].

Hydroxocobalamin: hydroxocobalamin can be used in the patients for treatment of vasoplegia in G6PD deficient patient or patients at risk of serotonin syndrome. Hydroxocobalamin is approved drug for cyanide toxicity. Mechanism of action of hydroxocobalamin in vasoplegia is because of its inhibitory action on NO synthase causing hypertension. Recommended dose of hydroxocobalamin is 5–10 g intravenously over 15 min [55]. Hydroxocobalamin has been used in liver transplant for treatment of vasoplegia with good results (Flowchart 23.2).

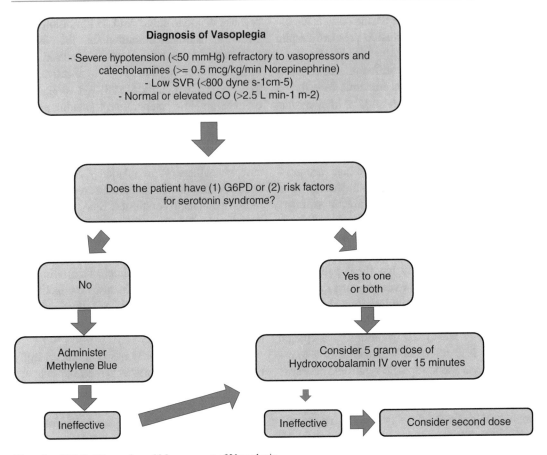

Flowchart 23.2 Diagnosis and Management of Vasoplegia

Other drugs which have been used or recommended for the treatment of vasoplegia:

Synthetic human Angiotensin II is an FDA approved drug for the treatment of vasoplegia from any cause. Angiotensin II administration replenishes the angiotensin in vasoplegic conditions which are usually associated with depleted angiotensin II level. It has been successfully used in combined liver and heart transplant. Notable side effect of Angiotensin II is thrombo embolism. Recommended dose of angiotensin II is 20–80 ng/kg/min [56].

23.6.5 Air Embolism During Liver Transplantation

Air embolism during liver transplantation is reported in all phases of liver transplantation. It can arise due to injury to the vessels during liver transplantation surgery. Air can be sucked to the central volume from openings in the hepatic veins during dissection phase. Air embolism is facilitated by low central venous pressure which is maintained to lower portal pressure and decrease the blood loss. Other sources of air

Flowchart 23.3 Diagnosis of air embolism

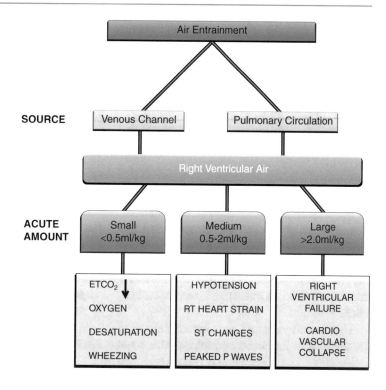

embolism are: veno-venous bypass, rapid transfusion of fluid, tubing and vascular unclamping during reperfusion phase. Incidence of air embolism depends upon the modality to diagnose the air embolism. TEE is the most sensitive monitor to diagnose air embolism (Flowchart 23.3).

23.7 Severe Post-Reperfusion Syndrome (PRS)

Reperfusion stage is the most critical step of surgery in which sudden metabolic and heamodynamic imbalances occur. These characterize PRS which was described in 1987. Hilmi described significant PRS as >30% drop in MAP or HR lasting more than 30 min, asystole, heamodynamically significant arrthymias or need of con-

tinuous infusion of vassopressors during intraoperative period. Overall incidence of PRS varies ranging from 8% to 30%. Incidence may vary in LDLT and cadeveric transplants and type of clamping technique being applied.

Changes during unclamping include decrease in MAP, HR, SVR & CI, increase in CVP, PAP, PVR leading to right ventricular failure and cardiovascular collapse in severe cases. Acidosis, hyperkalaemia, hypocalcaemia worsen during reperfusion stage with prolonged fibrinolysis and release of vasoactive substances like cytokines, reactive oxygen species, TNF-α, NO, bradykinins by the recipient.

Management and prevention of severe postreperfusion syndrome should ideally be guided by TEE. This includes (1) Hyperkalaemia and acidosis correction. (2) Vasopressors, e.g., small dose of epinephrine (10–20 μg) or phenylephrine (100 μg) with continuous infusion of norepinephrine/vasopressin. (3) Methylene blue. (4) Hydroxocobalamin. (5) Magnesium sulphate: Magnesium administration before reperfusion of the transplanted liver has been shown to significantly reduce blood lactate levels, suggesting that it may protect against ischemia-reperfusion injury [57]. Pretreatment with magnesium sulfate also has been shown to attenuate PRS in patients undergoing living donor liver transplantation.

Magnesium correction should be simultaneous as its levels decline during dissection and anhepatic phase of liver transplant [58]. It is a powerful vasodilator which should be avoided in hepatic encephalopathy [59]. (6) Ischemic Preconditioning: no conclusive evidence of its beneficial effect.

Hence well-managed post reperfusion stage results in less incidence of postoperative renal dysfunction, less bleeding and decrease in systemic inflammatory response.

23.7.1 Dynamic LVOT Obstruction (LVOTO)

LVOTO (pressure gradient >36 mmHg) should be ruled out in all cases of refractory cases of hypotension during LT. Incidence of LVOTO is 0.2% of the general population.

In chronic liver disease patients have hypertrophied ventricles, low SVR and common use of diuretics making them more susceptible to LVOTO. It becomes more severe in presence of SAM of anterior mitral leaflet leading to fall in ejection of stroke volume and sudden drop in cardiac output. LVOTO is pronounced during anhepatic stage. TEE monitoring is essential to follow the degree of LVOTO and SAM.

Avoid hypovolemia (optimize preload) and treat hypotension with norepinephrine or vasopressin or volume. Bolus of phenylephrine 100 μg to be used to increase SVR (increase afterload). Use of β- Blocker (e.g., Esmolol) with slow correction of Ca^{2+} is done to prevent hypercontractability (inotropy). Epinephrine should not be used (Fig. 23.3).

23.7.2 Pulmonary Hypertension

Anaesthetic management is aimed to prevent pulmonary hypertension crises and right ventricle failure in acute decompensated pulmonary hypertension.

General Principles include:

1. Avoid hypoxic pulmonary vasoconstriction (FiO_2 0.6), acidosis ($PaCO_2$ 30–35), hypothermia (36–37 °C), high airway pressure (low tidal volume 6–8 mL/kg IBW).

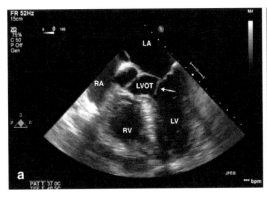 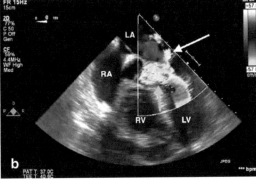

Fig. 23.3 Transesophageal 2 dimensional echocardiographic images showing ME 5 chamber view. (**a**) Systolic anterior motion of anterior mitral valve (arrow) leading to obstruction of the left ventricular outflow tract. (**b**) Turbulent flow in the left ventricular outflow tract (green arrow) and posteriorly directed regurgitant jet (white arrow). *LA* left atrium, *LVOT* left ventricular outflow tract, *RA* right atrium, *RV* right ventricle

2. Reduce RV afterload.
3. Maintain SVR.
4. Intravenous vasodialators: Milrinone (25–50 µg/kg bolus followed by infusion 0.5–0.75 µg/kg/min). Prostacyclin (4–10 ng/kg/min). Iloprost (1–3 ng/kg/min).
5. Selective pulmonary vasodialators: Nitric Oxide (5–40 ppm continuously). Inhaled Prostacyclin (25–50 µg diluted in 50 mL saline nebulized over 15 min repeated every hour).
6. Maintain sinus rhythm.
7. Inotropes: Adrenaline, dobutamine.

TEE or pulmonary artery catheter is used as a monitor. Aim to keep SBP > 90 mm of Hg, mean BP > 65 mm of Hg, MPAP, 35 mm of Hg, PVR/SVR < 0.5, cardiac index > 2.2l/min/m².

23.7.2.1 Arrhythmias

Commonly seen electrophysiological abnormalities in liver transplant are prolonged QT intervals, increased QT dispersion, chronotropic incompetence and electromechanical uncoupling.

Atrial fibrillation is the most common cardiac arrhythmia in liver transplant. The incidence in liver transplant candidates is higher than in the general population (4.5% vs. 0.8–1.5%), resulting in higher perioperative cardiac morbidity [60]. This results in prolonged hospital stay, increased incidence of AKI and low graft survival.

The risk factors contributing to arrhythmias in patients undergoing liver transplant include cirrhotic cardiomyopathy, cardiac ion channel remodelling, electrolyte imbalances, impaired autonomic function, hepatorenal syndrome, metabolic abnormalities, advanced age, inflammatory syndrome and comorbidities.

Intraoperative arrthymias lead to suboptimal ventricular rate, loss of atrial contraction and sympathetic activation.

23.7.2.2 Treatment

1. Rapid correction of electrolytes and acidosis.
2. Control of HR with β-blockers or i.v. Dilitizam which causes hypotension.
3. Amiodarone (150 mg bolus and then 15–30 mg/h intravenously)—controls rate with better hemodynamic stability but can cause QT prolongation.
4. Electrical Cardioversion (100–200 J) in hemodynamically unstable patients.

23.7.3 Miscellaneous

1. Related to vascular access: Intra-arterial lines—Temporary vascular occlusion, thrombosis, ischemia, haematoma, catheter related sepsis Advanced Venous Access, cordis 9Fr internal jugular venous cannulation—bleeding, haematoma, arterial/venous injury, incorrect placement in azygous vein (left sided), pneumothorax, haemothorax, pneumomediastinum and air embolism, arrthymias, sepsis, catheter fracture, PAC—pulmonary artery rupture due to overinflation of balloon, arrthymias.
2. TEE probe—bleeding from varices more common with gastric varices, infection.
3. Re-expansion pulmonary oedema: drainage of hydrothorax should be slow and not continuous otherwise can lead to re-expansion pulmonary oedema.
4. Complications related to patient positioning—Due to prolonged surgery in supine position: Pressure alopecia, ulnar nerve injury (wrist drop), foot drop, brachial plexus injury due to application of retractors or tight tucking with elbows not flexed causing compression between clavicle and first rib.
5. Retractors: commonly used retractors are Omni and Thompson. Higher compression can lead to loss of arterial waveform during retractor application. Other complications

include brachial plexus injury, diaphragmatic injury, basal atelectasis, rib #, liver or splenic tear and postoperative pain.

23.8 Conclusion

Intraoperative complications can take place in any phase but most of them occur in reperfusion phase.

Hemodynamic collapse because of bleeding or without obvious bleeding can take place in any phase.

TEE should be readily available to help in the differential diagnosis of cardiovascular collapse.

Point of care coagulation monitoring by Viscoelastic method should guide transfusion.

Care should be taken to maintain temperature, electrolytes and acid load.

It is difficult to predict intraoperative complications therefore adequate help in the form of additional manpower, adequate blood products and devices should always be available.

References

1. Massicotte L, Beaulieu D, Roy J-D, et al. MELD score and blood product requirements during liver transplantation: no link. Transplantation. 2009;87:1689–94.
2. Massicotte L, Sassine M-P, Lenis S, et al. Survival rate changes with transfusion of blood products during liver transplantation. Can J Anaesth. 2005;52:148–55.
3. Barbosa RR, Rowell SE, Sambasivan CN, Diggs BS, Spinella PC, Schreiber MA. A predictive model for mortality in massively transfused trauma patients. J Trauma. 2011;71:S370–4.
4. Diab YA, Wong EC, Luban NL. Massive transfusion in children and neonates. Br J Haematol. 2013;161(1):15–26.
5. Neff LP, Cannon JW, Morrison JJ, Edwards MJ, Spinella PC, Borgman MA. Clearly defining pediatric massive transfusion: cutting through the fog and friction with combat data. J Trauma Acute Care Surg. 2015;78(1):22–8; discussion 28–29.
6. Esmat Gamil M, Pirenne J, Van Malenstein H, Verhaegen M, Desschans B, Monbaliu D, et al. Risk factors for bleeding and clinical implications in patients undergoing liver transplantation. Transplant Proc. 2012;44:2857–60.
7. McCluskey SA, Karkouti K, Wijeysundera DN, Kakizawa K, Ghannam M, Hamdy A, Grant D, Levy G. Derivation of a risk index for the prediction of massive blood transfusion in liver transplantation. Liver Transpl. 2006;12:1584–93.
8. Massicotte L, Beaulieu D, Roy JD, Marleau D, Vandenbroucke F, Dagenais M, Lapointe R, Roy A. MELD score and blood product requirements during liver transplantation: no link. Transplantation. 2009;87:1689–94.
9. Mor E, Jennings L, Gonwa TA, Holman MJ, Gibbs J, Solomon H, et al. The impact of operative bleeding on outcome in transplantation of the liver. Surg Gynecol Obstet. 1993;176:219–27.
10. Massicotte L, Sassine MP, Lenis S, Roy A. Transfusion predictors in liver transplant. Anesth Analg. 2004;98:1245–51.
11. Li C, Mi K, Wen TF, Yan LN, Li B, Wei YG, Yang JY, Xu MQ, Wang WT. Risk factors and outcomes of massive red blood cell transfusion following living donor liver transplantation. J Dig Dis. 2012;13:161–7.
12. Noval-Padillo JA, León-Justel A, Mellado-Miras P, Porras-Lopez F, Villegas-Duque D, Gomez-Bravo MA, Guerrero JM. Introduction of fibrinogen in the treatment of hemostatic disorders during orthotopic liver transplantation: implications in the use of allogenic blood. Transplant Proc. 2010;42:2973–4.
13. Görlinger K. Coagulation management during liver transplantation. Hamostaseologie. 2006;26:S64–76.
14. Mangus RS, Kinsella SB, Nobari MM, Fridell JA, Vianna RM, Ward ES, Nobari R, Tector AJ. Predictors of blood product use in orthotopic liver transplantation using the piggyback hepatectomy technique. Transplant Proc. 2007;39:3207–13.
15. Fan ST, Yong BH, Lo CM, Liu CL, Wong J. Right lobe living donor liver transplantation with or without venovenous bypass. Br J Surg. 2003;90:48–56.
16. Nishida S, Nakamura N, Vaidya A, Levi DM, Kato T, Nery JR, Madariaga JR, Molina E, Ruiz P, Gyamfi A, Tzakis AG. Piggyback technique in adult orthotopic liver transplantation: an analysis of 1067 liver transplants at a single center. HPB (Oxford). 2006;8:182–8.
17. Busque S, Esquivel CO, Concepcion W, So SK. Experience with the piggyback technique without caval occlusion in adult orthotopic liver transplantation. Transplantation. 1998;65:77–82.
18. Gurusamy KS, Pamecha V, Davidson BR. Piggy-back graft for liver transplantation. Cochrane Database Syst Rev. 2011;(1):CD008258.
19. Hartmann M, Szalai C, Saner FH. Hemostasis in liver transplantation: pathophysiology, monitoring, and treatment. World J Gastroenterol. 2016;22(4):1541.
20. Schiefer J, Lebherz-Eichinger D, Erdoes G, Berlakovich G, Bacher A, Krenn CG, Faybik P. Alterations of endothelial glycocalyx during orthotopic liver transplantation in patients with end-stage liver disease. Transplantation. 2015;99:2118–23.

21. Broomhead RH, Patel S, Fernando B, O'Beirne J, Mallett S. Resource implications of expanding the use of donation after circulatory determination of death in liver transplantation. Liver Transpl. 2012;18:771–8.

22. Park C, Huh M, Steadman RH, Cheng R, Hu KQ, Farmer DG, Hong J, Duffy J, Busuttil RW, Xia VW. Extended criteria donor and severe intraoperative glucose variability: association with reoperation for hemorrhage in liver transplantation. Transplant Proc. 2010;42:1738–43.

23. Ozier Y, Tsou MY. Changing trends in transfusion practice in liver transplantation. Curr Opin Organ Transplant. 2008;13:304–9.

24. Hannaman MJ, Hevesi ZG. Anesthesia care for liver transplantation. Transplant Rev (Orlando). 2011;25:36–43.

25. Massicotte L, Lenis S, Thibeault L, Sassine MP, Seal RF, Roy A. Effect of low central venous pressure and phlebotomy on blood product transfusion requirements during liver transplantations. Liver Transpl. 2006;12:117–23.

26. Schroeder RA, Collins BH, Tuttle-Newhall E, Robertson K, Plotkin J, Johnson LB, Kuo PC. Intraoperative fluid management during orthotopic liver transplantation. J Cardiothorac Vasc Anesth. 2004;18:438–41.

27. Gurusamy KS, Li J, Vaughan J, Sharma D, Davidson BR. Cardiopulmonary interventions to decrease blood loss and blood transfusion requirements for liver resection. Cochrane Database Syst Rev. 2012;5:CD007338.

28. Vitin AA, Martay K, Vater Y, Dembo G, Maziarz M. Effects of vasoactive agents on blood loss and transfusion requirements during pre-reperfusion stages of the orthotopic liver transplantation. J Anesth Clin Res. 2010;1:104.

29. Hong SH, Park CS, Jung HS, Choi H, Lee SR, Lee J, Choi JH. A comparison of intra-operative blood loss and acid-base balance between vasopressor and inotrope strategy during living donor liver transplantation: a randomised, controlled study. Anaesthesia. 2012;67:1091–100.

30. Kozek-Langenecker SA, Afshari A, Albaladejo P, Santullan CA, De Robertis E, Filipescu DC, Fries D, Görlinger K, Haas T, Imberger G, Jacob M, Lancé M, Llau J, Mallett S, Meier J, Rahe-Meyer N, Samama CM, Smith A, Solomon C, Van der Linden P, Wikkelsø AJ, Wouters P, Wyffels P. Management of severe perioperative bleeding: guidelines from the European Society of Anaesthesiology. Eur J Anaesthesiol. 2013;30:270–382.

31. Henry DA, Carless PA, Moxey AJ, O'Connell D, Stokes BJ, Fergusson DA, Ker K. Anti-fibrinolytic use for minimising perioperative allogeneic blood transfusion. Cochrane Database Syst Rev. 2011;3:CD001886.

32. Hiippala ST, Myllylä GJ, Vahtera EM. Hemostatic factors and replacement of major blood loss with plasma-poor red cell concentrates. Anesth Analg. 1995;81:360–5.

33. Arshad F, Ickx B, van Beem RT, Polak W, Grüne F, Nevens F, Ilmakunnas MKoivusalo AM, Isoniemi H, StrengersPF GH, Hendriks HG, Lisman T, Pirenne J, Porte RJ. Prothrombin complex concentrate in the reduction of blood loss during orthotopic liver transplantation: PROTON-trial. BMC Surg. 2013;13:22.

34. Simpson E, Lin Y, Stanworth S, Birchall J, Doree C, Hyde C. Recombinant factor VIIa for the prevention and treatment of bleeding in patients without haemophilia. Cochrane Database Syst Rev. 2012;3:CD005011.

35. Ni Ainle F, Preston RJ, Jenkins PV, Nel HJ, Johnson JA, Smith OP, White B, Fallon PG, O'Donnell JS. Protamine sulfate downregulates thrombin generation by inhibiting factor V activation. Blood. 2009;114:1658–65.

36. De Kock M, Laterre PF, Van Obbergh L, et al. The effects of intraoperative intravenous clonidine on fluid requirements, hemodynamic variables, and support during liver transplantation: a prospective, randomized study. Anesth Analg. 1998;86(3):468–76.

37. Frenette L, Cox J, McArdle P, Eckhoff D, Bynon S. Conjugated estrogen reduces transfusion and coagulation factor requirements in orthotopic liver transplantation. Anesth Analg. 1998;86(6):1183–6.

38. American Society of Anesthesiologists Task Force on Perioperative Blood Transfusion and Adjuvant Therapies. Practice guidelines for perioperative blood transfusion and adjuvant therapies: an updated report by the American Society of Anesthesiologists task force on perioperative blood transfusion and adjuvant therapies. Anesthesiology. 2006;105:198–208.

39. Cap AP, Spinella PC, Borgman MA, Blackbourne LH, Perkins JG. Timing and location of blood product transfusion and outcomes in massively transfused combat casualties. J Trauma Acute Care Surg. 2012;73:S89–94.

40. Dzik WH, Blajchman MA, Fergusson D, Hameed M, Henry B, Kirkpatrick AW, Korogyi T, Logsetty S, Skeate RC, Stanworth S, MacAdams C, Muirhead B. Clinical review: Canadian National Advisory Committee on blood and blood products—massive transfusion consensus conference 2011: report of the panel. Crit Care. 2011;15:242.

41. Johansson PI, Stensballe J, Oliveri R, Wade CE, Ostrowski SR, Holcomb JB. How I treat patients with massive hemorrhage. Blood. 2014;124:3052–8.

42. Gologorsky E, De Wolf AM, Scott V, et al. Intracardiac thrombus formation and pulmonary thromboembolism immediately after graft reperfusion in 7 patients undergoing liver transplantation. Liver Transpl. 2001;7:783–9.

43. Lerner AB, Sundar E, Mahmood F, et al. Four cases of cardiopulmonary thromboembolism during liver transplantation without the use of antifibrinolytic drugs. Anesth Analg. 2005;101:1608–12.

44. Sakai T, Matsusaki T, Dai F, et al. Pulmonary thromboembolism during adult liver transplantation: incidence, clinical presentation, outcome, risk

factors, and diagnostic predictors. Br J Anaesth. 2012;108:469–77.

45. Dalia AA, Khan H, Flores AS. Intraoperative diagnosis of intracardiac thrombus during orthotopic liver transplantation with trans esophageal echocardiography: a case series and literature view. Semin Cardiothorac Vasc Anesth. 2017;21:245–51.

46. Badenoch A, Sharma A, Gower S, Selzner M, Srinivas C, Wąsowicz M, McCluskey SA. The effectiveness and safety of tranexamic acid in orthotopic liver transplantation clinical practice: a propensity score matched cohort study. Transplantation. 2017;101:1658–65.

47. Nicolau-Raducu R, et al. Epsilon-aminocaproic acid has no association with thromboembolic complications, renal failure, or mortality after liver transplantation. J Cardiothorac Vasc Anesth. 2016;30(4):917–23.

48. Sibulesky L, Peiris P, Taner CB, Kramer DJ, Canabal JM, Nguyen JH. Intraoperative intracardiac thrombosis in a liver transplant patient. World J Hepatol. 2010;2(5):198–200.

49. Heik SC, Kupper W, Hamm C, et al. Efficacy of high dose intravenous heparin for treatment of left ventricular thrombi with high embolic risk. J Am Coll Cardiol. 1994;24:1305–9.

50. Boone JD, Sherwani SS, Herborn JC, et al. The successful use of low dose recombinant tissue plasminogen activator for treatment of intracardiac/pulmonary thrombosis during liver transplantation. Anesth Analg. 2011;112:319–21.

51. Shanmugam G. Vasoplegic syndrome—the role of methylene blue. Eur J Cardiothorac Surg. 2005;28:705–10.

52. Mekontso-Dessap A, Houël R, Soustelle C, et al. Risk factors for post-cardiopulmonary bypass vasoplegia in patients with preserved left ventricular function. Ann Thorac Surg. 2001;71:1428–32.

53. Hosseinian L, Weiner M, Levin MA, Fischer GW. Methylene blue: magic bullet for vasoplegia? Anesth Analg. 2016;122:194–201.

54. Fukazawa K, Pretto EA Jr. The post-reperfusion syndrome (PRS): diagnosis, incidence and management. In: Liver transplantation-basic issues. University of Miami; 2012.

55. Roderique JD, VanDyck K, Holman B, Tang D, Chui B, Spiess BD. The use of high-dose hydroxocobalamin for vasoplegic syndrome. Ann Thorac Surg. 2014;97:1785–6.

56. Ortoleva JP, Cobey FC. A systematic approach to the treatment of vasoplegia based on recent advances in pharmacotherapy. J Cardiothorac Vasc Anesth. 2019;33(5):1310–4.

57. Kim JE, Jeon JP, No HC, et al. The effects of magnesium pretreatment on reperfusion injury during living donor liver transplantation. Korean J Anesthesiol. 2011;60:408–15.

58. Chung HS, Park CS, Hong SH, et al. Effects of magnesium pretreatment on the levels of T helper cytokines and on the severity of reperfusion syndrome in patients undergoing living donor liver transplantation. Magnes Res. 2013;26:46–55.

59. Bennett MW, Webster NR, Sadek SA. Alterations in plasma magnesium concentrations during liver transplantation. Transplantation. 1993;56:859–61.

60. Barger J, Trejo-Gutierrez JF, Patel T, Rosser B, Armanda-Michel J, Yataco ML, et al. Preexisting atrial fibrillation and cardiac complications after liver transplantation. Liver Transpl. 2015;21:314–20.

Part IV

Donor Issues: Liver Donor Hepatectomy and Organ Donation

Peri-Operative Assessment and Management of Live Donor for Donor Hepatectomy

24

Sangeeta Deka and Vijay Vohra

24.1 Introduction

Living donor transplant is an important component of liver transplant programme in the Asian countries. This is due to the lack of deceased donors in the Asian sub-continent. In India at present 80% of the transplants are live donor and 20% contribute to the deceased donor programme.

Living liver donor surgery is a major surgery and therefore all the implications of a major surgery are applicable here. Completely healthy individual undergoes surgical procedure for no health benefit. Liver is a very complex organ and the surgery of the liver is associated with fairly high incidence of major and minor complications. A crude morbidity of 31% is reported with donor hepatectomy [1]. One study reported a complication rate of 39% but most of the complications are mild in nature [2].

There is a large variation in the incidence of reported complications which is because the way these complications are defined. First successful living donor liver transplant (LDLT) was performed in 1989 in Chicago in a child with biliary atresia but following that there has been a huge progress made in LDLT in adults with right lobe liver grafts. Eastern countries like Japan and Korea have been leading the progress in this field.

There are a lot of inherent advantages of LDLT over deceased donor liver transplant (DDLT), the most apparent being that it can be performed in an elective manner most of the times. It gives an opportunity to time the surgery when the recipient's condition is optimized. As the donor and recipient's procedures go on at the same time, the cold ischaemia time of the liver is markedly reduced.

24.2 Donor Evaluation

The donor evaluation should start after initial screening is done. The initial screening involves knowing the blood group of the patient which needs to be compatible with the recipient, viral markers, and baseline biochemistry and coagulation status. If the initial screening does not reveal any prohibitive results like hepatitis B positive status, HIV positivity or severe anaemia, the assessment of the donor can proceed to the next level. The donors need to be between the ages of 18–55 years who explicitly consents to becoming a liver donor. The donor must be psychologically stable, informed of the risk of the surgery and also fully aware of the benefits and risk to the recipient. Every effort should be made that donors are not called for donation when the recipient condition is hopeless, i.e. a very high

S. Deka · V. Vohra (✉)
Liver Transplant, GI Anaesthesia and Intensive Care,
Medanta The Medicity, Gurgaon, India
e-mail: vijay.vohra@medanta.org

model for end-stage liver disease (MELD) score with serious systemic disease.

24.2.1 Phase 1

This phase involves besides the routine haematology and biochemistry, the donor undergoes lipid profile, thyroid function test, plane CT upper abdomen to assess the liver steatosis and estimation of liver attenuation index (LAI). An alternative to doing the CT is MR fat estimation, which is another modality to estimate the fat content in the liver. Generally up to 30% fat in the liver is considered acceptable for donation whereas 30–50% fat makes the liver borderline liver. The donor also undergoes triphasic CT scan and assessment of liver volume. The anatomy of liver is ascertained. If required magnetic resonance cholangiopancreatography (MRCP) is done to ascertain the biliary anatomy.

24.2.2 Phase 2

The next phase of donor assessment requires a thorough medical and laboratory assessment along with psychological assessment by a psychiatrist. The overall health status is assessed to rule out any major illness involving heart, kidney, and lungs. Diabetes and severe uncontrolled hypertension are also ruled out during this phase. Psychologists carry out an evaluation to assess the psychological status of the donor and identify any potential psychiatric issues. The donor must understand the procedure which is being undertaken and the implications of the surgical procedure. The implications of the surgical procedures (Donor hepatectomy) include loss of work for days to up to a month, possible morbidity like bile leak etc. All donors must have electrocardiogram (ECG) done, 2D echocardiography (2D ECHO)/stress echocardiography, chest X-ray, ultrasound abdomen, and pelvic and CT calcium score for donors >50 years.

24.2.3 Phase 3

In this phase clearance is obtained from gynaecology point of view by a gynaecology specialist, breast clearance in female donors and clearance from cardiac point of view with the help of a dedicated cardiologist.

24.3 Multidisciplinary Team Assessment

A multidisciplinary team, including Anaesthesia, Hepatology, Surgeon, Radiologist, and Psychiatry, take the responsibility of assessing the donor.

The objective of the assessment is as follows:

- General medical health of the donor.
- Liver function test and potential graft quality.
- Psychological status and capacity to give a valid consent.
- Motivation for donation—not under peer pressure.
- Anatomical issues (Surgical decision).

24.4 Pre-Anaesthetic Assessment

Pre-operative assessment is carried out keeping in mind the requirement of any major surgery with potential of large amount of blood loss. Donor is a person who is undergoing surgery for no direct benefit to his health.

ASA I/ II donors are only accepted to donate liver. The donor undergoes evaluation relating to the functioning of the liver as well as thorough systemic evaluation of the major organ systems.

History of previous surgery is recorded. Previous abdominal surgery can result in adhesions and may result in blood loss during the surgical procedure. Previous cholecystectomy makes the intraoperative cholangiogram, a difficult proposition. Any untoward episodes in relation to previous surgery is taken note of.

History of excessive post-operative nausea, vomiting (PONV) is enquired into. PONV is present, will require two or three drug combination (Ondasatron, Metoclopramide, and Dexamethasone) of anti-emetics in the post-op period. Abdominal surgery in a female patient is a high risk of PONV.

24.5 Systemic Assessment

Cardiovascular system evaluation is carried out in all donors; the intensity of the assessment varies depending on the age and other co morbid conditions. The assessment aims to investigate and reveal any underlying condition, which is not apparent. Older donors would undergo thorough history, examination, and relevant investigations like ECG, echocardiography, possibly stress echocardiography.

Those with diabetes and or hypertension may need to undergo carotid Doppler as well. Unstable cardiovascular status like angina or uncontrolled hypertension contraindicates donation. Hypertension which is well controlled without any end organ effects is not a contraindication for donation—Grade recommendation B1 [3].

Respiratory System—Evaluation is carried out to identify donors who are having risk factors, which makes them vulnerable to increased risk of post-operative pulmonary complication. Older donors with age more than 50 years, smoking history, asthma, along with prolonged upper abdominal surgery (> 3 h), intraoperative ventilation, are all factors for increased risk of pulmonary complications post-operatively [4]. History, examination, SpO$_2$, chest X-ray, and selected donors with pulmonary function tests are carried out in the donors. Severe restrictive dysfunction as seen in ankylosing spondylitis or severe asthma with pronounced obstruction would contraindicate donation as it jeopardizes the post-operative recovery [5–7]. Incentive spirometry is advised along with deep breathing exercises with adequate post-operative pain control to minimize post-operative pulmonary complications [8].

Haematological assessment is carried out as per the protocol of the center – some preferring to do more elaborate testing to rule out possibilities of hypercoaguable states. Procoagulant screening may not be done in all donors but is justified in donors who are donating to recipients who are donating to recipients with portal vein thrombosis or budd chiari syndrome [9]. Routine assessment will include complete blood count including platelet concentration, prothrombin time (PT) and activated partial thromboplastin time (APTT).

Pre-operative assessment is carried out in a protocolized manner so that all relevant investigations are done. The assessment is documented in a specially designed pre-operative assessment form (Fig. 24.1). Pre-operative anaesthetic evaluation also serves as a counselling session for the donor. The donor is appraised of the aspects of the procedure, the road map from assessment to surgery, post-operative course, and return to pre-operative status.

Post-operative pain management is discussed with the donor is made aware of the options available to control the post-operative pain. Thoracic epidural is probably the preferred method of pain relief post-operatively in most of the centres but the patient must consent to the procedure other options include intra venous narcotics, intrathecal morphine, fascial plane block—transversus abdominus plane (TAP block) have been used with variable success. Thoracic epidural if it is to be performed should be done while the patient is still awake before the start of anaesthesia. Some patients might find this daunting and may not agree to have an epidural while they are still awake. Performing epidural block under anaesthesia is not recommended as the morbidity with this procedure is higher. Certain adjuvants can be used in the local anaesthetic solution in the form of narcotics like fentanyl, morphine, etc. Various pre-medicants have also been used to improve post-operative analgesia—gabapentin and pregabalin.

Preoperative Assessment Of Donor Hepatectomy

Name: ______ Age:__ Sex:__ Weight:__ Height:__ BMI__

Name of the Recipient: ______ Relation: ______

Blood Group (RECIPIENT) ______ Blood Group (DONOR) ______

History

Cough/Exp	Any operation/anaesthesis/mishaps	Angina/CAD
COPD	Transfusion in Past	Hypertension
Kochs	Prolonged hospitalization	Dyspnoea
Bleeding Disorders	Allergy/Drug reaction	Exercise tolerance
G. Int Problem	Chronic Medicine Intake	Diabetes
Thyrotoxicosis/Hypothyroidism		Paralysis/Stroke/Seizures
		PIVD/Arthritis/Cervical Spondylosis

Personal History Alcohol Smoking Addiction Menstrual History

Drug History Present Past

General Examination

General Condition: Good/Fair/Sick looking/Toxic/Conscious/Drowsy/Unconscious

BP	Pulse	Resp Rate	Temp	Anaemia
Jaundice	Cyanosis	Oedema	Hydration	Clubbing

Cardiac Evaluation

- Echo : LVEF ECG
  PASP RWMA
  Valves
- Stress Echo
- Cardiology opinion

Respiratory Evaluation

- Breath Sounds/Air Entry
- SpO_2
- Pulmonary Function Test (PFT) Restrictive/Obstructive
- X-Ray Chest
- Pulmonologist Opinion
- P/A
- CNS

AIRWAY ASSESSMENT

Mouth Opening Teeth: Dentures: Loose tooth/teeth: Thyromental Distance:

Mallampatti Gr I II III IV

Haemotological Evaluation

Hb PCV TLC

DLC N L E M B

Platelets Blood Group

PT INR APTT

Liver Profile

Protein	S. Albumin
T. Billirubin	Conj. Billirubin
AST	ALT
ALK Phos	GGTT.

Biochemistry

S. Creatinine

BUN

Blood Sugar (R) F PP

Na/K/Ca/Mg/PO

Thyroid Profile

T3

T4

TSH

Viral Studies

Hbs Ag

Anti HBV

HCV RNA Genotype: Y/N

Anti HCV

HCV 1 & 2

CMV IgG: IgM:

Signature of Anaesthesiologist

Name of Anaesthesiologist

Date:

Time:

Issues:

Anasthesia Plan GA/LA/RA/MAC

Advice/Pre-OP Order

Fig. 24.1 Donor hepatectomy PAC Form

24.5.1 Assessment Day Before Surgery (Day −1)

This includes re-assessment and evaluation of recipient and donor scheduled for transplant surgery next day. A short physical examination of the patients is done. Repeat laboratory investigations, viz. complete blood count (CBC), liver function test (LFT), renal function test (RFT), coagulation profile, chest X-Ray (CXR), ECG, and 2D ECHO are done. If reports are acceptable, patient is cleared for surgery.

24.6 Anaesthetic Management

Awake epidural—After the patient is taken into the OR and routine standard monitors are connected, epidural catheter at mid-thoracic level (T6–T7) is placed in left lateral position after sedation with i.v. Midazolam 1–2 mg and i.v. fentanyl 25 μg. Catheter placement is checked and confirmed by injection of test dose of 3 mL of 2% lignocaine with adrenaline (15 μg).

Induction—After fixation of the epidural catheter, patient is made supine and induction of general anaesthesia done with i.v. Fentanyl 2 μg/mL, i.v. Propofol 2 mg/kg and tracheal intubation done after administration of a non-depolarizing muscle relaxant, usually i.v. cisatracurium 0.2 mg/kg. Under general anaesthesia, a radial arterial catheter, a central venous catheter (commonly in right IJV) and urinary catheter is placed. Patient position is done carefully, gel ring placed under head, limbs are padded to prevent pressure injury, and pneumatic pumps are applied in the lower limb for DVT prophylaxis. Normothermia is maintained with a forced air heating blanket (Bair-hugger) and room temperature maintained. Choice of intravenous fluid is a crystalloid, usually plasmalyte and the goal is to maintain mean arterial B.P. of >60 mmHg and a central venous pressure of <5 mmHg. 100–200 mL boluses of crystalloid is administered as and when required. Urine output is maintained greater than or equal to 0.5 mL/kg body weight.

24.6.1 Transfusion Requirement and Methods of Minimizing Blood Loss

Blood transfusion is associated with increased risk of infection and poor patient outcome.

Imamura et al. in a review of over one thousand hepatectomies for hepatocellular carcinoma found blood loss as a significant independnt factor for major complications [10]. The hospital stay and intensive care stay is also correlated with the transfusion requirement.

24.6.1.1 Low Central Venous Pressure (CVP)

CVP less than 5 mmHg is desirable while doing liver transection to minimize blood loss. Higher CVP causes back pressure in hepatic venous system resulting in more blood loss during liver parenchymal transection. Hence, low CVP allows a better control and haemostasis in case of inadvertent vessel injury [11]. There are various measures to lower CVP intraoperatively to reduce bleeding during transaction. Commonest practice is to restrict intravenous fluid administration. Fluid infusion rate of around 100–200 mL/h is maintained with intermittent boluses to keep MAP >60 mmHg. Epidural anaesthesia continued intraoperatively also helps in lowering CVP by venodilation. Few centres practice intraoperative phlebotomy without volume replacement to reduce the CVP. Intraoperative injection of a diuretic, commonly Frusemide (Lasix) has also been used for low CVP. Care must be taken to not lower the CVP too much as too low CVP (near zero) can cause air to enter through accidental venous tear or laceration during surgery resulting in air embolism. So one should be alert to this possibility which can be identified with sudden fall in end tidal etco2 in the presence of normal cardiac output.

24.6.1.2 Acute Normovolemic Hemodilution (ANH)

ANH is a method where patient's own blood is collected in one or more blood units just after anaesthesia and before commencement of surgery in the operating theatre and the blood volume taken out is replaced by simultaneous administration of crystalloid or colloid. The blood is stored in the operating theatre and is transfused at the end of surgery if there is blood loss and need of transfusion. ANH can be considered if patient's haemoglobin concentration is more than 12 g/dL. Risk of blood transfusion related immunologically mediated allergic reactions and transmission of viral illnesses can be eliminated. It is also safe to use in people with rare blood types.

24.6.1.3 Pre-Operative Autologous Blood Transfusion

Donor's blood is collected few weeks before scheduled date of surgery and stored in the blood bank. The last collection preferably should not be later than 72 h. The stored blood is then used and transfused back to the donor during surgery if required.

Cell saver technique or *intraoperative cell salvage* can be used wherein the blood lost during surgery is immediately returned to blood circulation with the help of a cell salvage machine which removes the impurities, wash the red cells and also add an anticoagulant to prevent it from clotting before transfusing it back into circulation. These are various methods which can be implemented to minimize blood transfusion in donor hepatectomy surgeries.

Metabolic acidosis is usually seen during donor surgery. It is primarily lactic acidosis due to reduced hepatic blood flow and hepatic dissection. Serial arterial blood gas analysis are done intraoperatively to check for acidosis and any abnormality is corrected.

All patients are preferably extubated in the operating theatre after the end of surgery and shifted to intensive care unit for overnight monitoring and optimization.

24.7 Post-Operative Care

Once the surgery is over the donor is shifted to either post-operative care unit or transferred straight to the intensive care unit. The family/attendant of the donor is informed and are encouraged to visit their patient. Chest X-Ray A/P view is done in all donors to view the lung fields and position of the central venous catheter. Complete blood count, electrolytes, blood sugar, PT, APTT, and arterial blood gas analysis (ABG) is done in all donors.

24.8 Pain Management

Donor hepatectomy surgery is associated with significant acute post-operative pain [12].

Optimal pain management of the living donor is a major challenge in the immediate post-surgical period.

Acute severe pain may be detrimental to post-operative outcome and recovery of the patient [13]. Therefore, it is pertinent to improve the quality of post-operative pain control and management. Thoracic epidural has been found to be the most effective mode of post-operative analgesia in donor hepatectomy surgery [14]. It also allows opioid sparing, restores gut motility, decreases incidence of development of chronic post-operative pain, and decreases post-operative morbidity [15].

In our practice, epidural catheter is placed in almost all patients at mid-thoracic level of T6–7. A local anaesthetic infusion is continued throughout surgery. After reversal of anaesthesia and extubation post-surgery in the operating theatre, a bolus of local anaesthesia (4 mL of Ropivacaine 0.2%) is administered and a continuous infusion of local anaesthetic and opioid combination (Ropivacaine 0.2% and Fentanyl 2mcg/mL) is started. Additional boluses of epidural local anaesthetic is also feasible via the patient control anaesthesia (PCA) machine. Pain intensity is monitored daily using the Visual analogue scale (VAS) by the dedicated pain nurse. Rescue analgesia (Inj. Tramadol 75–100 mg i.v.) is administered if the VAS score is greater than 5. Epidural catheter is removed on fourth post-operative day after prior checking of platelet count and INR. Side effects of epidural anaesthesia include failure of placement, dural puncture, and epidural hematoma in rare cases.

Safety of epidural catheter in major liver resection surgeries, especially in living donors, has been debated by many. Few studies have shown that it is a safe and effective method of post-operative pain control in donor hepatectomies [16, 17].

However, there are studies which have discouraged the use of epidural analgesia due to the derangement in coagulation status after liver resection which may cause epidural hematoma [18]. Choi et al. in their study found that platelet count decreased significantly immediately after surgery and decreasing trend remained till Post-operative day (POD) 6. There was also a significant rise in PT post-op and remained significant till POD 7. Coagulation status if deranged, should be normalized at the time of removal of epidural catheter. As per American Society of Regional Anaesthesia (ASRA) guidelines, epidural catheter can be removed if INR <1.5.

Intravenous analgesia in few patients, due to failure of insertion of epidural catheter and in few cases, patient's refusal for epidural analgesia, intravenous narcotic (Fentanyl/Morphine) infusion is continued intraoperatively and PCA is continued after conclusion of surgery. The choice of narcotic depends on the anaesthesiologist. Morphine has a longer duration of action and therefore fits into the profile if only patient control analgesia mode is to be used without basal infusion. There should be adequate monitoring for respiratory depression and a cut off of eight breaths per minute should warrant dose adjustment.

24.8.1 Abdominal Wall Blocks

Many studies have been conducted where multimodal approach of pain control after donor hepatectomy have been observed. Abdominal wall blocks such as lateral and subcostal transversus abdominis plane (TAP) blocks, rectus sheath block with liposomal bupivacaine have worked well and provided analgesia for a significant duration in post-operative period which is comparable to analgesia provided by epidural [19]. Adelmann et al. in their study found that continuous bilateral Erector spinae plane block with catheters in situ significantly reduced the dose of opioid and gabapentin consumption in post-operative period.

24.8.2 Multi Modal Analgesia

There is current trend to minimize the use of narcotics in the post-operative period due to possible detrimental effects like respiratory depression, nauseas, vomiting, gastric motility as well as possible narcotic dependence and abuse. Multi-modal analgesia requires combination of various modalities available—the most common being use of gabapentinoids pre-operatively, non-steroidal anti-inflammatory drugs, acetaminophen, low dose ketamine, and abdominal wall blocks. There have been studies on the use of non-traditional modalities like acupuncture in the donors [20].

24.9 DVT Prophylaxis

Deep vein thrombosis is a common complication after prolong surgery. In up to 10% of the patients DVT can translate into pulmonary embolism which can be fatal [21].

Sequential compression devices are used in the post-operative period to prevent deep vein thrombosis. This is continued till the patient Starts getting out of bed, which is normally 24–48 h post-surgery. Other modes of DVT preventions can also be carried out—compression stockings, leg exercises, and low molecular weight heparin (LMWH). LMWH in the dose of 0.2–0.4 ml (20–40 mg), 12 hourly is used for 4–7 days till the donor is fully mobile [22]. Anticoagulant use increases the risk of bleeding in post-operative period, which must be weighed in context with the prophylaxis of DVT and possible pulmonary embolism.

24.10 Remnant Liver: Monitoring Its Function

Major hepatic resection has its own risks. One of them is post-hepatectomy liver failure (PHLF) which increases morbidity, mortality, and length of hospital stay in donors. PHLF is defined as failure of the remaining hepatocytes to compensate for the loss of existing hepatocytes in maintaining synthetic and excretory function

manifesting as hyperbilirubinemia, hypoalbuminemia, prolonged prothrombin time (PT), elevated serum lactate levels, and hepatic encephalopathy [23]. Many authors have defined PHLF but the one which is widely used in clinical practice includes a combination of prolonged PT (INR > 1.7), elevated serum total bilirubin (>50 μmol/L), hepatic encephalopathy, and/or ascites on fifth post-operative day [24]. A good remnant of liver volume is necessary to prevent liver failure. Studies have shown that a remnant volume of 30–40% is safe after resection [24]. Hence it is pertinent to assess the patient and evaluate liver volume and function in pre-operative period to prevent hepatic failure post hepatectomy.

24.11 Robotic Donor Hepatectomy

The first laparoscopic donor right hepatectomy was first reported in the year 2006 [25]. Most of the right lobe laparoscopy donor hepatectomy have been carried out using a hand assisted procedure and with a high conversion rate [26]. This led to development of robotic donor hepatectomy and the first robotic procedure was reported in 2012. The challenges offered for robotic surgery include positioning of the patient, limitation of access to the patient, respiratory effects of prolonged pneumoperitoneum, intra-abdominal organ perfusion (including liver), in presence of raised intra-abdominal pressure and maintenance of body temperature. Adequate precautions should be undertaken in positioning of the patient so that all the pressure points are adequately padded to prevent pressure necrosis or neurological damage (Fig. 24.2). Robotic surgery is associated with longer duration of procedure as docking and undocking of the robot takes time. Prolonged infusion of muscle relaxant and use of inhalational agent can affect the recovery of the patient post-operatively. Cisatracurium, desflurane, and short acting opioids like fentanyl are advocated for prompt recovery on completion of the surgery. Protection of pressure areas is of paramount importance. Skin loss and blister formation has been reported after the procedure.

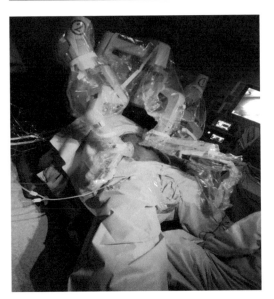

Fig. 24.2 Robotic donor hepatectomy

24.12 Liver Regeneration

Following donation, the liver regeneration process begins immediately and takes about 2–3 weeks for restoration of its function [27]. Liver regeneration occurs in three phases. In the first phase the liver grows rapidly within first 2 weeks after surgery. Second phase includes reversal of tissue oedema and normalization of volume which happens in 1–2 months. Liver regenerates slowly in the third phase and the volume reaches a steady state [28].

Gradual improvement in liver function test and coagulation profile is seen which also signifies the ongoing active regeneration of liver. However, it has been found that full regeneration of liver volume does not occur and the liver regenerates to about only 80% of original volume [29]. This study also states that liver volume recovers significantly faster than hepatocellular function.

24.13 Complications

Complications of donor hepatectomy surgery can be categorized into major and minor complications. Overall incidence of complications is around 40% and 1% incidence of residual disability, liver failure or death in living donors [30]. Major complications are those which require surgical or any other invasive intervention. Common major complications are surgical bleed requiring re-exploration, bile leak, biliary stricture, pleural effusion, deep venous thrombosis (DVT), pulmonary embolism due to DVT, collection of fluid in the abdomen (Table 24.1).

Minor complications include deranged liver function, wound infection and dehiscence, alopecia, thrombosis of internal jugular vein due to its cannulation, temporary neuropraxia, pressure sores in robotic donor hepatectomy due to prolonged duration of surgery. Late complications include development of incisional hernia at the incision site. Depression and other psychiatric illness is also observed.

Donor safety is of paramount of importance. The overall analysis of the LDLT donors shows a good safety profile but has a morbidity of up to 25% [31]. Careful selection of the donors is important and monitoring should continue into the post-operative period. Additionally post-operative psychological outcome as well as qual-

Table 24.1 Complications

Complications
Biliary complications: Biliary leak, biliary stricture
Infection: Wound infection, intra-abdominal infection, lung
Post-operative bleeding: Intra-abdominal bleeding, incision bleeding
Effusion: Pleural effusion, intra-abdominal effusion
Deep vein thrombosis: Pulmonary embolism

ity of life should be monitored. There is requirement of specialized patient care which is essential for the safety of living donors.

Key Points

- A liver donor is a healthy individual and donor hepatectomy surgery is a complex surgery with known morbidity and mortality. Hence, it is essential to select and evaluate them properly in order to minimize complications.
- Donor evaluation is done in three phases and includes thorough medical examination, laboratory tests and radiological assessment of liver.
- Pre-anaesthetic counselling is important in regards to post-operative pain management as donor hepatectomy surgery is associated with severe acute post-operative pain.
- CVP of less than 5 mmHg is desirable to minimize blood loss. Various methods include fluid restriction, diuretic administration, phlebotomy, autologous normovolemic hemodilution, pre-operative autologous blood donation, etc. However, too low a CVP can result in dangerous air embolism.
- Epidural analgesia is a safe and effective method of post-operative pain control in donors. Derangement in coagulation has been observed post hepatectomy hence, monitoring of coagulation profile is mandatory till the epidural catheter is taken out.
- Remnant liver volume should be adequate (>30%) enough to prevent post hepatectomy liver failure.

References

1. Beavers KL, Sandler RS, Shrestha R. Donor morbidity associated with right lobectomy for living donor liver transplantation to adult recipients: a systematic review. Liver Transpl. 2002;8(2):110–7.
2. Pomfret EA, Pomposelli JJ, Gordon FD, Erbay N, Lyn Price L, Lewis WD, et al. Liver regeneration and surgical outcome in donors of right-lobe liver grafts. Transplantation. 2003;76(1):5–10.
3. UK guidelines for Directed Altruistic Organ Donation. British Transplantation Society (BTS). Operational Guidelines & Standards June 2014.2014
4. Moller JT, Wittrup M, Johansen SH. Hypoxemia in the postanesthesia care unit: an observer study. Anesthesiology. 1990;73(5):890–5.
5. Pedersen T, Eliasen K, Henriksen E. A prospective study of risk factors and cardiopulmonary complications associated with anaesthesia and surgery: risk indicators of cardiopulmonary morbidity. Acta Anaesthesiol Scand. 1990;34(2):144–55.
6. Craig DB. Postoperative recovery of pulmonary function. Anesth Analg. 1981;60(1):46–52.
7. Schwieger I, Gamulin Z, Suter PM. Lung function during anesthesia and respiratory insufficiency in the postoperative period: physiological and clinical implications. Acta Anaesthesiol Scand. 1989;33(7):527–34.
8. Restrepo RD, Wettstein R, Wittnebel L, Tracy M. Incentive spirometry. Respir Care. 2011;56(10):1600–4.
9. Hilmi IA, Planinsic RM. Live liver donors: are they at a higher risk for post-operative thrombotic complications? World J Transplant. 2012;2(1):1–4.
10. Imamura H, Seyama Y, Kokudo N, Maema A, Sugawara Y, Sano K, et al. One thousand fifty-six hepatectomies without mortality in 8 years. Arch Surg. 2003;138(11):1198–206.
11. Chen CL, Chen YS, de Villa VH, Wang CC, Lin CL, Goto S, et al. Minimal blood loss living donor hepatectomy. Transplantation. 2000;69(12):2580–6.
12. Holtzman S, Clarke HA, McCluskey SA, Turcotte K, Grant D, Katz J. Acute and chronic postsurgical pain after living liver donation: incidence and predictors. Liver Transpl. 2014;20(11):1336–46.
13. American Society of Anesthesiologists Task Force on Acute Pain Management. Practice guidelines for acute pain management in the perioperative setting: an updated report by the American Society of Anesthesiologists Task Force on Acute Pain Management. Anesthesiology. 2012;116(2):248–73.

14. Koul A, Pant D, Rudravaram S, Sood J. Thoracic epidural analgesia in donor hepatectomy: an analysis. Liver Transpl. 2018;24(2):214–21.

15. Rodgers A, Walker N, Schug S, McKee A, Kehlet H, van Zundert A, et al. Reduction of postoperative mortality and morbidity with epidural or spinal anaesthesia: results from overview of randomised trials. BMJ. 2000;321(7275):1493.

16. Choi SJ, Gwak MS, Ko JS, Kim GS, Ahn HJ, Yang M. The changes in coagulation profile and epidural catheter safety for living liver donors: a report on 6 years of our experience. Liver Transpl. 2007;13(1):62–70.

17. Siniscalchi A, Begliomini B, De Pietri L, Braglia V, Gazzi M, Masetti M, et al. Increased prothrombin time and platelet counts in living donor right hepatectomy: implications for epidural anesthesia. Liver Transpl. 2004;10(9):1144–9.

18. Salame E, Goldstein MJ, Kinkhabwala M, Kapur S, Finn R, Lobritto S, et al. Analysis of donor risk in living-donor hepatectomy: the impact of resection type on clinical outcome. Am J Transplant. 2002;2(8):780–8.

19. Amundson AW, Olsen DA, Smith HM, Torsher LC, Martin DP, Heimbach JK. Acute benefits after liposomal bupivacaine abdominal wall blockade for living liver donation: a retrospective review. Mayo Clin Proc Innov Qual Outcomes. 2018;2(2):186–93.

20. Jesse MT, Kulas M, Unitis J, Betran N, Abouljoud M. Acupuncture in living liver and kidney donors: a feasibility study. J Integr Med. 2019;17(1):3–7.

21. Sandler DA, Martin JF. Autopsy proven pulmonary embolism in hospital patients: are we detecting enough deep vein thrombosis? J R Soc Med. 1989;82(4):203–5.

22. Rydberg EJ, Westfall JM, Nicholas RA. Low molecular weight heparin in preventing and treating DVT. Am Fam Physician. 1999;59(6):1607–12.

23. Van den Broek MAJ, Olde Damink SWM, Dejong CHC, Lang H, Malago M, Jalan R, et al. Liver failure after partial hepatic resection: definition, pathophysiology, risk factors and treatment. Liver Int. 2008;28(6):767–80.

24. Guglielmi A, Ruzzenente A, Conci S, Valdegamberi A, Iacono C. How much remnant is enough in liver resection? Dig Surg. 2012;29(1):6–17.

25. Koffron AJ, Kung R, Baker T, Fryer J, Clark L, Abecassis M. Laparoscopic-assisted right lobe donor hepatectomy. Am J Transplant. 2006;6(10):2522–5.

26. Park JI, Kim KH, Lee SG. Laparoscopic living donor hepatectomy: a review of current status. J Hepatobiliary Pancreat Sci. 2015;22(11):779–88.

27. Marcos A, Fisher RA, Ham JM, Shiffman ML, Sanyal AJ, Luketic VA, et al. Liver regeneration and function in donor and recipient after right lobe adult to adult living donor liver trans- plantation. Transplantation. 2000;69(7):1375–9.

28. Haga J, Shimazu M, Wakabayashi G, Tanabe M, Kawachi S, Fuchimoto Y, et al. Liver regeneration in donor and adult recipients after living donor liver transplantation. Liver Transpl. 2008;14(12):1718–24.

29. Nadalin S, Testa G, Malago M, Beste M, Frilling A, Schroeder T. Volumetric and functional recovery of the liver after right hepatectomy for living donation. Liver Transpl. 2004;10(8):1024–9.

30. Abecasis MM, Fisher RA, Olthoff KM, Freise CE, Rodrigo DR, Samstein B, et al. Complications of living donor hepatic lobectomy—a comprehensive report. Am J Transplant. 2012;12(5):1208–17.

31. Lei J, Yan L, Wang W. Donor safety in living donor liver transplantation: a single-center analysis of 300 cases. PLoS One. 2013;8(4):e61769.

Brain Death and Organ Donation

25

C. Vasantha Roopan

25.1 Introduction

Organ transplantation is the only option in patients with end-organ failure. Renal, cardiac, and hepatic failures are some of the common end-organ failures requiring organ transplant with excellent outcomes and improving the survival rates and quality of life in the transplanted recipients. Cadaveric donors are the primary source of organs for these patients, particularly for organs like heart, lung, and cornea and for other organs where availability of living donor is scarce. Road traffic injuries are one of the leading ten causes of death worldwide [1] and a significant number of them may be potential brain-dead donors. Therefore, diagnosing brain death and caring of the brain-dead donor becomes very important in improving the quality of the organs retrieved and hence the outcome and quality of living in the recipient.

25.2 Organ Donation in India

Different countries have their own laws governing organ donation for both living and cadaveric donors in accordance with local beliefs, customs, and demand for organs. Some countries depend entirely on living donors, while some depend entirely on deceased ones. In India, the Transplantation of Human Organ Act was passed in 1994, amended in 2008 and 2011 and updated in 2014. It aims at streamlining living and cadaveric transplants and prevent organ trafficking and malpractices.

In India the deceased donor organ donation rates is around 0.65–0.8 pmp (in the year 2016–17) [2, 3], (Fig. 25.1). This is very low when compared to Spain (46.9 pmp), USA (31.96 pmp), and UK (23.05 pmp) in the year 2017 [2], (Fig. 25.2). Currently in India, only 13 of the 36 states and union territories have performed deceased donor organ transplants. Of these only 5 or 6 do it on a regular basis and have a proper system of organ donation in place [4], (Figs. 25.3 and 25.5]. Therefore, there is a huge gap between the necessity and availability of organs.

C. V. Roopan (✉)
Apollo Hospitals, Chennai, Tamilnadu, India

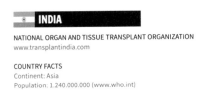

INDIA

NATIONAL ORGAN AND TISSUE TRANSPLANT ORGANIZATION
www.transplantindia.com

COUNTRY FACTS
Continent: Asia
Population: 1.240.000.000 (www.who.int)

INDIA
DECEASED
ORGAN DONOR
EVOLUTION

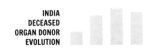

SELECT A YEAR   2020 | 2019 | 2018 | 2017 | 2005 | 2004 | 2003 | 2002 | 2001 | 2000 | 1999 | 1998 | 1997 | 1996 | 1995 | 1994 | 1993 |

ORGAN DONATIONS — 2020

	ACTUAL DECEASED DONORS		UTILIZED DECEASED DONORS		ACTUAL DCD DONORS		UTILIZED DCD DONORS		LIVING DONORS	
	NUM	PMP	NUM	PMP	NUM	PMP	NUM	PMP	NUM	PMP
	347	0.25	-	-	0	0	-	-	6457	4.67

ORGAN TRANSPLANTS — 2020

	KIDNEY		LIVER		PANCREAS		HEART		LUNG		HEART LUNG	
	NUM	PMP	NUM	PMP	NUM	PMP	NUM	PMP	NUM	PMP	NUM	PMP
DECEASED	516	0.37	291	0.21	14	0.01	89	0.06	67	0.05	-	-
LIVING	4970	3.60	1487	1.08								

52.8%

KIDNEY TRANSPLANTS — 2020

	LIVING		DECEASED		DOUBLE		KIDNEY PANCREAS	
	NUM	PMP	NUM	PMP	NUM	PMP	NUM	PMP
	4970	3.60	516	0.37	0	0	0	0

LIVER TRANSPLANTS — 2020

	LIVING		DECEASED		SPLIT		KIDNEY LIVER	
	NUM	PMP	NUM	PMP	NUM	PMP	NUM	PMP
	1487	1.08	291	0.21	0	0	0	0

TISSUE TRANSPLANTS — 2020

	CORNEA		SKIN		HEART VALVES		MUSCOLOSKELETAL		BLOOD VESSELS	
	NUM	PMP	NUM	PMP	NUM	PMP	NUM	PMP	NUM	PMP
	0	0	0	0	0	0	0	0	0	0

Fig. 25.1 Deceased donor statistics of India for the year 2020. (Image courtesy: International Registry in Organ Donation and Transplantation—IRODaT www.irodat.org)

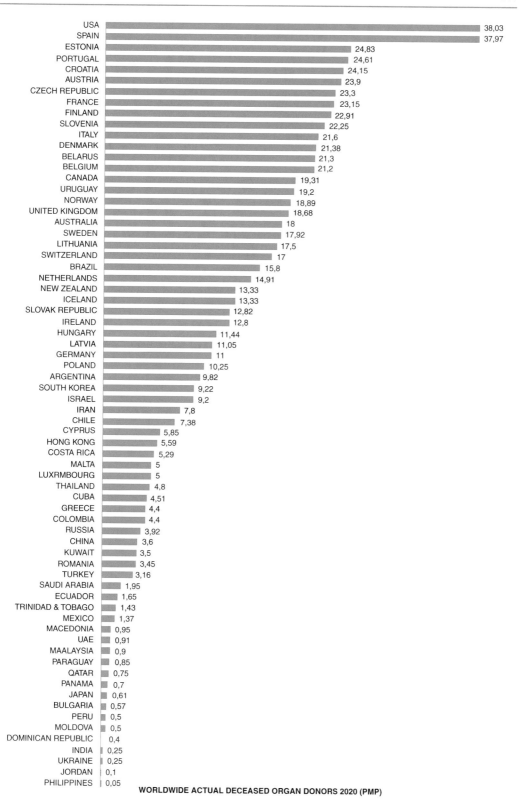

Fig. 25.2 Worldwide actual deceased organ donors in 2020 per million population (pmp). (Image courtesy: International Registry in Organ Donation and Transplantation—IRODaT www.irodat.org)

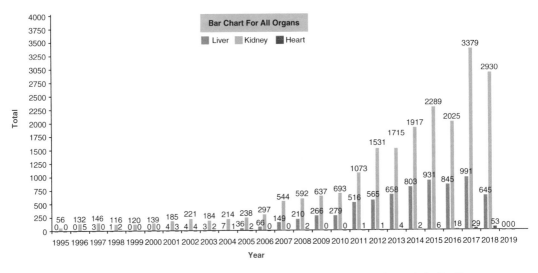

Fig. 25.3 Bar chart showing number of individual organ transplants performed each year in India. (Image courtesy: National Organ and Tissue Transplant Organization—NOTTO www.notto.gov.in)

25.3 Brain Death

25.3.1 Definition

Though almost all countries accept brain death as a form of death, there is no universally accepted definition for it. Also, the term brain death is not fully descriptive of the actual condition, where it can mean death of any part of brain like cerebrum, cerebellum or midbrain, but the most important criteria to define brain death would be the death of midbrain. Brain stem death would have been a better term. Brain death can be defined as "the irreversible cessation of all functions of the brain including brain stem."

25.3.2 Pathophysiology of Brain Death [5], (Fig. 25.4)

A variable period of raised intracranial pressure (ICP) always precedes brain death. The resulting physiological responses to raised ICP are super-

imposed on the patients' prior comorbidities and therapy.

25.3.3 Cardiovascular Changes

Due to raised ICP there is a variable period of hypertension with associated bradycardia. This is followed by a marked sympathetic stimulation due to an intense "catecholamine storm" leading to raised systemic vascular resistance and tachycardia. These are associated with central redistribution of blood volume, increased afterload, and visceral ischemia. The severity of changes depends in part on the speed of onset of brain death. In fact approximately 40% of the brain-dead donors develop echocardiographic evidence of myocardial dysfunction. After the catecholamine storm, there is a loss of sympathetic tone and peripheral vasodilatation. The resulting hypotension, if untreated, leads to hypoperfusion of all organs, including the heart, and may contribute to rapid donor organ loss. ECG

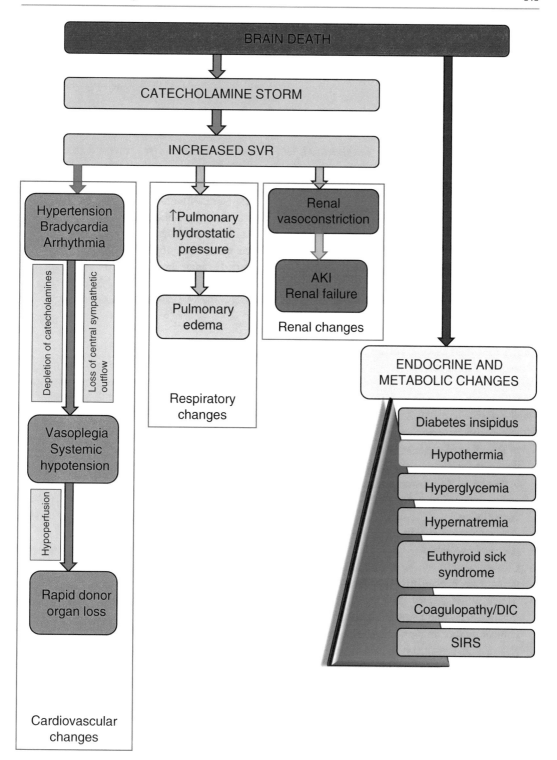

Fig. 25.4 Pathophysiological changes in brain stem death

abnormalities are also common, which include ST and T wave changes, arrhythmias and conduction abnormalities.

25.3.4 Pulmonary Changes

Raised pulmonary hydrostatic pressure leads to pulmonary edema, which is aggravated by endothelial damage due to raised levels of endogenous norepinephrine.

25.3.5 Endocrine, Metabolic, and Stress Response

Posterior pituitary function is very commonly lost in brain-dead donors, whereas anterior pituitary function may be variably lost due to its extradural blood supply. The common problems encountered are as follows:

- Diabetes insipidus due to depletion of antidiuretic hormone.
- Hypothermia: there may be a variable period of hyperthermia preceding it. Hypothermia is due to decreased metabolic activity, partly due to decreased TSH secretion, decreased peripheral conversion of T4 and intense vasodilation.
- Hyperglycemia due to insulin resistance and decreased secretion.
- Clinical picture similar to euthyroid sick syndrome seen in critically ill patients.
- Active inflammatory response due to mediators released from damaged brain producing a clinical picture similar to systemic inflammatory response syndrome (SIRS).
- Coagulopathy and Disseminated intravascular coagulation (DIC) due to the release of tissue thromboplastin from the damaged brain.

25.3.6 Diagnosis of Brain Death

It involves the early identification of brain death by establishing an etiology, after exclusion of all reversible causes of coma and confirmation of brain death by neurological testing for cranial reflexes and apnea test.

Early identification and diagnosis of brain death is an essential component of management of brain-dead donors as

- Brain death is frequently followed by a predictable pattern of complex multi-organ dysfunction.
- Early identification and support of potential brain-dead donors improves the quality of the procured organ and hence the outcome.
- Active management and support of the potential brain-dead organ donors should be initiated as soon as brain death is diagnosed irrespective of the consent. Therapy can be discontinued if consent is declined.

(a) Establishing an etiology:
    Conclusive proof of an etiology that can cause irreversible structural and functional damage to the brain should be identified.
(b) Exclusion of all reversible causes of coma:
    All known reversible causes of coma should be ruled out like
    - Severe hypothermia.
    - Metabolic and endocrine causes: hypoglycemia, hypothyroidism, panhypopituitarism, severe electrolyte disturbances, hepatic coma, etc.)
    - Poisoning or drug overdose: adequate time should be given for suspected drugs if any to clear out or antidotes be given. Sedation and paralysis if any, to be reversed.
    - Cardiovascular or respiratory causes: severe hypotension or sleep apnea syndrome.
(c) Neurological testing for diagnosing brain death:
    - The patient must have a persisting Glasgow Coma Score of 3 demonstrating the functional loss of the reticular activating system and any other centers of consciousness.
    - A formal apnea test demonstrating the lack of the capacity to breathe, and thereby the functional loss of the respira-

tory centers located in and associated with the medulla oblongata. The apnea test is preferably carried out after the examination of brain stem reflexes.

- The cranial nerves (with the exception of I, II, and the spinal component of XI) originate in the brainstem and the demonstration of their functional loss confirms the widespread damage to the brainstem and by association, the reticular activating system and medulla oblongata. All of the following brainstem derived cranial nerve reflexes are examinable and must be demonstrated to be absent:
  - Pupils should be fixed in diameter and unresponsive to light (Cranial Nerves II, III).
  - Nystagmus or any eye movement should not occur when each ear is instilled with ice cold water. Each eardrum should be clearly visualized before the test (Vestibulo–ocular reflex—Cranial Nerves III, IV, VI, VIII).
  - There should be no corneal reflex (Cranial Nerves V, VII).
  - There should be no facial or limb movement when supraorbital pressure is applied (Cranial Nerves V, VII).
  - There should be no gag reflex following stimulation to the posterior pharynx or cough reflex following suction catheter passed into the trachea (Cranial Nerves IX, X).
  - Oculocephalic reflex (Doll's head eye phenomenon). This test must not be performed in patients with an unstable cervical spine injury. The examiner keeps the patient's eyes open and the head is turned from the middle position to 90 ° on both sides. When the reflex is intact the eyes turn opposite to the side of head movement as if lagging behind. The reflex is absent when the eyes move with the head and do not move within the orbit. If cold caloric test can be performed, this test may be omitted.

25.3.6.1 Apnea Test [6]

This test should preferably done after the examination of brain stem reflexes. This test confirms the functional loss of brain stem function thereby confirming brain death. Before performing apnea test the physician should make sure the patient meets the prerequisites for performing the test namely

- Core temperature ≥ 36.5 °C or 97.7 °F.
- Hemodynamically stable: SBP ≥ 100 mmHg, with or without vasopressor/inotropic supports.
- Euvolemia.
- No hypoxia.
- Eucapnia.
- No prior evidence of CO_2 retention (severe COPD, morbid obesity, etc.).

After determining that the patient meets the above prerequisites, apnea test is conducted.

- A baseline arterial blood gas is done to determine the baseline PCO_2.
- Pre-oxygenate with 100% oxygen for at least 10 mins to raise the $PaO_2 > 200$ mmHg.
- Disconnect the ventilator.
- Insert an insufflation cannula through the endotracheal tube up to the level of carina and provide 100% oxygen through the cannula at a rate of about 6 L/min (apneic oxygenation).
- Observe closely for any respiratory efforts/ movements of the chest for a duration of 8–10 mins.
- Abort if SBP falls below 90 mmHg or SpO_2 falls below 85% for more than 30 s or cardiac arrhythmia develops.
- Retry the procedure, if possible (after stabilization of vital parameters) with T-piece, CPAP of 10 cm of H_2O and 100% O_2 at 12 L/min.
- If no respiratory drive is present, repeat the arterial blood gas after 8–10 mins.
- Apnea test is considered positive, when there is no respiratory effort after 8–10 mins of apneic oxygenation and there is a raise of >20 mmHg of PCO_2 from the baseline or arterial $PCO_2 \geq 60$ mmHg after apneic oxygenation.

- If the apnea test is inconclusive even after repeated attempts or is not possible then the ancillary diagnostic tests can be performed.

25.3.6.2 Ancillary Tests

Other confirmatory tests (also called as ancillary tests for brain stem death) like EEG, cerebral angiography, Transcranial doppler, radioisotope brain scanning, MRI, and MRA are not mandatory.

However, when the neurological examination and the apnea test cannot be performed due to hemodynamic instability, hypoxia or severe facial or chest trauma, EEG, and the four vessel cerebral angiography (considered the "gold standard") demonstrating no blood flow to the brain will be useful.

In children there remains uncertainty about the reliability of clinical brainstem testing. In neonates especially, organs for transplantation should not be removed in the first 7 days of life with beating hearts. Radioisotope brain scanning has been recommended under the age of 1 year when brainstem death certification is required.

25.3.7 Clinical Observations Compatible with the Diagnosis of Brain Death

The following observations are compatible with the diagnosis of brain death and should not be confused for the presence of brain stem function (Tables 25.1 and 25.2). Brain-dead patients can have

Table 25.1 Brain death guidelines [7]

Irreversible etiology
Neurologic exam
Coma
Brainstem reflexes absent
Apnea test positive
Ancillary tests
No electrical activity on EEG
No cerebral blood flow on angiography or transcranial doppler
No uptake of technetium on brain scan ("hollow skull phenomenon")

Table 25.2 Apnea testing prerequisites [7]

Absence of breathing drive is tested with a CO_2 challenge. Documenting a $PaCO_2$ increase to above normal is typical practice. Test requires preparation
Prerequisites
Normotensive
Normothermic
Euvolemic
Eucapnic (PCO_2 35–45 mm hg)
No hypoxia
No prior evidence of CO_2 retention (COPD, morbid obesity)

Procedure

- Adjust vasopressors so systolic blood pressure is 100 mmHg. Pre- oxygenate for at least 10 min with 100% oxygen so PaO_2 is 200 mmHg
- Reduce ventilator frequency to 10 breaths/min, to eucapnia. Reduce PEEP to 5 cm H_2O (oxygen desaturation with decreasing PEEP may suggest difficulty with apnea testing)
- If SpO_2 remains <95%, obtain a baseline arterial blood analysis
- Disconnect patient from ventilator
- Preserve oxygenation: Insert insufflation catheter through the endotracheal tube and close to the level of the carina, and deliver 100% O_2 at 6 L/min
- Watch for respiratory movements for 8–10 min. Respiration is defined as abdominal or chest excursions, and may include a brief gasp
- Abort if systolic blood pressure decreases to <90 mmHg
- Abort if SpO_2 is <85% for >30 s. redo test with T-piece, CPAP of 10 cm H_2O, and 100% O_2 at 12 L/min
- If no respiratory drive is observed, repeat arterial blood analysis after 8 min
- If respiratory movements are absent and $PaCO_2$ is 60 mmHg (or 20 mmHg increase in $PaCO_2$ over a baseline normal $PaCO_2$) the apnea test is positive (i.e., supports the diagnosis of brain death)
- If the test is inconclusive but the patient is hemodynamically stable during the procedure, the test can be repeated for 10–15 min after another pre-oxygenation

- Spontaneous "spinal" movements of the limbs (not to be confused with a pathological flexion or extension response).
- Respiratory-like movements (shoulder elevation and adduction, back arching or intercostal expansion without significant tidal volume.
- Sweating, blushing and tachycardia.
- Normal blood pressure without pharmacological support.

- Absence of diabetes insipidus (normal osmolar control mechanism).
- Deep tendon reflexes.
- Babinski's reflex.

25.3.8 Certification of Brain Death

The tests for brain stem death should be repeated again before certification of brain stem death. As per the THOA guidelines, the minimum time interval between the first and second testing will be 6 h in adults. In case of children 6–12 years of age, 1–5 years of age and infants, the time interval shall increase depending on the opinion of the experts certifying brain stem death. The time of second declaration (Apnea test) is taken as the time of death of the donor (Table 25.3).

THOA recommends that of the two physicians certifying brain stem death, at least one should preferably be a neurologist or neurosurgeon. Both the certifying physicians should not be involved in any way with the care of the patient or the transplant program. Where neurologist/neurosurgeon is not available, then any Surgeon or Physician and Anesthetist or Intensivist, nominated by Medical Administrator In-charge of the hospital shall be the member of the board of medical experts for brain stem death certification.

Table 25.3 Time interval between neurological examination and tests needed

Generally accepted minimum time interval between first and second testing for brain stem death		Confirmation of brain stem death by
Adults	6 h	Clinical examination[a]
Age: 2 months–1 year	24 h	Clinical examination[a] and EEG[b]
Age: 7 days–2 months	48 h	Clinical examination[a] and EEG[b]
Age: Less than 7 days	Not recommended	Not recommended

[a]Coma, absent brain stem reflexes and positive apnea test
[b]A repeat examination and EEG not necessary if a concomitant radionucleotide angiography demonstrates no visualization of arteries

THOA also recommends that once the patient is declared brain dead, the cost of maintaining the donor be borne by the prospective recipients or the hospital administration, which receives the organ for transplantation or the in house hospital through corpus funds. No other monetary benefits should be given to the donor family and donation should be purely voluntary.

25.4 Care of the Psychological Issues for Organ Donor Family and Treating Staffs

The death of a loved one has a very devastating psychological and emotional effects on the kith and kin of the family. In addition, the treating staffs and physicians may develop "caregiver stress" due to repeated exposures of death of varied reasons. All members of the caring team need to come together and support and care for each other's stress to cope up with the situation. Also they should respect the donor's family wishes and try to deal it with dignity. Decision to voluntarily donate at such times of emotional turmoil needs a great level of poise and this decision has to be respected and dealt with utmost empathy. The care of the family of the brain dead involves the role of the transplant coordinator, intensivists, primary physician, and social worker. Given the tremendous amount of emotional turmoil they undergo in accepting the brain death of their loved ones and the thought of surgical removal of the organs and the "mutilated" body after the retrieval requires lot of counseling and all the members of the organ procurement team play a great part in this. Updating them regularly and being in touch with them in each and every step of management is essential. Caring of the deceased organ donor can be demanding psychologically both in the clinical management of the donor as well as in dealing with their relatives. Junior medical and nursing staff particularly need education and support for appropriate management of the patient and also for skilled and appropriate communication with the relatives [8].

25.5 Conclusion

When the need for transplant organs is exponentially increasing, corresponding wise utilization of the available organs becomes a necessity. For that a proper well-oiled machinery for donor identification and care is essential to improve the number and quality of the organs, so that even marginal donors can be wisely utilized without wastage of organs. Legislations and monitoring committees are an invaluable part of the system to curb any malpractices and keep a check on the system. Though India is rapidly progressing towards such a state still a lot has to be done to achieve international donor rates and utilization of the organs (Fig. 25.5).

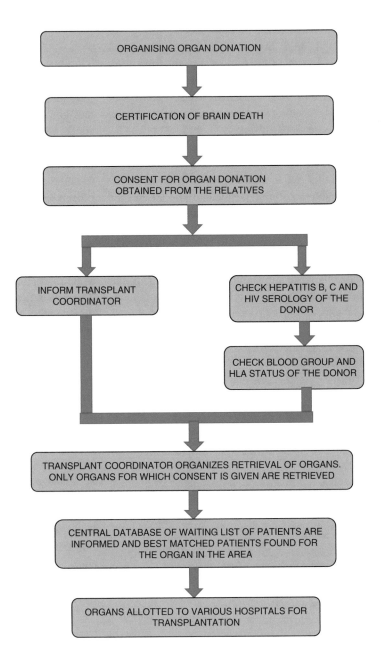

Fig. 25.5 Work-flow in deceased organ procurement

Key Points

- Diagnosing brain death and caring of the brain-dead donor becomes very important in improving the quality of the organs retrieved and hence the outcome and quality of living in the recipient.
- There is no universally accepted definition for brain death.
- Brain death can be defined as "the irreversible cessation of all functions of the brain including brain stem".
- The catecholamine storm associated with raised ICP and the associated endocrine and metabolic changes associated with brain death lead to the resultant pathophysiological changes seen in it.
- Early identification and diagnosis of brain death is an essential component of management of brain-dead donors.
- Confirmation of brain death is done by neurological testing for cranial reflexes and apnea test.
- If the apnea test is inconclusive even after repeated attempts or is not possible then the ancillary diagnostic tests can be performed.
- In children there remains uncertainty about the reliability of clinical brain-stem testing.
- There are some clinical observations that are compatible with the diagnosis of brain death and should not be confused for the presence of brain stem function.
- Each country has its own laws and legislations regarding organ donation and transplantation.
- In India, the Transplantation of Human Organ Act (THOA) was passed in 1994, amended in 2008 and 2011 and updated in 2014.
- As per THOA guidelines there is a specific time interval to be followed between first and second testing for brain death.
- THOA recommends that of the two physicians certifying brain stem death, at least one should preferably be a neurologist or neurosurgeon. Both the certifying physicians should not be involved in any way with the care of the patient or the transplant program.

Appendix

FORM 10
FOR CERTIFICATION OF BRAIN STEM DEATH
(To be filled by the board of medical experts certifying brain-stem death)
[Refer rules 5(4)(c) and 5(4)(d)]

We, the following members of the Board of medical experts after careful personal examination hereby certify that Shri/Smt./Km. .... aged about .... son of /wife of / daughter of .... Resident of.. is dead on account of permanent and irreversible cessation of all functions of the brain-stem. The tests carried out by us and the findings therein are recorded in the brain-stem death Certificate annexed hereto.

Dated.................   Signature...................................

1. R.M.P.-Incharge of the HospitalIn which brain-stem death has occurred.
2. R.M.P. nominated from the panel of Names sent by the hospitals and approved by the Appropriate Authority.
3. Neurologist/Neuro-Surgeon
4. R.M.P. treating the aforesaid deceased person

  (where Neurologist/Neurosurgeon is not available, any Surgeon or Physician and Anaesthetist or Intensivist, nominated by Medical Administrator In-charge from the panel of names sent by the hospital and approved by the Appropriate Authority shall be included)

BRAIN-STEM DEATH CERTIFICATE

(A)   PATIENT DETAILS..

      1.   Name of the patient: Mr./Ms..

                S.O./D.O./W.O.   Mr./Ms..

                                         Sex..Age..

      2.   Home Address: ....

                                         ....

      3.   Hospital Patient Registration Number (CR No.) ....

      4.   Name and Address of next of kin or person responsible for the patient (if none exists, this must be specified)

                ....

      5.   Has the patient or next of kin agreed to any donation of organ and/or tissue?

                ....

      6.   Is this a Medico-legal Case? Yes............................No.....................

(B)   PRE-CONDITIONS:

      1.   Diagnosis: Did the patient suffer from any illness or accident that led to irreversible brain damage? Specify details.........................
                ....
                Date and time of accident/onset of illness...
                Date and onset of non-reversible coma...

      2.   Findings of Board of Medical Experts:
                First Medical Examination...
                Second Medical Examination..

                (1) The following reversible causes of coma have been excluded:
                        Intoxication (Alcohol)
                        Depressant Drugs
                        Relaxants (Neuromuscular blocking agents)
                        Primary Hypothermia
                        Hypovolaemic shock
                        Metabolic or endocrine disorders
                        Tests for absence of brain-stem functions

References

1. World Health Organisation. The top causes of death. 2018. https://www.who.int/news-room/fact-sheets/detail/the-top-10-causes-of-death.
2. IRODaT. International Registry of Organ Donation and Transplantation. 2018. https://www.irodat.org/?p=database&c=IN#data.
3. Suriyamoorthi S. National Data—deceased organ donation and transplantation. Indian Transpl Newsl. 2017;16(50). https://www.itnnews.co.in/indian-transplant-newsletter/issue50/National-Data-Deceased-Organ-Donation-and-Transplantation-587.htm.
4. Shroff S. Twenty-five years of transplantation law in India—progress and the way forward. Indian J Transplant. 2019;13(3):151–3.
5. Smith M. Physiologic changes during brain stem death—lessons for management of the donor. J Heart Lung Transplant. 2004;23(9 Supplement):S217–22. https://doi.org/10.1016/j.healun.2004.06.017.
6. Wijdicks EFM, Varelas PN, Gronseth GS, Greer DM. Evidence-based guideline update: determining brain death in adults: report of the quality standards subcommittee of the American Academy of neurology. Neurology. 2010;74(23):1911–8. https://doi.org/10.1212/WNL.0b013e3181e242a88.
7. Scott JB, Gentile MA, Bennett SN, Couture M, MacIntyre NR. Apnea testing during brain death assessment: a review of clinical practice and published literature. Respir Care. 2013;58(3):532–8. https://doi.org/10.4187/respcare.01962.
8. Colreavy F, Dwyer R. Medical management of the adult organ donor patient. In: ICSI A4 Guide; 2010. p. 9–14.

Donation After Circulatory Death

26

M. N. Chidananda Swamy

Abbreviations

CIT	Cold ischaemia time
DBD	Donation after brain death
DCD	Donation after circulatory death
DWIT	Donor warm ischaemia time
FWIT	Functional warm ischaemia time
HMP	Hypothermic machine perfusion
MP	Machine perfusion
NMP	Normothermic machine perfusion
Normothermic	Ex vivo machine perfusion
NRP	Normothermic regional perfusion
THOA	Transplantation of Human Organs Act
WIT	Warm ischaemia time

Dr. Starzl the father of Liver Transplantation had written that 'what was inconceivable yesterday, and barely achievable today, often becomes routine tomorrow'.

Thomas E. Starzl, MD, PhD, known as the 'Father of Transplantation'—laid the ground-work for an entire new field of medicine. The above statement has been very true with regard to Donation after Cardiac Death (DCD).

Organ transplantation is the only option to improve the quality of life and improve the life expectancy in patients with end-stage organ failure. With advances in transplant technology, immunosuppression and intensive care, there is an ever-increasing demand for organ transplantation.

Suitable organs for transplantation can be obtained either from a living donor or a deceased donor. Living donor programmes pose an inherent risk to the donors and a suitable matching donor may not always be available. Living donor programmes may also be a harbouring ground, for illegal organ trade. Organ donation can also be done after death either after death by the neurological criteria (Donation after Brain Death [DBD]) or death by the cardiorespiratory criteria [Donation after Cardiac Death (DCD)].

In order to understand the process of DCD one needs to understand the definition of death which forms the cornerstone in understanding the legal aspects of organ donation by either criterion.

26.1 Definition of Death

The traditional definition of death in India, as in many other countries, is an 'irreversible cessation of circulatory and respiratory functions'.

M. N. C. Swamy (✉)
Neurocritical Care Unit, Brunei Neuroscience Stroke and Rehabilitation Center, Pantai Jerudong Specialist Centre, Jerudong, Brunei Darussalam

© The Author(s), under exclusive license to Springer Nature Singapore Pte Ltd. 2023
V. Vohra et al. (eds.), *Peri-operative Anesthetic Management in Liver Transplantation*,
https://doi.org/10.1007/978-981-19-6045-1_26

In 1981, the Uniform Determination of Death Act was enacted in the US. It said that 'An individual who has sustained either (1) irreversible cessation of circulatory and respiratory functions or (2) irreversible cessation of all functions of the entire brain, including the brain stem, is dead. A determination of death must be made with accepted medical standards' [1, 2].

Under Section 2(e) of The Transplantation of Human Organs Act, 1994, a deceased person is a person in whom there is a 'permanent disappearance of all evidence of life, by reason of brain stem death or in a cardio-pulmonary sense at any time after live birth has taken place' [1, 3].

Prior to the introduction of legislation defining brainstem death, all deceased donor transplants were performed using non-heart beating donors. 'Non-heart beating donor (NHBD)' was the initial terminology for these donors to differentiate them from brain-dead donor where the heart is still beating. This was later replaced by 'Donation after Cardiac Death' to include cardiac factor for death in the terminology.

NHBD was the very first method of organ donation and only kidneys were recovered due to a variety of limitations including surgical technique, ischemia and available methods of preservation. In the present situation any organ or tissue including kidneys, liver, pancreas, lungs and hearts can all be recovered and successfully transplanted. Tissues such as bone, cornea, heart valves, veins and soft tissues have always been recovered from patients following pronouncement of cardiac death.

With the introduction of successful cardiac transplantation, the terminology was changed to 'Donation after Circulatory Death' (DCD) to reflect the correct status of heart which can still be viable and used.

By convention 'Brain-Dead Donors' have lost all functions of the brain, but cardiac function is intact to circulate blood to all organs and organ donation can be a controlled action. In contrast in the 'Non-Heart Beating Donors' circulation has ceased leading to loss of blood supply to organs. Hence in this situation, organ retrieval must be an urgent procedure and pref-erably within the next 60 min to preserve the viability of the organs proposed to be retrieved. There are two broad categories of non-heart beating donors according to the circumstances of cardiac arrest.

1. Uncontrolled—Where cardiac arrest occurs suddenly and is unexpected. The time taken to retrieve organs and put them in ice (Warm ischaemic time) from these uncontrolled non-heart beating donors is prolonged.
2. Controlled—Where elective withdrawal of ventilation in an end of life situation leads to cardiac arrest. The warm ischemia time in these donors is much less and can be controlled, therefore are better suited for this type of donation [4].

The need to maximise deceased donation is included under the World Health Organisation (WHO) Guiding Principles for Human Cell, Tissue and Organ Transplantation (Cruzado WHO GP). The critical pathway (Fig. 26.1) of deceased donation provides a systematic approach to the organ donation process, considering both donation after cardiac death and donation after brain death [5].

The critical pathway as published by World Health Organisation (WHO) (Fig. 26.1) also provides guidelines and helps in identifying the challenges faced and aids in maximising deceased donation. It also reaffirms that the 'Dead Donor Rule' [6, 7], the requirement that organ retrieval must not result in the death of the patient—must be always respected.

The acceptance of the Harvard criteria for diagnosis of brain death, in 1968 and with the associated improvement in outcomes of organ transplantation led to a decline in the DCD programmes. However, with the ever-widening gap in the availability of organs and the patients on the waiting list has produced a resurgence of interest in DCD process. Thus, there is an essential need to understand the process of DCD and to address the ethical aspects thereof, and to establish proper institutional protocols and criteria for clinical practice [8].

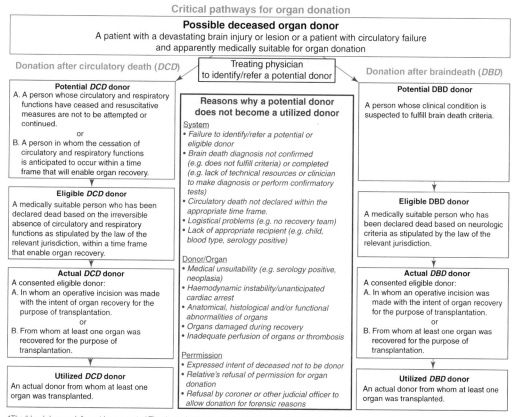

Fig. 26.1 The WHO critical pathway for organ donation [5]

26.2 Ethical and Legal Issues in Donation After Cardiac Death (DCD) [8–13]

As the numbers of patients awaiting suitable donor organ increases, it is imperative that donation by the DCD criteria will also increase. This increasing need for DCD necessitates the development of appropriate guidelines and protocols and establishing professional training and education programmes. These guidelines and protocols should holistically encompass the principles of 'end of life care', the 'dead donor rule', the legal, ethical, moral and professional aspects of DCD and should be universally acceptable.

The American Society of Anaesthesiologists (ASA) [9, 14] 'Statement on Controlled Organ Donation after Circulatory Death' is a valuable resource guide for development of policies and procedures for controlled DCD and also to address the ethical issues associated with DCD. Accordingly, the following protocols and ethical guidelines concerning controlled DCD need to be addressed:

1. First and foremost, the legally valid autonomous wishes of the patient to donate their organs must always be respected.
2. The ethical principle of beneficence (to prevent and remove evil or harm and do or promote good) and the ethical principle of nonmaleficence (not to cause harm) is reflected in preventing pain and suffering of the donor.
   (a) The principle of double effect in which an act that has an intended beneficial

effect (relieving a patient's pain) must not be performed with the intention to cause an adverse effect (hastening death).

3. The principle of social justice—the fair distribution of benefits and burdens to all members of a society.

4. The roles of the team members need to be well defined, to prevent any perceived, actual or potential conflict of interest between the interests of the potential DCD donor and the recipient.

5. The risks and benefits of organ procurement and transplantation as well a complete disclosure of the outcomes of DCD programmes on organ transplant should be discussed with recipients and potential DCD donors or their surrogate decision-makers as applicable.

6. There must be respect for the Dead Donor Rule [7, 8], which does not allow the procurement of organs from patients who are not declared dead and prohibits killing patients for organ procurement.

7. Informed consent must be obtained and documented in the medical record for antemortem procedures performed on potential controlled DCD donors.

8. Physicians whose values or religious beliefs do not align with the patient's wishes may recuse themselves from participating in the care of the patient.

9. The treating intensivist should be responsible for providing care to the potential donor, including administration of medications to ease pain and suffering without hastening the death, withdrawing the life sustaining therapy, declaring death and recording the time of death. The treating intensivist should in no way be involved in the process of organ procurement, transplantation of the organs or care of the recipient.

10. The discussion on organ donation and the consent for the same should be made by the local organ procurement organisation or authority and separate informed consent should be obtained. Consent also needs to be obtained for any ante mortem procedures (cannulation, administration of medications, bronchoscopy, etc.) and appropriate documentation is done in the medical records with instructions for 'Do not Resuscitate' orders.

11. The consent for withdrawal of life sustaining treatment should be independent and made before any consideration for organ donation and should be documented in the medical records.

12. End of life care to the potential donor takes priority in providing comfort with medications (narcotics and/or sedatives before extubation) without hastening the process of death. Also, efforts should be made to preserve the privacy, dignity, and religious or spiritual sentiments of the donor and the family.

The modified Maastricht classification [15] (Table 26.1) most widely used to categorise DCD process, based on the site of death, the locations where DCD can be practiced depending on the site of death, nature of death and the type of DCD process applicable to each category.

Patients who have sustained significant neurological injuries but who do not fulfil criteria for brain death can be ideal candidates for controlled DCD and patients with other diagnoses and who are under ICU care, and in whom a decision is made to withdraw treatment. In these patients consent/authorisation is obtained from the family and from the patient also especially if a premorbid declaration is in place.

Uncontrolled DCD presents separate challenges as in the control of warm ischemic injury, assessment of donation potential, mobilisation of retrieval services and approaching the family for consent and authorisation to proceed. Due to logistical reasons uncontrolled DCD is restricted only to kidney retrieval and limited to only transplant centres or centres where a retrieval team is readily available.

Table 26.1 The modified Maastricht Classification (2013) [15]

Category	Circumstances	Controlled/ uncontrolled	Location of care
Category-I: Uncontrolled	Dead on Arrival	Uncontrolled	ED in a transplant centre
	1A. Out of Hospital		Sudden cardiac arrest, unanticipated, No resuscitation efforts. WIT as per standard guidelines
	1B. In Hospital		
Category-II: Uncontrolled	Unsuccessful resuscitation	Uncontrolled	ED in a transplant centre. Sudden cardiac arrest, unanticipated, Unsuccessful resuscitation efforts.
	1A. Out of Hospital		
	1B. In Hospital		
Category-III: Controlled	Withdrawal of life sustaining therapy (WLST)	Controlled	ICU and ED in both Transplant and Nontransplant centres. Planned withdrawal of life sustaining therapy
Category-IV: Controlled	Cardiac arrest in a brain-dead donor	Uncontrolled/ Controlled	ICU in transplant centre. Sudden cardiac arrest while awaiting testing for brain death or management of potential brain-dead donor
Category-V	Unexpected cardiac arrest in ICU patient	Uncontrolled	ICU in a transplant centre

26.3 Process of DCD [15, 16]

The potential donor in DCD is the one in whom 'imminent death' is anticipated. These are the individuals in whom death is not confirmed by neurological criteria, but they are maintained on assisted mechanical ventilation and a decision is made to withdraw treatment and death can happen in the next 4 h.

Donation after circulatory death involves removal of organs from the voluntary donor with residual neurological activity and thus is ineligible for donation based on neurological criteria as applied to donation after brain death. Patients with other diagnoses in whom withdrawal of treatment is planned may also be considered for DCD. The process of donation involves withdrawal of all life sustaining treatment and allowing circulatory arrest to occur and retrieving organs after the mandatory short wait is completed as applicable. The process of DCD is summarised in Fig. 26.2.

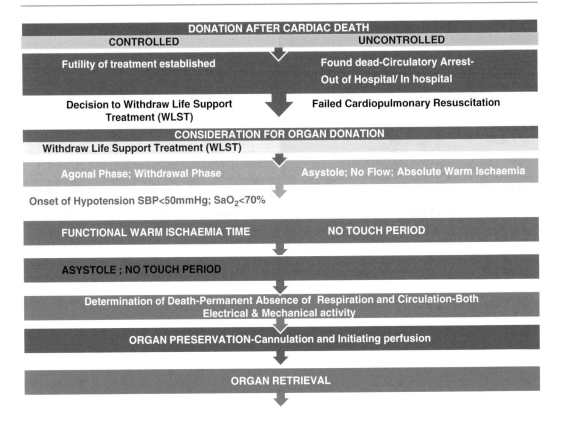

Fig. 26.2 Process of Donation after Cardiac Death (DCD)

26.4 Acceptable Time Limits in DCD

Controlled DCD	Uncontrolled DCD
Functional WIT starts when Systolic BP is below 50 mmHg or 60 mmHg till cannulation and beginning of organ perfusion.	Warm Ischaemia starts from Asystole till cannulation and beginning of organ perfusion
Acceptable functional WIT < 30 min	

No flow—Kidney <30 min, Liver <15 min

CPR Duration—<30 min

No touch period—2–20 min, depending on local institutional/national protocols

Total WIT—120–150 min

Steps of DCD are as follows (shown in Fig. 26.3) [8, 15–17].

1. Discussion on futility of treatment leading to decision to discontinuation of treatment—this happens to be the most critical step and the trigger for further series of events culminating in donation of the organs.

2. Seeking consent from the family members for donation. This discussion has to happen only after the family has consented for termination of the life sustaining treatment. This has to be undertaken by the transplant coordination team and the treating intensivist. At no point any member from the transplant team should be involved in either the decision to withdraw treatment or in the process of obtaining consent for DCD.

3. Allocation of organs to prospective recipients

4. Management of the donor before withdrawing treatment—all supportive care needs to be continued. All measures to facilitate donation (like vasoactive drugs, increasing ventilatory support, insertion of intravenous lines) but without hastening death or causing harm to the donor can be continued.

Potential Donor
- Adult patient in ICU-Futility of treatment established due to nature of illness
  OR
- In ED -Dead on arrival, Unsuccessful resuscitation, Cardiac arrest while awaiting establishing brain death
- Establish medical suitability of donation,
- Futility of treatment established
- Consent for Withdrawal of Life Sustaining Treatment (WLST)

Authorisation for Donation
- Donor family approached by specialist staff in organ donation/Transplant Coordinator
- Consent for organ donation obtained
- Ensure haemodynamic stability till withdrawal of treatment
- Withdrawal of treatment (cardiorespiratory support) as per end of life care protocol
- Organ retrieval scheduled as per consent for various organs to be retrieved and ischaemic vulnerability of organs
- Withdrawal of treatment-in ICU / OR based on consent obtained, premortem interventions authorised

Declaration of Death
- Establish irreversible cessation of cardiorespiratory function
- Absence of central pulses
- Absent heart sounds
- Asystole on continuous ECG display
- Absent pulsatile flow on intraarterial pressure monitoring
- Absence of contractile function on echocardiography
- Absence of pupillary response to light, absent motor response, to painful stimulus
- Acceptable waiting period for cessation of circulation -60 min -4 h depending on institutional protocols

Documentation
- Time of withdrawal of life ustaining treatment
- Time when sysolic BP reduced below critical value (50 mmHg), Time when oxygen saturation decrease < 70% (ONSET OF FUNCTIONAL WARM ISCHEMIA)
- No touch Period 2 -20 minutes depending on country protocols; Standard criteria globally -5 min
- Time of death -after mandatory NO TOUCH PERIOD, after recording of irreversibly absent electromechanical criteria of circulatory function.

Post mortem interventions- Organ preservation
- Donor shifted to OR
- Measures to minimise warm ischaemia -rapid cannulation of femoral vesslels/ infra diaphragmatic aorta -Machine Perfusion or Standard Cold Storage
- Machine Perfusion -Normothermic Regional Perfusion /Normothermic Ex Vivo Machine Perfusion / Hypothermic Machine Perfusion
- Premortem cannulation of Femoral vessels, Heparinisation -Ethical and Legal concerns

Fig. 26.3 Summary of process of Donation after Cardiac Death (DCD)

5. Withdrawal of life sustaining treatment (WLST)—Once the retrieval teams are available, withdrawal of treatment is initiated either in the ICU or operating room as per the institutional or local protocol. Withdrawal in the ICU is preferable to minimise the ischemic time.

6. Withdrawal process includes administration of sedative and opioid medications as per end of life care guidelines, cessation of mechani-

cal ventilation and other medications and extubation. Proper documentation needs to be done for: (a) Time of withdrawal of treatment and (b) time of onset of hemodynamic instability with desaturation on pulse oximetry for accurate determination of the 'Functional Ischaemic Time'. If lung retrieval is also planned, then reintubation and recruitment should be done only after declaration of death.

7. Diagnosis of circulatory death—The most debatable point in DCD is the declaration of death after the cessation of circulation and respiration. Death should be declared at the earliest in a manner that is scientifically, ethically and professionally acceptable to minimise the warm ischaemia time while ensuring that the dead donor rule is not breached. Towards this the globally accepted circulatory criteria are applied. These include continuous cessation of spontaneous cardiorespiratory efforts for 5 min to ensure that risk of autoresuscitation has passed.

On completion of the mandatory waiting period, the continuous absence of circulation (both electrical and mechanical) needs to be demonstrated and documented before declaration of death in DCD:

1. Absence of central pulses
2. Absence of heart sounds
3. Continuous Asystole on ECG display
4. Absence of pulsatile flow on arterial pressure monitoring.
5. Absence of pupillary response, corneal reflex and absence of any motor response to painful stimuli (supra orbital pressure) should also be documented.

The time of death is also documented in the medical records.

The deceased donor is then shifted to the operating room (if WLST is performed in the ICU or if the proposed donor is from the ED) quickly and with respect and dignity for the retrieval process. The coordinator should ensure proper communication and documentation of all timings and consents with completion of WHO Safety checklist.

A variety of interventions may be necessary in the antemortem period to prevent, minimise, or reverse the ischaemic injury. These include the following:

1. Efforts towards optimisation of clinical parameters to improve the viability of organs by ensuring euvolemia, haemodynamic stability and normothermia till the time of withdrawal of support.
2. Ante mortem interventions as permitted under the local regulations of the state or institution (administration of heparin, steroids, vasodilators, cannulation and bronchoscopy)
3. Minimising the time interval between the diagnosis of death and organ retrieval (by withdrawing life support in the operating room, antemortem cannulation)
4. Post-mortem reperfusion of particularly vulnerable organs like liver
5. Early tissue typing to allow prompt identification and mobilisation of suitable recipients.

The warm ischemia time lasts from the point of asystole, till the end of mandatory no touch period. The duration of no touch period is essential to confirm cardiac death and varies in different countries. This mandatory no touch period is followed by cannulation of aorta and initiation of cold perfusion which is considered as the start of the cold ischemia time. This could vary but could last anywhere up to another 30–40 min.

Interventions or manoeuvres which may restore cerebral circulation like cardio-pulmonary resuscitation (CPR), full cardiopulmonary bypass, intubation and mechanical ventilation, institution of perfusion either regional or systemic (ECMO), should not be permitted during the mandatory waiting period. If any interventions are deemed necessary, complete exclusion of cerebral circulation must be achieved before instituting the modality.

The University of Wisconsin predictive tool (Table 26.2) [18] can be valuable in predicting the suitability for organ donation after cardiac death and predict the likelihood of death within a given time. Patients in the younger age group, non-triggered modes of ventilation, high FiO2,

Table 26.2 University of Wisconsin donation after cardiac death evaluation tool [18]

Criteria	Assigned points	Pt. score
Spontaneous respirations after 10 mm		
Rate >12	1	
Rate <12	3	
TV > 200 cm³	1	
TV < 200 cm³	3	
NIF < 20	3	
NIF > 20	1	
No spontaneous respirations	9	
Vasopressors/inotropes		
No vasopressors/inotropes	1	
Single vasopressor/inotropes	2	
Multiple vasopressors/inotropes	3	
Patient age		
0–30	1	
31–50	2	
51+	3	
Intubation		
Endotracheal tube	3	
Tracheostomy	1	
Oxygenation after 10 min		
02 Sat >90%	1	
02 Sat 80–89%	2	
02 Sat <79%	3	
Final score		
Time from extubation to expiration		

use of inotropes and a low arterial pH all indicate rapid circulatory collapse. Most patients considered for DCD die within 2 h of withdrawal of treatment. Any increase in the waiting period may lead to non-pursual of the retrieval and thus loss of suitable donor.

26.5   Ischaemia Reperfusion Injury (IRI) and Organ Preservation After DCD [15, 17, 19–24]

Organs retrieved from DCD donors are exposed to greater ischaemia as compared to DBD. It is well accepted that the rapidly increasing demands for organ transplantation has led to a severe shortage of transplantable organs. To overcome this deficiency, organs available by DCD, extended criteria donors (ECD) and marginal donors are being increasingly accepted. However, organs obtained by these procedures tolerate ischaemia poorly leading to increased incidence of IRI, and associated risk of early allograft dysfunction (EAD), primary non-function (PNF), poor long-term graft and patient survival and increased incidence of biliary complications in case of liver transplantation. This can be seen as 'declining DCD' in up to 40% patients on the grounds 'prolonged time to asystole' or deemed as medically unfit.

IRI is a result of the combined detrimental effects of (1) ischaemic period during organ retrieval and preservation and (2) reperfusion injury on transplantation. IRI is a multifactorial inflammatory state associated with hypoxia, metabolic stress, leukocyte extravasation, cellular death pathways and activation of the immune response. There is profound efflux of accumulated metabolic products formed during ischaemia leading to a profound inflammatory response during reperfusion and causing cellular injury. This cascade of changes is common in all donor organs obtained by DCD or ECD and the severity of effects depends on the different organs.

Different organs have different susceptibilities to ischaemic injury with irreversible loss of function. All organs retrieved for transplantation by DCD and ECD are exposed to prolonged donor warm ischaemia time (DWIT). There exists significant variation in the accepted definition and acceptable duration of DWIT. In addition, the concept of functional DWIT (FDWIT) also needs to be understood. This starts once the donor physiological values start decreasing below critically acceptable thresholds, and includes haemodynamic instability, mandatory wait period (No touch period), time from incision to cannulation of aorta and cross clamp all of which form the total DWIT and affect the outcome of the individual graft organs. The current acceptable thresholds include systolic blood pressure below 50 mmHg and oxygen saturation less than 70%. FDWIT ends with beginning of cold perfusion or cross clamp. As different organs have different susceptibilities to warm ischaemia, specific

Table 26.3 Functional donor warm ischaemia time for organ retrieved by Donation after Cardiac Death (DCD) [15]

Organ	Maximum functional donor warm ischaemia time (min)	Comments
Kidney	120	Kidneys obtained through DCD have higher incidence of delayed graft function, but long-term function is similar to those from DBD. Maximum acceptable time can be extended to another 120 min provided viability of organ can be demonstrated.
Liver	30	Acceptable outcomes seen with DCD livers but can be associated with higher incidence of postoperative morbidity, graft failure or biliary complications as compared with DBD organ.
Lung	60	Time to reinflation of the lungs (not recommencement of ventilation) is critical rather than the time to cold perfusion.
Pancreas	30	

thresholds for individual organs are accepted. If these thresholds are exceeded prior to retrieval, then retrieval itself may be abandoned or the organs may be discarded if it is post retrieval. Hence, correct recognition and documentation of the onset time for FDWIT is mandatory. There should be facility for immediate cannulation of the aorta and beginning of cold perfusion. Many of the events associated with DWIT are nonmodifiable as they occur prior to declaration of death. As a general rule organ retrieval time should be as minimum as possible, for liver it varies from 60 min (UK) to 90 min (Netherlands). The acceptable FDWIT for various organs commonly accepted by DCD process [16] are as given in Table 26.3. Standardisation of acceptance criteria for variables such as donor BMI, Age, CIT, FDWIT, procurement procedure times FDWIT, asystole to cross clamp time are all essential to reduce complications and improve graft viability.

Standard static cold storage (SCS) [22] remains the gold standard in graft preservation for all organs. This is achieved through cooling to 4 °C by perfusion with various organ preserving solutions (OPS), thus to reduce oxygen demand and allowing for survival of the organ in the hypoxic environment. IRI is a combination of oxidative stress, inflammatory signalling and structural changes contributing to poor organ function. The lack of perfusion during SCS leads to accumulation of cellular waste products, hypoxia induced alteration in enzymes necessary for breakdown of metabolic products and debris,

release of free radicals, aggravating microvascular and parenchymal cell injury and death.

This inefficient protection of the organs by SCS can be the main reason for large number of organs being discarded in the assumption of doubtful viability. Adopting techniques to assess, preserve and recover the marginal grafts ex vivo could dramatically increase the pool of available organs. Various strategies have been recommended and are being developed to help in the assessment, preservation and recovering the marginal organs which would have been discarded.

26.6 Machine Perfusion (MP) [19–24]

MP has shown the greatest potential in this aspect of organ preservation and various modifications of the same are currently being evaluated and applied in regular clinical practice. MP is expected to provide a physiological environment by circulation of an oxygen rich perfusate through the organ either through normothermia or hypothermia. MP has the potential to aid in (a) functional assessment of the organ viability and prediction of post-transplant outcome and (b) extending preservation time and thus reducing ischaemic time and attenuate reperfusion injury, (c) allow for recovery of organs initially considered unsuitable for transplant, (d) aid in organ repair thus resulting in better quality organ retrieval and (e) extending the time between organ retrieval and transplantation.

Table 26.4 Comparison of Normothermic Machine Perfusion (NMP) and Static Cold Storage (SCS) [21]

Factors	NMP	SCS
Preservation time (h)	12+	4–6
Temperature (°C)	37	4
Oxygenation	Normoxia	Hypoxia
Parenchymal preservation	Yes	Yes
Functional evaluation	Yes	No
Therapeutic intervention	Yes	No

Various strategies for MP have been utilised with a variety of temperature settings. Based on the temperature settings MP can be classified into hypothermic (temp 0–12 °C), subnormothermic (25–34 °C) and normothermic (35–38 °C).

The typical ex vivo MP circuit contains a humidified organ chamber, perfusion solution, reservoir for perfusion solution collection, oxygenator and optional leukocyte filter (used when blood is used as perfusion solution) connected via sterile tubing.

Principal components of MP used in liver preservation include blood reservoir, pumps (some circuits may comprise two pumps for hepatic artery and portal vein separately when used for liver perfusion), an oxygenator and a heat exchanger.

Normothermic MP (NMP) provides a near physiologic environment for assessing overall graft function, metabolic demand and viability, and may provide more accurate predictions for primary graft failure and post-transplant outcomes. Multiple trials in both laboratory and clinical setting have shown that NMP preserved grafts perform well, abolishing the negative effects of prolonged ischaemia and providing for extended preservation times. The probable advantages of NMP over SCS are as follows (Table 26.4):

26.7 Functional Assessment of Organs [21]

Numerous factors are of importance when considering any organ for transplant. These factors include but not limited to:

1. Donor cause of death
2. Process of Donation (DCD vs. DBD)
3. Donor age
4. Organ retrieval/explant time
5. Presence of graft injury or disease.

Of particular concern is assessment of these organs for viability. The functional assessment of these organs can be facilitated by utilising MP as given in Table 26.5.

Table 26.5 Evaluation of Donation after Cardiac Death (DCD) organ function and viability preserved by Normothermic Machine Perfusion (NMP) [21]

Organ	Proposed ischemic time on machine perfusion	Assessment factors
Heart	~4 h	1. Aortic pressure, Flow rate,
		2. Haemodynamic profile,
		3. Elevated lactate levels both arterial and venous, Noninvasive functional assessment,
		4. Coronary angiography,
		5. Functional echocardiographic assessment, Contrast echocardiography to assess coronary perfusion.
Lung	~4 h	1. Haemodynamic stability (Pulmonary artery pressure, flow, pulmonary vascular resistance)
		2. Perfusate haemogas and biochemical properties (arterial blood gas (ABG) values, lactate levels, pH)
		3. Gross organ anatomy (weight, consolidation, oedema)
		4. Ventilation (airway pressure, dynamic compliance)
		5. Oxygenation capacity (PaO2/FiO2, ΔPO2, ΔPCO2)
		6. Bronchoscopic and radiologic visualisation
		7. Bronchoalveolar lavage (BAL) fluid and tissue biopsies for microbiology, metabolic and molecular analysis.
		8. Research is on to identify specific biomarkers predictive of post-transplant graft outcome both in laboratory animal studies and human. Increased levels of glucose, and pyruvate/lactate ratios can lead to pulmonary oedema and poor lung function. Changes in inflammatory gene expression and cytokine levels also been studied. However, a clear consensus is yet to be agreed upon, for more specific criteria capable of predicting transplant outcomes need to be defined.
Liver	~8–12 h	Acceptable Viability criteria by MP include:
		1. Lactate levels below 2.5 mmol/L,
		2. Bile production,
		3. Acid base homeostasis,
		4. Pressure/flow parameters,
		5. Homogenous perfusion with 'soft' parenchymal consistency,
		6. Perfusion parameters,
		7. Perfusate properties,
		8. Perfusate pH to assess liver injury and function.
		9. Acidosis is indicative of metabolic disruption.
		10. Elevated levels of bicarbonate and Factor V indicate viable graft with preserved metabolic and synthetic function.
		11. Hepatocellular biomarkers include measurement of aspartate aminotransferase (AST), alanine aminotransferase (ALT), glutamate dehydrogenase (GLDH) and beta galactosidase enzymes can also be used to cellular injury and death.
		12. Circulating lactate levels and lactate clearance has been used as predictive indicator of liver evaluation.
		13. Volume of bile produced, bile content and specific properties are more significant. Bile production more than 30 g in 6 h of NMP indicates good graft function with low perfusate transaminase and potassium levels and decreased venous congestion and cell necrosis.
		14. Markers of cholangiopathy are also essential, and need to be monitored.
		15. Production of alkaline bile (pH >7.5) happens to be a good marker of cholangiocyte function.

26.8 Classification of Perfusion Techniques Based on Preservation Temperature [22]

Various strategies of MP and at different temperatures have been described. There are no standard criteria to describe the perfusion temperature or the technical details leading to wide variation in the studies. Most of these techniques have focused on liver perfusion but the same broad concepts are applicable to other organs.

26.9 Hypothermic Machine Perfusion (HMP) (0–12 °C)

Hypothermic MP is designed to provide perfusion with perfusate temperature at 4 °C. It has been well described in kidney transplantation and shown to improve early graft function and improved 1-year graft survival.

Perfusion by this technique and temperature is shown to reduce tissue metabolism and also through the preservative solution, provides the necessary metabolic substrates for ATP synthesis and removal of metabolic waste products by washing the parenchyma and endothelium.

Some of the proposed benefits of HMP are as follows:

1. Minimisation of cold ischaemic injury
2. Improved graft viability
3. Protection against biliary lesions
4. Restore mitochondrial redox activity and cellular energy status
5. Reduced inflammatory response by preventing activation of Kupffer cells, reduced activity of neutrophils and platelets during reperfusion.

It is considered safe technique as if the machine fails at any stage, the graft continues to be protected under the standard cold storage conditions. The main disadvantage of HMP is the inability to have a 'real time' assessment of liver function as the liver does not produce bile during hypothermia.

It has been shown to be successful in providing good quality DCD grafts as compared to non-perfused grafts with low incidence of biliary strictures or early allograft dysfunction.

26.10 Midthermic Machine Perfusion (13–24 °C)

Perfusion at these temperatures were proposed to achieve a balance between the adverse effects of cold ischaemia and the high metabolic demands of normothermia. In addition, exposure to normothermic temperatures after a period of cold storage can result in significant risk of oxidative stress.

Advantages of midthermic perfusion include:

1. Lower intravascular resistance,
2. Better preserved microcirculation
3. Stronger mitochondrial function
4. Higher energy charge
5. Better bile production.

Clinical evaluation of up to 3 h of midthermic (21 °C) perfusion has not shown any signs of liver injury or dysfunction when the grafts were gradually warmed to the final temperature over 1 h, in contrast significantly improved liver function was seen.

26.11 Subnormothermic Machine Perfusion (25–34 °C)

Subnormothermic machine perfusion can be feasible without the use of red blood cells as the respiratory chain activity of mitochondria is reduced and leading to reduced demand of cellular energy. This simplifies the procedure and could also reduce the costs. The benefits have been demonstrated in experimental setting seen as reduced hepatic and biliary injury, biliary improvements and lower serum alkaline phosphatase levels. Developing better preservation protocols have the potential to improve graft function from marginal donors thus increasing the donor pool.

Controlled oxygenated rewarming is the most recent application of the perfusion machine, where perfusion begins at hypothermic temperatures and gradually progressing to subnormothermia. Controlled oxygenated rewarming has been shown to be beneficial in clinical setting also, as seen by lower aspartate aminotransferase levels and 100% graft and patient survival at 6 months post transplantation. Subnormothermic ex vivo perfusion may be utilised as complimentary to other preservation techniques. One example of this can be 'super cooling' technique. In this technique prior to supercooling liver is loaded with cryoprotectants so also after post supercooling rewarming. Livers are loaded with nonmetabolizable glucose derivative (3-0methyl-D-glucose). Livers are supercooled avoiding intracellular ice formation and at the end of supercooling, 3 h of subnormothermic perfusion was performed to achieve an adequate recovery period for the liver before the transplantation.

26.12 Normothermic Machine Perfusion (35–38 °C) [22–24]

Normothermic MP is designed to provide full physiological cellular metabolism by facilitating perfusion of oxygenated blood-based solutions at body temperature. NMP has the potential to restore normal metabolic physiology, recondition marginal organs and allow for assessment of graft viability. Multiple options of the NMP have been developed and more widely used in liver perfusion and preservation. Functional markers to evaluate liver function include bile production and composition, lactate clearance, ability to maintain acid base balance (pH) and transaminases in the perfusate, glucose metabolism have all been recommended as surrogate markers of IRI, liver transplantability and graft performance after transplantation.

Normothermia usually refers to the physiological body temperature, 37 °C for humans. The idea associated with this technique is to replicate the normal metabolism of the liver outside the body, providing oxygen and essential substrates in an environment of normal temperature (37 °C), avoiding ischaemia and hypothermia altogether. One main advantage of NMP is the opportunity to evaluate the viability of the organ before transplantation by measuring the markers of hepatic metabolism (bile production, liver enzymes assay). The main difficulty is in providing sufficient oxygen and other necessary substrates to prevent graft deterioration and bacterial contamination. Typical perfusate used in NMP is composed of concentrates of red blood cells, plasma nutrients, cofactors and insulin, antibiotics, electrolytes and buffers, making NMP a complex and expensive procedure. Extracellular oxygen carriers or oxygen carrying plasma expanders are being proposed as alternative to usage of human blood products.

NMP is associated with the following benefits:

1. Mitigate the negative effects of simple cold storage
2. Beneficial in defatting by the addition of pharmacologic 'Defatting cocktail' which can stimulate lipid metabolism
3. Ability to extend graft preservation times up to 20–86 h.

First multicentric randomised trial of NMP vs. SCS in which 170 livers from NMP were compared with 164 preserved by SCS. The study revealed that there was a 50% reduction in organ rejection and 54% longer preservation time. However, there was no advantage in terms of major outcome measures like graft or patient survival or the frequency of biliary complications. Favourable results in terms of length of hospital stay or graft survival, in rejected livers exposed to varying periods of cold storage have also been reported.

In the coming years NMP can change the concept of organ preservation from being a method of treatment to that of repair of the organs. The use of these ex vivo perfusion techniques has changed the perspective of DCD transplantation and can act as stimulus to expand the organ retrieval process across all ICUs. Another outcome of this NMP is shift of priority to that of organ recovery. Organ recovery leads to better quality grafts and increasing the possibility of using organs which would have been normally considered non viable and unsuitable for transplantation.

The main challenges of NMP include providing good oxygen carrying (using blood and blood components) without encountering problems of thrombus formation, vascular damage and infection. The other concern is to provide not only sufficient oxygen carrying capacity but also other physiologic mediators (substrates and cofactors) essential for homeostasis in the organ ex vivo.

Normal blood can be the ideal perfusate for NMP but necessitates sophisticated technology to maintain oxygenation and adequate intravascular flow, without activating circulating blood cells, microthrombi and associated negative effects on microcirculation of the organ. Replacing the blood with synthetic solution with complete range of functions as blood is another challenge.

26.13 Normothermic Regional Perfusion (NRP) [23]

NRP involves in situ perfusion of subdiaphragmatic abdominal organs following isolation from the rest of the circulation. This in situ oxygenated perfusion is initiated after declaration of circulatory death and prior to organ procurement, thus resuscitate the organs and restore the intracellular energy stores. NRP necessitates use of either cardiopulmonary (CPB)/extra corporeal membrane oxygenator (ECMO) to recover the donor blood into a membrane oxygenator and then deliver it to the subdiaphragmatic aorta. This technique has been shown to be successful in both laboratory conditions and clinical usage and is being widely practiced in Europe and USA. The 1–2 year graft survival rates were more than 85.7% and 71.4%, respectively.

26.14 International DCD Programmes [7]

Many countries have actively adopted the DCD programme to increase the donor pool and thus facilitate transplantation. The methods adopted to determine death, the definition and duration of the observation period after circulatory arrest vary amongst each country. Similarly, the process of consent either 'opt-in or opt-out' of DCD also varies between nations with most nations adopting a 'Opt-in' registration process. Controlled DCD is the most common mode in UK, whereas France, Spain and some centres in UK follow the Uncontrolled DCD model. The mandatory waiting period 'NO TOUCH period', varies according across the different countries and varies from 2 min in USA to maximum of 20 min in Italy, as against the universally accepted norm of 5 min.

26.15 Lessons from UK Success Story in Overcoming Ethical, Legal and Professional Challenges [25, 26]

Donation after circulatory death accounts for nearly 40% of all deceased donations in UK, and along with Netherlands they form the world leaders in DCD. The predominant form of DCD in UK is 'Category III-Awaiting cardiac arrest or the Controlled DCD'.

The number of donations by DCD has shown a rapid increase by 170% (200–539 donors) between the period from 2007 to 2012. More families seem to consent for DCD than DBD.

The reasons for this shift could be multifactorial, but the major contributory factor is the attempt to resolve the ethical, legal and professional challenges inherent to DCD. In 2008, the Organ Donation Task force made 14 recommendations, with the aim of increasing organ donation by 50% over 5 years.

Recommendation 3 of the Taskforce states that 'Urgent attention is required to resolve outstanding legal, ethical and professional issues in order to ensure that all clinicians are able to work within a clear and unambiguous framework of good practice. Additionally, an independent UK-wide Donation Ethics Group should be established'.

Accordingly, in 2008 seven major ethical, legal and professional guidances have been published relating to deceased donation and DCD in particular. This professional framework established in UK is the strongest in the world.

In any organ donation and transplantation programme, two key ethical, legal and professional principles 'Dead Donor Rule (DDR)' and 'Consenting Donor Rule' need to be understood and which have been well addressed in the guidelines. The term DDR was introduced in 1988 by John Robertson and in principle states that 'Organs be removed only from dead patients'. Over the years numerous alternate interpretations have been made. Arthur Caplan interpretation is the most widely accepted and states that 'Organs (vital organs) can be taken only from those who have been clearly, unequivocally pronounced dead. The limitation of such an interpretation was that even the minimal premortem interventions such as referral to an organ donation organisation, blood tests for tissue typing and virology, consent from the families for donation, delay in time and/or change of location for withdrawal of life sustaining treatment are not permissible for a successful implementation of DCD.

The 'Consenting Donor Rule (CDR)' addresses the legal standard required for consent for donation. Even in systems with 'hard presumed consent' the consent issue needs to be addressed by a societal or governmental decision rather than at an individual or the family level. In the UK, the Human Transplantation (Wales) Act 2013, came into force in December 2015, and is applicable only to all Welsh residents above 18 years age. This introduces the concept of 'Deemed Consent' a soft form of presumed consent. Under this unless a resident has opted out of the UK organ Donor Register their consent is deemed, but still the family will be approached, to ascertain that if the family is aware of any expressed objection by the individual for donation. The introduction of this 'Opt-Out/Deemed Consent' process significantly increased the deceased donation rates from an 18.0 pmp (per

million population) at the introduction of the act in 2015 to 28.9 pmp in 2019 and the DCD rates had increased from 44.4% in first quarter of 2016 to 76.5% in last quarter of 2018.

In addition, the seven guidelines (Annexure) published in the UK following the 2008 Task force recommendations to resolve the outstanding legal, ethical and professional issues related to organ donation and as response keeping in view the challenges of DDR and CDR principles have aided in better implementation of DCD and its resultant success.

26.16 DCD in India [4]

DCD is not practiced in India keeping in view the legal permissibility as per THOA criteria. THOA although recognises DCD as a mode of organ retrieval but fail to further delineate the exact process or the other ethical, moral and clinical aspects of DCD especially with regard to withdrawal of life sustaining treatment, etc. Also, there are no existing protocols or guidelines established by any institution or organisation with regards to the practice of DCD. DCD in the present mode is seen as applicable limitedly only to retrieval and transplantation of tissues. DCD can also happen only in instances where a confirmed brain-dead donor develops a sudden cardiac arrest while awaiting retrieval.

26.17 Outcomes From DCD [9]

The long-term outcomes from transplanted kidneys retrieved by DCD has been comparable in both DBD and DCD. In case of uncontrolled DCD, the organ function can be assessed by machine perfusion and assessment performed to identify the unsuitable organs. Similarly, for liver, the long-term outcomes are comparable when using cardiopulmonary bypass or ex vivo normothermic perfusion to establish perfusion to reverse ischaemia. For lung transplantation from DCD donors although results are good especially when used with ex vivo lung perfusion. Heart transplantation using a graft from DCD donor can be controversial as when death has been declared on cardiac criteria and when the same heart is restarted.

26.18 Future Trends and Directions for DCD [9, 19, 24, 25]

For patients with end-stage organ failure, solid organ transplantation offers a cost-effective treatment that increases both quality of life and life expectancy. There remains a discrepancy between the need for transplantation and the number of donors. This deficiency of availability of transplantable organs places increasing demand on donation following declaration of death either by the neurological criteria or circulatory criteria.

Accordingly, there is an increasing number of donations happening by the DCD criteria. This necessitates the development of appropriate guidelines and protocols and establishing professional training and education programmes. These guidelines and protocols should holistically encompass the principles of 'end of life care', the 'dead donor rule', the legal, ethical, moral and professional aspects of DCD and should be universally acceptable.

Theoretically, MP can simulate physiological condition ex vivo and aid in better preservation and evaluation of the graft by providing continuous circulation of oxygen, essential nutrients and adequate ATP stores to restore normal physiology, while flushing out metabolites and preventing their accumulation. NMP can also be costlier than SCS, and also be more challenging logistically.

Further studies will be needed to explore the long-term outcomes, late complications, outcomes in specific high-risk groups, viability biomarkers, optimum and maximum duration of perfusion, perfusate composition, organ specific directed therapeutic interventions during NMP.

Consideration for organ and tissue donation should be routine part of care in any ICU or ED. Emphasis should be placed on presumptive consent rather than opt in registration as exists in most countries, improving the quality of organs retrieved by permitting premortem interventions to minimise the warm ischaemia time, maintain-

ing cardiorespiratory stability till withdrawal of life sustaining treatment and implementing withdrawal of treatment in the operating room. The guidelines and protocols should also include measures to be initiated if the death does not occur within the acceptable time frame for donation and the further management of the patient thereof.

Important Terminologies: Donation after Cardiac Death (DCD)
- Donation after Brain Death (DBD)
- Donation after Cardiac/Circulatory Death (DCD)
- Dead Donor Rule (DDR)
- Warm Ischaemia Time (WIT)
- Functional Warm Ischaemia Time (f-WIT)
- No-Touch Period
- Machine Perfusion (MP)
- Normothermic Regional Perfusion (NRP)
- Normothermic Ex Vivo Machine Perfusion (NMP)
- Hypothermic Machine Perfusion (HMP)

Key Points
- Donation after cardiac death (DCD) is becoming increasingly popular amongst the transplant community. This resurgence has been the result of increasing number of hopeful recipients on the waiting list.
- Appropriate modifications in existing legislations to cover areas of ethical, legal and professional concerns regarding ethical, legal and professional standards involving DCD.
- Deemed (Presumed) consent and authorisation should become standard of care in all ICUs.
- End of life care and Organ donation should become a standard practice in all

hospitals and especially intensive care units.

- When considering DCD for a patient, care to be taken as regards the ethical, legal and moral principles of donation which itself is altruistic in nature and due diligence be essayed in providing 'end of life care'.

- The acceptance and implementation of DCD process should not become a deterrent for donations by the neurological criteria (DBD).

- DCD grafts should not be taken as interchangeable with DBD grafts. The degree of risk associated with each organ offered and the recipient situation need to be understood and balance situation needs to be established based on each individual centre.

- The process of DCD places special challenges as it differs from the process of donation after brain death (DBD).

- The limitations of SCS in organ preservation needs to be understood. As an alternative preservation strategy MP is emerging as an Ex vivo strategy to provide better solutions to protect and evaluate the organs before transplantation.

- NMP can provide a near normal physiologic environment for overall assessment of the graft function, and viability and predict post-transplant outcomes. Thus, by utilising NMP, the number of organs which were being discarded can be utilised thus improving the donor pool.

Annexure: Major Ethical, Legal and Professional Publications on Deceased Organ Donation, United Kingdom [26]

The following seven guidelines were published in the UK following the 2008 Task force recommendations to resolve the outstanding legal, ethical and professional issues related to organ donation and as response keeping in view the challenges of dead donor rule (DDR) and consenting donor rule (CDR) principles have aided in better implementation of donation after circulatory death (DCD) and its success.

The seven major UK Ethical, Legal and Professional Publications on Deceased Organ Donation since 2008 include:

1. **Guidelines by Academy of Medical Royal Colleges, Code of Practice for the Diagnosis and Confirmation of Death (2008)**—This was the revised version of the Code of Practice of 1976 and last amended in 1998 which provides guidance for the diagnosis of death using cardiorespiratory (circulatory) criteria as modified from neurological criteria. This guidance is designed to be applicable to all deaths, and not just diagnosis of death for the purpose of organ donation. This also reassured the intensive care doctors involved in DCD when to diagnose and confirm death after cardiorespiratory arrest and they were acting as per standard guidance.

2. **Legal Guidance from all Four UK Jurisdictions on DCD (2009–2011)**—It provides legal guidance to medical staff involved with DCD, and recognised the difference between DBD and DCD. The deceased donation guidelines in the UK Human Tissue Act 2004, and the Human Tissue (Scotland) Act 2006, were not applicable in patient's hours before death and potential DCD. This also justified the procedures related to DCD. It also clarified that the present and past wishes and feelings of the adult should be respected in addition to seeking the views of the nearest relative and the primary carer of the adult and deciding when an intervention is of benefit.

   The following steps were permitted to facilitate DCD:
   (a) Delaying withdrawal of life sustaining treatment
   (b) Changing the patient's location
   (c) Maintaining physiological stability

It also emphasises that 'anything that can harm or distress to the potential donor' is unlikely to be of benefit to the patient and should be avoided.

3. **General Medical Council Guidance: 'Treatment and Care towards the End of Life' (2010)**—End of Life guidance was issued by the General Medical Council (GMC) in 2010. This established a duty on UK doctors to follow the national guidelines and procedures for identifying potential donors at the end of life and where clinically appropriate to notify the local transplant coordinator.

4. **Joint Professional Statement from the Intensive Care Society and the British Transplantation Society (2010)**—This provides unambiguous professional support from the UK Intensive Care Society and more importantly provides support for admission to ICU purely for Organ Donation. This also provides guidance to intensive care physicians before and after patient's death and also safe practice guidance for lung DCD with resultant increase in lung DCD to 16%.

5. **Joint Professional Statement from the College of Emergency Medicine and the British Transplantation Society (2011)**—It is understood that up to 15% potential deceased donors come from the Emergency Department. This joint statement provides professional support for the identification of potential donors in the Emergency Department and support for managing organ donation from the Emergency Department itself if admission to ICU is not possible.

6. **Independent UK Donation Ethics Committee Guidance on DCD (2011)**—Established in January 2010, with support from all four UK governments and hosted by the Academy of Medical Royal Colleges, this provides independent advice and resolution on ethical aspects of organ donation and transplantation. The first major publication of UK DEC was ethical guidance for DCD in 2011.

This provides procedural and process ethical guidance for clinicians. UK DEC focuses on roles, responsibilities and conflicts of interest. Key statements by UK DEC include:

(a) Contact between the clinical team treating the potential donor and the Specialist Nurse for Organ Donation (SNOD)/ Transplant coordinator before the decision is made to withdraw life-sustaining treatment is ethically acceptable.

(b) SNODs should not provide medical care to the potential donor while they are still alive.

(c) Two senior physicians, with registration of more than at least 5 years, and at least one should be a consultant should verify that further active treatment is no longer of benefit to the patient.

(d) Care should be provided in an appropriate environment and by staff with appropriate skills and experience to deliver the end of life care plan.

(e) After death, it is acceptable for the treating clinician to take necessary actions to facilitate donation, e.g., tracheal reintubation for lung DCD.

7. **NICE Guidance on Organ Donation (2011)**—The 2011 NICE, Organ Donation for Transplantation: Improving Donor Identification and Consent Rates for Deceased Organ Donation Guidance: This recommends:

(a) A triggered referral to a SNOD if there is a:
   • Plan to withdraw life sustaining treatment
   • Plan to perform brain stem testing
   • Catastrophic brain injury (early referral), defined as absence of one or more cranial nerve reflexes, and a Glasgow Coma Score (GCS) of 4 or less not explained by sedation.

(b) While assessing the patient's best interest, the patient should be clinically stabilised in an appropriate critical care setting while the assessment for donation is performed.

(c) A collaborative approach to the family for organ donation involving:

- -A specialist nurse for organ donation.
- -A local faith representative if appropriate.

These seven guidelines help in resolving the legal, ethical and professional issues in deceased donation to ensure all clinicians are supported and are able to work within a clear and unambiguous framework of good practice.

References

1. Shroff S, Navin S. "Brain death" and "circulatory death": need for a uniform definition of death in India. Indian J Med Ethics. 2018;3(4):321–3.
2. Uniform Determination of Death Act. Chicago, Illinois; 1980. http://www.uniformlaws.org/shared/docs/determination%20of%20death/udda80.pdf. Accessed 31 Jul 2018.
3. Ministry of Law, Justice and Company Affairs, Govt of India. The Transplantation of Human Organs Act; 1994. https://mohfw.gov.in/sites/default/files/Act%20 1994.pdf. Accessed 30 Jul 2018.
4. Sharma A, Navin S. Donation after circulatory death – challenges in India. Indian Transpl Newsl. 2017;16(49):1.
5. Domínguez-Gil B, Delmonico FL, Shaheen FA, et al. The critical pathway for deceased donation: reportable uniformity in the approach to deceased donation. Transpl Int. 2011;24:373–8.
6. Sahay M. Transplantation of human organs and tissues act - "simplified". Indian J Transpl. 2018;12:84–9.
7. Robertson JA. The dead donor rule. Hast Cent Rep. 1999;29(6):6–14.
8. Jericho BG. Organ donation after circulatory death: ethical issues and international practices. Anesth Analg. 2019;128(2):280–5.
9. Sade RM. Brain death, cardiac death, and the dead donor rule. J S C Med Assoc. 2011;107(4):146–9.
10. Manara AR, Murphy PG, O'Callaghan G. Donation after circulatory death. Br J Anaesth. 2012;108(Suppl 1):i108–21.
11. de Tantillo L, González JM, Ortega J. Organ donation after circulatory death and before death: ethical questions and nursing implications. Policy Polit Nurs Pract. 2019;20(3):163–73.
12. Browne A. The ethics of organ donation after cardiocirculatory death: do the guidelines of the Canadian Council for Donation and Transplantation measure up? Open Med. 2010;4(2):e129–33.
13. Simon JR, Schears RM, Padela AI. Donation after cardiac death and the emergency department: ethical issues. Acad Emerg Med. 2014;21(1):79–86.
14. American Society of Anesthesiologists. Statement on controlled organ donation after circulatory death. Last amended October 25, 2017 (original approval October 25, 2017). http://www.asahq.org/quality-and-practicemanagement/standards-guidelines-and-related-resources/statement-on-controlled-organ-donation-after-circulatory-death.
15. Cota N, Burgess M, English W. Organ donation after circulatory death. Anaesth Tut Week. 2013;282. https://www.anaesthesiauk.com/https://resources.wfsahq.org/atotw/organ-donation-after-circulatory-death-anaesthesia-tutorial-of-the-week-282/.
16. Thuong M, Ruiz A, Evrard P, Kuiper M, Boffa C, Akhtar MZ, Neuberger J, Ploeg R. New classification of donation after circulatory death donors definitions and terminology. Transpl Int. 2016;29:749–59.
17. Croome KP, Taner CB. The changing landscapes in DCD liver transplantation. Curr Transpl Rep. 2020;7:1–11.
18. Lewis J, Peltier J, Nelson H, Snyder W, Schneider K, Steinberger D, Anderson M, Krichevsky A, Anderson J, Ellefson J, D'Alessandro A. Development of the University of Wisconsin donation after cardiac death evaluation tool. Prog Transpl. 2003;13(4):265–73.
19. Jia J, Nie Y, Li J, Xie H, Zhou L, Yu J, Zheng SS. A systematic review and meta-analysis of machine perfusion vs. static cold storage of liver allografts on liver transplantation outcomes: the future direction of graft preservation. Front Med. 2020;7:135.
20. Fernández AR, Sánchez-Tarjuelo R, Cravedi P, Ochando J, López-Hoyos M. Review: ischemia reperfusion injury-a translational perspective in organ transplantation. Int J Mol Sci. 2020;21(22):8549.
21. Pinezich M, Vunjak-Novakovic G. Bioengineering approaches to organ preservation ex vivo. Exp Biol Med. 2019;244(8):630–45.
22. Petrenko A, Carnevale M, Somov A, Osorio J, Rodríguez J, Guibert E, Fuller B, Froghi F. Organ preservation into the 2020s: the era of dynamic intervention. Transfus Med Hemother. 2019;46:151–72.
23. Schlegel A, Muller X, Dutkowski P. Machine perfusion strategies in liver transplantation. Hepatobiliary Surg Nutr. 2019;8(5):490–501.
24. Ceresa CDL, Nasralla D, Coussios CC, Friend PJ. The case for normothermic machine perfusion in liver transplantation. Liver Transpl. 2018;24(2):269–75.
25. Gardiner D, Charlesworth M, Rubino A, Madden S. The rise of organ donation after circulatory death: a narrative review. Anaesthesia. 2020;75:1215–22.
26. Dale G. How the UK Overcame the ethical, legal and professional challenges in donation after circulatory death. QUT Law Rev. 2016;16(1):125–34.

Management of Deceased Donor for Organ Donation

27

Seema Bhalotra and Annu Sarin Jolly

27.1 Introduction

The demand for organs from deceased donors is rapidly increasing all over the world. High rate of mortality in patients on waiting list for organs is clearly evident and impresses on the importance of strict institution of protocols and policies for management of a potential organ donor. It also emphasizes on the need for a multidisciplinary team approach so that all potential organs for transplant in the donor are maintained at their normal physiological condition till the time of retrieval to ensure the success of transplant. These measures will not only help in combating organ shortage by maximizing the organ yield from a donor but also ensure better graft survival after donation.

Early identification of a potential donor is very important and critical as it will lead to early institution of steps which can help in yield of better quality and quantity of organs. The role of critical care physicians in the management of organ donors is very vital. It extends from the identification of potential donors, declaration of brain death, and proper medical care to yield good quality grafts and thereby save the lives of those on the waiting list. There is no single protocol which is accepted world over for management of a deceased donor. Many countries have their own guidelines which may differ from others by few policies and practises. On the other hand, there are also many countries world over which still have no such protocols and guidelines in place. This chapter aims at summarizing the best protocols and practices followed in India and world over.

The process of deceased donor management is complex and has well defined steps which begin from donor identification and end up in successful organ retrieval and transplant surgery. They are summarized in Fig. 27.1.

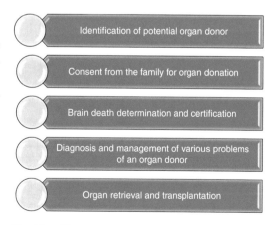

Fig. 27.1 The process of potential donor management

S. Bhalotra (✉)
Liver Transplant, GI Anesthesia and Critical Care, Mednata the Medicity, Gurugram, India

A. S. Jolly
Liver Transplant and General Anaesthesia, Narayana Superspeciality Hospital, Gurgaon, India

27.2 Pathophysiological Changes Due to Brain Death

For the definition purposes a **potential organ donor** is defined by the presence of either brain death or a catastrophic and irreversible brain injury that leads to fulfilling the brain death criteria [1]. It can also be defined as the irreversible loss of all brain functions, including the brain stem [2]. The brain death and the criteria to define it has been discussed in details in the previous chapter. A brief overview of the physiological changes due to brain death will be covered in this chapter as the management of the potential organ donor will primarily involve the use of supportive and therapeutic measures to reverse or mitigate the physiologic changes that occur after brain death, including potentially severe autonomic and inflammatory responses.

Brain has a central and primary role to play in the normal functioning of all the organ and organ systems of the body. Failure of the brain to function due to brain death is therefore a catastrophic physiological event which leads to significant deterioration in the function of various organs. There is loss of integrated neurological function and autonomic coordination and basic organ functions are also lost leading to cardio-respiratory deterioration and finally somatic death within days of brain death. Different clinical studies have shown that there is an interruption in hypothalamic-pituitary-adrenocortical regulation which leads to several pathophysiological alterations in haemodynamic, hormone balance, body temperature, and lung function [3, 4]. There is also a massive release of proinflammatory and anti-inflammatory cytokines and catecholamines due to the marked rise of intracranial pressure (ICP) secondary to the irreversible damage to the brain [5].

These changes can be witnessed usually in two phases—the early and late phase.

The **early phase** of the brain death is characterized by massive sympathetic outflow which is produced as a result of cerebral ischemia leading to Cushing's reflex which is a mixed picture of vagal and sympathetic overactivity. When blood supply is further compromised there is ischemia of the medulla oblongata which results in compensatory arterial hypertension followed with intense vasoconstriction, raised systemic vascular resistance, and tachycardia. This is known as the "catecholamine or autonomic storm" (Fig. 27.2).

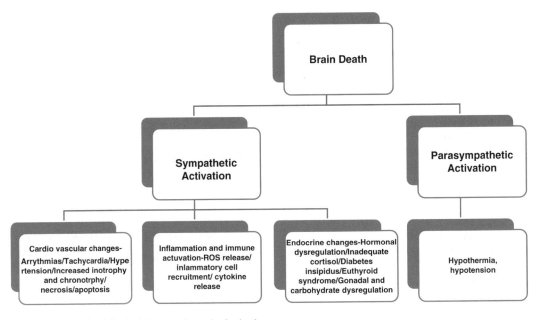

Fig. 27.2 Pathophysiological changes due to brain death

This is the adaptive response of the dying brain to maintain cerebral perfusion pressure and the sympathetic hormones and mediators thus released cause central redistribution of blood volume, increased afterload, and visceral ischemia having a detrimental effect on the tissue perfusion. If timely intervention is not done, the organs suffer an ischaemic insult during this phase due to intense vasoconstriction. The severity of injury is related directly with the speed of herniation. It has been observed that the rise in the level of catecholamines is dependent upon the rate of rise in intracranial pressure (ICP). If the rise in ICP is rapid, the catecholamine can show as much as 1000 fold elevation from baseline indicating the intensity of the so-called autonomic storm. This intense catecholamine surge can have marked adverse effects on the myocardium leading to injury, altered metabolism which is associated with depletion of adenosine triphosphate in the cardiac myocyte [6].

The early phase is followed by the **late phase**. As ischemia progress down the spinal cord, it impairs the function in the thoracic sympathetic chain with leads to severe hypotension due to marked reduction in afterload. The loss of autonomic tone results in profound vasodilatation and reduced supply to the organs. This reduced tissue perfusion can compromise the functioning of the various transplantable organs. Temperature changes and endocrine dysfunction is also seen due to ischaemic damage to the hypothalamus and pituitary. The mechanisms of these changes are not very well understood.

27.3 Approach to a Patient with Brain Death

Studies have revealed that if there is a delay in management of a donor it may lead to the loss of 10–20% of potential donor tissues due to the rapid progression from brain death to somatic death in them. Timely treatment of the donor is thus very crucial [1]. Therefore, institution of strict organ-protective intensive care strategies is the first step towards a successful transplant and in the treatment of the future organ recipient [3]. The care of the brain-dead donor is often difficult and complex. It may extend over several hours or even days.

The principles behind management of a deceased donor are maintaining haemodynamic stability and homeostasis thereby optimizing organ perfusion till they are retrieved (Fig. 27.3). Thus a successful organ donation may involve maintaining the hemodynamic variables and laboratory parameters within the normal ranges which

Fig. 27.3 The principles of donor management

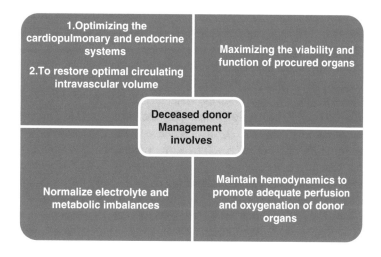

becomes a challenge due to the pathophysiological changes which occur due to the deceased brain.

A detailed assessment and evaluation of the donor is required. Care should be immediately initiated once we identify a potential donor as delay in initiation of proper management can render the organs non transplantable. A detailed medical history and complete physical examination is must to identify any comorbidities which can be optimized or any other systemic conditions which can act as a contraindication to the transplant of a particular organ or the patient as such. A thorough review of the patients cause of brain death and details of the hospital stay should be done to note the events or parameters which might affect our decision to retrieve the organs. Besides these general criteria, it is important to determine the intrinsic function of the organs to be transplanted and to ascertain that the illness has not impaired these organs irreversibly so an array of general and organ specific investigations should be carried out. It is also mandatory to screen for sepsis and malignancy. Once brain death is declared and authorization from the family for donation is obtained the transplant team is intimated.

Table 27.1 General care of a deceased donor

Category	Recommendation
General management	Central line insertion and monitoring
	Arterial line insertion and monitoring
	Nasogastric tube insertion
	Foley's catheter insertion
	Care of all lines and endotracheal tube, to be changed as per protocol
	Head of the bed at 30–40° elevation
	Regular position change side to side
	Warming blankets and warm fluids to maintain body temperature >35
	Pneumatic compression device for preventing deep vein thrombosis
	Eye protection
	Tracheal suctioning at frequent intervals
	Ulcer prophylaxis
	Broad spectrum antibiotics

27.4 General Care and Monitoring

A brain-dead person requires the same regular nursing care as any other patient in the intensive care unit. The regular routine nursing care can be summarized into Table 27.1.

These patients need meticulous monitoring as they are prone to organ dysfunction, electrolyte, and metabolic changes due to the systemic effects of brain death. The **routine monitoring** includes electrocardiography (ECG), blood pressure (BP), pulse oximetry, core temperature, urine output, and central venous pressure. Special monitoring to be instituted includes the following.

- Arterial line insertion for beat to beat BP and arterial blood gas monitoring (ABG)
- Use of a Swan-Ganz catheter for measurement of pulmonary capillary wedge pressure and pulmonary venous oximetry in case of unsta-

ble donors, who have persistent acidosis with evidence of tissue hypoperfusion
- Central venous pressure (CVP) monitoring to guide fluid administration
- Cardiac output (CO) and stroke volume variation (SVV) monitoring if available

The upper extremities are preferred for insertion of arterial and central venous lines as during the time of organ harvesting the femoral line readings can become inaccurate.

Previous laboratory parameters of the patient should be meticulously seen for abnormal values and trends. The parameters to be routinely monitored include the following:

- Blood chemistry- Complete blood count (CBC), liver function test (LFT), renal function test (RFT)
- Coagulation profile- Prothrombin time (PT), Activated partial thromboplastin time (APTT)
- Urine -Routine analysis and culture
- Blood group -Type and crossmatch
- Sputum - Gram stain and Culture
- Chest X-ray (CXR)
- Arterial blood gas analysis (ABG)
- Electrocardiography (ECG)
- Echocardiography (ECHO)

- Serum electrolyte
- Microbiological screening for hepatitis B, hepatitis C, HIV
- Cultures of blood and urine may be required, if there is evidence of infection or if the patient is hospitalized for more than 72 h [7]
- Some additional tests may be required for multiorgan donors e.g. bronchoscopy for lung transplantation.

Apart from the basic investigations some other laboratory parameters may require monitoring at frequent intervals for depending upon the condition and requirement of the patient, for example, ABG, chest X-ray, serum electrolytes, blood glucose levels, etc. (Pictures 27.1 and 27.2).

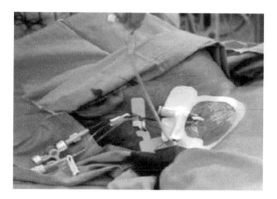

Picture 27.1   Central venous line insertion

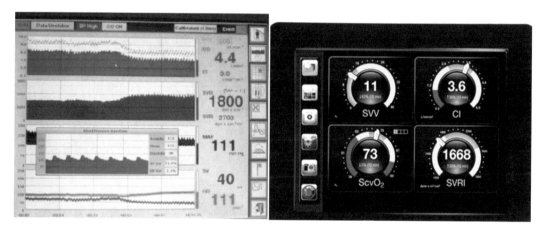

Picture 27.2   Cardiac output monitors

27.5   Specific Management

The process of preparation and maintenance of a deceased donor for organ retrieval is not a simple task as it requires balancing the interventions needed for the successful preservation of multiple organs. Interventions that improve the function of one organ may be detrimental to the function of other organs [8]. A very precarious balance has to be maintained while managing the donor so that the quality and quantity of the organs retrieved is not compromised. Each organ specific transplant team has their own stringent requirement. Where on one hand the renal transplant team would prefer the donor to be well hydrated and have good diuresis the team involved with harvesting the heart, lungs, liver, and pancreas would not prefer or permit aggressive hydration as it may lead to tissue oedema that may jeopardize the transplantability of these organs. There are studies which suggest that the restrictive fluid balance approach which is actually intended to improve lung graft function and viability has no substantial detrimental effect on the renal graft procurement or its function after transplant [9].

The rampant pathophysiological changes determine the management process. The incidence of these changes are mentioned in Table 27.2.

Table 27.2 Pathophysiological changes after brain death

S. No.	Pathophysiological changes	Incidence
1.	Hypotension	80
2.	Diabetes insipidus	60
3.	Disseminated intravascular coagulation	30
4.	Cardiac arrythmias	30
5.	Pulmonary oedema	20
6.	Acidosis	10

27.6 Cardiovascular Support

The goals in the management include the following:

- Maintenance of BP avoiding both hypertension and hypotension
- Optimizing the fluid management and to maintain normovolemia
- Maintenance of organ perfusion by optimizing cardiac output (CO)
- Minimize use of vasoactive agents

The haemodynamic parameters which are aimed at while providing cardiovascular support to these patients are mentioned in Table 27.3.

27.6.1 Hypotension

It has been observed that around 80–95% of brain-dead organ donors experience hypotension as the most common hemodynamic abnormality. It may lead to hypoperfusion of all organs including the heart. If proper treatment is not started timely, it may lead to rapid donor loss [10]. There are multiple factors which can be blamed for it which include damage to vasomotor centre, hypovolaemia, myocardial dysfunction, and endocrine failure. Additional factors which may contribute to hypotension include excessive use of osmotic diuretics, hyperglycaemia-induced osmotic diuresis, diabetes insipidus (DI), inadequate fluid resuscitation, ongoing haemorrhage due to trauma or coagulopathy, hypothermic "cold" diuresis and

relative adrenal insufficiency which may occur as a consequence of trauma, and critical illnesses [1].

Management includes checking for signs of any ongoing bleeding. Medications that may contribute towards hypotension, for example, antihypertensive drugs or diuretics should be avoided or wisely used. Three management strategies are commonly adopted and are instituted depending on the patient's clinical response. to them. These strategies include the following.

- Fluid resuscitation and volume expansion
- Vasopressors and inotropes
- Hormonal replacement

Fluid resuscitation is the cornerstone therapy for management of hypotension. The choice and selection of fluid whether colloid or crystalloid and which crystalloid or colloid is best still remains a matter of debate. There is no consensus on the appropriate fluid management therefore different centres all over the world have their local preferences in the use of crystalloids and colloids. However, the decision for fluid selection should be considered based on certain laboratory and haemodynamic parameters which include serum electrolytes, blood glucose levels, estimated volume deficiency, haematocrit and haemoglobin levels of the patient, and the polyuria from central diabetes insipidus.

The aim is to meet the haemodynamic goals while maintaining a haematocrit of around 25–30% or haemoglobin level of about 10 gm/dl and normal serum electrolyte and blood glucose levels in an effort to improve the compromised

Table 27.3 Haemodynamic goals

S. No.	Parameter	Desired goal
1.	Heart rate/rhythm	60–100 beats/min/sinus
2.	Mean arterial blood pressure (MAP)	60–80 mm of Hg
3.	Central venous pressure (CVP)	4–6 mm of Hg
4.	Pulmonary artery occlusion pressure (PAOP)	10–15
5.	Left ventricular ejection fraction (LVEF)	>45%
6.	Urine output	>/=1 ml/kg/h

microcirculation and tissue perfusion [11]. Two important aspects of fluid resuscitation are the choice of fluid and monitoring

27.6.1.1 Fluid

As hypernatremia is a very common finding and leads to reduced graft function it has been recommended to use crystalloids with balanced salt content to avoid it.

- 0.9% normal saline solution is seen to cause hyperchloremic acidosis when used for fluid resuscitation. It also increases renal vascular resistance and confounds base excess so is best avoided.
- 5% dextrose if used excessively is seen to worsen hyperglycaemia.
- 0.45% or half normal saline and lactated Ringer's solution are frequently used [12].
- Colloids, such as hydroxyethyl starches, need to be avoided in organ donors. They are seen to cause early graft dysfunction by damaging the renal epithelial cells [12].
- 4% and 20% albumin solutions can be used. It helps in reducing the fluid administration but

because of the high sodium content these solutions are only moderately effective [12].
- Lactated Ringer's solution, lactate free solutions like plasmaLyte or half-normal saline solution (0.45%), with the addition of sodium bicarbonate at 50 mmol/L, can be given if the donor has acidosis. It reduces the incidence of hypernatremia in the donors.

27.6.1.2 Monitoring

The volume status of the patient and the response to therapy can be judged by appropriate and sophisticated hemodynamic monitors available [8]. Serial or continuous measurements of central venous pressure, pulmonary arterial obstructive pressure, stroke volume, CO, cardiac index, and mixed venous oxygen saturation and stroke volume variation should also be meticulously done [8]. If fluid resuscitation and volume replacement is not effective in achieving haemodynamic stability, vasoactive drugs are given. Fluid therapy, pressor agents such as epinephrine and norepinephrine and dopamine, dobutamine can be added depending on the values of CVP, PAOP, SVR, and CI as shown in Fig. 27.4.

Fig. 27.4 Flow chart of management of haemodynamic instability

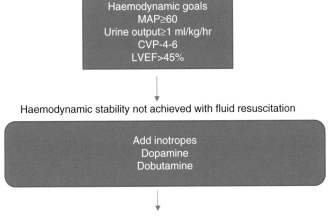

Haemodynamic goals
MAP≥60
Urine output≥1 ml/kg/hr
CVP-4-6
LVEF>45%

Haemodynamic stability not achieved with fluid resuscitation

Add inotropes
Dopamine
Dobutamine

Haemodynamic stability not achieved with inotropes

Pulmonary artery catheterization
Aim to maintain
Pulmonary capillary occlusion pressure=8-12 mm of Hg
Systemic vascular resiatance(SVR)-800-1200dynes/cm³
Cardia index= or > 2.4l/min/m²↓

No response initiate hormonal therapy

Vasopressor therapy—There is no prescribed best inotrope or pressor agents in these patients [13]. The donors will require vasopressor therapy when adequate fluid resuscitation does not help to restore haemodynamics. Approximately 80–90% of donors require inotropic and/or vasopressor support [14]. There is no world over consensus on the choice of vasopressor to be used. There are very few retrospective studies regarding the selection of catecholamines for use in organ-protective intensive care [15]. Noradrenaline, adrenaline, vasopressin, dopamine, and dobutamine are being used solely or in combination in accordance to the protocol of the institution.

Dopamine has been the first choice in many centres followed by dobutamine and isoproterenol. It is advisable to administer in doses less than 10 µg/kg/min as higher infusion rates can result in an increase in the incidence of acute tubular necrosis. It can also cause decrease in the perfusion of other organs due to splanchnic vasoconstriction [16]. Many transplant teams prefer not to use it as dopamine causes presynaptic modulation of norepinephrine release and a prolonged dopamine infusions may cause depletion of norepinephrine stores in the heart, possibly resulting in myocardial dysfunction after transplantation.

Dobutamine and isoproterenol are considered second line agents because of peripheral vasodilatation and poor tolerability [17]. Failure to achieve the target MAP and haemodynamic goals in the scenario of severe systemic vasodilatation warrants the use of norepinephrine (0.5–2.5 µg/kg/min) or epinephrine (2–4 µg/min). Vasopressin has also been used in such cases where there is severe catecholamine depletion.

Hormone resuscitation—If hypotension persists despite fluid loading and optimum dose of vasopressors and inotropes, hormonal resuscitation with methylprednisolone, triiodothyronine (T3) and vasopressin is instituted. The use of these three hormones is referred to as the triple therapy or hormonal resuscitation therapy. The use of triple therapy remains controversial. There are a number of studies which advocate the use of

this therapy as it is found to improve both hemodynamic stability in brain-dead patients, as well as the quality of the procured organs [18].

In a 10 year data analysis conducted by the United Network for Organ Sharing (UNOS) various hormone replacement modalities were evaluated and it was found that the combination of a thyroid hormone, corticosteroid, insulin, and an antidiuretic hormone had the most promising results in multiple organ procurement [19]. Hormone replacement therapy may be initiated if hemodynamic goals are not met and/or the left ventricular ejection fraction remains less than 45% [8].

The recommended replacements are:

1. Vasopressin: 1 U bolus followed by an infusion of 0.5–4.0 U/h,
2. Methylprednisolone: 15 mg/kg immediately after the diagnosis of brain death and every 24 h afterwards.
3. Insulin infusion to maintain blood glucose levels between 80 and 150 mg,
4. Thyroxine (T_4; 20 µg bolus) followed by infusions of 10 µg/h T_3, administered as a 4 µg bolus, followed by infusion of 3 µg/h T_4 improves hemodynamic status and prevents cardiovascular collapse in hemodynamically unstable organ donors.

27.6.2 Hypertension

Autonomic storm is usually short lived and is seen due to marked rise in ICP. It occurs at the time of brain stem herniation and leads to marked vasoconstriction causing severe hypertension, multiple tachyarrhythmias, and ischemic changes. Treatment is not required in most of the cases. In case one needs to lower the blood pressure or control the heart rate short acting agents are preferred. Anti-hypertensive like sodium nitroprusside and rapidly reversible β-adrenergic antagonists like esmolol are used. To control the arrythmias antiarrhythmics like lidocaine should be considered. Long acting agents are best avoided as it is difficult to titrate them and they have a negative inotropic effects [20].

27.6.3 Arrythmias

Atrial and ventricular arrhythmias and conduction defects are very often witnessed in a deceased donor. The causes of these arrythmias are multifactorial. They can occur because of hypotension with myocardial ischemia,electrolyte and arterial blood gas (ABG) disorders, hypothermia, inotropes infusion, and increased ICP [21]. They should be diagnosed and treated promptly. Prevention is the best policy and can be done by closely monitoring and maintain the electrolytes, BP, fluid volume, and body temperature within the acceptable range.

Treatment of arrythmias involves use of drugs like amiodarone or cardioversion. In case of bradyarrhythmia atropine is not useful and so drugs like adrenaline, isoprenaline are used. Pacing may be effective in refractory cases. The terminal arrythmia of these patients is resistant to therapy and requires use of cardiopulmonary resuscitation.

27.7 Respiratory Care and Ventilatory Support

Respiratory support forms an essential part of donor management. It involves:

- Maintaining adequate oxygenation by effective lung protective ventilatory strategies
- Vigorous tracheobronchial toilet and frequent suctioning

- Institution of all sterile precautions
- Head up positioning
- Pressure control ventilation or volume limited ventilation is generally the preferred mode of ventilation
- Recruitment maneuverers to be done frequently
- Minimize lung water by adequate hydration strategies
- Intensive chest physiotherapy with hourly gentle inflation of lungs and 2 hourly side-to-side turning
- Chest X-ray and ABG analysis as and when required
- Broad spectrum antibiotics

The goals of the standard management can be summarized in Table 27.4.

It has been found that the two main causes of hypoxemia which can render the lung non-transplantable are atelectasis and excessive fluid resuscitation. Proper use of alveolar recruitment strategies can help in treating atelectasis. Ventilatory support should be applied judiciously so as not to cause barotrauma to the lungs or affect the cardiac output thereby prevent complications and improve the organ yield.

Pulmonary oedema is very commonly seen in organ donors and the cause can be fluid overload, secondary to aspiration, cardiogenic or neurogenic. Treatment is generally supportive and involves judicious use of fluids with proper monitoring.

Table 27.4 Ventilatory goals

S. No.	Goals
1.	Tidal volume- volumes of 6–8 ml/kg
2.	$FiO < 0.6$ or lowest possible FiO_2 to maintain $SpO_2 > 92\%$ & $PaO_2 > 70$ mm of Hg
3.	Maintenance of normocapnia ($PaCO_2 \sim 30$–35)
4.	$PaO_2 > 70$ with minimum FiO_2
5.	$SaO > 95\%$
6.	PEEP < 5 cm H_2O adjusted to maintain $PaO_2 > 70$ mm of Hg
7.	Plateau pressure (<35 cm H_2O), peak pressure <40 cm of H_2O

27.8 Acid-Base Balance

Respiratory alkalosis secondary to mechanical hyperventilation is a common finding in deceased donors. It may occur due to institution of hyperventilation as a part of treatment protocol for elevated ICP. Lactic metabolic acidosis due to dehydration or tissue ischaemia may be another cause. It has a deleterious effect on tissue oxygen delivery. Treatment involves adjusting the ventilatory parameters and if it does not improve use of pharmacological agents is advocated to correct the calculated acid-base deficit.

27.9 Renal Support

Adequate systemic perfusion pressure and proper hydration are essential to maintain renal blood flow. A urine output (>1–2 ml/kg/h) is the primary goal in renal management of a deceased donor. This can be achieved by preventing haemodynamic instability using intensive monitoring and rapid action protocol.

Minimizing the use of vasopressors and adequate volume loading can contribute to good renal allograft function. If urine output falls despite of adequate volume loading, diuretic therapy should be used. Use of nephrotoxic drugs like aminoglycosides and agents that adversely affect renal perfusion like the NSAIDs should be avoided.

27.10 Endocrine Dysfunction

27.10.1 Central Diabetes Insipidus (CDI)

70% of the deceased donors develop CDI. It occurs due to inadequate amount of ADH secretion from the posterior pituitary. It leads to polyuria which causes obligatory loss of fluid and electrolytes from the body and needs aggressive management to prevent haemodynamic instability and electrolyte imbalance. The diagnostic criteria of this condition includes the following:

- Presence of polyuria (urine output >3–4 ml/kg/h),
- Hypernatremia (S.Na ≥150 mmol/L),
- Hyperosmolality (≥310 mOsm/L), and
- Low urine osmolality or inappropriately diluted urine (urine osmolality <300 mOsm/L).

The management of this condition requires the following.

1. Monitoring of urine output, serum electrolytes, glucose, and urinary electrolytes.
2. If urine output exceeds 300 ml/h or 4 ml/kg/h, desmopressin should be given. It is used in the dose of 1–4 μg 8–12 h.
3. Desmopressin is a synthetic analogue of vasopressin. It has enhanced antidiuretic potency, greatly diminished pressor activity and prolonged half-life as compared to Vasopressin.
4. Therapy is to be titrated to bring the urine output to ≤2 ml/kg/h.
5. Adequate volume replacement depending upon the urine output.
6. Maintain Na+ ≤ 155 mmol/lt with use of sodium free or low sodium intravenous fluids like 5% dextrose and N/2 saline.
7. Vasopressin in the dose of 1 U bolus and 0.5–4.0 U.h^{-1} infusion can be used in case of refractory hypotension (Table 27.5).

The common practice in CDI is to replace the previous hour's urine output with a hypotonic fluid. 5% Dextrose in 0.45% Normal saline is mostly administered. It is essential to closely monitor the serum electrolytes, especially serum

Table 27.5 Difference between desmopressin and vasopressin

Desmopressin	Vasopressin
Mild diuretic: Pressor = 2000–4000:1 Acts selectively on V2 receptors	Diuretic: Pressor = 1: 1 Acts on V1/V2 receptors
Long duration of action (6–24 h)	Short duration of action
Intra venous dose 2–6 μg 6 hourly	Dose-1 U IV bolus followed by 0.5–4 U/h
Intra nasal dose: 5–40 μg BD	No administration by intranasal route

sodium as hypernatremia has been found to be a risk factor for delayed or primary nonfunction of grafted organs.

27.10.2 Hyperglycaemia

Hyperglycaemia is a very common finding in brain-dead donors. It may be occur due to

- Stress,
- Catecholamine-induced insulin resistance,
- Steroid administration for treatment of cerebral oedema,
- Infusion of large amounts of dextrose-containing IV fluids.

Hyperglycaemia needs immediate treatment with insulin as it leads to osmotic diuresis and electrolyte disturbances. The aim of treatment should be to keep blood glucose between 120 and 180 mg/dl.

27.10.3 Thyroid Dysfunction

Rapid decline in T3 and ê TSH secretion is seen and it leads to:

- Decreased mitochondrial function and thus energy production
- Cardiac instability
- Labile blood pressure
- Anaerobic metabolism and acidosis

Studies have shown that the use of T3 in a deceased donor improves tissue and organ perfusion by improving the arterial BP. It also increases the left ventricular function and thereby the cardiac output. Replacement of thyroid hormones have shown to decrease the inotrope requirement in brain-dead donors. Thyroid hormone supplementation can be done in three forms. These include:

1. Intravenous T3 hormone administration –This form is found to be better and more potent; it

has a faster onset and a shorter duration of action (1.5 days). It is given as a bolus of 4 µg followed by an infusion given at a rate of at 3 µg/h
2. Intravenous levothyroxine administration - It is given in the dose of 20 µg bolus followed by an infusion given at a rate of 10 µg/h
3. Tab Thyroxine can also be given in case of nonavailability of intravenous preparation in a dose of 50–100 µg through the nasogastric tube.

27.10.4 Cortisol Replacement Is Must. It Is Vital to Administer It as It

- Improves donor organ function and graft survival
- Increase tissue oxygenation and donor lung recovery
- Attenuates the effect of proinflammatory cytokinin's released as a consequence of brain death [22]
- Recommended by UNOS
- Methylprednisolone is usually administered in the dose of 15–20 mg/kg. The use of methylprednisolone in brain-dead donors leads to improved short- and long-term outcomes for most transplanted organs. It improved oxygenation and reduces extravascular lung water thereby increasing the lung yield. It also reduces inflammation in the liver, heart, and kidney [23].

27.11 Temperature Regulation

The body becomes poikilothermic due to the loss of functioning of the thalamic and hypothalamic temperature regulation centre. This problem is further aggravated by systemic vasodilatation, administration of cold intravenous fluids, and blood products. Hypothermia has detrimental effects on the donor. It can not only preclude the certification of brain death but also lead to arrythmias due to cardiac irritability, coagulopathy and

Picture 27.3 Temperature maintained devices. (1) Hot air blanket (2) Fluid warmer

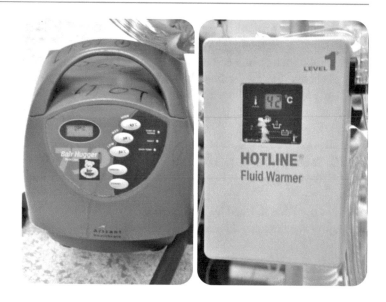

reduce oxygen delivery to tissues. As per guidelines the donor core temperature must be maintained ≥34 °C. Active measures must be taken to prevent hypothermia like using warming IV fluids, humidified, heated ventilator gases, and warming blankets and mattress. Convincing evidence suggests that mild therapeutic hypothermia of the donor can be adopted to reduce delayed graft function especially in the renal transplant recipient (Picture 27.3).

27.12 Coagulation System

Coagulopathy and disseminated intravascular coagulation (DIC) are often seen in brain-dead donors. The incidence is higher in head injury patients and is seen to occur due to release of thromboplastin from the injured brain [7]. Coagulopathy may result from various other causes like hypothermia, dilutional coagulopathy due to large volume resuscitation and massive blood transfusion. Treatment involves transfusion of appropriate blood components if the patient has clinically significant bleeding. Antifibrinolytic agents like Epsilon aminocaproic acid (EACA) are not used in organ donors, due to their potential of inducing microvascular thrombosis. This can render the organs potentially unsuitable for transplantation [20].

27.13 Infectious Disease Protection

The diagnosis of sepsis may be difficult in brain death. The signs of sepsis like elevated leukocyte count and tachycardia are non-specific and due to hypothalamic dysfunction the patient may not have fever. Antimicrobial therapy should be given based on the results of the various gram staining or cultures done. Nephrotoxic antimicrobials should be completely avoided. Preventive measures like having strict asepsis protocols, maintaining pulmonary hygiene, care of all invasive lines and catheters should be religiously followed.

27.14 Management of Nutrition

Nutrition should be continued based on standard ICU protocols. Enteral feeding should be instituted early as it has been found to have beneficial effects on organ functioning.

27.15 Ischaemia-Reperfusion Injury

Organ dysfunction induced by ischemia reperfusion injury is commonly witnessed in brain-dead patients. This occurs due to the low flow associated with severe vasoconstriction during the autonomic storm, followed by vasodilatation and reflow. Moreover it has been found that there is up-regulation of inflammatory cytokines and widespread microvascular and endothelial changes in these patients which may contribute to the injury mechanism [24]. Use of cytoprotective strategies with high dose steroids, N acetylcysteine, and p-selectine inhibitors has shown to improve short- and long-term recipient organ function. The donor management protocol can be summed up in Table 27.6.

Table 27.6 Treatment Protocol for Donor Management

S. No.	Condition	Recommendation
1.	Hypertension	Short acting anti-hypertensive drugs
2.	Hypotension	Restore circulatory volume and use vasoactive agents No response start hormonal therapy
3A	Fluids	Balanced crystalloid solution should be used 0.45% saline /lactated ringer preferred Avoid synthetic starch solutions 4%/20% albumin solution can be used Avoid excess volume loading
3B	Vasopressors	Norepinephrine/vasopressin/dopamine
3C	Blood and blood products	Consider need for blood, plasma, platelets to correct coagulopathy if there is active bleeding. Aim to keep Hb >10 g/dl
4.	Electrolytes	
	Serum sodium(Na)	Try to keep Na <150 meq/l, If Na levels are<150- use N/2 saline or 5% dextrose to reduce the levels
	Serum potassium(K)	K 3.5–4.5 mmol/L (target)
5.	Hyperglycaemia	Blood sugar to be 120–180 If >180 start insulin infusion
	Hypoglycaemia	Blood sugar-50–80 mg/dl-give 50% dextrose 10 ml IV If blood sugar <50 mg/dl-give 20 ml of 50% dextrose
6.	Steroid replacement	Methylprednisilone-15–20 mg/kg
7.	Diabetes insipidus	Vasopressin 20 U in 5% DW 500 ml mix UO >300 ml/h: IV infusion rate 3 ml/h UO 100–200 ml: keep the dose and maintain with 0.5–1 ml/h and HUO monitoring
8.	Thyroid replacement	Start with levothyroxine 150 μg daily or IV T3 after doing blood T3/T4 levels

27.16 Summary

The success of the transplant depends on the donor care. The organ yield and graft survival depends on the multidisciplinary approach at managing the donor, the meticulous monitoring and timely interventions done to reverse or slow down the normal sequalae of brain death. The aim is to support the body function with adequate oxygenation and tissue perfusion, till organs are retrieved. The therapeutic end-points for adequate tissue perfusion are the Rule of 100 as follows which when followed are seen to improve the organ yield.

Rule of 100's

- Systolic arterial pressure >100 mm Hg,
- Urine output >100 mL/h
- PaO$_2$ >100 mm Hg
- Haemoglobin concentration >100 g/L (10 gm/dL)
- Blood sugar 100 mg/dL

Avoiding lactic acidosis (pH = 7.35–7.45) and hypothermia (temperature >34 °C) [21, 25] (Fig. 27.5).

Key Points

- Early identification of a potential donor
- Immediate institution of Donor Management Protocol
- Meticulous monitoring and care in Intensive care unit
- Timely implementation of Hormonal therapy
- Early administration of Vasopressin for vasoplegia and Diabetes Insipidus
- Standardization of care and frequent audit

Critical Pathway for the Organ Donor

Patient name: _____

ID number: _____

Collaborative Practice	Phase I Referral	Phase II Declaration of Brain Death and Consent	Phase III Donor Evaluation	Phase IV Donor Management	Phase V Recovery Phase
The following professionals may be involved to enhance the donation process *Check all that apply* Physician Critical care RN Organ Procurement Organization (OPO) OPO coordinator (OPC) Medical Examiner (ME)/ Coroner Respiratory Laboratory Pharmacy Radiology Anesthesiology OR/Surgery staff Clergy Social worker	Notify physician regarding OPO referral Contact OPO ref: Potential donor with severe brain insult OPC on site and begins evaluation Time ____ Date ____ Ht ____ Wt ____ as documented ABO as documented ____ Notify house supervisor/ charge nurse of presence of OPC on unit	Brain death documented Time ____ Date ____ Pt accepted as potential donor MD notifies family of death Plan family approach with OPC Offer support services to family (clergy, etc) OPC/Hospital staff talks to family about donation Family accepts donation OPC obtains signed consent & medical/social history Time ____ Date ____ ME/Coroner notified ME/Coroner releases body for donation *Family/ME/Coroner denies donation—stop pathway—initiate post-mortem protocol—support family.*	Obtain pre/post transfusion blood for serology testing (HIV, hepatitis VDRL, CMV) Obtain lymph nodes and/or blood for tissue typing Notify OR & anesthesiology of pending donation Notify house supervisor of pending donation Chest & abdominal circumference Lung measurements per CXR by OPC *Cardiology consult as requested by OPC (see reverse side)* *Donor organs unsuitable for transplant—stop pathway—initiate post-mortem protocol—support family.*	OPC writes new orders Organ placement OPC sets tentative OR time Insert arterial line/ 2 large bore IVs Possibly insert CVP/Pulmonary Artery Catheter See reverse side	Checklist for OR Supplies given to OR Prepare patient for transport to OR IVs Pumps O₂ Ambu Flap valve Transport to OR Date ____ Time ____ OR nurse reviews consent form reviews brain death documentation checks patient's ID band
Labs/ Diagnostics		Review previous lab results Review previous hemody-namics	Blood chemistry CBC + diff UA C & S PT, PTT ABO A Subtype Liver function tests Blood culture X 2/ 15 minutes to 1 hour apart Sputum Gram stain & C & S Type & CrossMatch ____ # units PRBCs CXR ABGs EKG Echo Consider cardiac cath Consider bronchoscopy	Determine need for additional lab testing CXR after line placement (if done) Serum electrolytes H & H after PRBC Rx PT, PTT BUN, serum creatinine after correcting fluid deficit Notify OPC for ____ PT >14 ____ PTT <28 ____ Urine output ____ <1 mL/Kg/hr ____ >3 mL/Kg/hr ____ Hd < 30 / Hgb >10 ____ Na >150 mEq/L.	Labs drawn in OR as per surgeon or OPC request Communicate with pathology: Bx liver and/or kidneys as indicated
Respiratory	Pt on ventilator Suction q 2 hr Reposition q 2 hr	Prep for apnea testing; set FiO₂ @ 100% and antici-pate need to decrease rate if PCO₂ < 45 mm Hg	Maximize ventilator settings to achieve SaO₂ 98 - 99% PEEP = 5 cm O₂ challenge for lung placement FiO₂ @ 100%, PEEP @ 5 X 10 min ABGs as ordered VS q 1° ____	Notify OPC for ____ BP < 90 systolic ____ HR < 70 or > 120 ____ CVP < 4 or > 11 ____ PaO₂ < 90 or ____ SaO₂ < 95%	Portable O₂ @ 100% FiO₂ for transport to OR Ambu bag and PEEP valve Move to OR
Treatments/ Ongoing Care		Use warming/cooling blanket to maintain temperature at 36.5°C – 37.5°C NG to low intermittent suction	Check NG placement & output Obtain actual Ht ____ & Wt ____ if not previ-ously obtained		Set OR temp as directed by OPC Post-mortem care at conclusion of case
Medications			Medication as requested by OPC	Fluid resuscitation—con-sider crystolloids, colloids, blood products DC meds except pressors & antibiotics Broad-spectrum antibiotic if not previously ordered Vasopressor support to maintain BP > 90 mm Hg systolic Electrolyte imbalance consider K, Ca, PO₄, Mg replacement Hyperglycemia consider insulin drip Oliguria consider diuretics Diabetes insipidus con-sider antidiuretics Paralytic as indicated for spinal reflexes	DC antidiuretics Diuretics as needed 350 U heparin/kg or as directed by surgeon
Optimal Outcomes	The potential donor is iden-tified & a referral is made to the OPO.	The family is offered the option of donation & their decision is supported.	The donor is evaluated & found to be a suitable candi-date for donation.	Optimal organ function is maintained.	All potentially suitable, con-sented organs are recovered for transplant.

Fig. 27.5 UNOS protocol for donor management

References

1. Wood KE, Becker BN, McCartney JG, D'Alessandro AM, Coursin DB. Care of the potential organ donor. N Engl J Med. 2004;351:2730–9.
2. Goila AK, Pawar M. The diagnosis of brain death. Indian J Crit Care Med. 2009;13:7–11.
3. Powner DJ, Darby JM, Kellum JA. Proposed treatment guidelines for donor care. Prog Transplant. 2004;14:16–26.
4. Hahnenkamp K, Böhler K, Wolters H, Wiebe K, Schneider D, Schmidt HH. Organ-protective intensive care in organ donors. Dtsch Arztebl Int. 2016;113:552–8.
5. Amado JA, López-Espadas F, Vázquez-Barquero A, Salas E, Riancho JA, López-Cordovilla JJ, et al. Blood levels of cytokines in brain-dead patients: relationship with circulating hormones and acute-phase reactants. Metabolism. 1995;44:812–6.
6. Pinelli G, Mertes PM, Carteaux JP, Jaboin Y, Escanye JM, Brunotte F, et al. Myocardial effects of experimental acute brain death: evaluation by hemodynamic and biological studies. Ann Thorac Surg. 1995;60:1729–34.
7. Razek T, Olthoff K, Reilly PM. Issues in potential organ donor management. Surg Clin North Am. 2000;80:1021–32.
8. Kotloff RM, et al. Management of the potential organ donor in the ICU: Society of Critical Care Medicine/American College of Chest Physicians/Association of Organ Procurement Organizations Consensus Statement. Crit Care Med. 2015;43(6):1291–325.
9. Miñambres, et al. Impact of restrictive fluid balance focused to increase lung procurement on renal function after kidney transplantation. Nephrol Dial Transplant. 2010;25(7):2352–6.
10. Szabó G, Hackert T, Sebening C, Vahl CF, Hagl S. Modulation of coronary perfusion pressure can reverse cardiac dysfunction after brain death. Ann Thorac Surg. 1999;67:18–25.
11. Jenkins DH, Reilly PM, Schwab CW. Improving the approach to organ donation: a review. World J Surg. 1999;23:644–9.
12. Pandit RA, Zirpe KG, Gurav SK, Kulkarni AP, Karnath S, Govil D, et al. Management of potential organ donor: Indian Society of Critical Care Medicine: position statement. Indian J Crit Care Med. 2017;21:303–16.
13. Braunfeld MY. Cadaveric donors. Anaesthesiol Clin North Am. 2004;22:615–31.
14. Wood KE, Coursin DB. Intensivists and organ donor management. Curr Opin Anaesthesiol. 2007;20:97–9.
15. Plurad DS, Bricker S, Falor A, Neville A, Bongard F, Putnam B. Donor hormone and vasopressor therapy: closing the gap in a transplant organ shortage. J Trauma Acute Care Surg. 2012;73:689–94.
16. Goldberg LL. Cardiovascular and renal actions of dopamine. Potential clinical applications. Pharmacol Rev. 1992;24:1–29.
17. Scheinkestel CD, Tuxen DV, Cooper DJ, Butt W. Medical management of the (potential) organ donor. Anaesth Intensive Care. 1995;23:51–9.
18. Findlater C, Thomson EM. Organ donation and management of the potential organ donor. Anaesth Intensive Care Med. 2015;16:315–20.
19. Mi Z, Novitzky D, Collins JF, Cooper DK. The optimal hormonal replacement modality selection for multiple organ procurement from brain-dead organ donors. Clin Epidemiol. 2014;7:17–27.
20. Tropmann C, Dunn DL. Management of the organ donor. In: Irwin and Ripple's intensive care medicine. 5th ed. 2184-201.
21. Watts RP, Thom O, Fraser JF. Inflammatory signalling associated with brain dead organ donation: from brain injury to brain stem death and posttransplant ischaemia reperfusion injury. J Transp Secur. 2013;2013:521369.
22. Zaroff JG, Rosengard BR, Armstrong WF, et al. Consensus conference report: maximizing use of organs recovered from the cadaver donor; cardiac recommendations. Circulation. 2002;106:836–41.
23. Gelb AW, Robertson KM. Anaesthetic management of the brain dead for organ donation. Can J Anaesth. 1990;37:806–12.
24. Jassem W, Koo DD, Cerundolo L, Rela M, Heaton ND, Fuggle SV. Leucocyte infiltration and inflammatory antigen expression in cadaveric and living-donor livers before transplant. Transplantation. 2003;75:2001–7.
25. Selck FW, Deb P, Grossman EB. Deceased organ donor characteristics and clinical interventions associated with organ yield. Am J Transplant. 2008;8:965–74.

G. V. Prem Kumar, P. Balachandran, and K. Anusha

Static cold storage is the standard method for liver preservation. The detrimental effects of the concomitant cold ischemia are not suitable for high-risk livers because of which some potentially transplantable livers are being discarded. Normothermic machine perfusion of the liver is an alternative method of preservation that may reduce ischemia-reperfusion injury, biliary complications, early allograft dysfunction, and primary non-function and the clinical benefits are currently proved in various clinical trials. It allows functional assessment of the liver, termed "viability testing." The ability of the liver to reduce lactate in the perfusate is the most widely accepted marker of viability during normothermic machine perfusion, although clinical data are being generated.

28.1 Introduction

Liver transplantation offers the only effective definitive treatment modality for patients with end stage liver disease (ESLD). Shortage of donors limits the organ availability for ESLD patients, hence increasing the mortality in waitlisted patients. Rising incidence of alcohol-related liver disease, viral hepatitis, non-alcoholic fatty liver disease (NAFLD), and non-alcoholic steatohepatitis (NASH) has resulted in increase in number of waitlist candidates for liver transplantation. Hence, the criteria for organ donors have been expanded, to include marginal donors (Table 28.1).

Grafts from extended criteria donors are prone to a higher incidence of severe ischemic reperfusion injury, primary non-function, delayed graft function, acute as well as chronic rejection and intrahepatic biliary stricture, which are more pronounced with static cold storage (SCS). Normothermic machine perfusion (NMP) enables graft preservation at near-physiological condition, thus negating the effects of SCS on hepatocytes and biliary epithelium. NMP provides the liver graft with oxygen and nutrition at 37 °C.

Table 28.1 Extended criteria donors [1, 2]

1	Donor age > 65 years
2	BMI >27 kg/m^2
3	Macrovesicular steatosis >30%
4	Use of high dose vasopressors
5	Hypotension >1 h
6	Hypernatremia (Na >155 meq/mL)
7	Cold ischemia time (CIT) >8 h
8	Warm ischemia time (WIT) >40 min
9	History of alcoholism
10	ICU stay >5 days
11	Donation after cardiac death (DCD)
12	Donors with infection

G. V. P. Kumar (✉) · P. Balachandran
AIG Hospitals, Hyderabad, Telangana, India

K. Anusha
Yashoda Hospitals, Secunderabad, Telangana, India

© The Author(s), under exclusive license to Springer Nature Singapore Pte Ltd. 2023
V. Vohra et al. (eds.), *Peri-operative Anesthetic Management in Liver Transplantation*,
https://doi.org/10.1007/978-981-19-6045-1_28

According to Organ Procurement and Transplantation Network (OPTN) in the USA almost 22% of procured livers are discarded before transplantation, due to the gross appearance of the organ, and donor characteristics [3]. In United Kingdom, this number doubled from 8.2% to 16.6% [4]. This is overcome by assessing the functional status of the liver by NMP, which avoids cold ischemic preservation, thereby improving the use of ECD livers.

28.2 Evolution of NMP

In 1935, Alexis Carell and Charles Lindbergh [5] demonstrated organ viability and preservation for several days, when perfused with oxygenated serum at 37 ° C using a normothermic perfusion chamber. Starzl pursued this work further in the 1960s and indeed the first successful human liver transplants were performed following the pretreatment of livers with machine perfusion of diluted oxygenated blood [6]. In 1968, with introduction of simple and effective static cold storage solutions, the interest on machine perfusion waned due to its complexity [7]. After 50 years, there is resurgence in machine perfusion, with increasing waitlist mortalities due to a large gap between demand and supply of organs, which led to usage of marginal donors. The development of the current NMP techniques began in the early 1990s. The first study demonstrating the potential of NMP was published in 2001 by Schon et al. [8] They found that normothermic extracorporeal liver perfusion (NELP) holds the potential to keep a mammalian liver outside the body completely functional, possibly for more than 4 h. NELP can be used for liver preservation before transplantation or for the use of organs from non-heart beating donors. Few studies have reported successful preservation of Donation after Brain Death (DBD) and Donation after Cardiac Death (DCD) livers for 24 h in NMP compared to SCS livers

[9, 10]. Butler et al. reported that it is possible to maintain a liver in a viable condition for a minimum of 72 h of extracorporeal perfusion. But such long preservation needs bile salt supplementation [11, 12]. Mammalian studies were performed on porcine and rodents due to their close resemblance to human physiology. Brockmann et al. observed that NMP perfused porcine DCD liver grafts have superior function and better survival compared with SCS [13]. NMP proved to be superior to cold storage in porcine DCD livers in terms of liver injury, synthetic graft function, cytokine and proinflammatory response, and survival [14]. Two experimental studies demonstrated that NMP caused defatting of steatotic livers and metabolic conditioning [15, 16].

Many trials were done to assess the safety of NMP. In these studies, they compared the NMP vs. SCS livers by assessing graft survival and viability after transplantation following NMP of donor livers as a primary outcome. They also measured liver functions as bilirubin, Aspartate transaminase (AST), Alanine Transaminase (ALT), Alkaline phosphatase (ALP), and International Normalized Ratio (INR) as markers of early allograft dysfunction for the first 7 days as a secondary outcome.

28.3 Organ Preservation
(Table 28.2)

Table 28.2 Organ preservation techniques

Static method	Dynamic method
University of Wisconsin solution (UW)	Hypothermic machine perfusion (HMP)
Euro Collins solution	Subnormothermic machine perfusion (SMP)
Histidine-tryptophan-ketoglutarate solution (HTK)	Normothermic machine perfusion (NMP)
Celsior solution	
Institute George Lopez-1 (IGL-1)	

28.3.1 Static

The composition and addition of specific ingredients aims to counteract the deleterious effects that occur during cold preservation.

Static type of preservation mainly consists of storage in preservative solutions.

Ideal preservative solution [17]

1. Prevention of hypothermia-induced cell swelling and interstitial edema,
2. Prevention of electrolyte imbalance,
3. Prevention of intracellular acidosis,
4. Reduction of oxidative damage by ROS, and
5. Providing substrates for cellular energy metabolism.

28.3.2 Dynamic

To mitigate injury and improve the quality of the donated organs, by continuous perfusion of graft.

28.3.3 Hypothermic Machine Perfusion (HMP)

HMP involves perfusion at a low temperature (4°–10 °C) with enough oxygen in the perfusate to decrease the metabolic rate. HMP has been shown to protect against mitochondrial and nuclear injury by establishing reduced mitochondrial activity prior to reperfusion, as well as to lessen endothelial injury.

28.3.4 Subnormothermic Machine Perfusion (SMP)

SMP has recently been proposed as an alternative to HMP and NMP. The first study by Vairetti et al. involving SMP showed that perfusion of healthy rat livers at 20 °C resulted in significantly improved preservation compared with CS upon simulated transplantation [18].

In 2012, SMP at both 20 °C and 30 °C was investigated in a rat DCD model, and was directly compared with both CS and NMP [19]. After transplantation, livers preserved with SMP showed high bilirubin levels and low bile production compared with NMP.

28.3.5 Normothermic Machine Perfusion (NMP)

Unlike SCS, HMP, and SMP techniques, NMP aims to maintain normal metabolic rates in an attempt to maintain normal physiological conditions. Normothermic machine perfusion (NMP) is used to minimize the duration of cold storage, and is applied either in situ (e.g.; in donors before procurement), known as normothermic regional perfusion [20], or ex situ during or after organ transport to the recipient center.

In this chapter, we will focus on role of NMP in preservation of grafts from the marginal donors.

Advantages
- Improvement of transplant logistics.
- Increases donor pool by utilizing ECD and DCD, thereby reducing the waitlist mortality.
- Real-time assessment of organ function and viability prior to transplantation.
- Attenuation of ischemia/reperfusion injury.
- Washout of toxins and anaerobic end products like lactic acid, reactive oxygen species (ROS).
- Provides nutrients, ATP, oxygen, glucose, bile salts, prostaglandins.
- Potential for pharmacological interventions to recondition livers, and subsequent transplantation.
- Pre-emptive correction of electrolyte and acid base imbalance.
- Endothelial protection.
- Ischemic reconditioning.
- Low early transaminases levels post-transplant.
- Extended preservation.
- Reduced incidence of primary non-function, delayed graft function.
- Maintenance of vasoconstriction.
- Ability to predict post-transplant outcome.

Disadvantages

- Cost.
- Lack of adequate randomized trials to validate its pros and cons.
- Bacterial and fungal infections.
- Complicated machinery.
- Complicated procedures.
- Additional personnel, especially during transportation.
- Risk of subjecting good grafts to ischemia due to twisting or catheter occlusion, leading to graft loss.

28.4   Machine

The machine is devised using components developed for cardiopulmonary bypass.

It consists of:

1. Blood reservoir,
2. Pump(s) (some circuits comprise two pumps, representing portal venous and hepatic arterial flow),
3. Oxygenator, and
4. Heat exchanger.

The different commercially available devices are as follows:

1. The OrganOx metra (OrganOx Ltd., Oxford, UK),
2. The Liver Assist (Organ Assist, Gronigen, the Netherlands),
3. OCS™ Liver System (Transmedics, Andover, Massachusetts), and
4. The Cleveland NMP circuit (Cleveland Clinic, Cleveland, Ohio).

The basic NMP principles are retained, all these machines differ with few technical variations with respect to arterial flow, pressure control, oxygen delivery method, battery life, temperature during perfusion, feasibility of transportation during preservation (portability),

degree of automation, substrate type and delivery, pressure and pulsatility of the recirculating perfusate, and hepatic arterial and portal vein flow targets.

Here, we will describe OrganOx metra machine (Figs. 28.1 and 28.2)**, the most widely used machine, with published clinical data.**

The OrganOx metra normothermic perfusion device incorporates a centrifugal pump, an oxygenator, oxygen concentrator, heat exchanger, reservoir, flow probes, pressure sensors, infusions and blood gas analyzer together with tubings and connector components.

Full informed consent of potential recipients is critical, when considering liver grafts from extended criteria donors.

After harvesting, the graft is flushed with a preservative solution (HTK/UW solution) at 4 °C, and kept in a static cold storage. The graft is cannulated using various color coded cannulae (blue for the Inferior Vena Cava (IVC), red for the Hepatic Artery, yellow for Portal vein).

Meanwhile, the machine circuit is primed using 3 units of Leucoreduced packed red blood cells (cross matched to donor blood group) along with 5% albumin or Gelofusin, calcium gluconate, heparin and antibiotic (e.g. Cefuroxime) (Fig. 28.3b).

A. Graft kept in SCS initially for cannulation of vessels and bile duct.
B. Priming of circuit.
C. Surrogate organ Y-piece within the liver bowl.
D. After disconnecting the organ Y- piece.
E. Reconnection with the respective color coded cannulae of the graft.

The perfusion solution is maintained at 37 °C. Pressures are set at a mean of 70 mmHg on the arterial and 11 mmHg on the portal side. Perfusion fluid is oxygenated through oxygenators. Before NMP and every 30 mins during NMP, samples of the arterial and venous perfusion fluid are taken for analysis of blood gas parameters (pH, partial pressure of oxygen [PO_2],

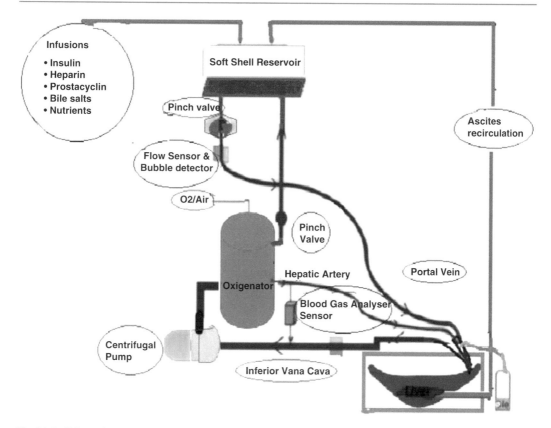

Fig. 28.1 Schematic diagram of organox metra machine

Fig. 28.2 Organox
metra machine

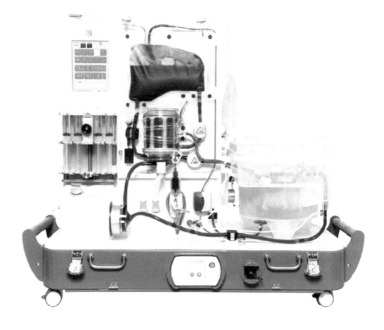

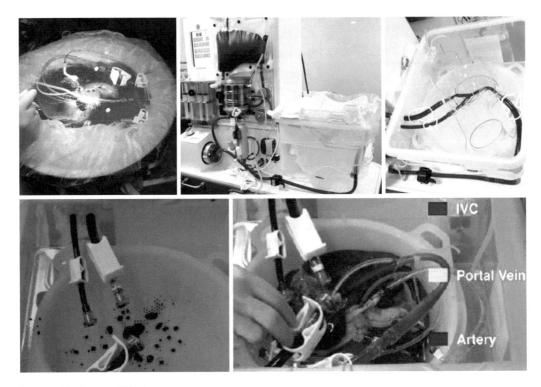

Fig. 28.3 Setting up of NMP

partial pressure of carbon dioxide [PCO$_2$], oxygen saturation [SO$_2$], bicarbonate [HCO3], lactate, glucose, and metHb). Bile samples are also collected to assess the adequacy of graft function (Fig. 28.4).

After priming, surrogate organ Y-piece within the liver bowl is disconnected. These circuits are reconnected to the respective color coded cannulae of the graft after deairing of the tubings. After ensuring proper connections, the machine perfusion is started.

Maintenance infusion solutions provided during the perfusion are Epoprostenol (prostacyclin), bile salts, insulin, heparin, nutrition including amino acids plus electrolytes. Sodium bicarbonate can be added if required during the perfusion, to maintain pH within physiological range of 7.35–7.45.

Bile produced by the liver is collected and measured every 30 mins.

Once the liver is placed on the device, the operation is fully automated with the exception of the manual glucose measurement. A graphical user interface (GUI) system displays several perfusion parameters during the operation: (Fig. 28.5).

- Flow rates: Arterial, Portal, and IVC, all in L/m.
- Pressures: Arterial, Portal, IVC, all in mmHg.
- Blood gases: pO$_2$, pCO$_2$, in kPa or mmHg (units can be changed by touching the GUI)
- pH.
- Blood temperature (°C).
- Bile production (mL/h).

The perfusate flows from reservoir to a hepatic artery through a high pressure system (low flow), and by gravity drainage to the portal vein, through a high flow system (low pressure). From the liver graft, the perfusate is pumped out of the inferior vena cava by a centrifugal pump. This is oxygenated and heated and collected back in reservoir bag.

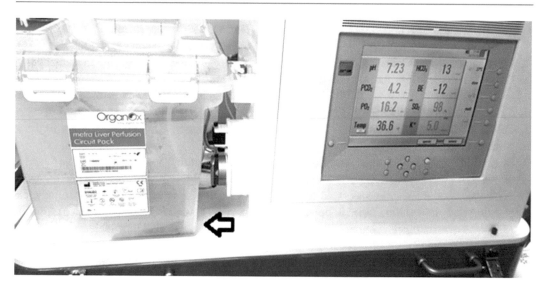

Fig. 28.4 Bile produced after machine perfusion, collected in liver bowl for assessment

Fig. 28.5 Graphical
user interface (GUI)
system

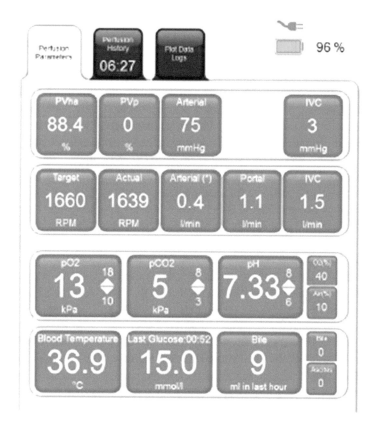

Organox machine benefits

1. Simple control panel.
2. Fully automated perfusion.
3. Rugged, robust design for ease of transport and safe storage.
4. Extended battery life for transportation.
5. Self-regulating oxygen supply.
6. Sterile disposable circuit which is pre-assembled, making it simple and rapid to prime.
7. All connectors are simple and rapid to use, ensuring that preparation time is minimal.
8. Maintains physiological temperature, flows, pressures, oxygenation and records bile production, all of which are displayed on the built in graphical user interface.

28.5 Patho-Physiology During Preservation

Preservation and optimization of the graft plays a key role in successful outcome of transplantation.

The main aim of preservation is to reduce the ischemic reperfusion injury (IRI) by maintaining the structural and functional integrity of the liver.

Static cold storage (SCS) is considered a gold standard for organ preservation. SCS when used to preserve organs after procurement slows metabolic processes. **Van't Hoff's rule**, cooling at 4 °C results in a metabolic rate approximately 10% of that at normal body temperature (37 °C). SCS at 4 °C is adequate for low risk livers. But in marginal livers, cold ischemia is poorly tolerated. It causes altered membrane potential due to altered ion distribution (++ intracellular Ca/Na) leading to cellular swelling, cytoskeletal disorganization, increased hypoxanthine, decreased ATP, cellular acidosis, and mitochondrial damage. This causes damage to hepatic sinusoidal endothelial cells and disruption of the microcirculation. These processes cannot be halted and invariably leading to damage of the organ during preservation and reperfusion.

During reperfusion, there is a rebound uptake of oxygen by cells leading to the release of free radicals, endothelial damage, intrahepatic inflammatory infiltration (leukocyte accumulation), and release of pro-inflammatory cytokines into circulation. Initiating cell death by necrosis, apoptosis, or autophagy. Ultimately, resulting in tissue damage.

The main rationale for normothermic machine perfusion is to mimic physiological conditions by maintaining physiological temperature, oxygenation enabling cellular metabolic function during organ storage, and avoiding depletion of cellular energy stores, eliminating metabolic waste products and finally preventing direct adverse events of hypothermia and static storage.

Many studies have shown beneficial effects of machine perfusion over static cold storage with respect to reduction of ischemic reperfusion (IR) injury.

Schlegel et al. [21] performed hypothermic oxygenated perfusion (HOPE) treatment through the portal vein, which led to a significant slowdown of mitochondrial respiration rate during 1 h machine perfusion. After reperfusion following low pressure HOPE, mitochondrial injury, nuclear injury, Kupffer cell activation and endothelial injury were significantly improved, as tested on an isolated liver perfusion model. In contrast, machine perfusion with deoxygenated perfusate showed no protection from hepatocyte injury and Kupffer cell activation. However, endothelial injury was also prevented by low pressure machine perfusion in the absence of oxygen. Perfusion with higher pressure provoked endothelial damage and Kupffer cell activation.

Imber et al. [9] observed that livers preserved with normothermic perfusion were significantly superior ($P = 0.05$) to cold-stored livers in terms of bile production, factor V production, glucose metabolism, and galactose clearance. Cold-stored livers showed significantly higher levels of hepatocellular enzymes in the perfusate and were found to have significantly more damage by a blinded histological scoring system.

28.6 Human Trials

The first-in-human normothermic machine perfusion of the liver (NMP-L) trial in 2013 confirmed the safety of the technology. In 20 patients transplanted with livers after NMP-L, there was 100% graft and patient survival at 6 months [22]. Laing et al. used hemoglobin-based oxygen carrier (HBOC)-201 and gelofusine for NMP [23].

Ravikumar et al. [22] compared NMP and SCS livers, observed initial 7 day transaminases levels and 30 day graft survival and concluded that NMP may be valuable in increasing the number of donor livers and improving the function of transplantable organs.

Selzner et al. [24] reported a safety and feasibility clinical NEVLP (Normothermic Ex Vivo Liver Perfusion) trial with human albumin–based Steen solution. They studied the transplant outcomes of ten human liver grafts that were perfused on the Metra device at 37 °C with Steen solution, plus 3 units of erythrocytes and compared with a matched historical control group of 30 grafts using cold storage (CS) as the preservation technique. Ten liver grafts were perfused for 480 mins (340–580 mins). They observed for lactate clearance and bile production during perfusion. Postoperatively, they monitored transaminases, bilirubin and INR, but didn't find significant difference between the two groups. They concluded that liver preservation with normothermic ex vivo perfusion with the Metra device using Steen solution is safe and resulted in comparable outcomes to CS after liver transplantation.

Bral et al. [25] presented a preliminary single-center North American experience using identical NMP technology. Out of ten grafts, 9 were transplanted and one was discarded due to portal vein cannulation issue. All transplanted livers functioned, and serum transaminases, bilirubin, international normalized ratio, and lactate levels corrected in NMP recipients similarly to controls. Graft survival at 30 days (primary outcome) was not statistically different between two groups. They found that Intensive care and hospital stays were significantly more prolonged in the NMP group. Their preliminary experience demonstrates feasibility as well as potential technical risks of NMP in a North American setting and highlighted a need for larger, randomized studies.

Nasralla et al. [26] did first randomized controlled trial to test the efficacy of machine perfusion against static cold storage in liver transplantation. They compared 170 NMP with 133 SCS livers. They observed that normothermic preservation is associated with a 50% reduction in graft injury, measured by hepatocellular enzyme release, despite a 50% reduction of organ discard and a 54% longer mean preservation time. They didn't find significant difference in bile duct complications, graft survival or survival of the patient. If NMP is applied to clinical practice, these results would have a major impact on liver transplant outcomes and waiting list mortality.

28.7 COPE Trial (Consortium for Organ Preservation in Europe)

First multicenter randomized controlled trial (RCT) comparing continuous NMP with SCS in human liver transplantation. This multi-national RCT was initiated by the Consortium for Organ Preservation in Europe [27], involving seven European transplant centers. They randomized adult DBD and type III DCD livers (1:1) to continuous NMP or SCS. Their primary end point was the difference in peak-AST, requiring 220 transplants (90% power to detect a 33% reduction). Secondary endpoints were organ utilization, preservation time, early allograft dysfunction (EAD), 6-month graft and patient survival and ischemic cholangiopathy on MRCP. They found that 272 livers (135 SCS, 137 NMP) were enrolled, consisting of 194 DBD and 78 DCD organs. 48 livers were discarded after retrieval (32 SCS vs. 16 NMP; $p = 0.01$), with two others declined but then transplanted by non-trial sites. NMP livers experienced significantly longer preservation times than SCS (11 h 39 min vs. 7 h 21 min; $p < 0.01$). Early graft function was superior in the NMP group with regard to peak AST

(974 IU/L SCS vs. 485 IU/L NMP; $p < 0.001$) and EAD (29.9% SCS vs. 12.6% NMP; $p = 0.002$). The magnitude of these effects was greater for DCD organs ($p = 0.02$). They concluded NMP livers show better early graft function than SCS as measured by peak-AST and EAD, both of which are surrogates for long-term graft outcomes. This is despite better organ utilization and longer preservation times in the NMP group.

VITTAL [28] trial is the first clinical trial designed to objectively assess function of declined livers using NMP-L and subsequently transplanting viable grafts. Laing RW et al. have conducted an open-label, non-randomized, prospective, single-arm trial designed to determine whether currently unused donor livers can be salvaged and safely transplanted. These livers are subjected to NMP following a period of static cold storage. Organs metabolizing lactate to $\leq$2.5 mmol/L within 4 h of the perfusion commencing in combination with two or more of the following parameters—bile production, metabolism of glucose, a hepatic arterial flow rate $\geq$150 mL/min and a portal venous flow rate $\geq$500 mL/min, a pH $\geq$7.30 and/or maintain a homogeneous perfusion—were considered viable and transplanted into a suitable consented recipient.

Their primary outcome measures are the success rate of NMP to produce a transplantable organ and 90-day patient post-transplant survival.

NICE: "More donor livers could be used for transplantation thanks to exciting new development"

January 16, 2019.

The National Institute for Health and Care Excellence (NICE) has approved the use in the NHS of ex vivo machine perfusion for preservation of livers donated for transplants. This procedure assessed by NICE has been hailed as an "exciting development" in increasing the number of livers which can be safely used for transplantation.

28.8 Parameters Assessed for Viability of Organ

NMP allows functional assessment of liver before transplantation, thereby reducing the incidence of PNF, EAD, Biliary complications, IRI, and PRS.

Mergental et al. [25] suggested criteria including perfusate lactate <2.5 mmol/L, bile production within 2 h of initiation of NMP, pH > 7.3, hepatic artery flow >150 mL/min, portal vein flow >500 mL/min, and homogenous graft perfusion with soft parenchymal consistency fulfilled within 3 h of initiation of NMP.

Viability criteria consisting of lactate clearance, pH maintenance, bile production, vascular flow patterns, and liver macroscopic appearance.

Mergental et al. suggested viability criteria (Table 28.3).

Biopsies were assessed for preexisting acute or chronic liver injury, large and small-droplet macrovesicular steatosis, coagulative necrosis, intrahepatic bile duct injury (apoptosis, vacuolation, and lifting of epithelium from the basement membrane), hepatocyte plate injury (hepatocyte loss of cohesion, detachment of hepatocyte plates from the sinusoidal lining), and glycogen depletion, which were recorded as percentages of cells affected [30].

During perfusion, two patterns of bile flow were identified: (1) steadily increasing bile production, resulting in a cumulative output of $\geq$30 g after 6 h (high bile output group), and (2) a cumulative bile production <20 g in 6 h (low bile output group). Concentrations of transaminases and

Table 28.3 Organ viability criteria

Perfusate lactate <2.5 mmol/L
Bile production within 2 h of initiation of NMP
pH > 7.3
Hepatic artery flow >150 mL/min
Portal vein flow >500 mL/min
Homogenous graft perfusion with soft parenchymal consistency

[a]Criteria to be fulfilled within 3 h of initiation of NMP

potassium in the perfusion fluid were significantly higher in the low bile output group, compared to the high bile output group. Biliary concentrations of bilirubin and bicarbonate were, respectively, 4 times and 2 times higher in the high bile output group. Livers in the low bile output group displayed more signs of hepatic necrosis and venous congestion, compared to the high bile output group. In conclusion, bile production could be an easily assessable biomarker of hepatic viability during ex vivo machine perfusion of human donor livers. It could potentially be used to identify extended criteria livers that are suitable for transplantation. These ex vivo findings need to be confirmed in a transplant experiment or a clinical trial [31].

28.9 Conclusion

In conclusion, this proof of concept that NMP is not only feasible, but that it may potentially improve the functional recovery of high-risk ECD livers compared with SCS. Although this is not an optimized protocol, this novel approach might be particularly beneficial for DCD organs. Normothermic machine perfusion is associated with a stable intraoperative hemodynamic profile postreperfusion, requiring significantly less vasopressor infusions and blood product transfusion after graft reperfusion and may have benefit to alleviate ischemia-reperfusion injury in liver transplantation. Further studies are needed to explore whether NMP confers other benefits.

References

1. Routh D, Naidu S, Sharma S, Ranjan P, Godara R. Changing pattern of donor selection criteria in deceased donor liver transplant: a review of literature. J Clin Exp Hepatol. 2013;3:337–46.
2. Nair A, Hashimoto K. Extended criteria donors in liver transplantation—from marginality to mainstream. Hepatobiliary Surg Nutr. 2018;7(5):386–8.
3. Feng S, Goodrich NP, Bragg-Gresham JL, Dykstra DM, Punch JD, DebRoy MA, et al. Characteristics associated with liver graft failure: the concept of a donor risk index. Am J Transplant. 2006;6(4):783–90.
4. NHSBT. Annual Report on Liver Transplantation. 2016.
5. Carrel A, Lindbergh CA. The culture of whole organs. Science. 1935;81:621–3.
6. Starzl TE, Groth CG, Brettschneider L, Moon JB, Fulginiti VA, Cotton EK, et al. Extended survival in 3 cases of orthotopic homotransplantations of the human liver. Surgery. 1968;63(4):549–63.
7. Belzer FO, Ashby BS, Gulyassy PF, Powell M. Successful seventeen-hour preservation and transplantation of human cadaver kidney. N Engl J Med. 1968;278:608–10.
8. Schon MR, Kollmar O, Wolf S, Schrem H, Matthes M, Akkoc N, et al. Liver transplantation after organ preservation with normothermic extracorporeal perfusion. Ann Surg. 2001;233:114–23.
9. Imber CJ, St Peter SD, Lopez de Cenarruzabeitia I, Pigott D, James T, Taylor R, et al. Advantages of normothermic perfusion over cold storage in liver preservation. Transplantation. 2002;73:701–9.
10. St Peter SD, Imber CJ, Lopez I, Hughes D, Friend PJ. Extended preservation of non-heart-beating donor livers with normothermic machine perfusion. Br J Surg. 2002;89:609–16.
11. Butler AJ, Rees MA, Wight DG, Casey ND, Alexander G, White DJ, et al. Successful extracorporeal porcine liver perfusion for 72 hr. Transplantation. 2002;73:1212–8.
12. Imber CJ, St Peter SD, de Cenarruzabeitia IL, Lemonde H, Rees M, Butler A, et al. Optimisation of bile production during normothermic preservation of porcine livers. Am J Transplant. 2002;2:593–9.
13. Brockmann J, Reddy S, Coussios C, et al. Normothermic perfusion: a new paradigm for organ preservation. Ann Surg. 2009;250(1):1–6.
14. Fondevila C, Hessheimer AJ, Maathuis MH, et al. Superior preservation of DCD livers with continuous normothermic perfusion. Ann Surg. 2011;254:1000–7.
15. Jamieson RW, Zilvetti M, Roy D, et al. Hepatic steatosis and normothermic perfusion-preliminary experiments in a porcine model. Transplantation. 2011;92:289–95.
16. Nagrath D, Xu H, Tanimura Y, et al. Metabolic preconditioning of donor organs: defatting fatty livers by normothermic perfusion ex vivo. Metab Eng. 2009;11:274–83.
17. Belzer FO, Southard JH. Principles of solid-organ preservation by cold storage. Transplantation. 1988;45:673–6.
18. Vairetti M, Ferrigno A, Rizzo V, Richelmi P, Boncompagni E, Neri D, et al. Subnormothermic machine perfusion protects against rat liver preservation injury: a comparative evaluation with conventional cold storage. Transplant Proc. 2007;39:1765–7.
19. Tolboom H, Izamis ML, Sharma N, Milwid JM, Uygun B, Berthiaume F, et al. Subnormothermic machine perfusion at both 20°C and 30°C recovers ischemic rat livers for successful transplantation. J Surg Res. 2012;175:149–56.

20. Oniscu GC, Randle LV, Muiesan P, et al. In situ normothermic regional perfusion for controlled donation after circulatory death—the United Kingdom experience. Am J Transplant. 2014;14:2181–6.

21. Schlegel A, Rougemont O, Graf R, Clavien PA, Dutkowski P. Protective mechanisms of end-ischemic cold machine perfusion in DCD liver grafts. J Hepatol. 2013;58:278–86.

22. Ravikumar R, Jassem W, Mergental H, Heaton N, Mirza D, Perera MT, et al. Liver transplantation after ex vivo normothermic machine preservation: a phase 1 (first-in-man) clinical trial. Am J Transplant. 2016;16:1779–87.

23. Laing RW, Bhogal RH, Wallace L, Boteon Y, Neil DAH, Smith A, et al. The use of an acellular oxygen carrier in a human liver model of normothermic machine perfusion. Transplantation. 2017;101:2746–56.

24. Selzner M, Goldaracena N, Echeverri J, et al. Normothermic ex vivo liver perfusion using Steen solution as perfusate for human liver transplantation: first north American results. Liver Transpl. 2016;22(11):1501–8.

25. Bral M, Gala-Lopez B, Bigam D, et al. Preliminary single center Canadian experience of human normothermic ex vivo liver perfusion: results of a clinical trial. Am J Transplant. 2017;17(4):1071–80.

26. Nasralla D, Coussios CC, Mergental H, Akhtar MZ, Butler AJ, Ceresa CDL, et al. A randomized trial of normothermic preservation in liver transplantation. Nature. 2018;557:50.

27. Nasralla D, et al. A randomized trial of normothermic preservation in liver transplantation. Nature. 2018;557(7703):50–6.

28. Laing RW, Mergental H, Yap C, et al. Viability testing and transplantation of marginal livers (VITTAL) using normothermic machine perfusion: study protocol for an open-label, non-randomised, prospective, single-arm trial. BMJ Open. 2017;7:e017733.

29. Mergental H, Roll GR. Normothermic machine perfusion of the liver. Clin Liver Dis. 2017;10(4):97.

30. Silva MA, Mirza DF, Murphy N, Richards DA, Reynolds GM, Wigmore SJ, Neil DA. Intrahepatic complement activation, sinusoidal endothelial injury, and lactic acidosis are associated with initial poor function of the liver after transplantation. Transplantation. 2008;85:718–25.

31. Sutton ME, Op Den Dries S, Karimian N, et al. Criteria for viability assessment of discarded human donor livers during ex vivo normothermic machine perfusion. PLoS One. 2014;9(11):e110642.

Role of ECMO in Liver Transplant

29

Jumana Yusuf Haji

J. Y. Haji (✉)
Department of Heart Transplantation and Advanced Cardiothoracic Surgery, Sir H. N. Reliance Foundation Hospital, Mumbai, Maharashtra, India
e-mail: drjyhaji@gmail.com

Abbreviations

ABG	Arterial blood gas
ACLF	Acute-on-chronic liver failure
ACT	Activated clotting time
ALF	Acute liver failure
APTT	Activated partial thromboplastin time
ARDS	Acute respiratory distress syndrome
CBC	Complete blood count
CCA	Cerebral circulatory arrest
CIT	Cold ischaemia time
CLD	Chronic liver disease
CNS	Central nervous system
DBD	Donation after brain death
DCD	Donation after cardiac death
ECLS	Extracorporeal life support
ECMO	Extracorporeal membrane oxygenation
ECPR	ECMO-assisted cardiopulmonary resuscitation
EEG	Electroencephalography
FDO_2	Fraction of sweep oxygen
FiO_2	Fraction of inhaled oxygen
HPS	Hepatopulmonary syndrome
IJV	Internal jugular vein
INR	International ratio
LDH	Lactate dehydrogenase
LFT	Liver function test
NMP	Normothermic machine perfusion
NRP	Normothermic regional perfusion
OP ECMO	Organ-preserving ECMO
$PaCO_2$	Arterial partial pressure of carbon dioxide
PaO_2	Arterial partial pressure of oxygen
PT	Prothrombin time
RFT	Renal function test
RP	Regional perfusion
SBP	Systolic blood pressure
TCD	Transcranial doppler
THOA	Transplantation of Human Organs Act
VA	Veno-arterial
VV	Veno-venous
WIT	Warm ischaemia time

29.1 Introduction

Extracorporeal membrane oxygenation (ECMO) is a form of extracorporeal life support (ECLS), which can take over the function of the heart or lung or both. The primary aim of ECMO is to rest these vital organs and take over their functions of oxygenation and delivery of oxygenated blood to the other vital organs, such as the kidney, liver, and brain.

Perioperative management of liver transplantation involves meticulous planning and stabilisation of the donor and recipient to achieve good results. Hence, a stable donor with good organs, minimal warm ischaemia time (WIT) to the organs, and a fit optimized recipient will greatly improve the post-transplant outcomes.

Liver transplantation can be a challenging proposition in certain situations as follows:

1. The potential donor, in a deceased donor transplant, is unstable.
2. WIT is prolonged due to delay in retrieval of organs.
3. The potential liver recipient, despite optimisation, remains in the fairly high-risk group due to comorbidities involving heart and lungs additionally.
4. The peri-operative and post-operative course is complicated by massive transfusions, reperfusion injury, and fluid overload which may lead to ARDS and/or cardiac decompensation.

ECMO plays a role in organ donation (to improve the quality of organs retrieved) where the focus is not on saving the patient but rather on preserving the viability of the organs. In transplant recipients, ECMO has a role when there is perioperative cardiac or pulmonary instability.

This chapter will introduce the reader to the various applications of ECMO in the liver transplant program.

29.2 ECMO Overview

ECMO, a form of ECLS, in its actual application is an evolution of the heart–lung machines used in cardiac surgery [1]. The first reported clinical application of extracorporeal support was in 1971 for respiratory failure in a young adult with post-traumatic ARDS. He underwent 2 days of veno-arterial support and survived. Interest in ECMO for adult respiratory failure following this case report resulted in a more widespread application. In 1975–1976, Bartlett et al. successfully applied bedside CPB to treat a new-born with meconium aspiration, marking the beginning of ECMO in critical care.

ECMO is now considered an extension of critical care, and the spectrum of indications is widening and becoming more dependent on the clinical picture at the time of presentation of the patient. With availability of improved technology and equipment, the contraindications to ECMO are decreasing. The patient who should ideally be considered for ECMO is an otherwise healthy person with no comorbidities who presents with life-threatening hypoxia and/or circulatory collapse. However, the window of opportunity to salvage such terminally ill patients is small, and if delayed till very late, it may become a futile exercise. Although ECMO has the capability to support cardiorespiratory function temporarily, it is not a cure for the underlying disease. It is a safety net that takes over the function of the heart/lung while the diseased organ rests and heals. In addition, ECMO has potential to halt further damage to other vital organs such as kidney, liver, brain due to hypoxia and low cardiac output state.

Depending on its configuration, ECMO can be either venovenous (VV) or venoarterial (VA) and is used to support respiratory function, circulation, or both. This treatment provides a bridge to aid in healing of these organs or as long-term support in those awaiting heart or lung transplantation. ECMO-assisted cardiopulmonary resuscitation (ECPR) has become an accepted norm in many countries, and the usage of ECMO in this case is either as a bridge to recovery or if futile a bridge to decision. If there is a wish to donate, then in such patients, ECMO can be bridge to organ donation [2, 3].

29.3   ECMO Components [4]

- **Centrifugal pump**: This helps to circulate blood volume from the patient to the oxygenator and back to the patient after gas exchange (Fig. 29.1). A minimum of 60% of the cardiac output needs to be circulated to meet ECMO goals. Newer pumps are efficient, with minimal reservoir volumes, and unlike roller pumps used in cardiopulmonary bypass machines, they cause less damage to blood cells, reducing the need for anticoagulation.

- **Membrane oxygenator**: (Fig. 29.2) This is made of multiple hollow fibres creating channels, with fibres of polymethyl pentene, a special material that selectively allows only gas to move across and is impermeable to liquids. The channels are crosslinked into a mesh of two sets of channels: one carrying blood and the second carrying water from the heater unit

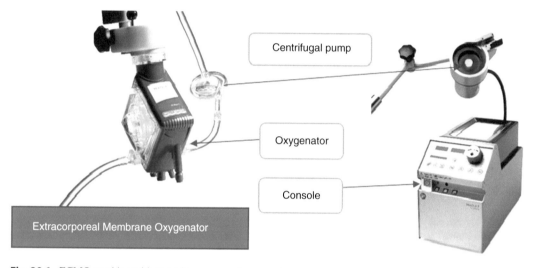

Fig. 29.1 ECMO machine with console, pump, and oxygenator

Fig. 29.2 Cross-section of an oxygenator showing the blood and water channels at right angle plane with gas flowing between the channels. Heater cooler unit supplies water through the channels and is essential to maintain blood temperature during transit through the oxygenator

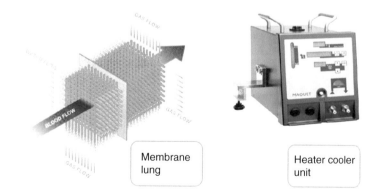

to prevent temperature fluctuations of blood during transit, and the space between the channels carries the gas (sweep gas), which could be oxygen or a mixture of air and oxygen for gas exchange.

29.4 Functions

Oxygenation The FiO_2 of the sweep gas (FDO_2) and the blood flow determine the oxygenation function of the membrane lung.

CO_2 Removal The rate of sweep gas flow determines the CO_2 elimination and is usually started at half the blood flow rate and titrated up to normalize the PCO_2. CO_2 elimination is easy, and in lungs with good compliance, a sweep flow as low as 1 L/min can also enable adequate CO_2 removal.

Heat Exchanger This is to prevent a drop in the temperature of the blood in the extracorporeal

circuit. Sometimes, patients are maintained slightly hypothermic to reduce their metabolic needs and oxygen requirement. The controlled temperature may mask any fever and thus, the first sign of sepsis.

Cannulas (Fig. 29.3) The cannulas are placed in the major blood vessels either peripherally or centrally into the major blood vessels to access blood flow into the membrane lung and return oxygenated blood back to the patient. Arterial cannulas are available in sizes of 19 and 21F, and venous cannulas are usually 150 cm long, with diameters of 19, 23, and 27F.

They are wire reinforced to prevent kinking and large enough to allow adequate blood flow and may also be anticoagulant coated. The access (venous) cannula in peripheral ECMOs are long and placed in a femoral vein. The return (arterial) cannula is short, and the vessel chosen for return cannula determines the configuration of ECMO.

Fig. 29.3 The arterial and venous cannulas inserted are wire reinforced and antikink large bore

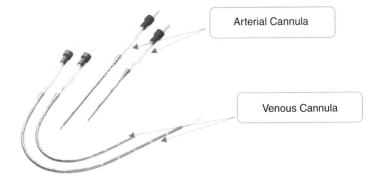

Arterial Cannula

Venous Cannula

29.5 ECMO Configurations:
Fig. 29.4

29.5.1 Venoarterial ECMO (VA ECMO)

Used for cardiac and circulatory support. It is achieved by placing the return cannula into a peripheral artery such as the femoral artery or the axillary artery such that blood is returned towards the heart through the artery and then the aorta carries it to the rest of the body. The VA configuration creates a parallel circulation to the heart bypassing the heart and hence is independent of the ejection fraction.

Clinical Picture Warranting VA ECMO [5]

Urgent	Cardiac index <2 l/min/m²
	Inotrope score is >50–100
	Inotrope score = dose of dopamine (mcg/kg/min) + dobutamine (mcg/kg/min) + 100 (dose of adrenaline (mcg/kg/min) + noradrenaline (mcg/kg/min)
	The rate of inotrope escalation is more important than the dose
	With or without intra-aortic balloon pump (IABP) support
Emergency	Resuscitation ongoing without adequate cardiac pump function

Indications for VA ECMO

Reversible Cardiac Conditions with Excellent Recovery

- Intractable Arrhythmias (Ventricular tachycardia/Fibrillation)
- Viral Myocarditis
- Pulmonary embolism with right heart failure
- Cardiac stunning from poisoning/drugs, for e.g., amlodipine overdose.

29.5.2 Venovenous ECMO (VV ECMO)

Used for gas exchange and lung support. It is achieved by placing the return cannula into a major vein like the internal jugular vein (IJV) or the femoral vein.

Clinical Picture Warranting VV ECMO

- Mortality risk >80%:
- $PaO_2/FiO_2 < 80$ with $FiO_2 > 0.9$.
- Murray score 3–4 (Table 29.1).

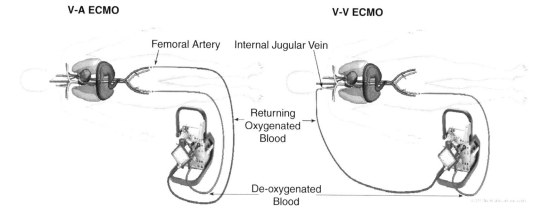

V-A ECMO   **V-V ECMO**

Femoral Artery   Internal Jugular Vein

Returning Oxygenated Blood

De-oxygenated Blood

Fig. 29.4 Shows the configuration of Venoarterial and venovenous cannula placement of cannulas. When blood is returned to an artery it results in a venoarterial configuration. Blood returned from oxygenator to a major vein as shown results in a venovenous configuration

Table 29.1 The Murray score calculator

Murray score	0 points	1 point	2 points	3 points	4 points
Chest Xray (quadrants with consolidation)	n.0	n.1	n.2	n.3	n.4
Hypoxaemia (PaO$_2$/FiO$_2$)	>300	225–299	175–224	101–174	<100
PEEP (cm H$_2$O)	<5	6–8	9–11	12–14	>15
Compliance (mL/cm H$_2$O)	>80	60–79	40–59	20–39	<19

The final score is calculated as the sum of the component parts divided by 4

Indications for VV ECMO

Direct Lung Injury

Common
- Pneumonia
- Aspiration

Uncommon
- Reperfusion injury
- Fat embolism

Indirect Lung Injury

Common
- Sepsis
- Massive transfusion

Uncommon
- Acute pancreatitis

29.5.3 Management of Patient on ECMO

Anticoagulation It is essential to prevent clotting of blood in the extracorporeal circuit. Usual regime used is unfractionated heparin bolus (100–150 U/kg) at initiation and continued as an infusion (10–15 U/kg/hr) to maintain activated clotting time (ACT) 1.5 times normal level (at 180–200 s or activated partial thromboplastin time (APTT) 1.5 times the reference level at 45–65 s or antithrombin time (AT) III 80–120% while keeping the platelet count and fibrinogen levels in the normal range. Using surface coated circuits help to run the ECMO with lower systemic heparinisation. Viscoelastic tests such as TEG and ROTEM help with better management of anticoagulation in especially in coagulopathic patients.

Investigations Table 29.2 describes the investigations needed to assess ECMO candidacy, achievement of goals, and anticipation of complications.

29.5.4 Complications

Table 29.3 These can be expected to occur at any time during the ECMO run and can be due to anticoagulation, circuit-related, cannulation-related, or equipment-related factors. Knowledge of complications is important as it will help understand contraindications and potential challenges of initiating ECMO on a CLD/post-transplant patient.

All patients will need periodic detailed examination for neurological complications, vascular complications, bleeding complications, haemolytic complications, and complications due to super added infections.

29.5.5 ECMO in Liver Transplantation

ECMO in liver transplantation does not follow conventional indications, contraindications, and management principles. This chapter will cover various types of ECMO applications, as follows:

29.5.5.1 In Donors

1. Brain-dead donor (DBD) who when becomes unstable, the donor management becomes difficult in view of haemodynamic instability and enhanced oxygen requirement and is stabilized with ECMO – Organ preserving (OP) ECMO.
2. In Donation after cardiac death (DCD) assisted with ECMO to ensure good functional organs with minimal warm ischaemia time.

Table 29.2 Investigations and their frequency and clinical value during ECMO run to assess patient

Haematological	Hb	Often to assess for bleeding Maintain Hb > 10 if ECMO goals not met and during cannulation
	Haematocrit	>30
	WBC count	Daily to look for sepsis as patient on ECMO may not spike temperature due to temperature control
	Peripheral smear LDH Plasma free Haemoglobin	Daily to look for haemolysis especially if running at higher flows
Coagulation profile	ACT—hourly	To titrate heparin need
	APTT—6 hourly	To titrate heparin need
	Platelet count—daily	Maintain >50,000
	Fibrinogen—daily	Maintain normal levels 200–400 mg/dl
	TEG/ROTEM	Useful in coagulopathic patients to assess blood product requirements
Metabolic parameters	Lactate	As needed for assessing ECMO goals, metabolic needs, liver function
	ABG	As needed for titrating FiO_2 and sweep gas to maintain oxygenation pH and CO_2 clearance
	$SCVO_2$	To assess oxygen delivery (DO_2) versus consumption (VO_2)
	Sugar	As needed to maintain blood sugar levels in normal range
	Electrolytes	As required
Organ function testing	Heart	Daily echocardiogram, ECG to guide ECMO configuration, maintenance and decannulation strategies
	Lung	Daily X-ray chest for cannula position and to assess lungs Thoracic CT scan for assessing lung only if needed as difficult to move patient on ECMO
	Liver	LFT daily
	Kidney	RFT daily
	Brain	EEG, TCD, and CT as indicated to assess function if clinical examination inconclusive NIRS- to assess brain oxygenation
Predicting secondary infections	Cultures Procalcitonin CRP	Maintain high degree of suspicion as ECMO patients are prone to line sepsis and septic markers may be masked due to controlled temperature

3. Patients on ECMO in ICU and progress as donors after brain death- As ECMO is an extension of critical care, more patients will receive ECMO but when the ECMO runs become futile and progress to brain death, they may be considered as potential donors.

These points necessitate careful clinical, ethical, and medicolegal evaluation.

29.5.5.2 In Recipients

Patients with acute liver failure (ALF), acute on chronic liver failure (ACLF) or chronic liver disease (CLD) while awaiting transplantation, may decompensate and develop perioperative respiratory failure due to hepatopulmonary syndrome (HPS), or acute respiratory distress syndrome (ARDS) or concomitant cardiac decompensation (primary or secondary to liver failure) and/or circulatory failure (sepsis) can be suitable candidates for ECMO.

The detailed discussion on indications, contraindications, and challenges of ECMO management in a liver transplantation program are discussed as below.

Table 29.3 Complications to anticipate on ECMO and troubleshooting/treating the complications

Complications	Effect		Solution
Heparinisation related	Bleeding	Local	Titrate heparin and watch for bleeding from cannula sites, mouth, and nose Avoid any insertion or removal of lines while on ECMO Decrease heparinisation
		Systemic	Monitor Hb HCT Monitor BP CVP PPV U/O Monitor neurology for intracranial bleed Decrease/stop heparinisation
	Clotting	Oxygenator	Measure pre-, post-, and transmembrane pressures Increase heparinisation Change oxygenator
		Circuit	Check for clots with adequate direct light. Monitor limbs and neurology for any ischaemic embolic complications especially when on VA ECMO Change circuit Increase heparinisation
Circuit related	Chattering or bobbing of the tubings carrying the blood to and from the oxygenator	Flow fluctuations	Look for kinks in tubings
	Clots	Risk of embolization	Change circuit
	Air in circuit	Air embolism will stop the pump	Hand crank, resuscitate patient, de-air circuit
Cannula related	Inadequate flows		Use larger cannulas Add another access
	Recirculation		Access and return cannula too close, causing recirculation of ECMO oxygenated blood without circulating in the patient in VV ECMO
	Vascular injury		Ultrasound guidance Surgeon-assisted open/semi open techniques Imaging peri and post procedure
	Arterial circulation to the limb distal to the femoral arterial cannula can be compromised		Insertion of distal reperfusion cannula
Equipment related	Equipment failure		Back up console Resuscitate patient and manage conventionally till replacement or manual hand cranking can be initiated

29.6 ECMO for Transplant Donors

Globally, ECMO has been applied in organ donors, but the rules and ethical, legal, financial, and logistic considerations vary in every country. India is yet to explore this uncharted territory, with its huge potential in the transplant program.

With the growing demand and a low donation rate every potential organ available for donation is accepted. This may lead to poor quality or marginal organs especially if the brain-dead donor has been unstable. The increasing demand for transplantation has led to a significant expansion of acceptance criteria for donors after brain death

(DBD) and an increase in utilization of donors after circulatory death (DCD). As the number of patients on ECMO increases, this makes them a potential donor especially if they progress to brain death.

Organ donation in India is acceptable only after testing for brain death and following certification as per the Transplantation of Human Organs Act (THOA) 1994 and its amendments of 2014. This act defines and legalizes the concept of brain death testing and certification. Donation after circulatory death is still not an accepted mode unless it is in a Maastricht type IV where a brain-dead patient suffers a circulatory collapse in the hospital.

The role of ECMO in organ donation can be considered under the following conditions:

- Brain-dead ECMO patient as a potential donor.
- OP ECMO for unstable DBD donors.
- Regional perfusion (RP) and normothermic regional perfusion (NRP) for DCD donors.

29.7 Brain Dead ECMO Patient as Potential Donor

Intracerebral bleed or thromboembolic infarction is a major potential complication in a patient on ECMO. In such a situation withdrawal of ECMO support is advised even if the primary ECMO goals are met (stabilisation of heart and lungs). Such a patient could then be considered for organ donation.

Ethics considering withdrawal of ECMO in a brain-dead patient is similar to which affects discontinuing ventilator care.

Bronchard et al. found that brain-dead donors on ECMO were younger and had more severe intensive care medical conditions (haemodynamic, renal, biological, and liver insults), but there was no significant difference in graft survival, and they were hence considered suitable for organ procurement [6].

The challenge in this scenario is proving brain death. Patients on ECMO cannot be assessed by traditional apnoea testing definitively, unless a

few prerequisites are met and fallacies are understood.

29.7.1 Declaring Brain Death on ECMO [7–10] Can Be Considered Under the Following

1. Neurological testing
2. Apnoea testing on ECMO
3. Ancillary tests

29.8 Prerequisites for Testing for Brain Death

29.8.1 Establish Irreversible and Proximate Cause of Death

Exclude the presence of a CNS depressant drug, as most ECMO patients might be on high doses of sedatives, hypnotics, and muscle relaxants to decrease interference with ECMO flows due to patient movement.

29.8.2 Correct Any Severe Electrolyte, Acid/Base, and Endocrine Disturbance

Achieve normal core temperature, as many ECMO patients are deliberately maintained at lower temperatures to decrease metabolic demands. Hence, it becomes essential to correct to normal body temperature prior to brain stem testing.

Achieve acceptable blood pressure, preferably a baseline MAP >65 mm HG.

29.8.2.1 Neurological Examination
After prerequisites are met a detailed neurological examination can be done by one or two physicians at specified time intervals as per the protocol.

Demonstrate the absence of any response to noxious stimuli except spinally mediated ones.

Demonstration of absence of all brain stem reflexes including pupillary response to light, oculocephalic reflex, oculovestibular reflex, corneal reflex, gag and cough reflex.

29.8.2.2 Apnoea Testing on ECMO: Fig. 29.5

- Eliminating the factors causing instability and fallacies—various measures can be adopted to aid the Apnoea testing, these include:
- Giving CPAP through a ventilator or T tube or with a rebreathing bag to prevent collapse hypoxia during apnoea testing.
- Using higher O_2 insufflation up to 10 L/min to prevent hypoxia: this could lead to some CO_2 elimination.
- Using lower O_2 to prevent CO_2 elimination through the ET tube inadvertently.
- Carbon dioxide augmentation and elevation of the CO_2 level prior to apnoea testing. Introduction of CO_2 at a rate of 1 L/min into the circuit markedly reduces the observation time compared with conventional apnoeic oxygenation. Intentional elevation of baseline CO_2 to shorten apnoea test time.
- No disconnection, but to continue ventilation with carbogen at 2–4 breaths/min, to prevent loss of PEEP and lung collapse due to de-recruitment.

Thus, most patients undergoing apnoea testing for establishing a diagnosis brain death may have an inconclusive test. Multiple testing fallacies exist, and these methods are not standardized but maybe necessary to maintain donor stability.

Hence, alternative ancillary tests may become essential to prove brain death.

29.8.2.3 Ancillary Tests

The study declaring brain death on ECMO demonstrated variations in practices in brain death declaration, especially with regards to apnoea testing, in patients on ECMO. Most centres used more than one test along with clinical examination to declare brain death. Standardization is needed to assure consistent, accurate brain death pronouncement to facilitate organ procurement when appropriate. Brain death guidelines are yet to include ECMO patients.

Electroencephalography: Electroencephalography (EEG) may be mandatory, especially in the face of an inconclusive apnoea test and may necessitate other ancillary tests if EEG also becomes inconclusive.

Cerebral circulatory arrest: The Italian medical guidelines state that the accepted and recommended diagnostic tests to demonstrate cerebral circulatory arrest (CCA) can be any of the following, either independently or in combination:

Pretesting	Testing	End points	Fallacies
• Systolic pressure > 100 mm Hg with vasopressors	• Disconnect patient from ventilator	• ABG after 10 min of absent respiratory movements with $PaCO_2 > 60$ mmHg or 20mm Hg above baseline is considered as positive test	• $PaO_2 > 200$ not achievable in patients on VV ECMO
• Preoxygenate with 100% oxygen for 10 mins or $PaO_2 > 200$	• Insufflation catheter through ET tube (100% O_2 at 6 L/min)		• Patients on VA ECMO may not have pulsatile flow and/or systolic BP of 100 mm
• Reduce respiratory rate to 10/min	• Off sweep O_2 or decrease to 1L/min	• Abort if $SPO_2 < 85\%$ or SBP < 90 for more than 30s	
• Reduce PEEP to 5 cm H_2O	• Look for spontaneous respiratory movements for 8–10 min	• If test inconclusive but patient is stable, continue for 10–15 min	• Sweep flow of 1 L/min can cause adequate CO_2 clearance to render test inconclusive
• Obtain baseline ABG if $SPO_2 > 95\%$			

Fig. 29.5 Steps of Apnoea testing on ECMO [7]

cerebral angiography, brain scintigraphy, transcranial doppler (TCD), or CT angiography.

Transcranial Doppler: TCD signal disappearance during continuous TCD monitoring strongly suggests evolution to a condition of BD and prompts further evaluations. In France, it cannot be the sole confirmatory test as the test window may be limiting [11].

Ancillary tests too have been inadequately tested on ECMO patients. The alterations in blood flow patterns, oxygenation, and ventilation that are created by ECMO may affect the usefulness of ancillary tests used for the diagnosis of brain death while patients are on ECMO.

29.8.3 Role of ECMO in Deceased Donor Management

Donation After Brain Death Brain death is often associated with cardiac failure and/or arrhythmias, which may necessitate high-dose inotropes and can progress to lactic acidosis. Fluid resuscitation, ventilator-associated pneumonias, and development of ARDS is common, especially with prolonged ventilation with high PEEP. All these may lead to haemodynamic instability and hence loss of a potential donor or poor organ perfusion if hypotension is pronounced.

Indication for ECMO in such a donor would be an organ preserving ECMO if poor LV function is resulting in severe metabolic acidosis, increasing inotrope score, inability to maintain satisfactory haemodynamics. Patients with ARDS, low PaO2/FiO2 ratio, those needing high PEEP can also be candidates for OP ECMO if brain death testing is positive.

OP ECMO: OP ECMO is the use of ECLS with the primary aim to preserve organs for transplantation and not for saving life [12].

Dave et al. in their paper discussed the ethical considerations of using OP-ECMO in donation after determination of brain death to avoid the loss of organs for transplantation [13].

The various ethical dilemmas of OP ECMO that need to be addressed include:

- Timing: ECMO in patients who are yet to be declared brain dead (including those who have not yet been tested for brain death) may potentially accelerate death due to the risk of potential intracranial bleed. If post initiation, brain death testing is negative, then it is a wasted cost and morbidity and discomforting to the patient. Hence, consent for ECMO initiation should be done after determination of brain death and not for the determination of brain death. If done for brain stem death testing, it should not be organ preserving and consent should be for determination of brain death not for OP ECMO.
- Cannulation: Cannulation can be considered invasive but not as invasive as the organ donation process itself. Cannulation requires heparinisation, which could lead to potential bleeding. Adequate pain relief should be provided even following brain death declaration.
- Consent: If pre-existing consent for organ donation is available in the national registry or in countries permitting presumed consent, the failure to opt out can itself be considered as consent for OP ECMO. However, in the absence of any such declaration of a patient's wish, consent from next of kin is required prior to the initiation OP ECMO.
- Cost and resources: ECMO is an expensive and resource-intensive procedure necessitating expertise and specialized equipment. Hence, many questions need to be addressed as regard the cost of the treatment. Liver transplant itself being an expensive program, the added cost of ECMO may be justified if it leads to a good outcome and definitely not at the cost of depriving a therapeutic ECMO in another needy patient.

29.8.4 Donation After Cardiac Death (DCD) [14]

DCD has not been implemented systematically in India because of the lack of clarity about it either in the original THOA or its subsequent amendments. However, the point worth mentioning is that there is nothing mentioned against performing such donations. In India, DCD can happen only in category II B and IV patients (Table 29.4). Considering Category III patients for DCD may be questionable as it involves withdrawal of life support in end-of-life situations and, there are no clear guidelines for this practice at present [15].

Steps of DCD are as shown in Fig. 29.6. The ischemia time known as functional ischemia time begins from the time patient is disconnected from the ventilator and also withdrawal of inotrope support. At this time the patient's blood pressure and oxygenation starts dropping and organ hypoxia begins. The warm ischemia time lasts from the point of asystole, till the end of mandatory no touch period. The duration of no touch period to confirm cardiac death varies in different countries. The standard duration of no touch period can range from minimum of 5 min up to 20 min as in Italy.

This mandatory no-touch period is followed by rushing the donor to an adjoining OT, followed by incision and cannulation of the aorta and initiation of cold perfusion, which is considered as the start of cold ischemia time (CIT). This could vary but could last anywhere up to another 30–40 min.

Table 29.4 The modified Maastricht classification of DCD in Paris 2013 [15]

Maastricht classification	Presentation of death	DCD situation
Category I	Found dead I A. Out-of-hospital sudden unexpected irreversible cardiac arrest with unsuccessful resuscitation I B. In—hospital sudden unexpected irreversible cardiac arrest with unsuccessful resuscitation	Uncontrolled
Category II	Witnessed cardiac arrest II A. Out of hospital II B. In hospital	Uncontrolled
Category III	Planned withdrawal of life sustaining therapy	Controlled
Category IV	Cardiac arrest in brain dead donor	Uncontrolled

DCD Protocol

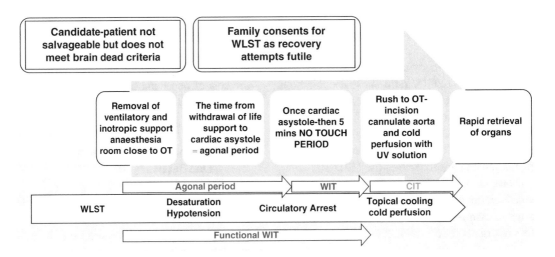

Fig. 29.6 Steps of DCD

The extended WIT results in rapid cell ischemia and ATP depletion, which can be slowed down by cold perfusion but cannot be reversed. Hence, if the delay in cold perfusion causes the ATP depletion to reach a critical level, the organ is rendered unusable due to cell death, and the outcomes would be poor if it were to be transplanted (Fig. 29.7).

ECMO on the other hand allows for replenishment of ATP by perfusing the organs with oxygenated blood, while they are being retrieved and this delays the critical point and can thus prevent cell death.

DCD has been discussed in detail elsewhere, thus the discussion here will remain limited to ECMO assisted DCD (EDCD)/Extracorporeal Interval Support for Organ Retrieval (EISOR).

- Steps of EDCD
- Results of EDCD
- Challenges of EDCD

The steps of EDCD are as shown in Fig. 29.8. Here, the withdrawal of life support is possible in the ICU itself or in the OT, depending on the cannulation and clamping laws of the country. The patient's femoral artery and vein are cannulated or guide wires are placed, and the patient is prepped for ECMO cannulas either prior to starting DCD process or after the no-touch period.

The blood flow returning to the aorta needs to be limited to below the diaphragm to prevent the reanimation of the heart and brain. This can be done by directly clamping the aorta after incision and inserting ECMO cannulas directly into the abdominal aorta and inferior vena cava. This is the procedure adopted for EDCD in the UK, where no intervention is permissible on a patient prior to the end of the no-touch period post withdrawal of life support. The UK additionally only allows clamping of the abdominal aorta to prevent the resumption of circulation to the heart and lungs. The no touch period in UK is 5 min. Italy on the other hand has a long no touch period of 20 min. Pre-mortem cannulation is allowed, and hence, withdrawal of life support can be done in the ICU. The cannulation requires heparinization, which can potentially lead to a bleeding risk and hasten death; hence, some countries allow only the insertion of guide wires and prepping, and cannulas are ready to be inserted post-mortem. The aortic cut-off to separate the abdominal circulation is achieved by retrograde endovascular balloon occlusion of the aorta (REBOA) (Fig. 29.9). Most countries that use pre-mortem percutaneous cannulation use REBOA. However, there is a potential risk of balloon malfunction leading to circulation through upper body. This may cause reanimation and lead to confusion regarding the diagnosis of death,

Fig. 29.7 Depletion pattern of ATP during WIT and CIT during retrieval of organs during DCD and EDCD

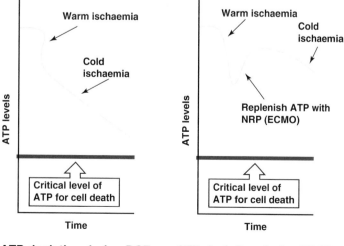

ATP depletion during DCD   ATP depletion during EDCD

EDCD Protocol

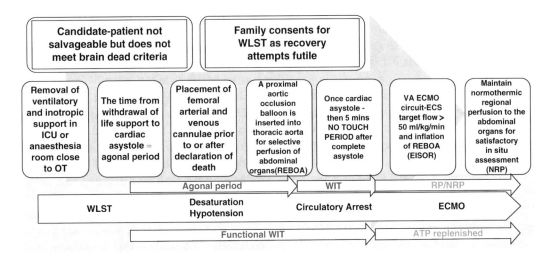

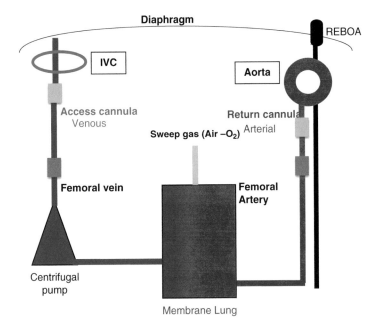

Fig. 29.8 Steps of EDCD

Fig. 29.9 Placement of cannulas in femoral vein femoral artery and of REBOA in aorta at the level of the diaphragm to limit ECMO circulation to abdominal organs and prevent reanimation of heart and brain

which could be very distressing to the family and physicians. Hence, REBOA is not used routinely by all nations.

Regional perfusion (RP) DCD: ECMO is initiated at the point when profound hypotension sets in, to provide cold circulation through the abdominal organs, thereby helping with the replenish-ment of ATP, while the thoracic organs are retrieved or remain at normal body temperature (normothermic). NRP is continued for several hours while assessing the organs for appearance, function, and biochemistry. This allows time to resuscitate the organ and establish confidence that the organs are fit for transplant. Dual temperature NRP with abdominal normothermic perfusion and concomitant cold lung flushing allows a rapid removal of the lungs with preservation of the abdominal normothermic circulation throughout the thoracic procurement [16]. Normothermic machine perfusion (NMP) uses this principle by cannulating the liver alone and circulating UV solution with nutrients while assessing the function of the organ [17]. However, the time needed to retrieve and cannulate the organ translates to longer WIT and CIT, although currently, there is no evidence of long-term results of NRP versus NMP.

While NRP can be continued on an average of up to 4 h, the abdominal organ appearance and functions are assessed as described in Table 29.5 and Fig. 29.10.

Results of EDCD: RP by ECMO is increasingly being advocated as a useful remedy for the effects of ischemia/reperfusion injury, and it has been reported to enable the transplantation of organs from donors previously deemed unsuitable. In a systematic review, Shapey et al. reported the outcomes of 482 kidneys and 79 livers that were transplanted from regional perfusion-supported donors after circulatory death (RP-DCD) sources [18, 19].

The 1-year patient and graft survival rates for RP-DCD kidney transplantation were better than the rates with standard DCDs and were comparable to, if not better than, the rates with DBDs. Most studies reported PNF rates of 0%, with the remainder reporting rates comparable to those for DBDs older than 60 years. The rates of acute rejection in all RP-DCD groups were lower than the rates with other donor types.

The 1-year graft survival was lower with uncontrolled RP-DCD liver transplantation, whereas 1-year patient survival was similar. Primary nonfunction and ischemic cholangiopathy were significantly more frequent with RP-DCDs versus DBDs, but there was no difference in postoperative mortality between the two groups. Controlled normothermic regional perfusion supported donors after circulatory death (NRP-DCDs), reported a rate of 91% for 1-year patient and graft survival (10/11), better than that with standard DCDs. Patient survival was similar to that for DBD but was significantly better than that for DCD recipients.

29.8.5 Challenges and Ethical Issues of EDCD [20]

The challenges of EDCD are ethical, financial, and logistic. Although EISOR looks promising, it presents several ethical challenges, specifically, the dignity of death and questionability of the pre-mortem and post-mortem interventions. The ethical issues need to be resolved by legislation clearly outlining candidature, timing, consent, and resource allocation to an EDCD program.

The confounding issues or challenges can be as in Table 29.6.

The ethical and legal framework of each country is different, and no common worldwide consensus is possible due to different social, economic, and religious beliefs regarding organ transplantation. It is easier to implement EDCD in countries that maintain a national register or have an opt-out policy for organ donation (Fig. 29.11).

29.8.6 Logistic, Economic, and Social Questions

ECMO is a cost intense programme and also necessitates trained manpower for successful

Table 29.5 The various laboratory indicators of organ viability during NRP

Liver	Kidney	Pancreas
Bile production	Urine output	S-amylase
LFT evolution	Urine chemistry	
Improving lactates on serial measurements		
Post-perfusion gross appearance		
Normalizing pH		

Venous Gases

Time	pH	H+	pCO2	pO2	HCO3	BE	Na+	K+	Ca2+	Gluc	Lact	Hct	Hb	Sats
0														
30'														
60'														
90'														
120'														

Biochemistry

Time	Bili	ALP	ALT	AST	Urea	Creat	Hb	WCC	Plat	Blood Cultures
0										
30'										X
60'										X
90'										X
120'										

Time	Flow mls/min	Pressures (mmHg)		Reservoir volume	Temp °C	Notes*
		Venous	Arterial			

Fig. 29.10 NRP charting of ECMO flow, temperature, volumes, and pressures. Organ function biochemistry and blood gases are noted, and the trend shows if organ function is good or there are markers of cell death

Table 29.6 The ethical issues that can arise the drawbacks and advantages or alternative methods to overcome the issues are outlined

Consent	Individuals may consent by designating the decision on a driver's license, in advance directives and wills, or through an online donor registry. If no previous consent by a patient exists, a surrogate will usually have to give consent if the patient is unable	Individuals who consent to organ donation may not understand the dying process or be aware of the ethical dilemmas involved in organ donation
Conflict of interest	Organ donation should be considered after decision for WLST	Consent for donation to be taken by a trained individual not part of the care team after decision to withdraw life support has been made else there may be a bias
	Organ procurement teams and transplant surgeons are not to be involved in the decisions or act of withdrawing support or declaring death	There may be bias in decision to withdraw life support if the team caring for donor and treating recipient are the same
The challenges of EDCD are ethical, financial, and logistic	The challenges of EDCD are ethical, financial, and logistic	The challenges of EDCD are ethical, financial, and logistic
Although EISOR looks promising, it presents several ethical challenges, specifically, the dignity of death and questionability of the pre-mortem and post-mortem interventions. The ethical issues need to be resolved by legislation clearly outlining candidature, timing, consent, and resource allocation to an EDCD program	Although EISOR looks promising, it presents several ethical challenges, specifically, the dignity of death and questionability of the pre-mortem and post-mortem interventions. The ethical issues need to be resolved by legislation clearly outlining candidature, timing, consent, and resource allocation to an EDCD program	Although EISOR looks promising, it presents several ethical challenges, specifically, the dignity of death and questionability of the pre-mortem and post-mortem interventions. The ethical issues need to be resolved by legislation clearly outlining candidature, timing, consent, and resource allocation to an EDCD program
The ethical issues are as below	The ethical issues are as below	The ethical issues are as below
The challenges of EDCD are ethical, financial, and logistic	The challenges of EDCD are ethical, financial, and logistic	The challenges of EDCD are ethical, financial, and logistic

(continued)

Table 29.6 (continued)

Although EISOR looks promising, it presents several ethical challenges, specifically, the dignity of death and questionability of the pre-mortem and post-mortem interventions. The ethical issues need to be resolved by legislation clearly outlining candidature, timing, consent, and resource allocation to an EDCD program	Although EISOR looks promising, it presents several ethical challenges, specifically, the dignity of death and questionability of the pre-mortem and post-mortem interventions. The ethical issues need to be resolved by legislation clearly outlining candidature, timing, consent, and resource allocation to an EDCD program	Although EISOR looks promising, it presents several ethical challenges, specifically, the dignity of death and questionability of the pre-mortem and post-mortem interventions. The ethical issues need to be resolved by legislation clearly outlining candidature, timing, consent, and resource allocation to an EDCD program

implementation of ECMO. Some of the logistic, economic, and social questions which need to be addressed when considering implementation of ECMO care in transplantation programme include:

Cost of ECMO: The question of who will bear the added cost of the ECMO especially when the organs cannot be used for transplantation.

More trained teams are needed for successful ECMO: Specialized ECMO team with cannulation and perfusion knowledge are required and at unpredictable times.

The priority in using ECMO should be primarily for a therapeutic ECMO candidate rather than an organ. ECMO for organ preservation can be supplemented using NMP after rapid retrieval.

Transport of donor exclusively to a specialist centre with ECMO facility and transplant program to support EDCD may not be acceptable.

29.8.7 Challenges in the Use of ECMO for Organ Donation Specific to India

Currently, in India, there are no specific guidelines for withdrawal of life support in patients who are not brain dead; thus, DCD is possible only in Maastricht category IV patients. Indian experience in DCD is very limited. PGI Chandigarh is the only centre which has reported DCD in five cases, where CPR was initiated after mandatory 5 min non touch period following asystole and rapid recovery was done in OT. Only the kidneys were used, and all donors were in hospital witnessed arrest uncontrolled Maastricht type [21].

DCD and OP ECMO are resource intensive may come up for consideration at unpredictable times of the day necessitating availability of specially trained team. There is no clarity on the legal implications of OP ECMO in unstable braindead donors.

ECMO program in India is new and families need detailed counselling for therapeutic ECMO. In such situations, counselling a family for organ donation after brain death on ECMO becomes more challenging. Acceptance and standardisation of procedure for brain stem testing for a patient on ECMO is lacking the world over.

However, as the deceased organ donation rates in India are very dismal, necessitating a need for expanding the inclusion criteria for organ donors which should also include patients on ECMO and donation after circulatory death.

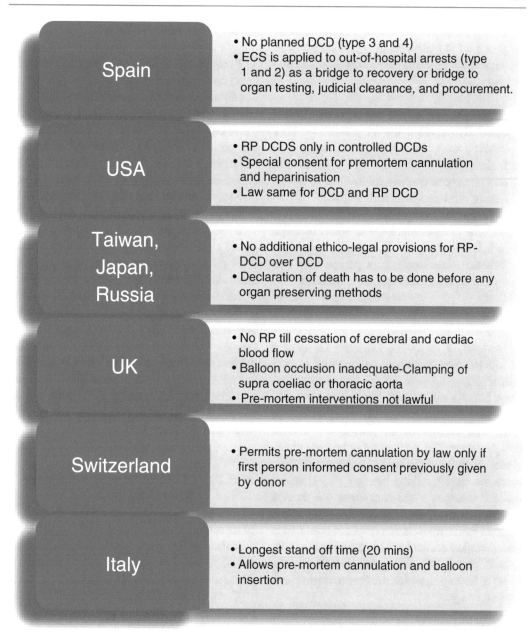

Fig. 29.11 Practices in various countries based on the legal provisions

29.8.8 ECMO in Liver Transplant Recipients: Who Would Benefit?

Patient selection criteria for ECMO are very important. Liver transplant recipients with additional cardiac and/or respiratory failure could be considered for ECMO.

Multiple organ involvement is common in liver disease. Most CLD patients may have more than one associated system decompensation such as hepatorenal syndrome, hepatic encephalopathy (even coma) coagulopathy (low platelets, high INR, low fibrinogen), and GI bleed, all of which are relative contraindications for the use of ECMO [22–24].

The challenges for instituting ECMO successfully in a CLD patient awaiting transplant or in the immediate post-transplant period could be as follows:

- Instrumentation of the major neck vessels, especially in post-transplant patients or those awaiting transplant would be challenging
- Anticoagulation for ECMO in patients who may already be coagulopathic
- Risk of bleeding (local and internal)
- Exposure to blood products.
- Vascular complications (local vessel damage, limb ischaemia).
- Infection (line sepsis) in a patient who will receive immunosuppressant medications
- Cost considerations/Manpower considerations

However, a review of literature shows that ECMO has been attempted successfully in liver failure patients who are too sick to undergo transplant. ECMO aids in stabilising them preoperatively to make them transplant-worthy or salvage them with ECMO postoperatively in case of complications. The availability of bedside viscoelastic tests of coagulation, improved ECMO machines, and bio-lined tubing's and cannulas make it easier to avoid anticoagulation in sick coagulopathic patients. Another advantage is that all other extracorporeal therapies can be added in series while maintaining haemodynamics with ECMO, thereby alleviating the need for harmful doses of inotropes, which can lead to further end-organ damage.

The situations where ECMO has been considered in liver failure patients are

- Acute liver failure
- Hepato-pulmonary syndrome
- Poor cardiac functional status
- Porto-pulmonary hypertension
- Post-transplant ARDS

29.8.9 Acute Liver Failure

ALF may present as a complex situation with multi-organ involvement and features of extreme coagulopathy and/or encephalopathy. However, it presents abruptly with varied aetiologies, in otherwise young and fit individuals with no past comorbidities. Many extracorporeal therapies such as continuous renal replacement therapy (CRRT), plasma exchange, and molecular adsorbent recirculating system (MARS) have all been used in the past either to aid in recovery or to bridge patients to transplant.

ECMO is expected to be beneficial in cases of severe circulatory collapse with rapidly escalating inotrope score or pulmonary complications due to fluid overload and VAP. In these patients, ECMO may help to stabilize the patient, who would otherwise be too sick to transplant. The largest reported series is from King's Hospital, London where they were able to salvage two patients who presented with cardiogenic shock and ALF on ECMO without transplant. They successfully bridged five patients who were deemed too sick to transplant of which only one survived to hospital discharge [25].

29.8.10 ECMO in Hepatopulmonary Syndrome

Hepatopulmonary syndrome (HPS) is a triad of liver disease, intrapulmonary vascular dilatation, and abnormal gas exchange, and it is found in 10–32% of patients with liver disease.

The algorithm for the management of severe HPS consists of various supportive therapies, as shown in Fig. 29.12 [26].

Patients with HPS are acclimatized to very low blood oxygen levels due to large shunts in the lung due to neovascularisation.

Most reported cases of HPS and ECMO are in patients that have had superadded ARDS or fluid overload complicating the hypoxia.

Fig. 29.12 Algorithm of management of HPS with severe hypoxia preoperatively

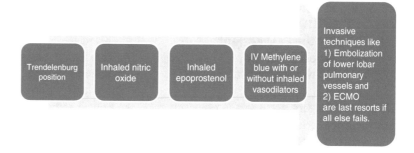

There are isolated case reports of the successful use of ECMO as a bridge to liver transplant in an extremely hypoxemic cirrhotic HPS patient with ARDS [27].

Early liver transplant, which helps in the reversal of blood shunting in the lungs by hypoxic pulmonary vasoconstriction, is the only definitive treatment of hepatopulmonary syndrome. There are concerns that ECMO in the post liver transplant setting may potentially reverse hypoxic pulmonary vasoconstrictive responses by flooding the lungs with oxygen-rich blood and delay the reversal of shunting. However, this is only a theoretical concern as there are reports of successful use of ECMO [28, 29].

29.8.11 Perioperative ECMO

This application of ECMO has been described in patients with poor cardiac functional status. There is a case report of successful liver transplant in a patient with severe mitral regurgitation, severe tricuspid regurgitation, dilated left atrium and left ventricle, cardiac insufficiency, pulmonary arterial hypertension, and hypoxemia [30]. The patient underwent LT from a cardiac deceased donor. The surgery was completed by venoarterial ECMO. The femoral vessels were cannulated after the dissection of the patient's liver and before venous clamping. The venous cannula was positioned below the renal vein, while the arterial cannula was up to the common iliac artery.

VA ECMO can also be an intraoperative rescue option in case of myocardial decompensation

to stabilize the heart [31]. Porto pulmonary hypertension recognized during liver transplantation was addressed by ECMO and has been reported by Martucci et al. [32]. An interesting case of ECMO as a bridge to lung transplantation in a patient with persistent severe portopulmonary arterial hypertension following liver transplantation has also been reported by Wiklund et al. [33].

Post-Liver Transplant There are many occasions when a patient presents with ARDS in the immediate post-transplant period due to fluid overload, massive transfusion, or with septic shock. This situation is difficult as decision to salvage these patients with ECMO can be fraught with multitude of challenges as they are immune compromised which makes them susceptible to line sepsis. They present additional challenges like limited vascular access, coagulopathy, kidney decompensation after major surgery and a new graft which needs time to reverse the chronic liver failure. Hence it is important to consider ECMO only if there is a clear involvement of lungs or heart with a reversible treatable cause. Post liver transplant patients in multi organ failure should not be considered for ECMO. The survival of patients who received ECMO for septic shock in adults was 25% and review of literature shows that the survival of adult LT recipients with refractory septic shock was 25% (2 of 8) despite ECMO support though the study cohort was small [34, 35]. Hence septic shock in an immunocompromised post-operative patient is a poor indication for ECMO.

29.8.12   In Summary, When Should ECMO Be Offered for the CLD Patient Awaiting Liver Transplantation? [36, 37]

HPS with refractory hypoxaemia, especially due to superadded insults of ARDS/volume overload preoperatively, perioperatively, or post-liver transplant, as deemed necessary.

ALF with MOF

Patients with cardiac conditions who may not tolerate the stress of liver transplant

Post-operative ARDS

Younger recipients below 60 years of age

When both ECMO and liver transplant services are available in the same centre.

29.9   Conclusion

ECMO has become an extension of therapies to stabilize heart and lung in critically ill ICU patients failing conventional therapy. ECMO and transplant programs with their multidisciplinary team and advanced critical care knowledge requirement would tend to be available in the same hospital setups. Hence it is vital to understand the applications of this technology in transplant patients. While ECMO can be a bridge to heart and lung transplants, for liver transplant it has a good potential to expand the donor pool and improve the organ outcomes. For perioperative liver transplant patient stabilisation with ECMO careful patient selection and planning could potentially yield better outcomes in patients deemed too ill to transplant. For this a better understanding of ECMO principles and their applications is vital.

Statements of Ethical Compliance

- The author has no relevant financial or non-financial interests to disclose.
- The author has no conflicts of interest to declare that are relevant to the content of this article.
- The author certifies no affiliations with or involvement in any organization or entity with any financial interest or non-financial interest in the subject matter or materials discussed in this manuscript.
- The author has no financial or proprietary interests in any material discussed in this article.
- Ethical approval not required

Acknowledgements Dr. Jumana Haji would like to acknowledge.

Dr. Chidanand Swamy Consultant intensivist Neurocritical care unit Brunei Neuroscience stroke and rehabilitation centre for expert inputs and editing.

Dr. Ramanathan K R Director ICU fellowship program, National University hospital Singapore for expert inputs.

Dr. Naveen Ganjoo, Consultant Liver disease and transplantation at SSNMC super specialty Hospital.

Dr. Pallavi Marghade Specialist anaesthesiologist at Kings College Hospital London- UAE Chief editor JACCR.

References

1. https://www.elso.org/Portals/0/ELSO%20 Guidelines%20General%20All%20ECLS%20 Version%201_4.pdf. Guidelines for ECMO from ELSO.Org.
2. Mancini M, Diekema D, Hoadley T, Kadlec K, Leveille M, McGowan J, et al. Part 3: ethical issues. Circulation. 2015;132(18 Suppl 2):S383–96.
3. Casadio M, Coppo A, Vargiolu A, Villa J, Rota M, Avalli L, et al. Organ donation in cardiac arrest patients treated with extracorporeal CPR: a single Centre observational study. Resuscitation. 2017;118:133–9.
4. Lequier L, Horton S, McMullan D, Bartlett R. Extracorporeal membrane oxygenation circuitry. Pediatr Crit Care Med. 2013;14:S7–S12.
5. Zangrillo A. The criteria of eligibility to the extracorporeal treatment. HSR Proc Intensive Care Cardiovasc Anesth. 2012;4(4):271–3.
6. Bronchard R, Durand L, Legeai C, Cohen J, Guerrini P. Bastien brain-dead donors on extracorporeal membrane oxygenation. Crit Care Med. 2017;45(10):1734–41. https://doi.org/10.1097/CCM.0000000000002564.
7. Kreitler KJ, et al. Declaring brain death on ECMO. Jefferson Digital Commons. 2015. https://jdc.jefferson.edu/jhnj/vol12/iss1/7/.
8. Bein T, Müller T, Citerio G. Determination of brain death under extracorporeal life support. Intensive Care Med. 2019;45:364–6.
9. Pirat A, Komurcu O, Yener G, Arslan G. Apnea testing for diagnosing brain death during extracorporeal

membrane oxygenation. J Cardiothorac Vasc Anesth. 2014;28:e8–9.

10. Migdady I, Stephens R, Price C, Geocadin R, Whitman G, Cho S. The use of apnea test and brain death determination in patients on extracorporeal membrane oxygenation: a systematic review. J Thorac Cardiovasc Surg. 2021;162(3):867–877.e1.

11. Cestari M, Gobatto ALN, Hoshino M. Role and limitations of transcranial doppler and brain death of patients on veno-arterial extracorporeal membrane oxygenation. ASAIO J. 2018;64(4):e78. https://doi.org/10.1097/MAT.0000000000000720. PMID: 29135481.

12. Christopher D, Woodside K. Expanding the donor pool. Crit Care Med. 2017;45(10):1790–1.

13. Dalle Ave A, Gardiner D, Shaw D. The ethics of extracorporeal membrane oxygenation in brain-dead potential organ donors. Transpl Int. 2016;29(5):612–8.

14. Haji JY. Role of ECMO for organ donation [Internet]. J Anaesth Crit Care Case Rep. 2019;5(2):1–3.

15. Thuong M, Ruiz A, Evrard P, Kuiper M, Boffa C, Akhtar M, et al. New classification of donation after circulatory death donors definitions and terminology. Transpl Int. 2016;29(7):749–59.

16. Oniscu G, Siddique A, Dark J. Dual temperature multi-organ recovery from a Maastricht category III donor after circulatory death. Am J Transplant. 2014;14(9):2181–6.

17. Bowen G, Quintini C. Normothermic machine perfusion (NMP) for human liver transplantation in the United States. Transplantation. 2017;101:S83.

18. Shapey I, Muiesan P. Regional perfusion by extracorporeal membrane oxygenation of abdominal organs from donors after circulatory death: a systematic review. Liver Transpl. 2013;19(12):1292–303.

19. Oniscu G, Randle L, Muiesan P, Butler A, Currie I, Perera M, et al. In situ normothermic regional perfusion for controlled donation after circulatory death-the United Kingdom experience. Am J Transplant. 2014;14(12):2846–54.

20. Dalle Ave A, Shaw D, Bernat J. Ethical issues in the use of extracorporeal membrane oxygenation in controlled donation after circulatory determination of death. Am J Transplant. 2016;16(8):2293–9.

21. Sharma A, Singh S, Kumar S, Dasgupta S, Kenwar D, Rathi M, et al. A single-center experience of kidney transplantation from donation after circulatory death: challenges and scope in India. Indian J Nephrol. 2017;27(3):205.

22. Haji JY, et al. www.jaccr.com. J Anaesth Crit Care Case Rep. 2019;5(3):3–6.

23. Levesque E, Salloum C, Feray C, Azoulay D. The utility of ECMO, not just after but also during liver transplantation. Transplantation. 2019;103(10):e319–20.

24. Taieb A, Jeune F, Lebbah S, Schmidt M, Deransy R, Vaillant J-C, et al. Emergency abdominal surgery outcomes of critically ill patients on extracorporeal membrane oxygenation: a case-matched study with a propensity score analysis. World J Surg. 2019;43(6):1474–82.

25. Auzinger G, et al. Extracorporeal membrane oxygenation before and after adult liver transplantation: worth the effort? Crit Care. 2014;18(Suppl 1):P203. https://doi.org/10.1186/cc13393.

26. Nayyar D, Man HSJ, Granton J, et al. Proposed management algorithm for severe hypoxemia after liver transplantation in the hepatopulmonary syndrome. Am J Transplant. 2015;15:903–13.

27. Monsel A, Mal H, Brisson H, et al. Extracorporeal membrane oxygenation as a bridge to liver transplantation for acute respiratory distress syndrome-induced life-threatening hypoxaemia aggravated by hepatopulmonary syndrome. Crit Care. 2011;15:R234. https://doi.org/10.1186/cc10476.

28. Fleming GM, et al. Hepatopulmonary syndrome: use of extracorporeal life support for life-threatening hypoxia following liver transplantation. Liver Transp. 2008;14(7):966–70. https://doi.org/10.1002/lt.21477.

29. Kumar L, Varghese R, et al. Extracorporeal membrane oxygenation for posttransplant hypoxaemia following very severe hepatopulmonary syndrome. BMJ Case Rep. 2017;2017:bcr2017221381.

30. Sun X, et al. Utilization of extracorporeal membrane oxygenation for a severe cardiocirculatory dysfunction recipient in liver transplantation: a case report. Medicine. 2018;97(37):e12407.

31. Lauterio A, De Carlis R, Cannata A, Di Sandro S, De Gasperi A, Russo C, et al. Emergency intraoperative implantation of ECMO for refractory cardiogenic shock arising during liver transplantation as a bridge to myocardial surgical revascularization. Transplantation. 2019;103(10):e317–8.

32. Martucci G, Burgio G, Lullo F, et al. Veno-arterial extracorporeal membrane oxygenation as an intraoperative rescue option in case of portopulmonary hypertension recognized during liver transplantation. Minerva Anestesiol. 2017;83:1336–7.

33. Wiklund L, Haraldsson A, et al. Extracorporeal membrane oxygenation as a bridge to lung transplantation in a patient with persistent severe Porto-pulmonary arterial hypertension following liver transplantation. Eur J Cardiothorac Surg. 2011;39(5):777–8.

34. Lee KW, Cho CW, et al. Extracorporeal membrane oxygenation support for refractory septic shock in liver transplantation recipients. Ann Surg Treat Res. 2017;93(3):152–8.

35. Park TK, Yang JH, Jeon K, Choi S-H, Choi J-H, Gwon H-C, et al. Extracorporeal membrane oxygenation for refractory septic shock in adults. Eur J Cardiothorac Surg. 2015;47(2):e68–74.

36. Braun HJ, Pulcrano ME, Weber DJ, Padilla BE, Ascher NL. The utility of ECMO after liver transplantation: experience at a high-volume transplant center and review of the literature. Transplantation. 2019;103(8):1568–73.

37. Choi N-K, Hwang S, Kim K-W, Park G-C, Yu Y-D, Jung S-H, et al. Intensive pulmonary support using extracorporeal membrane oxygenation in adult patients undergoing liver transplantation. Hepato-Gastroenterology. 2012;59(116):1189–93.

Part V

Acute Liver Failure

Critical Care Management of Acute Liver Failure

30

CH. Balasubrahmanyam and Palepu B. Gopal

30.1 Introduction

Acute liver failure (ALF) is a severe and complex condition that results from acute and massive hepatocellular destruction with very poor prognosis, with an approximately 80% mortality rate in historical series. ALF is an infrequent condition, with an incidence of 1–8 cases per million inhabitants, and it is responsible for 6% of deaths due to liver disease and up to 7–8% of liver transplants [1]. ALF mainly affects young adults, with a peak age between 35 and 45 years. Women account for approximately 60% of cases [2]. The development of cerebral oedema, sepsis and multiple organ failure are the main causes of mortality [3].

30.1.1 Definition and Classification

Acute liver failure was first described by Trey C and Davidson [4] as "hepatocellular dysfunction of such severity that encephalopathy occurs within eight weeks of appearance of first symptoms in the absence of pre-existing liver disease." In 1993, O'Grady et al. [5] based on data from King's College subdivided ALF into hyperacute, acute, and sub-acute presentation depending on the interval from onset of disease to onset of encephalopathy. The most widely accepted definition is by American association of study of liver disease [6] who in 2005 defined ALF as a clinical syndrome characterized by evidence of coagulopathy (international normalized ratio [INR] >5) and any degree of altered mental status in a patient without pre-existing liver disease and duration of illness <26 weeks. Hepatic encephalopathy (HE) is usually considered the hallmark of Hyderabad, Telangana, India this disease and differentiates ALF patients from those with acute liver injury [7] (Fig. 30.1).

O'Grady's classification possesses the advantage of having prognostic value [5] (Fig. 30.2). Thus, the time between the presentation of jaundice and the onset of HE subdivides patients into three categories (hyperacute, acute, and sub-acute), which are useful to define the prognosis. The hyperacute form has a better prognosis but a higher incidence of cerebral oedema. On the other hand, acute and sub-acute presentations have a worse prognosis, but a lower incidence of cerebral oedema [8].

Critical care management of acute liver failure can be sub-divided into etiological and organ specific management (Table 30.1).

CH. Balasubrahmanyam · P. B. Gopal (✉)
Critical Care Medicine, Citizen's Hospital,
Hyderabad, Telangana, India

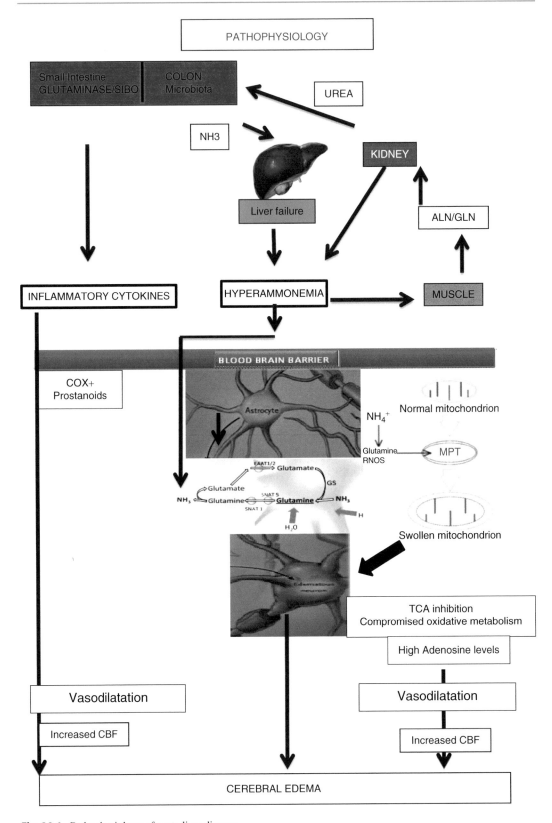

Fig. 30.1 Pathophysiology of acute liver disease

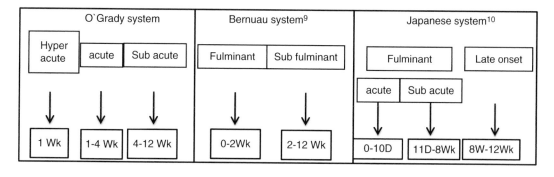

Fig. 30.2 Classification systems of acute liver failure

Table 30.1 Etiological management of acute liver failure

Category	Etiology	Common c/f	Treatment
Viral hepatitis	Hepatitis A virus	Hyperacute presentation; ALF is more common in older patients or those with underlying liver disease	Supportive
	Hepatitis B virus ± delta virus		Entecavir (taken on an empty stomach) or tenofovir at standard renal adjusted Doses
	Hepatitis E virus	History of travel to endemic areas or those with exposure to porcine farm animals; has a higher risk during pregnancy, especially in the third trimester	
	Herpes simplex virus	Immuno compromised patient	Acyclovir: 10 mg/kg IV every 8 hours (using IBW) adjusted for kidney Function
	Varicella zoster virus	Manifested by a vesicular rash	
	Cytomegalovirus	Rare and controversial as to the potential for causing ALF	Ganciclovir: 5 mg/kg IV every 12 h (using IBW) adjusted for kidney function
	Epstein–Barr virus		
	Human herpesvirus-6		
	Adenovirus, coxsackie B virus, hemorrhagic fever virus	Rare causes of ALF	

Table 30.1 (continued)

Category	Etiology	Common c/f	Treatment
Drugs	Idiosyncratic reactions	Isoniazid, nonsteroidal anti-inflammatory drugs, carbamazepine	
	Dose-dependent hepatotoxicity	Acetaminophen, sulfonamides, tetracycline	Oral NAC: 140 mg/kg loading dose, then 70 mg/kg every 4 h
			IV NAC: 150 mg/kg loading dose, then 50 mg/kg IV over 4 h, then 100 mg/kg IV over 16 h as a continuous infusion
	Herbal supplements	Patients' families must be asked about treatment history	
Vascular diseases	Right heart failure		
	Sinusoidal obstruction syndrome	Most common following systemic chemotherapy in preparation for bone marrow transplantation	
	Budd-Chiari syndrome		TIPS/anticoagulation/liver transplantation
	Ischemic hepatitis (shock liver)		
Toxins	Amanita phalloides toxin	Acute gastroenteritis; renal failure and pancreatitis	Charcoal: via NGT every 4 h alternating with silymarin Penicillin G: 1 g/kg/day IV and NAC (Dosing as for acetaminophen overdose) Silymarin: 300 mg PO/NGT every 12 h Legalon-SIL: 5 mg/kg/day IV (given in 4 divided doses) or 5 mg/kg IV Loading dose followed by 20 mg/kg/day via continuous infusion
	Bacillus cereus toxin	Fried rice syndrome	
	Carbon tetrachloride		
	Yellow phosphorus		
Metabolic diseases	Wilson disease	Younger patients; Coombs negative hemolytic anemia, hypouricemia, and a low alkaline phosphatase level with a high bilirubin level	
	Reye syndrome	Occurs in young children with viral syndrome and salicylate ingestion	
	Acute fatty liver of pregnancy	Associated with defects in fetal and maternal mitochondrial long-chain 3-hydroxyacyl coenzyme A dehydrogenase	Delivery of fetus
Malignant infiltration	Metastatic breast cancer	The most common solid organ metastasis to cause liver failure	
	Lymphoma		
Autoimmune diseases	Autoimmune hepatitis		Methylprednisolone: 60 mg/day IV

30.2 Intracranial Hypertension (ICH), Hepatic Encephalopathy in ALF and Management

The most lethal complication associated with ALF is the *development of Hepatic encephalopathy (HE) and cerebral edema.* (CE) As a consequence of cerebral edema and increased intracranial pressure (ICP), CNS complications may range from ischemic and hypoxic injury to uncal herniation and death. ICH accounts for 20–35% of the mortality in ALF [9]. The presence of severe HE is associated with a high frequency of ICH (25–35% in grade III and up to 75% in grade IV) [8]. ICH (defined as an ICP above 20–25 mmHg for >15 min) is one of the most severe complications of ALF and is associated with a poor prognosis [10]. Additional factors that may worsen the neurological outcome are the coexistence of infection or presence of inflammation without sepsis alongside the presence of other organ failure [10–12].The risk of developing intracranial hypertension (ICH) is higher in female and younger patients with severe liver failure (MELD >32), presenting in acute or hyperacute state [5] with renal failure, ionotropic therapy, and ammonium concentrations above 200 mmol/L [11, 13, 14].

30.2.1 ICP Monitoring

The rationale for ICP measurement is based on retrospective trials that showed a prevalence of over 50% of ICH in ALF patients and an association with elevated mortality risk [15]. Nonetheless, there is no randomized data available to evaluate the benefit of ICP monitoring [15–17].

30.2.2 Methods of ICP Monitoring

Direct and Invasive:-Invasive ICP monitoring can be obtained through two different approaches: intraparenchymal microtransducers and direct catheters (intraventricular, subdural or epidural). Epidural transducers are a relatively safe method [17]. However, it has a less-than-optimal degree of precision compared with other methods due to the damping effect of the surrounding dura mater. ICP evaluated by an intraparenchymal catheter has a good correlation with values obtained with intraventricular catheters [18]. The rates of infection from intraparenchymal catheters are minimal but are associated with a bleeding rate of 7% and bleeding-related deaths of approximately 3% [15], but there was no 21-day mortality benefit in acetaminophen-related ALF and a worse prognosis in the non-acetaminophen group [15]. Therefore, placement of ICP devices remains a matter of intense debate, with their use reserved for patients at high risk of ICH, and in centers with large neurosurgical experience in ALF management [19–21].

All Indirect and Non-invasive techniques are complex and demonstrate considerable *"inter and intra-assay" variability.* Changes in CBF reflecting ischemia and vasodilation of the cerebral circulation and resistance to flow, with increased ICP, can be assessed using MCA Doppler [22]. An increase in CBF usually precedes the rise of ICP. Indirect data can be obtained by monitoring reverse jugular vein oxygen saturation; values over 80% usually indicate hyperemia and under 55% relative ischemia. The latter suggests a scenario where cerebral oxygen consumption is in excess of supply due to epileptiform activity (increased demand) or inadequate supply (hyperventilation and hypocapnia, inadequate blood pressure or cardiac index). The measurement of optic nerve sheath diameter is also representative of ICP, according to a recent assessment [23].The optic nerve sheath is anatomic continuity to meninges, is distensible and the ICP influences its diameter [24]. Thus, literature suggests the utility of ONSD measurement as screening method to ICH diagnosis, with a cut-off of 5.7 mm measured 3 mm behind the globe. CT and MRI may show radiological signs of brain oedema. However, the absence of these signs does not rule out ICH [25].

30.2.3 Therapeutic Interventions

30.2.3.1 General Supportive Strategies

- Head end elevation to 30 degree with neck in neutral position.
- Intubation and mechanical ventilation in grade III and IV HE.
- Use propofol and low-dose fentanyl, and if needed cisatracurium once intubated [26]. Intermediate or long acting benzodiazepines should be avoided [27].
- Deploy low-tidal volume lung protective strategy to prevent ARDS. High-intrathoracic pressures result in cerebral venous outflow obstruction [28].
- For non-invasive approach for BP monitoring in suspected ICH - target a higher mean arterial pressure goal (>80 mmHg).
- In case of concern of seizure activity, EEG monitoring should be undertaken and antiepileptic drugs administered;
  - Phenytoin has traditionally been the medication of choice; however, agents without risk of hepatotoxicity and more easily achieved therapeutic levels such as levetiracetam or lacosamide are now more frequently utilized.
- Avoid acid-base and electrolyte disturbances.
  - Hypokalemia, and metabolic acidosis which increases renal proximal tubule ammoniagenesis [29].
  - Metabolic alkalosis promotes formation of NH3+ from (NH4+) augmenting its passage across the blood–brain barrier [30].
  - Hyponatremia, which is a risk factor for cerebral edema via reduced extracellular osmolarity [31],
- Prevent hypoglycemia by initiating 10% or 20% dextrose infusion in central line.

30.2.4 Specific Strategies

30.2.4.1 Strategies to Reduce Hyperammonemia

Lactulose: It is a nonabsorbable disaccharide. It is metabolized in caecum by enteric bacteria to lactate and acetate. This in turn lowers the cecal pH leading to increased fecal nitrogen excretion and decrease in serum ammonia levels [32, 33]. However, there have been no studies showing mortality benefit in ALF [34]; avoid lactulose via oral or NG route in ALF as it may cause bowel distention, worsening ileus, and complicating transplant surgery. If used, it is safer to be given rectally.

Rifaximin: It is an oral antibiotic with a broad spectrum activity against enteric bacteria. Its possible benefit in lowering ammonia in patients with ALF has not yet been explored [34].

LOLA & LOPA: LOLA (L ornithine L aspartate) is a stable salt of the amino acids ornithine and aspartic acid. These two amino acids get converted to glutamate in the muscles and hepatocytes. Glutamate is the substrate on which the enzyme glutamine synthase (present in the muscle as well as liver), acts and combines it with ammonia to make glutamine and thereby reduces blood ammonia levels [35]. A recent placebo controlled double blind RCT [36] in ALF showed that LOLA did not decrease ammonia levels, and improved neither encephalopathy nor survival. In the above mentioned study ammonia levels were measured for 6 days among patients receiving LOLA as well as placebo, however, the rate of decline of ammonia was also similar between the two arms. Peculiarly, patients receiving LOLA had more frequent seizures. Very high glutamine levels in the systemic circulation are found in ALF [37, 38]. LOLA could theoretically further increase ammonia detoxification by the skeletal muscle by increased glutamine synthesis. This glutamine is recirculated back to the intestine and kidney where it is broken down to ammonia and glutamate by glutaminase, thus LOLA is ineffective in reducing the ammonia levels.

LOPA (L ornithine phenyl acetate):- Phenyl acetate combines with glutamine to form phenylacetyl glutamine which is water soluble and is excreted in urine, but human studies are yet to find a beneficial effect and is contraindicated in renal failure.

Renal replacement therapy: Continuous renal replacement therapy (CRRT) is recommended over intermittent hemodialysis [39] because of lower fluctuations in ICP and improved hemodynamic stability in the setting of AKI and other conventional indication for dialysis therapy (e.g., metabolic acidosis and hyperkalemia) [40, 41]. CRRT using continuous veno venous hemofiltration with high-filtration volume (90 ml/kg/h) has been shown to be an effective method of rapidly lowering serum plasma ammonia levels [42, 43]. Early CRRT helps to maintain euvolemia, augment ammonia clearance [42, 43], correction of electrolyte and in acidosis correction. Initiating CRRT with isotonic dialysate in patient with intracranial hypertension and induced hypernatremia can cause rebound edema from dialysis disequilibrium syndrome and precipitate brain herniation, so use hypertonic dialysate or hypertonic saline infusion in post filter return arm of CRRT.

30.2.5 Prophylactic Strategies

- Hypertonic saline used to prophylactically elevate serum sodium level between 145 and 155 meq/l has been demonstrated to reduce the incidence and severity of intracranial hypertension in grade 3 and 4 hepatic encephalopathy patients is a single center study [44]. Prophylactic hyperventilation does not provide a benefit in terms of reducing the incidence of cerebral oedema [45].
- The prophylactic use of antiepileptic drugs is not warranted [46].
- Prophylactic antibiotics have been shown to reduce the risk of infection that later stages of encephalopathy are associated with increased incidence of cerebral edema, and that fever may worsen intracranial hypertension [47].
- Recently, the role of prophylactic hypothermia was evaluated in a randomized trial. This study [48] included 46 patients with intracranial pressure monitoring that were randomized to hypothermia (targeted temperature of 33–34 °C) or normothermia (36 °C) treatments. Interestingly, although the target temperature was consistently achieved in both groups, there was no difference in the incidence of sustained elevation of ICP (35% vs.

27% in intervention and control group, respectively) or in overall survival.

30.3 Specific Strategies to Reduce Cerebral Edema and ICH

ICP should be maintained below 20–25 mmHg and the difference between MAP and ICP (cerebral perfusion pressure, CPP) should remain above 50 mmHg [49]. Sustained surges in ICP (>25 mmHg) or development of clinical signs should be treated immediately, with Osmotherapy.

Hypertonic saline with sodium goal of 145–150 meq/l can be used either as:

1. Continuous infusion: 3% NaCl titrated between 30 and 100 ml/h or.
2. Intermittent bolus dosing: 200 ml of 3% sodium chloride.

Mannitol reduces brain water through its osmotic effect and improves cerebral perfusion through RBC rheological effect, in a dose of 0.5–1 g/kg bodyweight bolus. It should be avoided if plasma osmolarity >320 mOsm/l or osmolar gap >20 mOsm/l. High doses can result in acute renal failure and damage to the BBB. Mannitol [50] works best in mild to moderate intracranial hypertension and is less effective when the ICP is greater than 60 mmHg.

Hyperventilation [51] produces cerebral vasoconstriction secondary to CSF alkalosis, reduces vascular inflow, and eventually decreases ICP although its effect is short-lived and cerebral vasoconstriction can generate areas of cerebral ischemia, which can potentially worsen cerebral edema by causing cerebral hypoxia [52]. Based on available evidence, there is no role for prophylactic hyperventilation in patients with ALF. If life-threatening ICH is not controlled with osmotherapy and other general management, hyperventilation may be instituted acutely to delay impending herniation; beyond this acute situation, forced hyperventilation cannot be recommended as routine management.

Hypothermia reduces CBF and the entry of ammonia into the brain, decreases the availability of glutamate in the cerebral extracellular space, and diminishes anaerobic glycolysis [53]. In 1999, Jalan et al. [54] showed that a temperature reduction to 32–33 °C was associated with a significant decrease in ICP. A recent retrospective study [55] showed that therapeutic hypothermia had no impact on overall or transplant-free survival. However, this warrants an RCT to evaluate the role of hypothermia on overall survival. Also, hypothermia has not been compared to normothermia in a controlled trial, and has not been shown to improve transplant-free survival. Potential deleterious effects of hypothermia [56] include increased risk of infection, coagulation disturbance, and cardiac arrhythmias; while concern about the effect of hypothermia on hepatic regeneration [57] has also been raised. Its utility in controlling ICP remains an attractive and useful intervention in the ICU, and perhaps should be reserved for refractory intracranial hypertension or refractory hyperammonemia. Considering the risk and benefits, a reasonable approach [58] would be to use a milder goal for hypothermia starting at 35 °C. Though literature reports that hypothermia decreases ICP there is no beneficial effect on mortality.

Indomethacin inhibits endothelial cyclooxygenase, produces cerebral vasoconstriction, and decreases CBF. Toefteng et al. [59] evaluated the effect of indomethacin ICP in 12 ALF patients and reported significant reduction in ICP and an improvement in CPP. While further studies are awaited its use may be considered in refractory cases. A Randomized Control Trial [60] ALF patients corticosteroids failed to improve cerebral edema or survival, and is not advocated. Based on head injury data, IV thiopental [61] was assessed in 13 patients with Fulminant Hepatic Failure complicated by unresponsive intracranial hypertension. The ICP was reduced in all cases, and in eight cases thiopentone infusion achieved stable normal intracranial and cerebral perfusion pressure. Five patients made a complete recovery. The recommended dose of pentobarbital is a loading dose of 3–5 mg/kg (maximum 500 mg) over 15 min, followed by a continuous infusion of 0.5–2.0 mg/h. Barbiturate therapy must be used with simultaneous continuous ICP and arterial blood pressure monitoring.

Hepatectomy is a theoretical possibility as a bridging procedure to liver transplant for those patients with devastating and medically uncontrolled ICH in whom there is no perceived chance of spontaneous recovery.

30.4 Hemodynamic Derangement in ALF and Management

Cardiovascular and circulatory abnormalities are a common feature of ALF. ALF is characterized by a hyperdynamic circulation with high cardiac output, low MAP, and low systemic vascular resistance [62]. Troponin elevation [63, 64] is seen in approximately 60–70% of patients with ALF and is likely related to systemic stress versus true myocardial injury. Elevation of troponin in the setting of ALF did correlate positively with requirements for vasopressors, renal failure, and organ failure scores and did not correlate with evidence of cardiac dysfunction on ECHO studies [63].

The initial step in management of hemodynamic abnormalities is aimed at the restoration of effective circulating volume, as most patients are relatively volume depleted due to various causes.

Invasive monitoring devices are often used to optimize circulating volume and cardiac output [65]. Arterial pressure monitoring from a central artery is preferable. As intravascular volume assessment in ALF poses a challenge, dynamic measures utilizing echocardiography are superior to static hemodynamic measurements [66].

There is considerable data to suggest that a persistent positive fluid balance is associated with higher mortality in ALF. Elevated right sided cardiac pressures may be detrimental to liver venous outflow and hence liver function and regeneration, gut integrity and renal functions [67–69]. Therefore, volume overload should be avoided as much as volume depletion. The choice of fluid should be normal saline or balanced salt solutions, being guided by the patient's acid-base and electrolyte status with and preventing hyperchloremic acidosis, as it has been associated with an increased risk of renal failure and other morbidities [70, 71].

In case of increasing tissue and cerebral edema and need for volume therapy, albumin [72–74] infusion can be considered which will enhance plasma oncotic pressure and maintain intravascular volume.

Noradrenaline [75] is typically the vasopressor of choice as it effectively raises mean arterial pressure and can increase hepatic blood flow in parallel with less tachycardia. Vasopressin may augment noradrenaline effect and allow titrating down its dose, but vasopressin, according to animal studies [76], may exacerbate cerebral hyperemia, hyperammonemia, and consequent edema associated with ALF.

In 2007, Eefesen et al. [77] compared noradrenalin and terlipressin in ten ALF patients with ICP monitoring and cerebral microdialysis, and found terlipressin increased CPP without changing ICP, decreased brain lactate, and unchanged lactate/pyruvate ratio. In the absence of advanced hepatic encephalopathy a MAP of at least 65 mmHg, and with advanced encephalopathy and suspected intracranial hypertension, a MAP of at least 80 mmHg is recommended to maintain optimal CPP.

While ALF exhibits hyperdynamic circulation, those with hypoxic hepatitis may have both right and left sided cardiac dysfunction, with or without valvular heart disease. Minimizing right sided pressures, by treating PAH with pulmonary vasodilators (Prostaglandins and sildenafil) and ensuring adequate MAP should be the strategy. In patients with profound and reversible acute cardiac dysfunction, venoarterial extracorporeal membrane oxygenation [78] (VA ECMO) may be appropriate. Hypoxic hepatitis is a secondary form of ALF and as such, the primary presenting organ failure needs to be addressed and managed to facilitate liver recovery. Liver transplantation is not indicated.

About 62% of ALF exhibit adrenal insufficiency [79] which is not impacted by etiology and it correlate with the severity of illness. They are less responsive to the pressor effects of norepinephrine and which is restored when physio-

logic doses of hydrocortisone are added [80]. Thus patients with ALF who experience refractory hypotension should be evaluated for adrenal insufficiency and when adrenal insufficiency is identified, hydrocortisone should be administered at 200–300 mg daily in divided doses.

30.5 Nutritional and Metabolic Support in ALF

About half of ALF patients develop recurrent hypoglycemia due to glycogen depletion and defective glycogenolysis and gluconeogenesis [81], which can be sudden and can misinterpretation of mental changes. Blood sugar should be monitored at 2–3 h intervals and whenever it is lower than 60 mg/dl, an iv bolus of 50–100 ml of 50% dextrose administered. Glucose transport across the blood–brain barrier is increased because of upregulation of glucose carriers in ALF and hyperglycemia contributes to raised ICP because this increased glucose influx leads to cerebral lactic acid accumulation [82], thereby emphasizing the need for maintaining euglycemia. Low systemic blood pressure and poor systemic microcirculation in ALF result in a build-up of lactate, compounded by failing lactate metabolism. Hyperlactataemia [81] can not only aggravate hemodynamic instability, but also cause cerebral hyperemia and should be treated aggressively.

ALF increases energy requirements are by 60%, and further by complicating infection. Whole body protein catabolism may be increased up to four times the normal rate and results in massive amino acid losses in urine. Owing to the hypercatabolic state of ALF, nutrition is vital and enteral feedings should be initiated early. Only where enteral feeding is contraindicated, partial or total parenteral nutrition should be considered. Initially, combination of parenteral dextrose and lipid emulsions, with 40 gm protein/day can be administered. Lipid emulsions [83] may be used safely in patients with ALF. Avoid severe restrictions of protein [84] and provide normal protein intake of about 1 g/kg per day. Branched chain amino acids (BCAA) offer no additional advantage, except during frequent dialysis, in whom large BCAA losses may occur. Serum levels of phosphorus, potassium, and magnesium are usually low and should be supplemented. Critically ill patients with ALF are at high risk for GI bleeding. In patients who are ventilated or with severe coagulopathy related to hepatic dysfunction, initiation of GI prophylaxis with H$_2$ blockers or proton pump inhibitors is recommended [27].

30.6 Respiratory Derangement in ALF and Management

The earlier reported incidence [85, 86] of ALI in ALF is between 33 and 37%. Prevention and modern critical care management of ALI and ALF has resulted in current prevalence of ALI in ALF to 21%, though this does not have significant impact on outcomes [87].

Non-invasive ventilator (NIV) should be avoided in ALF patients at risk of hepatic, metabolic or septic high risk of encephalopathy, aspiration, and poor compliance. Invasive airway management to protect airway should be instituted in cases of high grade HE, followed by ventilatory support for hypoxia and respiratory failure.

Rapid sequence induction technique to minimize elevation in ICP using of nondepolarizing agents such as cisatracurium is preferred for endotracheal intubation. Cisatracurium is largely independent of renal or hepatic function for metabolism. Short acting opiate fentanyl for analgesia and propofol for sedation are usually preferred. Although propofol may decrease propofol in hypovolemic patients, it decreases cerebral metabolic rate and also acts as an anticonvulsant.

The balance of hypoxia, hypercarbia and risk of increased ICP are determining factors while choosing the modality of ventilation.

Protective ventilatory strategy with low tidal volumes [88] (6 ml/kg/ideal body weight) and appropriate levels of PEEP to maintain an open lung should be chosen. A target of pCO$_2$ between 34 and 41 mmHg is ideal. Judicious airway care, head up positioning and careful respiratory ther-

apy minimize risk of ventilator associated pneumonia. Protocol based microbiological cultures of endotracheal secretions and broncho-alveolar lavage should be followed.

Acute respiratory distress syndrome (ARDS) is uncommon ALF patients which may not impact mortality [89]. But in the unlikely patients who develop ARDS prone ventilation [90] does improve oxygenation and potentially decreases mortality, though fraught with the risk of increasing cerebral complications. High PEEP, i.e., >12, which can enhance ICP, can be monitored with middle cerebral artery Doppler. One can consider VV-ECMO in centers with expertise, keeping in view the increased risk of bleeding in ALF.

Hypoxemia is rather common and its etiological assessment is difficult. In some patients with hypoxic hepatitis there is evidence of hepatopulmonary syndrome [91] and this should be excluded with bubble ECHO. HPS is characterized by triad of chronic liver disease, gas exchange abnormalities with significant hypoxemia and/or increased A-a O2 gradient and evidence of right to left intrapulmonary shunt. In patients with intra-cardiac shunts, a small amount of contrast is usually recorded in the left chambers within 1 or 2 cardiac cycles after its appearance in the right side chambers. On the contrary, late arrival of contrast in the left atrium after a time delay of 4–8 cardiac cycles is diagnostic of intra-pulmonary shunt, and is due to the time required for passage through the pulmonary circulation [92].

There also may be evidence of a toxic liver syndrome with increased lung water and ARDS. Assessment of lung water, utilizing advanced hemodynamic monitoring such as volume view or PiCCO may optimize managing these patients.

30.7 Renal Derangement in ALF and Management

Etiology [93] of renal dysfunction in ALF is multifactorial with drug-induced nephrotoxicity, acute tubular necrosis, and abdominal compartment syndrome being the common causes.

Paracetamol [94] may also be one of the causes. The various other risk factors [95] for renal dysfunction in ALF are increased age, hypotension, systemic inflammatory response Syndrome [96] (SIRS), and infection.

Acute kidney injury also develops in 55–68% of all ALF patients and it resolves along with resolution of liver injury or with transplantation [97]. Early AKI develops due to direct injury pattern, whereas late onset typically is more akin to hepatorenal syndrome characterized by functional impairment [98, 99] which is due to a complex interplay between extrarenal vasodilation and renal arteriolar vasoconstriction coupled with inadequate cardiac output [100].

Avoiding nephrotoxic agents, aggressively handling infection and sepsis, deploying various techniques to maintain adequate renal perfusion and instituting timely renal replacement therapy are the mainstays of managing renal dysfunction in ALF [101]. Early targeted volume replacement and vasoactive agent administration, utilizing the hemodynamic management principles above, are keys to avoiding hypotension and to ensure adequate renal perfusion. Renal replacement therapy should be deployed judiciously and timely, rather than a last resort.

30.7.1 Renal Replacement Therapy

Although no study to date has clearly determined ideal and optimal timing for initiation of RRT, rational arguments for early initiation are favored by many liver centers. Studies [40] comparing CRRT versus IHD have noted greater variations in hemodynamic parameters and ICPs with IHD. This has led to the *preference for CRRT over IHD* in these patients and early initiation prevents or allows treatment of these disturbances with consequent complications. High dose CRRT [42] has been shown to decrease arterial ammonia as well. Low-urine output in spite of adequate intravascular volume, fluid overload, and rise in serum creatinine of 0.3 mg/dl have been advocated as indications [3] for CRRT in ALF and even post-transplant.

CRRT vs. IHD:-A retrospective analysis of 1604 patients in the U.S. ALFSG [15] showed that 70% of patients developed AKI with almost 30% requiring RRT. CRRT is recommended over intermittent hemodialysis, in most ALF patients, due to poor tolerance of HD owing to circulatory instability, sudden fluid shifts, and ICP rise [40]. Lactate free bicarbonate buffer as the dialysate and biocompatible dialysis membranes like polysulfone or polyacrylonitrile should only be used [93]. ALF patients require standard heparinization for dialysis in spite of the coagulopathy, due to coexisting antithrombin III deficiency. While cirrhotic patients tolerate citrate anticoagulation [102–104], those with acute and hyperacute ALF may not, due to deranged metabolism of citrate. If citrate is used, close monitoring of total calcium compared with ionized calcium is warranted. Full recovery of AKI is seen in most ALF patients either by the time of discharge or following liver transplantation [94]. Female gender, lower day three MELD scores, admission hypotension and lower grades of AKI are predictive factors for complete renal recovery following paracetamol induced ALF [96, 105].

30.8 Hemostasis in ALF and Management

Since liver synthesizes majority of coagulation factors and proteins required for fibrinolysis, disordered coagulation is an essential diagnostic component of ALF. Deranged international normalized ratio (INR) and prothrombin time are common and are essential to the diagnosis of ALF. Thrombocytopenia [106] is a frequent feature of ALF and is associated with increased incidence of multisystem organ failure and death. In spite of this, clinically significant bleeding events are rare and are seen only in 5% of ALF patients [107]. In depth analysis of coagulation pathophysiology in patients with ALF suggests that they have *"rebalanced hemostasis"* and despite prolongation of measured INR or PT they have a "normal coagulation state," and a significant proportion are actually hypercoagulable. This is due to significant increases in endogenous heparinoids, procoagulant microparticles, von Willebrand factor and factor VIII, reduced pro- and anticoagulant factors and release of "younger" more reactive platelets in patients with ALF [108–112]. In cases of both acute and chronic liver failure, decreased synthetic capacity of the liver results in decreased production of both procoagulant and anticoagulant proteins [113]. Compared to CLD and cirrhosis, ALF patients have more pronounced reductions in levels of factors II, V, VII, and X with increased levels of factor VIII, likely owing to acute inflammation and tissue factor-mediated consumption of these factors (with the exception of factor VIII) [114].

Recent studies [112] in ALF have identified platelet derived microparticles as being potentially responsible for thrombocytopenia, which may create a hypercoagulable state in the microcirculation and lead to systemic complications and poor outcomes. The "rebalanced state of hemostasis" [115, 116] of ALF can be measured by thromboelastography and thrombin generation studies which explains the low rate of bleeding complications.

Monitoring of coagulation in ALF requires standard and extended laboratory techniques (thrombin generation, factor VIII, etc.), in addition to thromboviscous technology, which is becoming a standard method in many liver centers.

The balanced hemostasis concept reinforces the recommendation that prophylactic correction of deranged coagulation or platelets is unnecessary. It may adversely affect prognostication as well as increase the risk of thrombosis or transfusion related acute lung complications. However, there are two situations that require such measures. (1) ICP monitor insertion requires correction of coagulation and platelet deficiencies, as guided by neurosurgical specialist societies. Some suggest prophylactic recombinant factor VIIa, without any evidence of mortality benefit, but an increased risk of thrombosis [15, 16, 111, 117]. (2) Significant active hemorrhage also necessitates correction, apart from source control of the hemorrhage. Although indications in the specific setting of ALF are not available, it seems reasonable to target plasma fibrinogen levels 1.5–2 g/L by infusing fibrinogen concentrate at an initial dose of 25–50 mg/kg body weight, and a platelet count >60,000 [118]. Supportive therapies such as tranexamic acid can also be considered. Hemoglobin level of 7 g/dl is usually acceptable, though packed cell transfusion may be considered in severe cardiorespiratory failure or subarachnoid hemorrhage [119]. Finally, vitamin K (5–10 mg) should be considered in all patients with ALF, because its deficiency can occur in >25% of patients.

30.9   Infection and SIRS in ALF

ALF is associated with dynamic immune dysfunction. An altered balance between opposing systemic pro- and anti-inflammatory immune profiles can contribute to organ failure and death in ALF [120]. Any type of liver injury leads to activation of the innate immune system, altered macrophage and neutrophil function, initial activation and subsequent reduction of complements, impaired phagocytosis and opsonization resulting in functional immunoparesis.

Liver cell death leads to a release of pro-inflammatory mediators, with elimination of pathogens and tissue regeneration, which may also initiate propagation of further tissue damage. This may lead to "spill over" phenomenon of chemotactic mediators and pro-inflammatory cytokines, with subsequent recruitment of monocytes, lymphocytes, and polymorphonuclear leukocytes [112]. They secrete vasoactive mediators, which by activating platelets and coagulation cascade, increase vascular permeability alongside microcirculatory failure and thrombosis [112] and eventual SIRS. Release of damage associated molecular patterns, e.g., HMGB1, from injured hepatocytes may also contribute to the development of SIRS [121]. SIRS leads to a vicious cycle wherein an increase in vascular permeability further contributes to tissue injury. Over time, the balance tilts towards the anti-inflammatory response, which is associated with immune suppression, recurrent infections, sepsis, and death [122].SIRS appears to be involved in the worsening of HE, reduces the chances of transplantation, and confers a poorer prognosis, independent of infection [123].

ALF patients are at increased risk of developing infections, sepsis, and septic shock. Though bacteremia is not independent predictor of mortality in ALF [124], infectious complications [125] are a leading cause of death. Bacterial infections [126] are seen in 60–80% of ALF patients, commonest being pneumonia (50%), followed by urinary tract infections (22%), intravenous catheter-induced bacteremia (12%), and spontaneous bacteremia (16%). Gram-negative enteric bacilli and Gram-positive cocci are the most common pathogens. Fungal infections [127] occur in about one-third of ALF patients requiring prolonged critical care, mostly with candida species, with concurrent bacterial infections. Viral infections and reactivation of CMV [128] is common in ALF patients.

30.9.1 Biomarkers

High level of clinical suspicion of infection should be maintained in patients with ALF. Diagnosis of infection in ALF patients poses many challenges. Clinical features are non-specific and lab indicators like C reactive protein [129] and procalcitonin [130] measurements are unreliable. Routine microbiologic surveillance may aid early detection and treatment of infections [126]. Frequent screening of blood, urine, and representative samples for cultures should be performed as indicated. Admission HE and SIRS score >2 are significant predictors of bacteremia. Deterioration of mental status, unexplained fever, and leukocytosis may herald the onset of infection [124]. Deterioration in hepatic coma grade after initial improvement, pyrexia unresponsive to antibiotics, established renal failure, and marked elevation in white cell count should prompt aggressive investigation for fungal, bacterial, or viral infection. This is especially important in patients already on broad spectrum antibiotics. Use of biomarkers for fungal infection [131] should be utilized, while recognizing

their high false positive rate, but low risk of false negative results.

Empirical broad spectrum antibiotics should be administered to ALF patients with SIRS, refractory hypotension or unexplained worsening of hepatic encephalopathy [132]. Though prophylactic [133] parenteral antimicrobial therapy reduces the incidence of infection in certain groups of ALF patients, resultant survival benefit has not been shown. Selective digestive decontamination [134] using nonabsorbable antibiotics and parenteral antibiotics also does not impact survival. There are no controlled trials confirming that the use of prophylactic antimicrobials decreases the likelihood of progression of HE or the development of raised ICP. Therefore, there is no sufficient data to support a generalized antibiotic prophylactic [133] practice in ALF. Empiric antibiotics are recommended for patients listed for super-urgent liver transplantation, since the development of infection and sepsis may prompt delisting. Decisions surrounding antimicrobial choice should be based on knowledge of local microbiological data.

30.9.2 Prognosis and Liver Transplantation

Liver transplantation has improved survival in ALF. The 1-year post-LT survival in ALF in less than that of elective LT performed for chronic liver disease. This is primarily due to increased ICH and sepsis resulting in increased mortality in the first 3 months following LT in ALF. Beyond the first year, ALF patients have better long-term survival [135].

Both whole organ deceased donor and living donor LT have been performed in ALF with great success. Another type of LT is auxiliary transplantation in which the recipient liver is left in place and a partial left or right lobe from the donor is transplanted, thus providing hepatic function until the native liver regenerates. Good survival rates of 60–65% have been reported with this procedure and immunosuppression can be withdrawn in 65–85% of patients at the end of 1-year post-LT.

Prognostic factors in ALF assist in the early identification of patients who would benefit from liver transplantation. They also help identify patients who may recover on their own with supportive care without the need for transplantation. Unfortunately, despite the presence of numerous clinical indicators and prognostic models, a successful prognostic scoring system has yet to be determined. This is mainly due to the varying etiologies of ALF and the variability in the course and complications of ALF.

The Kings College Criteria (KCC) was the first validated scoring system (introduced in 1989) and is currently one of the most widely used prognostic tools for ALF (Table 30.2). Modern medical management has modified KCC performance proven with its dropping sensitivity to studies done after 2005 (46–71%) compared with studies before 1995 (76–82%) [136]. Arterial blood lactate [137] greater than 3.5 mmol/L is an early predictor of mortality in APAP associated ALF (sensitivity 67%, specificity 95%, positive predictive value 79%, negative predictive value 91%) and when added may increase the predictive accuracy of the KCC.

In a systematic analysis [138] of the MELD (modified end stage liver disease) score in ALF, 526 patients with ALF from six studies (all did not have LT support) were included and overall 304 died (58%). By using a MELD score cut-off of 30.5–35, the pooled sensitivity was 77% (95% CI, 72–82%) and specificity was 72% (95% CI, 62–80%).

In a meta-analysis done by Mcphail et al. [136] comparing KCC and MELD score for predicting outcome in ALF, found that The Diagnostic Odds Ratio (DOR) for KCC in cases of AALF was 10.4(4.9–22.1) and for MELD 6.6 (2.1–20.2) whereas for NAALF the DOR for KCC was 4.16 (2.34–7.40) and 8.42 (5.98–11.88) for MELD. Concluding that Although KCC performs better for AALF, MELD has improved prognostic accuracy in NAALF.

Accordingly, the American Gastroenterological Associates [139] suggests using the MELD score rather than the KCC as a prognostic scoring system in patients presenting with ALF (a cut-off MELD score of 30.5 should be used for prognosis and higher scores predict a need for LT). A more recent European Association for the Study of the Liver guideline [7] recommends that LT be considered in those patients fulfilling either the KCC or Clichy criteria. A factor V level of less than 20% may indicate a poor prognosis necessitating consideration of LT in patients of 30 years of age or younger, and a higher threshold of less than 30% is of equivalent significance in older patients [139].

Important prognostic variables for predicting the lack of spontaneous recovery and the need for liver transplantation include: (1) advanced grades 3 and 4 HE and (2) severe coagulopathy defined as an INR >6.5. Additional unfavorable prognostic variables include unfavorable etiologies (e.g., AIH, WD, HSV, and HAV) and the rate of disease progression.

More recently, a retrospective analysis [140] done by the US Acute Liver Failure Study Group (ALFSG) developed a logistic regression model to predict transplant-free survival using admission variables include hepatic encephalopathy (HE) grade, ALF etiology, vasopressor use, bilirubin, and International Normalized Ratio showed good performance characteristics (C-statistic 0.84, specificity 95%, sensitivity 37.1%) in 1974 patients in the ALFSG registry (Fig. 30.3).

Table 30.2 King's college criteria for transplantation in acute liver failure – Acetaminophen induced and Non-acetaminophen induced

Acetaminophen-induced ALF	Nonacetaminophen-induced ALF
Arterial pH <7.30 after fluid resuscitation	Prothrombin time >100 s (INR >6.5)
Or all of the following:	*Or* any 3 of the following:
• Prothrombin time >100 s (INR >6.5)	• Non-A, non-B viral hepatitis, drug-induced or indeterminate etiology of ALF
• Serum creatinine >3.4 mg/dL	• Time from jaundice → encephalopathy >7 days
• Grade 3 or 4 hepatic encephalopathy	• Age <10 years or >40 years
	• Prothrombin time >50 s (INR >3.5)
	• Serum bilirubin >17.4 mg/dL

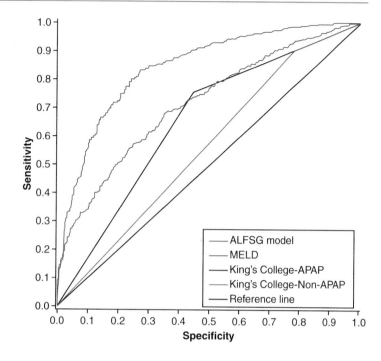

Fig. 30.3 ALFSG model, King's college model (APAP and Non-APAP) and MELD as prognostic models in acute liver failure

The latest model from the King's Liver Intensive Care Unit is a dynamic outcome prediction model [141] developed and validated for use in patients with paracetamol-induced ALF. It is based on prospective data including analysis of more than 20 daily variables sequentially assessed for 3 days after ICU admission in 912 un-transplanted patients between 2000 and 2012. The variables included in the final models to predict death-included age, hepatic encephalopathy, cardiovascular failure, INR, creatinine, and arterial pH on admission and dynamic variables of changing arterial blood lactate and INR. On validation in independent datasets from four transplant centers, the models showed good discrimination between survivors and non-survivors, improving with the inclusion of changes in INR and Lactate over time. Innovative in this approach was its access though a dedicated website and the generation of continuous survival estimates rather than a binary survival outcome, with the intention that the model should act as a decision-support tool to support clinical judgment rather than a sole arbiter as to proceeding with transplantation.

Platelet count has been shown to be closely linked to outcome. In a recent study [142] from the USALFSG, the evolution of thrombocytopenia was closely associated with development of multiorgan failure and a poor outcome in ALF. Recent studies [143] suggest that in some non-paracetamol etiologies, loss of liver volume in adults to less than 1000 cm³ may indicate irreversible damage and serve as an early indicator of poor prognosis, often in advance of the development of encephalopathy.

Apart from these scoring systems, other serum laboratory parameters (e.g., alfa-fetoprotein [144], galectin-9 [145], procoagulant microparticles [112] soluble CD163 [146], and liver-type fatty acid binding protein [147]) for predicting outcomes [148] in ALF have also been proposed.

Finally, it is important to emphasize that prognostic models should be only part of the overall functional evaluation of the very sick patient with ALF and an experienced multi-disciplinary team in an intensive care setting is required for correct interpretation. Rather than providing an absolute arbiter, these models should support decision making and the multifactorial team assessment.

30.10 Liver Support Devices in Acute Liver Failure [149]

Many ALF patients die either waiting for a donor liver or they are not suitable for transplantation. Extracorporeal liver support devices (LSD) have been developed to support this kind of patients. These devices help to either stabilize the patient while liver is recovering from insult or act as a bridge to liver transplantation. An effective artificial liver support device should be able to do three functions, namely, detoxification, synthesis of proteins, and regeneration. An ideal LSD would also replace the need for transplantation and may offer chronic replacement for end stage liver disease, but such support device is not yet available in market.

The liver support devices are classified into two basic groups as artificial liver support devices and bio-artificial liver support devices. While the artificial liver support devices are purely mechanical devices or non-cell based liver support devices, the bio-artificial liver support devices are cell-based liver support devices and have a cellular component such as primary hepatocytes or hepatic cell line. The artificial liver support devices only detoxify while the cellular component in bio-artificial liver support devices try replacing liver functions such as oxidative detoxification, biotransformation, excretion, and synthesis (Table 30.3).

Table 30.3 Characters of liver assist devices

Type of device	Artificial liver support	Bio-artificial liver support
Cellular component	No	Yes
Functions achieved	Detoxification only	All hepatic functions
Cost	Comparatively less	High cost
Ease of use	Relatively easier	Complexity of maintaining living components
Efficacy	Limited	Expected results more promising

30.11 Artificial Liver Support Devices (Non-cell Based)

Molecular adsorbents recirculating system (MARS), fractionated plasma separation and adsorption (Prometheus), single pass albumin dialysis (SPAD), and selective plasma filtration therapy (SEPET) are the current non-cell based artificial liver support devices.

Human blood contains toxins which are either water soluble (ammonia, aromatic amino acids, creatinine, interleukin, Interleukin-6, GABA, urea, tryptophan) or bound to albumin (bilirubin, bile acids, cytokines, protoporphyrin, middle and short-chain fatty acids, para-cresol, protoporphyrin, nitric oxide) toxins. Since hemodialysis and hemofiltration remove only water soluble toxins, albumin has been added to existing dialysis devices to remove albumin bound toxins, as in MARS and SPAD. Large pore filters have also been used to retain cellular components and separate plasma proteins including albumin as in Prometheus and SEPET. The filtrate either undergoes readsorption and then cleans the toxin-attached albumin, which is recycled in MARS and Prometheus or discarded in SPAD and SEPET.

MARS (Gambro GmbH, Hechingen, Germany) was introduced in 1990s, which is a combination of conventional hemodialysis against an Albumin dialysate solution over an Albumin impermeable membrane, and consists of a blood circuit and a secondary circuit. Blood passes through a high flux dialyzer over albumin impermeable membrane against 600 ml of 20% Human Albumin dialysate in the secondary circuit. The secondary circuit refreshes albumin by passing through anion-exchange resin and activated charcoal columns. A meta-analysis looking at four RCTs of MARS in ALF did not show any survival benefit, while mortality rates of MARS patients without transplantation are about 78–100%. MARS decreases bilirubin levels and encephalopathy, but may worsen coagulopathy. MARS does not improve non-transplantation ALF survival and can be used as a bridge to transplantation.

Prometheus, the Fractional plasma separation and adsorption (FPSA, Bad Homburg, Germany) system has a 250 kDa pore size filter and albumin-permeable membranes, the albumin-bound toxins diffuse across and the filtrate which is then passed over two columns of neutral resin and anion-exchange and returned to the patient. Prometheus provides higher clearance for most albumin liver Toxins, compared to MARS. When studied in alcoholic liver disease, MAP and SVR were better preserved compared to MARS.

Single pass albumin dialysis (SPAD) uses 5% albumin concentration which is discarded against a single countercurrent pass against the patient's blood in a hemofilter and is comparable to MARS in clinical and laboratory parameter efficiency. Selective plasma filtration therapy (SEPET) deploys a membrane pore size, allowing passage of molecules of less than100 kDa, size and thus preserves immunoglobulins, complement proteins, clotting factors and hepatocyte growth factor, but albumin is lost and is replaced along with FFP and electrolytes. Clinical trials of SEPET are underway currently.

30.12 Bio-Artificial Liver Support Devices (Cell-Based)

The systems of BAL, which are currently under clinical evaluation, include HepatAssist, Extracorporeal Liver Assist Device (ELAD), Modular Extracorporeal Liver support (MELS), Bio-artificial Liver support system (BLSS), and Amsterdam Medical Centre Bio-artificial Liver (AMCBAL).

The aim of BALs is to provide both detoxification and synthetic functions. Human hepatocytes may be the best cells for use in BAL, but their lack of availability, decreased efficacy in cell culture and inability to readily regenerate in vitro, limits their use. The alternatives are immortal cell lines such as C3A human hepato-blastoma cell lines and porcine hepatocytes. However, there are concerns oncogenesis and xenozoonosis. Moreover, hepatoblastoma cells (C3A) do not exhibit normal metabolic efficiency like ureagenesis and are inferior to primary hepatocytes in metabolic activity.

HepatAssist by Arbios has a hollow fiber extracorporeal bioreactor loaded with cryopreserved porcine hepatocytes. Overall safety was demonstrated across all groups while survival benefit was shown only in subgroup of patients with fulminant or subfulminant hepatic failure. Extracorporeal Liver Assist Device (ELAD) by Vital Therapies (San Diego, California, USA) utilizes hollow fiber cartridges loaded with C3A human hepatoblastoma cell lines. ELAD shas shown improvement in ammonia, bilirubin in HE, survival benefit is yet to be demonstrated through a large multicenter trial. The Modular Extracorporeal Liver support (MELS) system.

(Charite Berlin, Germany) utilizes hollow fibers with fresh porcine hepatocytes. A limited sample study in ALF has shown its safety as a bridge to transplant. Bio-artificial Liver Support System (BLSS) by Excorp Medical (Minneapolis, Minnesota, USA) is under phase II and III studies, which utilizes porcine hepatocytes in a single hollow fiber cartridge. Amsterdam Medical Center Bio-artificial Liver (AMC-BAL) utilizes porcine hepatocytes bound to a spiral-shaped polyester fabric with integrated hollow fiber, which showed some promise in preliminary studies, but larger trials are yet to be done.

In conclusion, excellent evidence proved critical care practices and progress in liver transplantation have improved the survival of ALF significantly. Clarity in definition and classification of ALF have aided in targeting therapies of for ALF subsects. Artificial liver assist devices and coming in are the scope for current research and possible future therapy of ALF.

Key Points

- Although etiological management is important organ supportive management also plays a pivotal role in ALF management.
- For worsening intracranial hypertension with hyperammonemia early continuous renal replacement therapy is the major salvage tool.
- "Rebalanced homeostasis" should always be born in mind warranting judicious use of blood products to correct prolonged clotting parameters.
- Though a lot of prognostic scoring systems are available still one universal prognostic score is still yet to be concluded.
- An ideal liver support device is still impractical at this point.

References

1. Germani G, Theocharidou E, Adam R, Karam V, Wendon J, O'Grady J, et al. Liver transplantation for acute liver failure in Europe: outcomes over 20 years from the ELTR database. J Hepatol. 2012;57:288–96.
2. Donnelly MC, Davidson JS, Martin K, Baird A, Hayes PC, Simpson KJ. Acuteliver failure in Scotland: changes in aetiology and outcomes over time (the Scottish Look-Back Study). Aliment Pharmacol Ther. 2017;45:833–43.
3. Stravitz RT, Kramer DJ. Management of acute liver failure. Nat Rev Gastroenterol Hepatol. 2009;6:542–53.
4. Trey C, Davidson CS. The management of fulminant hepatic failure. Prog Liver Dis. 1970;3:282–98.
5. O'Grady JG, Schalm SW, Williams R. Acute liver failure: redefining the syn-dromes. Lancet. 1993;342:273–5.
6. Polson J, Lee WM. AASLD position paper: the management of acute liver failure. American Association for the Study of Liver Disease. Hepatology. 2005;41(5):1179–97.
7. Wendon J, Panel members, Cordoba J, Dhawan A, Larsen FS, et al. European Association for the Study of the Liver. Electronic address:easloffice@easloffice.eu; Clinical practice guidelines panel, EASL Clinical Practical Guidelines on the management of acute (fulminant) liver failure. J Hepatol. 2017;66:1047–1081.
8. Ostapowicz G, Fontana RJ, Schiødt FV, Larson A, Davern TJ, Han SHB, et al. Results of a prospective study of acute liver failure at 17 tertiary care centers in the United States. Ann Intern Med. 2002;137:947–54.
9. Bernuau J, Rueff B, Benhamou JP. Fulminant and subfulminant liver failure: definitions and causes. Semin Liver Dis. 1986;6:97–106. https://doi.org/10.1055/s-2008-1040593.
10. Mochida S, Takikawa Y, Nakayama N, Oketani M, Naiki T, Yamagishi Y, et al. Diagnostic criteria of acute liver failure: a report by the Intractable Hepato-Biliary Diseases Study Group of Japan. Hepatol Res. 2011;41:805–812. https://doi.org/10.1111/j.1872-034X.2011.00860.x.
11. Bernal W, Hall C, Karvellas CJ, Auzinger G, Sizer E, Wendon J. Arterial ammonia and clinical risk factors for encephalopathy and intracranial hypertension in acute liver failure. Hepatology. 2007;46:1844–52.
12. Larsen FS, Wendon J. Alternative pathway therapy for hyperammonemia in liver failure. Hepatology. 2009;50:3–5.
13. Clemmesen JO, Larsen FS, Kondrup J, Hansen BA, Ott P. Cerebral herniation in patients with acute liver failure is correlated with arterial ammonia concentration. Hepatology. 1999;29:648–53.
14. Bhatia V, Singh R, Acharya SK. Predictive value of arterial ammonia for complications and outcome in acute liver failure. Gut. 2006;55:98–104.
15. Karvellas CJ, Fix OK, Battenhouse H, Durkalski V, Sanders C, Lee WM, et al. Out-comes and complications of intracranial pressure monitoring in acute liver failure: a retrospective cohort study. Crit Care Med. 2014;42:1157–67.
16. Vaquero J, Fontana RJ, Larson AM, Bass NM, Davern TJ, Shakil AO, et al. Complications and use of intracranial pressure monitoring in patients with acute liver failure and severe encephalopathy. Liver Transpl. 2005;11:1581–9.
17. Blei AT, Olafsson S, Webster S, Levy R. Complications of intracranial pressure monitoring in fulminant hepatic failure. Lancet. 1993;341:157–8.
18. Gelabert-González M, Ginesta-Galan V, Sernamito-García R, Allut AG, Bandin-Diéguez J, Rumbo RM. The Camino intracranial pressure device in clinical practice. Assessment in a 1000 cases. Acta Neurochir (Wien). 2006;148:435–41.
19. Wendon JA, Larsen FS. Intracranial pressure monitoring in acute liver failure. A procedure with clear indications. Hepatology. 2006;44:504–6.
20. Bernuau J, Durand F. Intracranial pressure monitoring in patients with acute liver failure: a questionable invasive surveillance. Hepatology. 2006;44:502–4.
21. Fortea JI, Banares R, Vaquero J. Intracranial pressure in acute liver failure: to bolt or not to bolt-that is the question. Crit Care Med. 2014;42:1304–5.
22. Larsen FS, Strauss G, Moller K, Hansen BA. Regional cerebral blood flow autoregulation in patients with fulminant hepatic failure. Liver Transpl. 2000;6:795–800.

23. Krishnamoorthy V, Beckmann K, Mueller M, Sharma D, Vavilala MS. Perioperative estimation of the intracranial pressure using the optic nerve sheath diameter during liver transplantation. Liver Transpl. 2013;19:246–9.

24. Helmke K, Hansen HC. Fundamentals of transorbital sonographic evaluation of optic nerve sheath expansion under intracranial hypertension I. Experimental study. Pediatr Radiol. 1996;26:701–5.

25. Wijdicks EF, Plevak DJ, Rakela J, Wiesner RH. Clinical and radiologic features of cerebral edema in fulminant hepatic failure. Mayo Clin Proc. 1995;70:119–24.

26. Raghavan M, Marik PE. Therapy of intracranial hypertension in patients with fulminant hepatic failure. Neurocrit Care. 2006;4:179–89.

27. Kandiah PA, Olson JC, Subramanian RM. Emerging strategies for the treatment of patients with acute hepatic failure. Curr Opin Crit Care. 2016;22(02):142–51.

28. Citerio G, Vascotto E, Villa F, et al. Induced abdominal compartment syndrome increases intracranial pressure in neurotrauma patients: a prospective study. Crit Care Med. 2001;29:1466–71.

29. Weiner ID, Wingo CS. Hypokalemia–consequences, causes, and correction. J Am Soc Nephrol. 1997;8(7):1179–88.

30. Taboada J, Dimski DS. Hepatic encephalopathy: clinical signs, pathogenesis, and treatment. Vet Clin North Am Small Anim Pract. 1995;25(2):337–55.

31. Iwasa M, Sugimoto R, Mifuji-Moroka R, et al. Factors contributing to the development of overt encephalopathy in liver cirrhosis patients. Metab Brain Dis. 2016;31(5):1151–6.

32. Rabinowich L, Wendon J, Bernal W, Shibolet O. Clinical management of acute liver failure: results of an international multicentre survey. World J Gastroenterol. 2016;22(33):7595–603.

33. Quero Guillén JC, Carmona Soria I, García Montes JM, Jiménez Sáenz M, Herrerías Gutiérrez JM. Hepatic encephalopathy: nomenclature, pathogenesis and treatment. Rev Esp Enferm Dig. 2003;95(02):135–42, 127–134.

34. Cordoba J. Hepatic encephalopathy: from the pathogenesis to the new treatments. ISRN Hematol. 2014:236–68.

35. Olde Damink SW, Deutz NE, Dejong CH, Soeters PB, Jalan R. Interorgan ammonia metabolism in liver failure. Neurochem Int. 2002;41:177–88.

36. Acharya SK, Bhatia V, Sreenivas V, Khanal S, Panda SK. Efficacy of L-ornithine L-aspartate in acute liver failure: a double-blind, randomized, placebo-controlled study. Gastroenterology. 2009;136:2159–68.

37. Clemmesen JO, Kondrup J, Ott P. Splanchnic and leg exchange of amino acids and ammonia in acute liver failure. Gastroenterology. 2000;118:1131–9.

38. Rosen HM, Yoshimura N, Hodgman JM, Fischer JE. Plasma amino acid patterns in hepatic enceph-alopathy of differing etiology. Gastroenterology. 1977;72:483–7.

39. Gupta S, Fenves AZ, Hootkins R. The role of RRT in hyperammonemic patients. Clin J Am Soc Nephrol. 2016;11(10):1872–8. https://doi.org/10.2215/CJN.01320216.

40. Davenport A, Will EJ, Davidson AM. Improved cardiovascular stability during continuous modes of renal replacement therapy in critically ill patients with acute hepatic and renal failure. Crit Care Med. 1993;21:328–38.

41. Lee WM, Larson AM, Stravitz T. AASLD position paper: the management of acute liver failure: update 2011. Baltimore, MD: American Association for the Study of Liver Diseases; 2011. http://www.guide-line.gov/content.aspx?Id=36894.

42. Slack AJ, Auzinger G, Willars C, et al. Ammonia clearance with haemofiltration in adults with liver disease. Liver Int. 2014;34:42–8.

43. Cordoba J, et al. Determinants of ammonia clearance by hemodialysis. Artif Organs. 1996;20:800–3.

44. Murphy N, Auzinger G, Bernel W, et al. The effect of hypertonic sodium chloride on intracranial pressure in patients with acute liver failure. Hepatology. 2004;39:464–70.

45. Ede RJ, Gimson AE, Bihari D, et al. Controlled hyperventilation in the prevention of cerebral oedema in fulminant hepatic failure. J Hepatol. 1986;2:43–51.

46. Bhatia V, Batra Y, Acharya SK. Prophylactic phenytoin does not improve cerebral edema or survival in acute liver failure–a controlled clinical trial. J Hepatol. 2004;41:89–96.

47. Kodakar SK, Gopal PB, Wendon JA. Intracranial pressure is related to body temperature in acute liver failure. Liver Transpl. 2001;7:C87.

48. Bernal W, Murphy N, Brown S, Whitehouse T, Bjerring PN, Hauerberg J, et al. A multicentre randomized controlled trial of moderate hypothermia to prevent intracranial hypertension in acute liver failure. J Hepatol. 2016;65:273–9.

49. Helbok R, Olson DM, Le Roux PD, Vespa P, Participants in the International Multidisciplinary Consensus Conference on Multimodality Monitoring. Intracranial pressure and cerebral perfusion pressure monitoring in non-TBI patients: special considerations. Neurocrit Care. 2014;21:S85–94.

50. Munoz SJ. Difficult management problems in fulminant hepatic failure. Semin Liver Dis. 1993;13:395–413.

51. Strauss GI. The effect of hyperventilation upon cerebral blood flow and metabolism in patients with fulminant hepatic failure. Dan Med Bull. 2007;54:99–111.

52. Curley G, Kavanagh BP, Laffey JG. Hypocapnia and the injured brain: more harm than benefit. Crit Care Med. 2010;38:1348–59.

53. Vaquero J, Rose C, Butterworth RF. Keeping cool in acute liver failure: rationale for the use of mild hypothermia. J Hepatol. 2005;43:1067–77.

54. Jalan R, Olde Damink SW, Deutz NE, Hayes PC, Lee A. Moderate hypothermia in patients with acute liver failure and uncontrolled intracranial hypertension. Gastroenterology. 2004;127:1338–46.

55. Karvellas CJ, Todd Stravitz R, Battenhouse H, Lee WM, Schilsky ML, US Acute Liver Failure Study Group. Therapeutic hypothermia in acute liver failure: a multicenter retrospective cohort analysis. Liver Transpl. 2015;21:4–12.

56. Schubert A. Side effects of mild hypothermia. J Neurosurg Anesthesiol. 1995;7:139–47.

57. Munoz SJ. Hypothermia may impair hepatic regeneration in acute liver failure. Gastroenterology. 2005;128:1143–4.

58. Nielsen N, Wetterslev J, Cronberg T, Erlinge D, Gasche Y, Hassager C, et al. Targeted temperature management at 33 degrees C vs. 36 degrees C after cardiac arrest. N Engl J Med. 2013;369:2197–206.

59. Tofteng F, Larsen FS. The effect of indomethacin on intracranial pressure, cerebral perfusion and extracellular lactate and glutamate concentrations in patients with fulminant hepatic failure. J Cereb Blood Flow Metab. 2004;24:798–804.

60. Rakela J, Mosley JW, Edwards VM, Govindarajan S, Alpert E. A double- blind randomized trial of hydrocortisone in acute hepatic failure. Dig Dis Sci. 1991;36:1223–8.

61. Forbes A, Alexander GJ, O'Grady JG, et al. Thiopental infusion in the treatment of intracranial hypertension complicating fulminant hepatic failure. Hepatology. 1989;10:306–10.

62. Siniscalchi A, Dante A, Spedicato S, Riganello L, Zanoni A, Cimatti M, et al. Hyperdynamic circulation in acute liver failure: reperfusion syndrome and outcome following liver transplantation. Transplant Proc. 2010;42:1197–9. https://doi.org/10.1016/j.transproceed.2010.03.097.

63. Jaber S, Paugam-Burtz C. Acute liver failure and elevated troponin-I: controversial results and significance? Crit Care. 2013;17:102.

64. Parekh NK, Hynan LS, De Lemos J, et al. Elevated troponin I levels in acute liver failure: is myocardial injury an integral part of acute liver failure? Hepatology. 2007;45:1489–95.

65. Møller S, Bernardi M. Interactions of the heart and the liver. Eur Heart J. 2013;34:2804–11.

66. Olson JC, Wendon JA, Kramer DJ, et al. Intensive care of the patient with cirrhosis. Hepatology. 2011;54:1864–72.

67. Legrand M, Dupuis C, Simon C, Gayat E, Mateo J, Lukaszewicz AC, et al. Association between systemic hemodynamics and septic acute kidney injury in critically ill patients: a retrospective observational study. Crit Care. 2013;17:R278.

68. Mitchell KH, Carlbom D, Caldwell E, Leary PJ, Himmelfarb J, Hough CL. Volume overload: prevalence, risk factors, and functional outcome in survivors of septic shock. Ann Am Thorac Soc. 2015;12:1837–44.

69. Chen H, Wu B, Gong D, Liu Z. Fluid overload at start of continuous renal replacement therapy is associated with poorer clinical condition and outcome: a prospective observational study on the combined use of bioimpedance vector analysis and serum N-terminal pro-B-type natriuretic peptide measurement. Crit Care. 2015;19:135.

70. Young P, Bailey M, Beasley R, Henderson S, Mackle D, McArthur C, et al. Effect of a buffered crystalloid solution vs. saline on acute kidney injury among patients in the intensive care unit: the SPLIT randomized clinical trial. JAMA. 2015;314:1701–10.

71. Yunos NM, Bellomo R, Glassford N, Sutcliffe H, Lam Q, Bailey M. Chloride liberal vs. chloride-restrictive intravenous fluid administration and acute kidney injury: an extended analysis. Intensive Care Med. 2015;41:257–64.

72. Finfer S, Myburgh J, Bellomo R. Albumin supplementation and organ function. Crit Care Med. 2007;35:987–8.

73. Finfer S, Bellomo R, Boyce N, French J, Myburgh J, Norton R, et al. A comparison of albumin and saline for fluid resuscitation in the intensive care unit. N Engl J Med. 2004;350:2247–56.

74. Caironi P, Tognoni G, Masson S, Fumagalli R, Pesenti A, Romero M, et al. Albumin replacement in patients with severe sepsis or septic shock. N Engl J Med. 2014;370:1412–21.

75. Lee WM, Stravitz RT, Larson AM. Introduction to the revised American Association for the Study of Liver Diseases Position Paper on acute liver failure 2011. Hepatology. 2012;55:965–7. https://doi.org/10.1002/hep.25551.

76. Chung C, Vaquero J, Gottstein J, et al. Vasopressin accelerates experimental ammonia-induced brain edema in rats after portacaval anastomosis. J Hepatol. 2003;39:193–9.

77. Eefsen M, Dethloff T, Frederiksen HJ, et al. Comparison of terlipressin and noradrenalin on cerebral perfusion, intracranial pressure and cerebral extracellular concentrations of lactate and pyruvate in patients with acute liver failure in need of inotropic support. J Hepatol. 2007;47:381–6.

78. Auzinger G, Willars C, Loveridge R, Best T, Vercueil A, Prachalias A, et al. Extracorporeal membrane oxygenation for refractory hypoxemia after liver transplantation in severe hepatopulmonary syndrome: a solution with pitfalls. Liver Transpl. 2014;20:1141–4.

79. Harry R, Auzinger G, Wendon J. The clinical importance of adrenal insufficiency in acute hepatic dysfunction. Hepatology. 2002;36:395–402.

80. Annane D, Bellissant E, Sebille V, et al. Impaired pressor sensitivity to noradrenaline in septic shock patients with and without impaired adrenal function reserve. Br J Clin Pharmacol. 1998;46:589–97.

81. Wang DW, Yin YM, Yao YM. Advances in the management of acute liver failure. World J Gastroenterol. 2013;19:7069–77.

82. Murphy ND, Kodakat SK, Wendon JA, et al. Liver and intestinal lactate metabolism in patients with acute hepatic failure undergoing liver transplantation. Crit Care Med. 2001;29:2111–8.

83. Nagayama M, Okuno M, Takai T, et al. Effect of fat emulsion in patients with liver disorders. Nutrition. 1991;7:267–70.

84. Montejo González JC, Mesejo A, Bonet Saris A. Guidelines for specialized nutritional and metabolic support in the critically-ill patient: update. Consensus SEMICYUCSENPE: liver failure and liver transplantation. Nutr Hosp. 2011;26(Suppl 2):27–31. https://doi.org/10.1590/S0212-16112011000800006.

85. Baudouin SV, Howdle P, O'Grady JG, et al. Acute lung injury in fulminant hepatic failure following paracetamol poisoning. Thorax. 1995;50:399–402.

86. Trewby PN, Warren R, Contini S, et al. Incidence and pathophysiology of pulmonary edema in fulminant hepatic failure. Gastroenterology. 1978;74(5 Pt 1):859–65.

87. Audimoolam VK, McPhail MJ, Wendon JA, et al. Lung injury and its prognostic significance in acute liver failure. Crit Care Med. 2014;42:592–600.

88. Malhotra A. Low-tidal-volume ventilation in the acute respiratory distress syndrome. N Engl J Med. 2007;357:1113–20.

89. Audimoolam VK, McPhail MJ, Wendon JA, Willars C, Bernal W, Desai SR, et al. Lung injury and its prognostic significance in acute liver failure. Crit Care Med. 2014;42:592–600.

90. Gattinoni L, Pesenti A, Carlesso E. Body position changes redistribute lung computed-tomographic density in patients with acute respiratory failure: impact and clinical fallout through the following 20 years. Intensive Care Med. 2013;39:1909–15.

91. Fuhrmann V, Madl C, Mueller C, Holzinger U, Kitzberger R, Funk GC, et al. Hepatopulmonary syndrome in patients with hypoxic hepatitis. Gastroenterology. 2006;131:69–75.

92. Gudavalli A, Kalaria VG, Chen X, Schwarz KQ. Intrapulmonary arteriovenous shunt: diagnosis by saline contrast bubbles in the pulmonary veins. J Am Soc Echocardiogr. 2002;15:1012e4.

93. Devauchelle P, Page M, Brun P, Ber CE, Crozon J, Baillon JJ, Allaouchiche B, Rimmelé T. Continuous haemodialysis with citrate anticoagulation in patients with liver failure: three cases. Ann Fr Anesth Reanim. 2012;31:543–6. https://doi.org/10.1016/j.annfar.2012.01.036.

94. O'Riordan A, Brummell Z, Sizer E, Auzinger G, Heaton N, O'Grady JG, et al. Acute kidney injury in patients admitted to a liver intensive therapy unit with paracetamol-induced hepatotoxicity. Nephrol Dial Transplant. 2011;26:3501–8.

95. Tujios SR, Hynan LS, Vazquez MA, Larson AM, Seremba E, Sanders CM, et al. Risk factors and outcomes of acute kidney injury in patients with acute liver failure. Clin Gastroenterol Hepatol. 2015;13:352–9.

96. Leithead JA, Ferguson JW, Bates CM, et al. The systemic inflammatory response syndrome is predictive of renal dysfunction in patients with non paracetamol- induced acute liver failure. Gut. 2009;58:443–9.

97. Moore K. Renal failure in acute liver failure. Eur J Gastroenterol Hepatol. 1999;11:967–75.

98. Davenport A. Management of acute kidney injury in liver disease. Contrib Nephrol. 2010;165:197–205.

99. Munoz SJ. The hepatorenal syndrome. Med Clin North Am. 2008;92:813–37, viii–ix. https://doi.org/10.1016/j.mcna.2008.03.007.

100. O'Brien Z, Cass A, Cole L, et al. RENAL Study Investigators and the Australian and New Zealand Intensive Care Clinical Trials Group. Higher versus lower continuous renal replacement therapy intensity in critically ill patients with liver dysfunction. Blood Purif. 2018;45(1–3):36–43.

101. Leventhal TM, Liu KD. What a nephrologist needs to know about acute liver failure. Adv Chronic Kidney Dis. 2015;22(05):376–81.

102. Schultheiss C, Saugel B, Phillip V, Thies P, Noe S, Mayr U, et al. Continuous venovenous hemodialysis with regional citrate anticoagulation in patients with liver failure: a prospective observational study. Crit Care. 2012;16:R162.

103. Slowinski T, Morgera S, Joannidis M, Henneberg T, Stocker R, Helset E, et al. Safety and efficacy of regional citrate anticoagulation in continuous venovenous hemodialysis in the presence of liver failure: the Liver Citrate Anticoagulation Threshold (L-CAT) observational study. Crit Care. 2015;19:349.

104. Patel S, Wendon J. Regional citrate anticoagulation in patients with liver failure time for a rethink? Crit Care. 2012;16:153.

105. Moore JK, Love E, Craig DG, Hayes PC, Simpson KJ. Acute kidney injury in acute liver failure: a review. Expert Rev Gastroenterol Hepatol. 2013;7:701–12.

106. Stravitz RT, Ellerbe C, Durkalski V, et al. Thrombocytopenia is associated with multiorgan system failure in patients with acute liver failure. Clin Gastroenterol Hepatol. 2016;14(4):613–620.e4.

107. Munoz SJ, Stravitz RT, Gabriel DA. Coagulopathy of acute liver failure. Clin Liver Dis. 2009;13:95–107.

108. Hugenholtz GC, Adelmeijer J, Meijers JC, Porte RJ, Stravitz RT, Lisman T. An unbalance between von Willebrand factor and ADAMTS13 in acute liver failure: implications for hemostasis and clinical outcome. Hepatology. 2013;58:752–61.

109. Lisman T, Bakhtiari K, Adelmeijer J, Meijers JC, Porte RJ, Stravitz RT. Intact thrombin generation and decreased fibrinolytic capacity in patients with acute liver injury or acute liver failure. J Thromb Haemost. 2012;10:1312–9.

110. Stravitz RT, Lisman T, Luketic VA, Sterling RK, Puri P, Fuchs M, et al. Minimal effects of acute liver injury/acute liver failure on hemostasis as assessed by thromboelastography. J Hepatol. 2012;56:129–36.

111. Agarwal B, Gatt A, Riddell A, Wright G, Chowdary P, Jalan R, et al. Hemostasis in patients with acute

kidney injury secondary to acute liver failure. Kidney Int. 2013;84:158–63.

112. Stravitz RT, Bowling R, Bradford RL, Key NS, Glover S, Thacker LR, et al. Role of procoagulant microparticles in mediating complications and outcome of acute liver injury/acute liver failure. Hepatology. 2013;58:304–13.

113. Lisman T, Leebeek FW, de Groot PG. Haemostatic abnormalities in patients with liver disease. J Hepatol. 2002;37:280–7.

114. Kerr R, Newsome P, Germain L, et al. Effects of acute liver injury on blood coagulation. J Thromb Haemost. 2003;1:754–9.

115. Lisman T, Porte RJ. Rebalanced hemostasis in patients with liver disease: evidence and clinical consequences. Blood. 2010;116:878–85.

116. Habib M, Roberts LN, Patel RK, Wendon J, Bernal W, Arya R. Evidence of rebalanced coagulation in acute liver injury and acute liver failure as measured by thrombin generation. Liver Int. 2014;34:672–8.

117. Munoz SJ, Rajender Reddy K, Lee W, Acute Liver Failure Study Group. The coagulopathy of acute liver failure and implications for intracranial pressure monitoring. Neurocrit Care. 2008;9:103–7.

118. Kozek-Langenecker SA, Afshari A, Albaladejo P, Santullano CA, De Robertis E, Filipescu DC, et al. Management of severe perioperative bleeding: guidelines from the European Society of Anaesthesiology. Eur J Anaesthesiol. 2013;30:270–382.

119. Lelubre C, Vincent JL, Taccone FS. Red blood cell transfusion strategies in critically ill patients: lessons from recent randomized clinical studies. Minerva Anestesiol. 2016;82:1010–1.

120. Antoniades CG, Berry PA, Wendon JA, Vergani D. The importance of immune dysfunction in determining outcome in acute liver failure. J Hepatol. 2008;49:845–61.

121. Antoine DJ, Jenkins RE, Dear JW, Williams DP, McGill MR, Sharpe MR, et al. Molecular forms of HMGB1 and keratin-18 as mechanistic biomarkers for mode of cell death and prognosis during clinical acetaminophen hepatotoxicity. J Hepatol. 2012;56:1070–9.

122. Possamai LA, Antoniades CG, Anstee QM, Quaglia A, Vergani D, Thursz M, et al. Role of monocytes and macrophages in experimental and human acute liver failure. World J Gastroenterol. 2010;16:1811–9.

123. Bernal W, Wendon J. Acute liver failure. Curr Opin Anaesthesiol. 2000;13:113–8.

124. Karvellas CJ, Pink F, McPhail M, Cross T, Auzinger G, Bernal W, et al. Predictors of bacteraemia and mortality in patients with acute liver failure. Intensive Care Med. 2009;35:1390–6.

125. Vaquero J, Polson J, Chung C, Helenowski I, Schiodt FV, Reisch J, et al. Infection and the progression of hepatic encephalopathy in acute liver failure. Gastroenterology. 2003;125:755–64.

126. Rolando N, Philpott-Howard J, Williams R. Bacterial and fungal infection in acute liver failure. Semin Liver Dis. 1996;16:389–402.

127. Rolando N, Harvey F, Brahm J, Philpott-Howard J, Alexander G, Casewell M, et al. Fungal infection: a common, unrecognised complication of acute liver failure. J Hepatol. 1991;12:1–9.

128. Lopez Roa P, Hill JA, Kirby KA, Leisenring WM, Huang ML, Santo TK, et al. Coreactivation of human herpesvirus 6 and cytomegalovirus is associated with worse clinical outcome in critically ill adults. Crit Care Med. 2015;43:1415–22.

129. Silvestre JP, Coelho LM, Povoa PM. Impact of fulminant hepatic failure in creactive protein? J Crit Care. 2010;25:e7–e12.

130. Rule JA, Hynan LS, Attar N, Sanders C, Korzun WJ, Lee WM, et al. Procalcitonin identifies cell injury, not bacterial infection, in acute liver failure. PLoS One. 2015;10:e0138566.

131. Farmakiotis D, Kontoyiannis DP. Emerging issues with diagnosis and management of fungal infections in solid organ transplant recipients. Am J Transplant. 2015;15:1141–7.

132. Bernal W, Auzinger G, Dhawan A, Wendon J. Acute liver failure. Lancet. 2010;376:190–201.

133. Karvellas CJ, Cavazos J, Battenhouse H, Durkalski V, Balko J, Sanders C, et al. Effects of antimicrobial prophylaxis and blood stream infections in patients with acute liver failure: a retrospective cohort study. Clin Gastroenterol Hepatolol. 2014;12:1942–11949.

134. Rolando N, Gimson A, Wade J, Philpott-Howard J, Casewell M, Williams R. Prospective controlled trial of selective parenteral and enteral antimicrobial regimen in fulminant liver failure. Hepatology. 1993;17:196–201.

135. Fontana RJ, Ellerbe C, Durkalski VE, et al. Two-year outcomes in initial survivors with acute liver failure: results from a prospective, multicentre study. Liver Int. 2015;35(2):370–80.

136. McPhail MJ, Farne H, Senvar N, Wendon JA, Bernal W. Ability of King's College Criteria and model for end-stage liver disease scores to predict mortality of patients with acute liver failure: a meta-analysis. Clin Gastroenterol Hepatol. 2016;14(4):516–525.e5.

137. Bernal W, Donaldson N, Wyncoll D, et al. Blood lactate as an early predictor of outcome in paracetamol-induced acute liver failure: a cohort study. Lancet. 2002;359(9306):558–63.

138. Herrine SK, Moayyedi P, Brown RS Jr, et al. American Gastroenterological Association Institute technical review on initial testing and management of acute liver disease. Gastroenterology. 2017;152(3):648–64.e5.

139. Flamm SL, Yang YX, Singh S, et al. American Gastroenterological Association Institute guidelines for the diagnosis and management of acute liver failure. Gastroenterology. 2017;152(3):644–7.

140. Koch DG, Tillman H, Durkalski V, Lee WM, Reuben A. Development of a model to predict transplant-free survival of patients with acute liver failure. Clin Gastroenterol Hepatol. 2016;14(8):1199–1206.e2.

141. Stravitz RT, Ellerbe C, Durkalski V, et al. Thrombocytopenia is associated with multi-organ system failure in patients with acute liver failure. Clin Gastroenterol Hepatol. 2016;14(4):613–20.

142. Shakil AO, Jones BC, Lee RG, Federle MP, Fung JJ, Rakela J. Prognostic value of abdominal CT scanning and hepatic histopathology in patients with acute liver failure. Dig Dis Sci. 2000;45(2):334–9.

143. Schmidt LE, Dalhoff K. Alpha-fetoprotein is a predictor of outcome in acetaminophen-induced liver injury. Hepatology. 2005;41(1):26–31.

144. Rosen HR, Biggins SW, Niki T, et al. Association between plasma level of Galectin-9 and survival of patients with drug-induced acute liver failure. Clin Gastroenterol Hepatol. 2016;14(4):606–12.e3.

145. Moller HJ, Gronbaek H, Schiodt FV, et al. Soluble CD163 from activated macrophages predicts mortality in acute liver failure. J Hepatol. 2007;47(5):671–6.

146. Karvellas CJ, Speiser JL, Tremblay M, Lee WM, Rose CF, US Acute Liver Failure Study Group. Elevated FABP1 serum levels are associated with poorer survival in acetaminophen-induced acute liver failure. Hepatology. 2017;65(3):938–49.

147. Ichai P, Samuel D. Etiology and prognosis of fulminant hepatitis in adults. Liver Transpl. 2008;14(Suppl 2):S67–79.

148. Puri P, Anand AC. Liver support devices. Medicine update; 2012. p. 489–3.

149. Mochida S, Takikawa Y, Nakayama N, Oketani M, Naiki T, Yamagishi Y, et al. Diagnostic criteria of acute liver failure: a report by the Intractable Hepato-Biliary Diseases Study Group of Japan. Hepatol Res. 2011;41:805–12. https://doi.org/10.1111/j.1872-034X.2011.00860.x.

Assessment for Transplanting Acute Liver Failure Patient

31

Ameya Panchwagh

Abbreviations

AKI	Acute kidney injury
ALF	Acute liver failure
APACHE II	Acute Physiology and Chronic Health Evaluation II
ARDS	Acute respiratory distress syndrome
CBG	Cortisol binding globulin
CPP	Cerebral perfusion pressure
CRRT	Continuous renal replacement therapy
CT	Computed tomography
EASL	European Association for the Study of the Liver
EVLW	Extravascular lung water
FC	Free cortisol
FiO_2	Fraction of inspired oxygen
HE	Hepatic encephalopathy
HPS	Hepatopulmonary syndrome
ICH	Intracranial hypertension
ICP	Intracranial pressure
INR	International normalized ratio
KCC	King's College criteria
LT	Liver transplantation
MELD	Model for end-stage liver disease
$PaO2$	Partial pressure of oxygen in arterial blood
PEEP	Positive end-expiratory pressure
PT	Prothrombin time
SIRS	Systemic inflammatory response syndrome
SOFA	Sequential organ failure assessment
TC	Total cortisol

A. Panchwagh (✉)
Liver Transplant and HPB Anaesthesia, Sir H. N.
Reliance Foundation Hospital and Research Centre,
Mumbai, India
e-mail: dr.ameya88@gmail.com

31.1 Introduction

Acute liver failure (ALF) is a life threatening illness defined as 'evidence of coagulation abnormality, usually an international normalized ratio above 1.5, and any degree of mental alteration (encephalopathy) in a patient without pre-existing liver disease and with an illness of less than 26 weeks duration' [1]. It is often a syndrome comprising of multi-organ dysfunction with a wide range of aetiologies and accounts for 8% of indications for liver transplantation in Europe and 7% in the USA [2, 3]. Advances in the field of Intensive care and liver transplantation have significantly improved the survival of patients with ALF [4, 5]. Nevertheless, close, careful, and continual assessment of these patients prior to transplant by a multidisciplinary team is extremely important to ensure good outcomes. In this chapter we discuss the assessment of ALF patients prior to transplantation in this challenging clinical scenario.

31.2 Assessing Patients with ALF for Liver Transplantation

Whilst assessing a patient of ALF for transplantation, in addition to the battery of tests to search for an etiologic diagnosis, the following issues need careful consideration.

31.2.1 Assessing the Need for Transplant

When assessing the need for transplant, it is important to identify patients who are likely to die without liver transplantation (LT). Various prognostic models are used worldwide with variable accuracies and limitations.

The King's College Criteria (KCC) [6] (Table 31.1), described in 1989, continue to be widely used and have a high degree of specificity but low sensitivity and negative predictive value. Few meta-analyses have reported overall specificity of 82% for non-paracetamol aetiologies and 92–95% for paracetamol-related ALF with a sensitivity of 68% [7–9]. Thus, the use of KCC in ALF patients predicts patients in need of LT with good accuracy. However, it will select some patients who would otherwise have survived without LT. Also, it does not guarantee survival for patients not meeting criteria. Dynamic application of criteria leads to an increase in both, sensitivity and specificity [7]. To improve the predictive value of the KCC, the measurement of lactate as an indicator of tissue dysfunction has been added to the criteria in the UK. An arterial lactate >3.0–3.5 mmol/L after fluid resuscitation is a marker of poor prognosis [10].

The Clichy criteria were described in 1986, from the study of a cohort of patients with fulminant hepatitis B [11] (Table 31.1), which makes use of factor V level as a guide to selection as liver transplant candidate. Studies have shown that Clichy criteria are less accurate than originally reported. Validation studies found less accuracy than for the KCC, with a positive predictive value of 89%, but a negative predictive value of 36% [12].

Table 31.1 King's College and Clichy criteria

King's College criteria [6]	
Paracetamol-related ALF	Non-paracetamol-related ALF
pH < 7.3 (irrespective of grade of encephalopathy)	PT > 100 s (INR > 6.5) (irrespective of grade of encephalopathy)
Or all three of the following • Grade III–IV encephalopathy • PT > 100 s (INR > 6.5) • Serum creatinine >300 μmol/L (3.4 mg/dL)	Or any three of the following • Age <10 or >40 years • Aetiology: (non-A, non-B hepatitis, halothane, idiosyncratic drug reaction, Wilson disease) • Period of jaundice to encephalopathy >7 days • PT > 50 s (INR > 3.5) • Serum bilirubin >300 μmol/L (17.5 mg/dL)
Clichy criteria [11]	
Presence of hepatic encephalopathy and Factor V level of <20% (if patient's age <30 years) OR <30% (if patient's age >30 years)	

In search of better alternatives to KCC and Clichy criteria various other scores have been evaluated.

With the rationale that patients with ALF have a severe inflammatory response, various non-liver specific scores such as Sequential Organ Failure Assessment (SOFA), and the Acute Physiology and Chronic Health Evaluation II (APACHE II) have also been evaluated. Some studies have focused on the use of model for end-stage liver disease (MELD) score to predict outcomes in ALF patients. However, advantage using MELD has not been conclusively demonstrated [13]. In a study comparing KCC, APACHE II, SOFA, and MELD to predict outcome in patients with ALF, KCC had the most specificity (83%) but lowest sensitivity (47%) and MELD had the highest sensitivity (89%) but the lowest specificity (25%). Compared to the other three scoring systems, the SOFA had the highest discriminative ability [14]. In another study APACHE II score was shown to have similar sensitivity and specificity as KCC [15]. The Acute Liver Failure Study Group index, based on International normalized ratio (INR), Coma grade, Bilirubin, Phosphorus level and an apoptotic marker M30 outperformed MELD and KCC, with a sensitivity of 86% and specificity of 65% [16]. A wide variety of blood markers have been proposed including: Gc-globulin levels, α-fetoprotein, serum phosphate, apoptosis, and necrosis markers and monocyte HLA-DR expression. However, due to lack of validation and easy availability their application in the prognostication of ALF patients is limited at present.

By far, the KCC and Clichy criteria are most widely used. Transplantation should be considered in those patients fulfilling Clichy or Kings College criteria (evidence level II-2, grade of recommendation 1) according to EASL Clinical Practical Guidelines on the management of acute liver failure [17]. It is important that these criteria be applied dynamically whilst assessing the patient for LT.

In paediatric population, criteria for LT are different from those in adults. INR is considered the best predictor of survival. An INR >4 and total bilirubin >17.6 mg/dl irrespective of Hepatic encephalopathy is the currently accepted criteria for LT in children [18, 19]. Special mention needs to be made about patients with Fulminant Wilson's disease who have high mortality without LT. The King's Wilson index which incorporates bilirubin, INR, AST, white blood cell count, and albumin at presentation is useful in identifying patients with high risk of mortality. A score of 11 or more indicates high mortality, with 93% sensitivity and 98% specificity with a positive predictive value of 93% [20].

31.2.2 Assessing Various Organ Systems

Acute liver failure is frequently associated with multi-organ failure. Assessing various organ systems of the ALF patient prior to transplantation is of paramount importance for knowing the severity of illness, preoperative optimization, to anticipate possible problems as well as to know the preparation required in the operating room during the transplant.

31.2.2.1 Central Nervous System

Hepatic encephalopathy (HE) is the hallmark of ALF in adult patients. Its aetiology is multifactorial. However, principal mechanism involves accumulation of ammonia due to liver failure which crosses the blood-brain barrier eventually causing cerebral oedema and intracranial hypertension (ICH). Traditionally, raised intracranial pressure was a major cause of mortality in these patients. With advances in critical care the mortality is reducing. Assessing the central nervous system is important to know the degree of affection as well as to institute therapies to prevent rises in intracranial pressure (ICP) and brain death.

Classically, HE has been graded using the West Haven criteria [21]. Table 31.2 which classifies patients into four grades (Grade I–IV). Patients with >grade II HE require endotracheal intubation for protection of the airway from aspiration. Worsening HE heralds a poor prognosis. Grade IV HE precedes the development of cerebral oedema, consequent ICH, and transtentorial herniation. In patients with higher grades of HE, the Glasgow Coma Scale is a validated and useful tool for assessment [22].

Assessing pupillary function is important in grade III–IV HE. Pupillary light reaction usually progresses from normal to hyper-responsive in early in grade II–III HE and hypo-responsive in grade IV [23]. Loss of pupillary function and fixed dilated pupils may signify brain herniation. Unequal pupils may point towards a possible intracranial bleed. With the availability of automated pupillometers assessing pupillary reflexes has become less operator dependent and more reproducible. A quick look at the vital parameters may show a bradycardic and hypertensive response (Cushing's response) in patients with

Table 31.2 Grade of encephalopathy

Grade	Signs and symptoms
I	Mild confusion, sleep disturbance
II	Moderate confusion, lethargy
III	Marked confusion, incoherent speech
IV	Unresponsive

ICH. Reversal of brain herniation using osmotherapy is possible if detected early.

Development of ICH in ALF is multifactorial. As ammonia plays a central role in the pathogenesis of cerebral dysfunction and ICH in ALF, it is prudent to assess arterial ammonia levels. Levels more than 150–200 μmol/L are associated with the development of ICH in ALF. Continuous renal replacement therapy (CRRT) should be initiated once the arterial ammonia level is >150 μmol/L and should be continued with the aim of keeping ammonia levels <100 μmol/L [24]. For patients already on CRRT, periodic assessment of ammonia levels helps in knowing the adequacy of CRRT as well as indicates the risk of ICH in patients with persistently elevated levels. From the standpoint of intraoperative continuation, assessment of the mode and settings of CRRT in use is helpful.

Assessing the degree of ICH is necessary to institute corrective measures, to know their adequacy as well as to set about hemodynamic goals to maintain optimum cerebral perfusion pressure (CPP). Rarely, patients may have an ICP bolt in place. More commonly surrogate markers of ICP such as Jugular bulb oximetry, transcranial doppler, near infrared spectroscopy, optic nerve sheath diameter are assessed to know the status of ICP and cerebrovascular haemodynamics as per availability and expertise. It is equally important to assess the various neuroprotective measures instituted for the patient for providing continuity of care whilst undergoing LT.

Lastly, in patients with ICH, computed tomography (CT) of the head can give useful information about cerebral oedema, intracranial bleed or transtentorial herniation whenever suspected. In the author's institute, it is a routine practice to get at CT scan of the head done en-route transfer to the operating room if not done prior, to rule out any contraindication to LT.

31.2.2.2 Cardiovascular System

Cardiac dysfunction in the form of arrythmias is relatively common in ALF patients. This may be attributed to therapeutic hypothermia or electrolyte imbalance in this patient population. A baseline check by an electrocardiogram and checking for electrolyte abnormalities may help diagnose and treat these issues.

Cardiac dysfunction in the form of reduced contractility is relatively uncommon, though some diseases with multisystemic involvement such as viral illnesses, phosphorous poisoning, Wilson's disease may present with such issues. It is useful to perform an echocardiograph to rule out such cardiac dysfunction.

Circulatory failure is common in patients with ALF, mostly attributable to the 'toxic liver syndrome' and the ensuing massive systemic inflammatory response syndrome (SIRS). Assessing parameters on advanced hemodynamic parameters is essential. ALF patients usually have a low mean arterial pressure, high cardiac output, normal or reduced cardiac contractility, and a low systemic vascular resistance. Assessment of the dose of various vasopressors is of paramount importance.

Around 60% patients with ALF have a relative adrenal insufficiency [25]. Measured total cortisol levels do not truly reflect the status of free cortisol levels due to low levels of cortisol binding globulin. Assessment of free cortisol levels can be made by measuring the total cortisol (TC) and cortisol binding globulin (CBG) levels and calculating the levels of free cortisol (FC) by the free cortisol index [26]:

$$\text{Free cortisol}\left(\text{mmol}/\text{L}\right) = \left(0.0167 + 0.182\left(CBG - TC\right)\right)[2] + \left(0.0122 \times TC\right)0.5$$
$$- \left(0.0167 + 0.182\left(CBG - TC\right)\right)$$

However, corticosteroid therapy is often started empirically on requirement of escalating doses of vasopressors.

31.2.2.3 Respiratory System

Patients with ALF are usually intubated and ventilated in view of airway protection.

Approximately 30% patients with paracetamol poisoning develop acute lung injury and acute respiratory distress syndrome (ARDS) [27]. ARDS develops secondary to increased permeability due to massive SIRS and release of inflammatory mediators which may be exacerbated by massive fluid transfusion during the resuscitation phase. In about half of these patient's tracheal aspirates are positive for gram-negative organisms [28] which puts them at risk of ventilator associated pneumonias. Hepatopulmonary syndrome (HPS) is also known to occur in ALF. A combination of all these factors may cause hypoxemia in these patients.

Assessment involves checking arterial blood gases and a chest X-ray. CT scan of the chest may be helpful in discerning fluid from consolidation, when in doubt. A bubble echocardiograph may be helpful in making the diagnosis of HPS. Patients with ARDS are usually on lung protective ventilation strategies. Assessment of the ventilator settings, oxygen requirement and degree of hypoxemia gives an insight about the degree of respiratory dysfunction. A look at the PaO_2/FiO_2 may throw light on the severity of Acute lung injury or ARDS. Extravascular lung water (EVLW) is now possible on newer advanced hemodynamic monitors, which may be helpful as well, in assessing the severity of ARDS.

31.2.2.4 Renal System and Acid-Base, Fluid, Electrolyte Balance

Acute kidney injury (AKI) is common in patients with ALF with an incidence of 40–85% [29]. Aetiology is multifactorial. Assessing serum creatinine and urine output may give an idea of the degree of renal dysfunction. More often, these patients require CRRT for renal and non-renal indications. It is important to assess CRRT flow rates, dialysate composition, anticoagulation in use, overall fluid balance, and electrolyte imbalances (notably hypokalaemia, hypomagnesemia, hypophosphatemia, serum sodium levels) for requirement of corrective measures.

31.2.2.5 Coagulation System

Assessment of traditional parameters of coagulation such as prothrombin time (PT) and INR is essential from a prognostic standpoint. However, it is now an established fact that coagulation status of these patients is rebalanced and hence assessing coagulation status by using viscoelastic tests (Thromboelastography, Rotational Thromboelastometry) is the norm.

31.2.2.6 Other Considerations

Increasing requirement of glucose to maintain normoglycemia and upward trending lactates usually point towards worsening liver function.

In addition, it would be useful to make a note of presence of various invasive lines and suitable sites for vascular access for use, if deemed necessary in the operating room.

Note should also be made the sedation/paralysis protocol in use and doses of all other medications in use. A review of antibiotics in use and recent culture reports is essential to formulate further plan of action.

In all the evaluation process, it is needless to say that a multidisciplinary team plays a special role. Also important is to evaluate the patient dynamically and to go by trends of various parameters rather than absolute numbers at a given point in time.

31.2.3 Assessment for Presence of Contraindications to LT

At times patients with ALF are deemed 'too sick to transplant'. Assessment should focus on actively looking for possible contraindications to LT as follows:

(a) Irreversible brain injury: Fixed dilated pupils for >2 h; CT showing of transtentorial herniation, loss of middle cerebral artery flow [17], two consecutive electroencephalograms showing absence of cerebral activity [30] may indicate irreversible brain injury which is an absolute contraindication for LT.

(b) Severe cardiopulmonary dysfunction: Low cardiac contractility, right heart failure, severe pulmonary hypertension (mean pulmonary artery pressure >50 mmHg), circulatory instability despite high dose of vasopressors, uncontrolled ARDS requiring high PEEP (>10–15 cm H$_2$O) or high inspired concentrations of oxygen (FiO$_2$ >0.8), appearance of a pneumonic patch may preclude LT.

(c) Uncontrolled sepsis: Bacteremia occurs in about 20–30% patients with ALF. It is wise to delay transplant till about 24 h exposure to targeted antibiotics and there is appropriate response to treatment. Uncontrolled sepsis with increasing vasopressor support may be considered as a potential contraindication.

(d) Haemorrhagic pancreatitis

(e) Systemic diseases which are not an indication for LT [17]: Hypoxic hepatitis, Haemophagocytic lymphohistiocytosis, malaria, dengue, rickettsiosis, malignant infiltrations of liver or widespread mitochondrial failure following certain drug ingestions are not indications for LT. Management in these situations focuses on treating the cause.

31.3 Conclusion

It is akin to walking a tightrope whilst assessing ALF patients for transplantation who give only a small 'window of opportunity' before they become 'too sick' for transplant. Careful evaluation by a multidisciplinary team is essential for ensuring good outcomes.

Key Points

- ALF is a multisystemic disease, often causing multi-organ failure.
- KCC and Clichy are the most widely used criteria in making a decision to transplant in ALF.
- Irreversible brain injury is an absolute contraindication for liver transplant.
- Patients need to be assessed for severe cardiopulmonary dysfunction, uncontrolled sepsis and certain systemic diseases causing ALF which may preclude transplantation.

- The specialist anaesthesia team must thoroughly assess relevant organ systems to know the severity of affection, to guide for optimisation, to arrange for requisite personnel and equipment for the intra-operative period and to get a realistic idea about post-operative course and recovery.
- The need of a multidisciplinary team approach and dynamic assessment of these patients cannot be overemphasized.
- It is important to go by trends of various parameters rather than absolute numbers at a given point in time.

References

1. Lee WM, Larson AM, Stravitz RT. AASLD position paper: the management of acute liver failure: update. 2011.
2. Adam R, Karam V, Delvart V, O'Grady J, Mirza D, Klempnauer J, et al. Evolution of indications and results of liver transplantation in Europe. A report from the European Liver Transplant Registry (ELTR). J Hepatol. 2012;57:675–88.
3. 2009 Annual report of the US organ procurement transplant network and scientific registry of transplant recipient; transplant data 1999-2008.
4. Bernal W, Hyyrylainen A, Gera A, Audimoolam VK, McPhail MJ, Auzinger G, et al. Lessons from lookback in acute liver failure? A single centre experience of 3300 patients. J Hepatol. 2013;59:74–80.
5. Germani G, Theocharidou E, Adam R, Karam V, Wendon J, O'Grady J, et al. Liver transplantation for acute liver failure in Europe: outcomes over 20 years from the ELTR database. J Hepatol. 2012;57: 288–96.
6. O'Grady J, Alexander G, Hayllar K, Williams R. Early indicators of prognosis in fulminant hepatic failure. Gastroenterology. 1989;97:439–45.
7. McPhail MJW, Wendon JA, Bernal W. Meta-analysis of performance of King's College Hospital Criteria in prediction of outcome in non-paracetamol induced acute liver failure. J Hepatol. 2010;53:492–9.
8. Craig DGN, Ford AC, Hayes PC, Simpson KJ. Systematic review: prognostic tests of paracetamol-induced acute liver failure. Aliment Pharmacol Ther. 2010;31:1064–76.
9. Bailey B, Amre D, Gaudreault P. Fulminant hepatic failure secondary to acetaminophen poisoning: a systematic review of the meta-analysis of prognostic

criteria determining the need for liver transplantation. Crit Care Med. 2003;31:299–305.

10. Bernal W, Donaldson N, Wyncoll D, Wendon J. Blood lactate as an early predictor of outcome in paracetamol-induced acute liver failure: a cohort study. Lancet. 2002;359:558–63.

11. Bernau J, Godeau A, Poynard T, Dubois F, Lesage G, Yvonnet B, Degott C, et al. Multivariate analysis of prognostic factors in fulminant hepatitis B. Hepatology. 1986;6:648–51.

12. Pawles A, Mostefa-Kara N, Florent C, Levy VG. Emergency liver transplantation for acute liver failure: evaluation of London and Clichy criteria. J Hepatol. 1993;17:124–7.

13. Mendizabal M, Marciano S, Videla MG, Anders M, Zerega A, Balderramo DC, et al. Changing etiologies and outcomes of acute liver failure: perspectives from 6 transplant centers in Argentina. Liver Transpl. 2014;20:483–9.

14. Chologitas E, Theochardiou E, Vasianopoulou, et al. Comparison of the sequential organ failure assessment score with the King's College Hospital criteria and the model for end-stage liver disease score for the prognosis of acetaminophen-induced acute liver failure. Liver Transpl. 2012;18(4):405–12.

15. Mitchell I, Bihari D, Chang R, Wendon J, Williams R. Earlier identification of patients at risk from acetaminophen-induced acute liver failure. Crit Care Med. 1998;26:279–84.

16. Rutherford A, King LY, Hynan LS, Vedvyas C, Lin W, Lee WM, Chung RT. Development of an accurate index for predicting outcomes of patients with acute liver failure. Gastroenterology. 2012;143:1237–43.

17. EASL. Clinical practical guidelines on the management of acute (fulminant) liver failure. J Hepatol. 2017;66:1047–81.

18. Dhawan A. Etiology and prognosis of acute liver failure in children. Liver Transpl. 2008;14:S80–4.

19. Sundaram V, Shneider BL, Dhawan A, Ng VL, Im K, Belle S, et al. King's College Hospital criteria for non-acetaminophen induced acute liver failure in an international cohort of children. J Pediatr. 2013;162:319–23.

20. Dhawan A, Taylor RM, Cheeseman P, De Silva P, Katsiyiannakis L, Mieli-Vergani G. Wilson's disease in children: 37-year experience and revised King's score for liver transplantation. Liver Transpl. 2005;11:441–8.

21. Ferenci P, Lockwood A, Mullen K, et al. Hepatic encephalopathy– definition, nomenclature, diagnosis, and quantification: final report of the working party at the 11th World Congresses of Gastroenterology, Vienna, 1998. Hepatology. 2002;35:716–21.

22. Bernal W, Wendon J. Acute liver failure. N Engl J Med. 2014;370(12):1170–1.

23. Yan S, Tu Z, Lu W, Zhang Q, He J, Li Z, Shao Y, Wang W, Zhang M, Zheng S. Clinical utility of an automated pupillometer for assessing and monitoring recipients of liver transplantation. Liver Transpl. 2009;15(12):1718–27.

24. Slack AJ, Auzinger G, Willars C, et al. Ammonia clearance with haemofiltration in adults with liver disease. Liver Int. 2014;34(1):42–8.

25. Harry R, Auzinger G, Wendon J. The clinical importance of adrenal insufficiency in acute hepatic dysfunction. Hepatology. 2002;36(2):395–402.

26. Coolens JL, Van Baelen H, Heyns W. Clinical use of unbound plasma cortisol as calculated from total cortisol and corticosteroid-binding globulin. J Steroid Biochem. 1987;26(2):197–202.

27. Baudouin SV, Howdle P, O'Grady JG, Webster NR. Acute lung injury in fulminant hepatic failure following paracetamol poisoning. Thorax. 1995;50(4):399–402.

28. Karvellas CJ, Pink F, McPhail M, et al. Predictors of bacteraemia and mortality in patients with acute liver failure. Intensive Care Med. 2009;35(8):1390–6.

29. Betrosian AP, Agarwal B, Douzinas EE. Acute renal dysfunction in liver diseases. World J Gastroenterol. 2007;13(42):5552–9.

30. Samuel D, Saliba F, Ichai P. Changing outcomes in acute liver failure: can we transplant only the ones who really need it? Liver Transpl. 2015;21:S36–8.

Bridging Therapies in Acute and Acute on Chronic Liver Failure

32

Swapnil Dhampalwar and Sanjiv Saigal

32.1 Introduction

Liver is a multifunctional organ that plays crucial role in digestive, immune, metabolic, synthetic and excretory, and functions of the body [1]. Although the liver's functional reserve and regenerative capacity are great, these could be hindered in the face of severe acute liver injury. Rationale of bridging therapies is to support these multiple functions for a transient period as shown in Fig. 32.1.

Liver failure can develop as acute liver failure (ALF) in the absence of pre-existing liver disease, ACLF of known or unknown underlying chronic liver disease, or a chronic decompensation of an end-stage liver disease. ACLF should be clinically distinguished from ALF and decompensated liver disease. AASLD defines ALF as "acute hepatic injury characterized by evidence of coagulopathy, usually INR ≥ 1.5, and any degree of encephalopathy in a patient without pre-existing cirrhosis and with an illness of <26

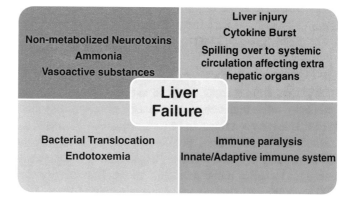

Fig. 32.1 Pleiotropic functions of liver and rationale of using bridging therapies in liver failure

S. Dhampalwar
Hepatology and Liver Transplantation, Medanta–The Medicity, Gurugram, India

S. Saigal (✉)
Hepatology and Liver Transplant, Centre for Liver and Biliary Sciences, Centre of Gastroenterology, Hepatology and Endoscopy, Max Super Speciality Hospital, Saket, New Delhi, India

weeks' duration" [2]. Acute-on-chronic liver failure (ACLF) may occur either in decompensated or in compensated cirrhosis after an acute insult and is associated with organ failures and high short-term (28-day) mortality. ACLF has been defined differently by different consortia.

32.2 Bridging Therapies

The aim of bridging therapies is to provide adequate liver function and maintain the patient well enough until recovery of native liver function occurs (bridge-to-recovery) or until a graft is found (bridge-to-transplant). Bridging therapies can be broadly classified into two categories: (1) artificial liver support system (ALSS); (2) experimental therapies like regenerative and cell-based therapies. The artificial liver support system (ALSS) includes: (a) therapeutic plasma exchange, (b) artificial liver support, and (c) bio-artificial liver support. The key concept is to remove harmful toxins, support the liver for spontaneous regeneration, and reduce the ongoing inflammatory injury.

32.3 Therapeutic Plasma Exchange (TPE)

The removal of patient's plasma and replacing it with plasma from a donor using an extracorporeal device refers to therapeutic plasma exchange (TPE). This has been found to be a very effective method of attaining blood purification in liver failure patients [3]. This increases hepatic blood flow and decreases blood ammonia levels. The TPE in addition also has the advantage of providing deficient clotting factors and albumin in these patients. TPE can cause hypocalcemia, metabolic acidosis, pulmonary and cerebral complications. Nevertheless, TPE continues to be one of the most frequently used methods of liver support for patients with acute hepatic failure.

Larsen et al. [4] in 2016 described the role of high-volume plasma exchange (HVP), defined as exchange of 8–12 or 15% of ideal body weight with fresh frozen plasma in a RCT of 182 patients with ALF. Patients received either standard medical therapy (SMT; 90 patients) or SMT plus HVP for 3 days (92 patients). It was shown that treatment with HVP improves outcome in patients with ALF by increasing liver transplant-free survival. This was attributable to attenuation of innate immune activation and amelioration of multi-organ dysfunction.

32.4 Liver Support System/Assist Devices

The liver assist devices can be classified into two major groups: artificial liver support devices and bioartificial liver support devices [5]. Artificial liver support devices are non-cell-based devices that mainly carry out the function of blood detoxification and blood purification. Human blood toxic substances can be classified into water soluble (ammonia, creatinine, interleukins (ILs), etc.) or protein bound (bilirubin, benzodiazepines, nitric oxide, etc.). Conventional techniques such as hemodialysis or hemofiltration remove only the water-soluble toxins. The protein-bound toxins can be removed only by addition of albumin to the dialysate or the use of large-pore filters [6].

Bioartificial liver support devices are cell-based liver support devices. They have a cellular component such as primary hepatocytes or hepatic cell lines. In majority of these devices, the hepatic cell lines are derived from porcine hepatocytes or from tumor cell line or harvested from organs that are deemed unsuitable for transplant. The former two cell lines raise safety concerns regarding infection and malignancy transmission. Human hepatocytes harvested from organs are in scarcity and stem cell research holds a promising future in this regard. The cellular components in these devices are intended to replace the important liver functions such as synthesis, detoxification, biotransformation, and excretion (Fig. 32.2).

Fig. 32.2 Types of bridging therapies

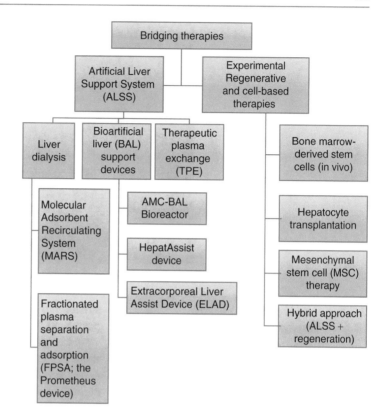

32.5 Molecular Adsorbent Recirculating/Recycling System

Molecular adsorbent recirculating system (MARS) combines conventional dialysis against an albumin dialysate followed by a conventional dialysis procedure to remove the toxins from the dialysate. MARS system consists of two circuits: the blood circuit and the secondary circuit. The blood circuit passes the patient's blood over an albumin impermeable membrane through a high-flux dialyzer. The opposing side of the membrane contains 600 ml of 20% albumin in the secondary circuit. The toxins will diffuse across the membrane and bind to the albumin on the other side. The albumin in the secondary circuit is then cleared of toxins by anion exchange resin and activated charcoal columns [7].

MARS has been found to reduce bilirubin levels, encephalopathy, pruritus, and serum copper levels in Wilson's disease. Improvement in renal function, cerebral blood flow, and varied effects on intracranial pressure (ICP) have also been reported [8]. The overall effect of MARS on mortality seems inconclusive. MARS may be used to stabilize patients prior to transplantation and for allograft dysfunction after transplantation till the liver recovers. It may not improve survival without transplantation [9] (Fig. 32.3).

Fig. 32.3 Molecular
adsorbent recirculating
system

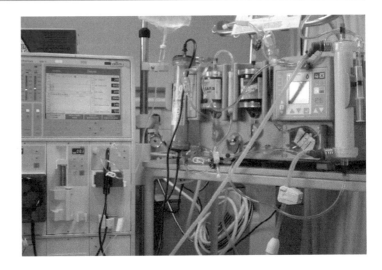

32.6 Fractionated Plasma Separation and Adsorption (Prometheus)

The Prometheus system uses purified blood without the use of exogenous albumin. In this system, the blood is passed over the AlbuFlow 250 kDa membrane which is permeable to albumin. The albumin-bound toxins pass through the albumin permeable membrane and the filtrate is passed through a column of neutral resin and anion exchange resin and returned to the patient. This removes the toxins from the albumin and is returned to the patient. The water-soluble, low molecular weight toxins are removed down-stream with a high-flux hemodialysis [10]. It is postulated that patients treated with Prometheus would be detoxified much more effectively than those treated with MARS. However, the clinical experience with this system is limited and no definite conclusions can be made as of now [11].

In one study comparing MARS versus Prometheus in patients with alcoholic hepatitis or alcoholic cirrhosis, it was found that mean arterial pressure and systemic vascular resistance improved better with MARS in comparison to Prometheus. However, bleeding complications with Prometheus are rare and there might even be the need to use anticoagulation during the procedure [12] (Fig. 32.4).

Fig. 32.4 Fractionated plasma separation and adsorption (Prometheus)

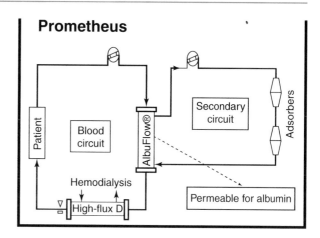

32.7 Single-Pass Albumin Dialysis

Single-pass albumin dialysis (SPAD) is a simple and inexpensive technique of blood purification where additional circuits are not needed. It is a simple veno-venous hemodialysis where the dialysate solution contains low concentration albumin (4.4%). The albumin toxin complexes are then discarded and not recycled. A single randomized controlled study has shown that MARS and SPAD were equally effective in reducing plasma bilirubin levels [13]. However, only MARS affected other paraclinical parameters such as serum bile acids, albumin-binding capacity, creatinine, and urea levels. Preliminary clinical experience shows that SPAD has a promising future with its simplicity and low cost [14].

32.8 Extracorporeal Liver Assist Device

Extracorporeal liver assist device (ELAD) is based on hepatoblastoma C3A cell line. This device was initially evaluated in King's College Hospital in London. The original device was assessed in 24 patients with acute liver failure. The device consisted of exposing the patient's whole blood for duration of about 3–168 h to the hepatocytes. The functioning cell mass was estimated to be about 80–90 g based on the rate of oxygen consumption of the device. The study, however, proved inconclusive in terms of survival rate [15].

Subsequently, modifications were done in the device to improve its efficiency and properties. These include increasing the functional cell mass to 300–400 g in adults, introducing oxygenation and nutritional components in the circuit to improve cell viability, whole blood exposure was replaced with ultra-filtrate exposure, and increasing pore size of the membrane to facilitate free movement of molecules in the device. This improved device was then evaluated in 25 patients who fulfilled criteria for liver transplant. The ELAD-treated and control patients had a similar 30-day survival rate. However, among the 19 patients who were listed for transplant, the ELAD-treated patients had a much higher 30-day survival rate of 81% in comparison to 56% in the control group [16].

32.9 Experimental Regenerative and Cell-based Therapies

Liver has the unique capability for regeneration; in fact, the liver failure is the failure of regeneration. This impressive regenerative power of liver is compromised in ACLF. The definitive therapy, i.e., liver transplant is confounded by lack of donor, resource, expertise, and high medical costs. Cellular therapies such as hepatocyte, stem cell transplantation, and non-cellular therapies using growth factors for liver regeneration augmentation, and Bone Marrow Stem Cell (BMSC) mobilization are emerging alternatives.

32.10 Bone Marrow-derived Stem Cells (In Vivo)

It is a simple and novel method of mobilizing BMSCs using growth factor. Patients receiving Granulocyte-Colony Stimulating Factor (G-CSF) treatment showed significant improvement in survival as well as reduction in MELD and SOFA scores as well as the complications such as HRS, HE, and sepsis. It is supported by studies in HBV-ACLF cohort as well as severe alcoholic hepatitis with ACLF. The selection of patient for considering this therapy is crucial. Garg et al. [17] considered all patients of ACLF but mostly ethanol-related ACLF, and in similar way Singh et al. [18] considered patients, whereas Duan et al. [19] selectively considered HBV-reactivation cohort. The therapy is continued with a close monitoring for organ failure and worsening of clinical parameters, which needs early consideration for transplant.

Combination of growth factors, i.e., G-CSF and darbepoetin alfa has been shown to be effective in patients of decompensated cirrhosis and may be an attractive option to be extrapolated into ACLF cohort [20].

32.11 Hepatocyte Transplantation

Clinical use of adult hepatocyte and fetal hepatic progenitor cells have shown transient clinical benefit in metabolic liver diseases and ALF but with very limited benefits in CLD and ACLF [21]. Recently, Wang et al. [22] have shown significant improvement in the survival of ACLF patients with intrasplenic hepatocyte transplantation.

32.12 Mesenchymal Stem Cell (MSC) Therapy

Use of autologous BM-MSC in ACLF is not possible due to the time constraint in sicker patients to derive any benefit. A solitary study using umbilical cord-derived MSC in ACLF has demonstrated decrease in MELD scores, increased platelet counts and prothrombin activity with survival benefit [23].

Hybrid Approach (ALSS + Regeneration) Combination of ALSS to remove toxins and use of G-CSF to augment liver regeneration is an innovative concept and was published as a single case report. This could be a new approach in managing these patients. G-CSF therapy should be considered in a potential liver transplant candidate when transplantation is not feasible. It helps in prevention of sepsis and organ failure besides augmenting hepatic regeneration in a failing liver. It is not suitable for all patient groups and should be avoided in ACLF patients in the presence of AKI, ongoing sepsis, macrophage activation syndrome or hemolysis, hepatocellular carcinoma (HCC), portal vein thrombosis, multi-organ dysfunction, grade 3 or 4 HE (as per West Haven criteria) [24].

32.13 Role in ALF

The aim of bridging therapies in ALF is to provide adequate liver function and maintain the patient well enough until recovery of native liver function occurs or until a graft is found. Summary of important studies has been given in Table 32.1.

Table 32.1 Studies using ALSS in ALF

Study	No of patients	Device	Biochemical improvement	Cardio-vascular improvement	CNS improvement	Survival
Schmidt et al. [25]	13	MARS	Yes	Yes	N/A	No
El Banayosy et al. [26]	27	MARS	No	N/A	N/A	Yes (50% vs 32%)
Kantola et al. [27]	159	MARS	Yes	N/A	Yes	No
Saliba et al. [28]	102	MARS	Yes	N/A	N/A	No
Larsen et al. [4]	182	HVP	Yes	Yes	Yes	Yes
Gerth et al. [29]	73	MARS	Yes	N/A	N/A	No
Komardina et al. [30]	39	Prometheus	Yes	Yes	N/A	No

32.14 Role in ACLF

ACLF is a distinct clinical syndrome character-ized by progressive liver failure due to an acute hepatic injury on an underlying chronic liver dis-ease. As per EASL-CLIF Consortium [31], ACLF is defined as acute decompensation (AD) of cir-rhosis associated with organ failure (OF) and high short-term mortality (28-day mortality ≥15%).

As per APASL [32], ACLF is defined as an acute hepatic insult manifesting as jaundice (serum bilirubin level of ≥5 mg/dL) and coagu-lopathy (INR of ≥1.5 or prothrombin activity of <40%), complicated within 4 weeks by ascites and/or encephalopathy in patients with previ-ously diagnosed or undiagnosed chronic liver disease (including cirrhosis) and is associated with high 28-day mortality. Important studies of ALSS in patients with ACLF have been sum-marized in Table 32.2. When to consider bridg-ing therapies in ACLF has been shown in Fig. 32.3.

Table 32.2 Studies using ALSS in ACLF

Study	No of patients	Device	Biochemical improvement	Cardio-vascular improvement	CNS improvement	Survival
Hessel et al. [33]	149	MARS	N/A	N/A	N/A	Yes
Kribben et al. [34]	145	Prometheus	Yes	N/A	N/A	Yes
Bañares et al. [35]	156	MARS	Yes	Yes	Yes	No
Xu et al. [36]	171	TPE	Yes	Yes	Yes	No
Gerth et al. [37]	101	MARS	Yes	N/A	Yes	Yes

32.15 Conclusion

Severe liver failure is associated with high mortality despite optimal medical treatment. Though, liver transplantation has emerged as a salvage therapy, many patients unfortunately die while waiting for transplant. Therefore, there is a clear need for a liver support system to provide a "bridge" to till recovery or transplant. Future large scale randomized trials are necessary before making recommendations regarding use of Bridge therapies in these high-risk group of patients with ALF and ACLF (Fig. 32.5).

Key Points
- ACLF has a burden of failing organ acutely as well as chronic liver failure
- Large number of ACLF have no identifiable trigger
- Bridging therapy can be bridge-to-recovery
- Bridging therapy could be bridging till a suitable donor liver is available leading to transplantation
- High-volume plasma exchange has limited role in ACLF
- Liver dialysis by MARS or Prometheus has a role in ACLF management
- Bioartificial liver support devices—AMC-BAL, Hepat Assist device, ELAD are being investigated
- Stem cells based therapies are in experimental stage at present.

Fig. 32.5 Scope of bridging therapy in ACLF, modified from Choudhary et al. [38]

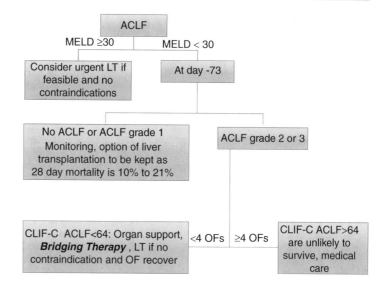

References

1. Mushlin PS, Gelman S. Hepatic physiology and pathophysiology. In: Miller RD, editor. Miller's anesthesia. 7th ed. Philadelphia: Churchill Livingstone; 2010. p. 412–24.
2. Lee L, Stravitz. AASLD position paper: the management of acute liver failure: update 2011. Hepatology. 2011;41(5):1179–97.
3. Iwai H, Nagaki M, Naito T, Ishiki Y, Murakami N, Sugihara J, et al. Removal of endotoxin and cytokines by plasma exchange in patients with acute hepatic failure. Crit Care Med. 1998;26:873–6.
4. Larsen FS, Schmidt LE, Bernsmeier C, Rasmussen A, Isoniemi H, Patel VC, et al. High-volume plasma exchange in patients with acute liver failure: an open randomised controlled trial. J Hepatol. 2016;64:69–78.
5. Phua J, Lee KH. Liver support devices. Curr Opin Crit Care. 2008;14:208–15.
6. Puri P, Anand AC. Liver support devices. Med Update. 2012;22:489–93.
7. Stange J, Mitzner SR, Risler T, Erley CM, Lauchart W, Goehl H, et al. Molecular adsorbent recycling system (MARS): clinical results of a new membrane-based blood purification system for bioartificial liver support. Artif Organs. 1999;23:319–30.
8. Bachli EB, Schuepbach RA, Maggiorini M, Stocker R, Müllhaupt B, Renner EL. Artificial liver support with the molecular adsorbent recirculating system: activation of coagulation and bleeding complications. Liver Int. 2007;27:475–84.
9. Mitzner SR, Stange J, Klammt S, Koball S, Hickstein H, Reisinger EC. Albumin dialysis MARS: knowledge from 10 years of clinical investigation. ASAIO J. 2009;55:498–502.
10. Rifai K, Ernst T, Kretschmer U, Bahr MJ, Schneider A, Hafer C, et al. Prometheus – a new extracorporeal system for the treatment of liver failure. J Hepatol. 2003;39:984–90.
11. Rifai K, Manns MP. Review article: clinical experience with Prometheus. Ther Apher Dial. 2006;10:132–7.
12. Krisper P, Stauber RE. Technological insight: Artificial extracorporeal liver support – how does Prometheus compare with MARS? Nat Rev Nephrol. 2007;3:267–76.
13. Sponholz C, Matthes K, Rupp D, Backaus W, Klammt S, Karailieva D, et al. Molecular adsorbent recirculating system and single-pass albumin dialysis in liver failure – a prospective, randomised crossover study. Crit Care. 2016;20:2.
14. Boonsrirat U, Tiranathanagul K, Srisawat N, Susantitaphong P, Komolmit P, Praditpornsilpa K, et al. Effective bilirubin reduction by single-pass albumin dialysis in liver failure. Artif Organs. 2009;33:648–53.
15. Ellis AJ, Hughes RD, Wendon JA, Dunne J, Langley PG, Kelly JH, et al. Pilot-controlled trial of the extracorporeal liver assist device in acute liver failure. Hepatology. 1996;24:1446–51.
16. Millis JM, Cronin DC, Johnson R, Conjeevaram H, Conlin C, Trevino S, et al. Initial experience with the modified extracorporeal liver-assist device for patients with fulminant hepatic failure: system modifications and clinical impact. Transplantation. 2002;74:1735–46.
17. Garg V, Garg H, Khan A, Sarin SK, et al. Granulocyte-colony stimulating factor mobilizes CD34? Cells and improves survival of patients with acute-on-chronic liver failure. Gastroenterology. 2012;142:505–12.
18. Singh V, Sharma AK, Sharma N, Sharma R. Granulocyte colony stimulating factor in severe alcoholic hepatitis: a randomized pilot study. Am J Gastroenterol. 2014;109:1417–23.

19. Duan XZ, Liu FF, Tong JJ, Hu JH. Granulocyte-colony stimulating factor therapy improves survival in patients with hepatitis B virus-associated acute on-chronic liver failure. World J Gastroenterol. 2013;19(7):1104–10.

20. Kedarisetty CK, Anand L, Bhatia V, Sarin SK. Combination of granulocyte colony-stimulating factor and erythropoietin improves outcomes of patients with decompensated cirrhosis. Gastroenterology. 2015;148(7):1362.

21. Dhawan A, Puppi J, Hughes RD, Mitry RR. Human hepatocyte transplantation: current experience and future challenges. Nat Rev Gastroenterol Hepatol. 2010;7(5):288–98.

22. Wang F, Zhou L, Ma X, Ma W, Wang C, Lu Y, Chen Y, et al. Monitoring of intrasplenic hepatocyte transplantation for acute on-chronic liver failure: a prospective five-year follow-up study. Transplant Proc. 2014;46(1):192–8.

23. Shi M, Zhang Z, Jin L, Liu Z, Wang FS, et al. Human mesenchymal stem cell transfusion is safe and improves liver function in acute-on-chronic liver failure patients. Stem Cells Transl Med. 2012;1(10):725–31.

24. Piscaglia AC, Arena V, Passalacqua S, Gasbarrini A. A case of granulocyte-colony stimulating factor/plasmapheresis-induced activation of granulocyte-colony stimulating factor-positive hepatic progenitors in acute-on-chronic liver failure. Hepatology. 2015;62(2):649–52.

25. Schmidt LE, Wang LP, Hansen BA, Larsen FS. Systemic hemodynamic effects of treatment with the molecular adsorbents recirculating system in patients with hyperacute liver failure: a prospective controlled trial. Liver Transpl. 2003;9:290–7.

26. El Banayosy A, Kizner L, Schueler V, Bergmeier S, Cobaugh D, Koerfer R. First use of the molecular adsorbent recirculating system technique on patients with hypoxic liver failure after cardiogenic shock. ASAIO J. 2004;50:332–7.

27. Kantola T, Koivusalo AM, Hockerstedt K, Isoniemi H. The effect of molecular adsorbent recirculating system treatment on survival, native liver recovery, and need for liver transplantation in acute liver failure patients. Transpl Int. 2008;21(9):857–66.

28. Saliba F, Camus C, Durand F, et al. Albumin dialysis with a noncell artificial liver support device in patients with acute liver failure: a randomized, controlled trial. Ann Intern Med. 2013;159(8):522–31.

29. Gerth HU, Pohlen M, Tholking G, Pavenstadt H, Brand M, Wilms C, et al. Molecular adsorbent recirculating system (MARS) in acute liver injury and graft dysfunction: results from a case-control study. PLoS ONE. 2017;12(4):e0175529.

30. Komardina E, Yaroustovsky M, Abramyan M, Plyushch M. Prometheus therapy for the treatment of acute liver failure in patients after cardiac surgery. Kardiochir Torakochirurgia Pol. 2017;14(4):230–5.

31. Moreau R, Jalan R, Gines P, et al. Acute-on-chronic liver failure is a distinct syndrome that develops in patients with acute decompensation of cirrhosis. Gastroenterology. 2013;144:1426–37.

32. Sarin SK, Kedarisetty CK, Abbas Z, et al. Acute-on-chronic liver failure: consensus recommendations of the Asian Pacific Association for the Study of the Liver (APASL) 2014. Hepatol Int. 2014;8:453–71.

33. Hessel FP, Bramlage P, Wasem J, Mitzner SR. Cost-effectiveness of the artificial liver support system MARS in patients with acute-on-chronic liver failure. Eur J Gastroenterol Hepatol. 2010;22(2):213–20.

34. Kribben A, Gerken G, Haag S, Herget-Rosenthal S, Treichel U, Betz C, et al. Effects of fractionated plasma separation and adsorption on survival in patients with acute-on-chronic liver failure gastroenterology. Gastroenterology. 2012;142(4):782–9.

35. Banares R, Nevens F, Larsen FS, Jalan R, Albillos A, Dollinger M, et al. Extracorporeal albumin dialysis with the molecular adsorbent recirculating system in acute-on-chronic liver failure: the RELIEF trial. Hepatology. 2013;57(3):1153–62.

36. Xu X, Liu X, Ling Q, Wei Q, Liu Z, Xu X, et al. Artificial liver support system combined with liver transplantation in the treatment of patients with acute-on-chronic liver failure. PLoS ONE. 2013;8(3):e58738.

37. Gerth HU, Pohlen M, Tholking G, Pavenstadt H, Brand M, Husing-Kabar A, et al. Molecular adsorbent recirculating system can reduce short-term mortality among patients with acute-on-chronic liver failure-a retrospective analysis. Crit Care Med. 2017;45(10):1616–24.

38. Choudhary NS, Saraf N, Saigal S, Soin AS. Liver transplantation for acute on chronic liver failure. J Clin Exp Hepatol. 2017;7:247–52.

Anaesthetic Management of Acute Liver Failure for Liver Transplant

33

Prachi Gokula and Vijay Vohra

Abbreviations

ALF	Acute liver failure
CPP	Cerebral perfusion pressure
CRRT	Continuous renal replacement therapy
CSF	Cerebrospinal fluid
FFP	Fresh frozen plasma
ICP	Intracranial pressure
IVC	Inferior vena cava
MAP	Mean arterial pressure
OLT	Orthotopic liver transplant
t-PA	Tissue plasminogen activator
VVB	Venovenous bypass

33.1 Background

Acute liver failure represents a rare but complex syndrome, characterised by acute liver dysfunction without evidence of any underlying chronic liver disease. It comprises of coagulopathy of liver aetiology and altered mentation due to hepatic encephalopathy, and may progress to multi-organ dysfunction.

ALF has been defined as the severe acute liver injury with encephalopathy and impaired synthetic function (INR of 1.5 or higher) in a patient without cirrhosis or pre-existing liver disease and with an illness of fewer than 26 weeks duration [1].

Although, with improved critical care therapy rate of transplant free survival has shown significant improvement in recent years, still liver transplant remains to be the only definite remedy available for patients with acute liver failure who do not improve with conservative management.

Early identification of acute liver failure and its aetiology with major advancements in intensive care therapy and identifying potential candidates for liver transplantation have greatly improved the survival rate of patients with ALF—Liver assist devices have too contributed as a "bridging therapy" to liver transplant or spontaneous recovery.

Identification of patients who are too sick to survive liver transplantation surgery or carry a guarded prognosis for postoperative recovery is as important, to avoid futile liver transplants and thereby improve outcome figures.

Liver transplantation for acute liver failure poses varied challenges for the perioperative anaesthesiologist in terms of the urgency of surgery, underlying multi-organ dysfunction and possible use of marginal grafts in emergency surgery where waiting for an optimum graft could jeopardise the patient outcome.

Protocols have been described to aid in the intensive care management of patients with acute

P. Gokula · V. Vohra (✉)
Department of Liver Transplant, GI Anaesthesia
& Intensive Care, Medanta The Medicity,
Gurgaon, Haryana, India
e-mail: vijay.vohra@medanta.org

liver failure. The literature pertaining to intraoperative management of these patients is limited, but it is in essence continuation of critical care management-especially avoiding manoeuvres during the course of surgery which would raise intracranial pressure.

Comprehensive preoperative evaluation should include detailed past medical and surgical history often elicited from relatives (due to the presence of advanced hepatic encephalopathy) and clinical examination to rule out any condition that may impact the decision to proceed with emergency liver transplant.

33.2   Specific Concerns

Multi-organ dysfunction is a major cause of morbidity associated with acute liver failure. Presence of established extra-hepatic organ failure at the time of surgery makes the context for liver transplant for patients with acute liver failure different from elective orthotopic liver transplant. Understanding of the various systems involved, careful monitoring and appropriate management of organ dysfunction is essential for a successful outcome.

33.3   Central Nervous System

Acute cerebral oedema resulting in subsequent rise in intracranial pressure with a decrease in cerebral perfusion pressure resulting in brainstem herniation is one of the major causes of mortality in patients with acute liver failure.

Cerebral blood flow in patients with acute liver failure have altered response to both arterial pressure and partial pressure of CO_2.

These patients exhibit impaired cerebral autoregulation, wherein cerebral blood flow (CBF) varies passively with mean arterial pressure (MAP) [2, 3]. Larsen et al. described "*dissociated vasoparalysis*" [4]—suggesting that CBF has blunted response to hypercapnia but shows preserved response to hypocapnia (cerebral vaso-

constriction). These observations suggested that the brain vasculature in patients with ALF is in a state of *constant vasodilatation*.

Despite the state of "luxury perfusion" [5] brain hypoxia is still a possibility in cases of decreased cerebral perfusion pressure due to intracranial hypertension or episodes of severe systemic hypotension in the absence of cerebral autoregulation. In order to optimise neurological outcome, balance needs to be maintained between adequate cerebral blood flow to support brain metabolism as well as avoiding hyperperfusion that may lead to intracranial hypertension.

Brain injury as a consequence of acute rise in intracranial pressure during various phases of liver transplant can result in irreversible brain damage. Therefore, there is a need for continuous monitoring of ICP in the intraoperative period as an essential component of anaesthetic management.

33.4   Cardiovascular System

Circulatory dysfunction in patients with acute liver failure is characterised by a state of hyperdynamic circulation with high cardiac output, low mean arterial pressure (MAP), and low systemic vascular resistance (SVR) [6]. Hemodynamic derangements in these patients may be attributed to hypovolemia- due to poor oral intake or loss of fluids and decreased effective circulating volume due to systemic vasodilatation-as a result of toxins released from the failing liver or other inflammatory mediators [7]. Cardiac function is essentially well preserved in these patients, except in some cases of hypoxic hepatitis that may have evidence of both right and left sided cardiac dysfunction with or without valvular abnormalities.

Maintaining optimal hemodynamic parameters becomes imperative in the face of intracranial hypertension or compromised renal function as may be present in cases of acute liver failure. Patient volume status needs to be adequately assessed and corrected before administration of vasopressors.

33.5 Coagulation

Coagulopathy is an integral component of acute liver failure and is indicative of the key role liver plays in haemostatic pathway.

Conventional coagulation tests such as PT/INR are often misleading and can be misconstrued as haemorrhagic tendency, thereby leading to unwarranted transfusion of blood products [8].

Most coagulation factors including fibrinogen and factors II, V, VII, IX, X, XI, and XII—synthesised by the hepatocytes—are markedly decreased except for factor VIII and vWF which are derived from endothelium, and are substantially increased [9, 10]. Decreased production of procoagulants as well as short half-life of these coagulation factors contribute towards underlying coagulopathy in cases of acute liver failure. Simultaneously, there is a decreased synthesis of anticoagulant factors by the liver such as protein C, protein S, protein Z, protein Z-dependent protease inhibitor, antithrombin, heparin cofactor II, and α2-macroglobulin, that may help offset the effect of depleted procoagulant factors [11].

Therefore, decreased synthesis of procoagulants, anticoagulant factors, impaired fibrinolytic system and platelet dysfunction- all contribute towards impaired haemostasis in acute liver failure [12]. Any disturbance in this fine balance can lead to either bleeding or thrombotic complications.

33.6 Renal Function

Renal dysfunction is a frequent complication associated with acute liver failure [13, 14]. Acute kidney injury(AKI) when present with ALF augurs a poor prognosis and is associated with increased length of hospital stay and mortality. Cause of renal insufficiency is often multifactorial, ranging from hypotension caused from volume depletion, hepatorenal syndrome or acute tubular necrosis. Risk factors for AKI include increased age, paracetamol-induced ALF, hypotension, the presence of the systemic inflammatory response syndrome (SIRS) and infection [15, 16].

33.7 Too Sick To Be Considered for Liver Transplant

The only *absolute contraindication* to liver transplant is irretrievable brain injury and any signs suggestive of it-such as presence of bilateral dilated non-reactive pupils, absence of spontaneous respiratory efforts, loss of middle cerebral artery flow or evidence of uncle herniation on CT should be actively used out.

Progressive vasoplegic shock with increasing requirement of vasopressor support, presence extensive bowel ischemia, severe hemorrhagic pancreatitis and poorly controlled ARDS - are considered to be *relative contraindications* for liver transplant.

Presence of bacteraemia, responding to treatment is not considered to be a contraindication. Relative changes in the prognostic variables should be taken into consideration before proceeding for liver transplant [17].

33.8 Shifting from ICU to Operating Room

Patients with acute liver failure are nursed and managed in intensive care units while being prepared for liver transplantation. Thereby, proper communication with detailed handover between the intensivist and anaesthetist in regard to the preoperative management is imperative to continue the required care during intraoperative period as well.

Patients with ALF in view of advanced stage of hepatic encephalopathy are often mechanically ventilated and are maintained with continuous infusions of sedative, analgesic with/without paralysing agents, and vasopressor agents if needed.

Intracranial hypertension is one of the major causes of morbidity associated with ALF and its management is of paramount importance to prevent any acute surges in it, not only during intraoperative period but during transit to OR as well.

Different strategies to keep ICP in check ranges from specific ventilatory settings to use of osmotic therapy.

Use of portable ventilators should be preferred as opposed to manual ventilation to avoid any gross changes in pCO2, as well as maintaining head end elevation, thereby, minimising rise in ICP.

During transfer, adequate sedation, analgesia, and muscle paralysis should be ensured to minimise chances of patient bucking or coughing on ET tube.

Due care should be taken of all the vascular accesses along with vasopressor infusions to prevent cardiovascular instability during the transfer.

Special monitoring devices such ICP monitor, if present, should be carried to the OR to aid in intraoperative management.

Often, patients of ALF are managed with CRRT in the preoperative period and the decision to continue the same during intraoperative period is individualised on per case basis.

33.9   Anaesthetic Management

Most of the patients with acute liver failure arriving in the operating room are being mechanically ventilated. Continuous infusion of sedatives and muscle relaxants if already present can be continued in the intraoperative period as well. In cases where patients are not mechanically ventilated, anaesthesia is induced with rapid sequence induction with fentanyl 1–2 mcg/kg, propofol 1–2 mg/kg and a rapid onset muscle relaxant either suxamethonium 1–2 mg/kg or rocuronium 0.6–1.2 mg/kg.

Suxamethonium may cause transient rise in ICP and hyperkalemia [18], therefore should be avoided if feasible.

Due care needs to be taken to attenuate any acute rise in ICP associated with the stimulus of laryngoscopy and intubation.

Anaesthesia technique includes continuous infusion of fentanyl 1–2 mcg/kg/h, propofol infusion, non-depolarising muscle relaxant (preferably cis-atracurium since its metabolism is independent of hepatic function and does not produce laudanosine as in case of atracurium).

Propofol has long been used as a sedative agent in patients with intracranial hypertension due to its potential to decrease cerebral metabolic rate and oxygen demand [19]. Propofol reduces cerebral blood flow and subsequently lower the intracranial pressure in patients with acute liver failure [20]. Due to its shorter duration of action, anticonvulsant properties as well as potential to decrease intracranial pressure, it is used as an adjunct to inhalational agent.

Anaesthesia is maintained with air/oxygen/ isoflurane or sevoflurane.

Ability of isoflurane to preserve Hepatic artery buffer response and splanchnic blood flow has made it the preferred inhalational agent [21].

Primary volatile anaesthetic technique is discouraged due to their tendency to cause increase in cerebral blood flow over 1 MAC and thus leading to rise in intracranial pressure. Therefore, maintenance with volatile anaesthetic in combination with a sedative (propofol being used most commonly) is preferred.

Depth of Anaesthesia Bispectral index (BIS) monitoring has been used extensively to monitor the depth of general anaesthesia. It is a non-invasive modality based on frontal electroencephalographic parameters. Various studies have utilised BIS monitoring to evaluate the level of consciousness in patients of liver failure with hepatic encephalopathy in the peritransplant period.

Advanced hepatobiliary disease causes increased levels of endogenous opioid peptides, which in addition to altered neurotransmission caused by bilirubin contributes to decreased anaesthetic requirement in patients with liver disease [22, 23].

Patients with hepatic encephalopathy tend to have lower anaesthetic requirements which can be reflected by lower MAC required to attain BIS values of less than 60 [24, 25].

33.10 Vascular Access

Since liver transplant as a surgery is associated with major fluid shifts with risk of massive blood loss, adequate venous access is vital to facilitate multiple drug infusions as well as rapid fluid

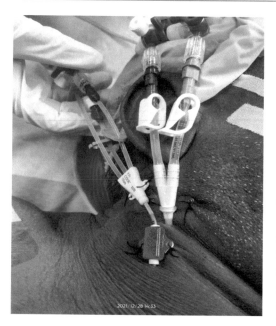

Fig. 33.1 Central venous catheter and Dialysis catheter inserted in IJV

infusion when necessary. For this purpose, two central venous catheters are placed- triple lumen 7Fr catheter- used for drug infusion, and advanced venous access/HD catheter (double lumen 11Fr) for rapid infusion of fluids. USG guided right sided IJV cannulation is preferred (Fig. 33.1).

In paediatric patients, two central venous catheters of the same size (appropriate for age) can be used.

Radial artery is frequently used for invasive blood pressure monitoring. In event of extreme hemodynamic instability or vasodilation, radial artery may underestimate central aortic pressure, in such instances, femoral artery cannulation may be contemplated.

33.11 Hemodynamic Monitoring and Management

Apart from clinical assessment, other invasive techniques should be used to assess the need for volume therapy/vasopressors in these patients. Use of invasive monitoring (such as pulmonary artery catheter or pulse contour analysis) provides measures of cardiac index. Due to invasive-

ness of pulmonary artery catheter (PAC) and its potential hazards, PAC should be reserved for high risk patients with significant cardiac co-morbidities. Non-invasive cardiac output monitors using pulse power analysis through the pulse CO algorithm or arterial pressure-based cardiac output (APCO) method for continuous cardiac output monitoring are commonly used.

In recent times, trans-oesophageal echocardiography (TEE) has emerged as an invaluable tool for intraoperative hemodynamic monitoring. TEE provides direct measurement of the cardiac filling therefore allowing real time assessment of fluid status during the surgery. It offers additional benefit of diagnosing intraoperative complications such as pulmonary embolism, myocardial ischemia or strain. Despite its advantages, absence of technical skill and expertise to operate TEE precludes its routine use.

Waveform analysis allowing continuous measurements of stroke volume variation (SVV) and pulse pressure variation (PPV) helps in assessment of volume status and allows prediction of the likely response to fluid challenge.

Persistent positive fluid balance has been found to be associated with higher mortality patients in many cohorts. Fluid overload can cause elevated venous pressure that may lead to tissue oedema and impaired microcirculatory flow [26–28]. Therefore, it is important to avoid volume overload as much as volume depletion.

Vasopressors are recommended in event of severe hypotension (SBP < 90 mmHg or MAP<65 mmHg) or in order to maintain a cerebral perfusion pressure of more than 50 mmHg.

Norepinephrine is the preferred vasopressor since it provides a more consistent and predictable increase in cerebral perfusion [29]. Epinephrine may decrease mesenteric blood flow and therefore compromise hepatic blood flow in cases of ALF. Vasopressin and its analogues are not routinely recommended in cases of acute liver failure due to their potential to cause celebrate vasodilatation and thereby exacerbating underlying intracranial hypertension. Although, this risk has not been substantiated in recent studies [30].

There is no general consensus on the target MAP but in patients without pre-existing hypertension MAP>60 mmHg is considered to be adequate. In patients with chronic hypertension who are at a risk of developing renal dysfunction, maintaining a MAP>75 mmHg should be considered [31]. Due to underlying impaired cerebral autoregulation, intraoperative hypertension should also be avoided to prevent cerebral hyperaemia that may worsen intracranial hypertension.

33.12 Neurologic Monitoring and Management

Different phases of liver transplant are associated with changes in ICP and can lead to catastrophic consequences if such changes go unrecognised and untreated.

Dissection and reperfusion phase are associated with rise in ICP and consequently decreased cerebral perfusion pressure, whereas anhepatic phase shows a decrease in intracranial pressure [32].

Intraoperative neurologic management in cases of ALF ranges from certain general supportive measures to specific targeted therapies to attenuate any overt surge in ICP. ICP should maintained below 25 mmHg. Mean arterial pressure should be optimised to ensure cerebral perfusion pressure between 50–80 mmHg. Higher cerebral perfusion pressures can cause cerebral hyperaemia, thereby worsening intracranial hypertension.

33.13 ICP Monitoring

It is imperative to monitor changes in icp intraoperatively to detect any untoward surges in intracranial pressure which otherwise may remain undetected and cause irreversible brain damage and cerebral herniation. The objective of ICP monitoring is to maintain ICP < 25 mmHg as well as ensure adequate cerebral perfusion pressure.

ICP monitors require implantation of catheters in the epidural, subdural-subarachnoid or intraventricular spaces through a burr hole. They provide real time as well as continuous data. Although invasive intracranial pressure monitors are considered to be the gold standard, overall survival benefit with their use has not been proven [33]. Due to their potential hazards, are no longer considered to be the standard of care.

Due to safety concerns associated with invasive ICP monitors, non-invasive modalities to monitor ICP have gained popularity and are commonly being used for intraoperative monitoring. Various modalities that have been used in this regard are-.

Optic nerve sheath diameter (ONSD) Optic nerve sheath is a continuation of dura mater of the brain, with the subarachnoid space of optic nerve communicating with subarachnoid space of the brain. Therefore, any pressure changes in CSF in cranial cavity are reflected in optic nerve sheath diameter (ONSD). A linear correlation has been observed between ICP and ONSD measurements (Fig. 33.2). Recent studies have suggested that an estimated increase in ONSD in the range of 4.5–5.5 mm is indicative of increased ICP (>20 mmHg) [34].

Transcranial Doppler (TCD) Klingelhofer et al. [35] first described relationship between ICP and TCD derived flow velocities. They correlated an increase in ICP with a decrease in TCD

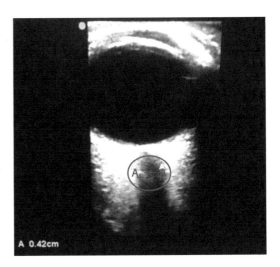

Fig. 33.2 Optic nerve sheath diameter

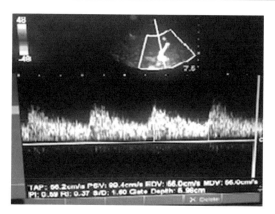

Fig. 33.3 Transcranial Doppler—*Calculation of Pulsatility index*

derived flow velocities and increase in *Pourcelot index* or *resistance index (RI)*. Middle cerebral artery is most commonly used for TCD measurement and Gosling pulsatility index (PI) (Fig. 33.3), most commonly used formula is PI = (systolic flow velocity − diastolic flow velocity)/(mean flow velocity).

Bellner et al. [36] proposed an equation to predict ICP values from pulsatility index and found that predicted ICP value was within ±4.2 mm Hg of the actual ICP, with a 95% confidence interval, in the ICP range of 5–40 mm Hg.(Equation-ICP = 10.972 × PI-1.284).

Operator dependent factors such as the ability to locate an acoustic window obtain a strong pulse signal with adequate depth and angle of insonation limit the reliability of TCD derived values. Reproducibility of the TCD also continues to be a limitation. Since TCD-ICP uses PI, which is a measure of systolic, diastolic and mean flow velocity, presence of anaesthetic agents can directly affect cerebral arteries and consequently the PI.

Electroencephalogram (EEG) This can be helpful in identifying seizure activity which occurs in up to 30% of patients and leads to characteristic change in EEG seen with increased intracranial pressure [37, 38]. Estimation of ICP from EEG is based on identification of slow high-voltage waves. Since most anaesthetic agents promote formation of delta or slow waves, identification of increased ICP levels under anaesthesia becomes difficult. Therefore, EEG is not routinely used in the intraoperative period.

Jugular Venous Oxygen Saturation (SJvO2) SJvO2 has been used as surrogate marker for cerebral metabolism and brain oxygenation. Measurement of jugular bulb oxygen saturation helps to assess the arterio-venous oxygen difference (AVDO2), which in turn indicates metabolic demand in comparison to oxygenation. It involves placement of a retrograde catheter in internal jugular vein with tip at jugular venous bulb. In situations where cerebral oxygen demand exceeds supply, greater amount of oxygen is extracted by the brain, therefore, causing a decrease in SJvO2. Conversely, SJvO2 increases when supply exceeds metabolic demands. Under physiological conditions, ranges from 55% to 75%. In ALF, consistent values of SJvO2 <60% or >80% are associated with raised intracranial pressure [39].

Decrease in SJvO2 can be caused by reduced cerebral perfusion pressure as in acute surge in ICP [39], whereas increased values in SJvO2 are indicative of cerebral hyperaemia. In situation, where both ICP and SJvO2 are elevated, management should be aimed at reducing cerebral blood flow [40]. SJvO2 has been shown to have a utility in managing ALF patients with moderate hypothermia [41]. Similarly SJvO2 has been utilised in managing ALF patients using hyperventilation to lower the intracranial pressure [42].

Cerebral oximetry It is a non-invasive method based on near infrared spectroscopy (NIRS) which measures haemoglobin saturation of arterial, venous, and capillary blood in the cerebral tissue. It is a new modality and is still awaiting validation through randomised control trials. Its use in acute liver failure is based on correlation of cerebral tissue oxygen saturation (SctO2) with increase in intracranial pressure. *Cerebral desaturation*—decrease in SctO2 can be the result of diminished oxygen supply to the brain or increase in oxygen demand by the brain tissue. The cause of change in SctO2 has to be ascertained before management of cerebral desaturation can be initiated.

This modality has been studied more in patients undergoing cardiac surgery in the operat-

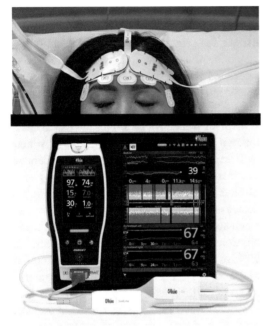

Fig. 33.4 Cerebral Oximeter

Fig. 33.5 Pulpillometer

ing theatre. Cerebral oximetry guided therapy led to improved patient outcome in comparison to the control group [43]. This study of 1034 cardiac patients showed diminished incidence of stroke postoperatively in protocol guided maintenance of $Scto_2$ at or near the pre-induction baseline. Although preliminary results are encouraging, still there is no definite studies showing short-term and long-term outcome benefits (Fig. 33.4).

Pupillometry Pupillary examination and light reflex has very poor reliability. Pupillary reactivity can be more accurately assessed using a commercially available pupillometer (Fig. 33.5). Pupillary reactivity <10% correlates with raised ICP [44]. A case series of neurosurgical patients by Papangelou A et al. [45] revealed abnormal pupillometry observation in 73% of clinical herniation episodes and these were identifiable 7.4 h (median interval) before the event. The main advantage of pupillometry is that it can be performed quickly and frequently. Further studies are required to validate these findings in ALF patients.

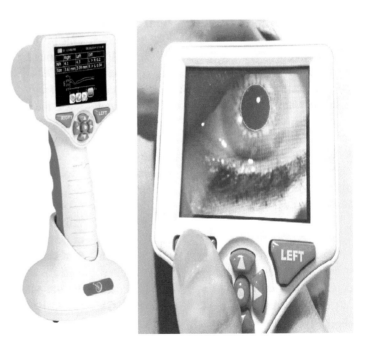

33.14 Strategies to Reduce Intracranial Pressure

- *Positioning*: Patients should be positioned with head end elevated to ~30° (to improve venous and CSF drainage) with head and neck in neutral position (to avoid compromise of jugular venous drainage).
- *Ventilation*: Lung protective ventilatory strategies should be adopted, although hypercapnia needs to be avoided to prevent any cerebral vasodilatation. $PaCO_2$ levels between 30 and 45 mmHg should be targeted. Hyperventilation causes pre capillary vasoconstriction and help in decreasing cerebral blood flow and ICP [46]. Hyperventilation has also been shown to restore impaired cerebral autoregulation in ALF, though this effect may be short-lived. Although, hyperventilation plays a key role in management of acute episodes intracranial hypertension, overzealous and prolonged periods of hypocapnia is discouraged as it can lead to cerebral ischemia. Therefore, despite being an indispensable tool in managing cerebral oedema, hyperventilation should be reserved only as an emergency rescue measure to terminate episodes of intracranial hypertension/imminent herniation.
- *Temperature regulation*: Hypothermia plays a neuro-protective role by decreasing cerebral metabolic rate and cerebral blood flow, thus reducing intracranial pressure. In acute liver failure, protective mechanism of hypothermia is multifactorial. Jalan et al. [47] demonstrated the beneficial role of moderate hypothermia (32–33 °C) in patients with refractory intracranial hypertension-unresponsive to mannitol or ultrafiltration therapy.

Subsequent studies by Karvellas et al. [48] and Bernal et al. [49], however, failed to demonstrate any benefit of moderate hypothermia over 36 °C on prevention of intracranial hypertension.

Potential complications associated with hypothermia include risks of infection, bleeding due to worsening of underlying coagulopathy and platelet dysfunction, arrhythmias,

electrolyte imbalance as well as altered drug metabolism [50].

These adverse effects are generally more common in event of severe hypothermia (<32 °C), and less severe at temperature <35 °C. Routine induction of hypothermia temperature <34 °C is, therefore, no longer recommended as a standard of care and should be considered only in management of refractory intracranial hypertension. In the absence of refractory intracranial hypertension, the reasonable approach, therefore, is to maintain normothermia (core body temp-35–36 °C) as well as avoid hyperthermia/fever [51].

- *Osmotic therapy*: Osmotherapy with mannitol, in the bolus dose of 0.25–0.5 g/kg over 10 min, can be effectively used in case of acute rise in ICP (>25 mmHg) intraoperatively. Lower doses of mannitol have proven to be equally efficacious, with reduced incidence of severe osmotic disequilibrium and dehydration. Hypertonic saline has also been successfully used in critical care settings in patients with intracranial hypertension, still data regarding its role in intraoperative setting is limited. Hyponatremia, of short duration, although is not a contraindication for using hypersonic saline, rate of correction should be inversely proportional to the duration of hyponatremia.

33.15 Pre-emptive Hepatectomy

Pro-inflammatory cytokines released by the "failing liver" have been postulated to contribute towards cerebral hyperaemia and cerebral oedema. Pre-emptive hepatectomy (in the absence of a donor liver) has been reported in few cases to prevent neurological/cerebrovascular collapse [52]. This, however, provokes various ethical dilemmas. Although, in cases where donor liver is available, expeditious clamping of portal vein can be performed, rendering the patient anhepatic. This helps to stabilise the neurological as well cardiovascular status of the patient [53, 54].

In such scenarios, temporary portocaval shunt can be considered that prevents splanchnic congestion and helps to main portal venous return, thereby minimising systemic consequences associated with prolonged portal vein clamping.

33.16 Venovenous Bypass (VVB) and IVC Clamping

Due to lack of adequate collateral venous circulation in these patients, conventional caval clamping technique may lead to profound hemodynamic instability and thereby cause a significant impairment in cerebral and renal perfusion. In order to maintain required hemodynamic parameters, often large volume replacement is done which can further aggravate underlying cerebral oedema. Use of veno-venous bypass has been postulated to be associated with decrease in neurological sequelae due to cerebral oedema. Few authors, however, did not find any evidence of adverse neurological outcome in patients undergoing OLT without VVB. They demonstrated that with use of vasoconstrictors, MAP and CPP could be well maintained, deeming VVB unnecessary [55, 56].

33.17 Managing the Coagulopathy

Intraoperatively evidence of coagulopathy is evident by increased bleeding from cut surfaces and delayed clot formations.

Conventional coagulation parameters often poorly predict the risk of bleeding in such patients, pre-emptive correction of PT/INR values without any evidence of apparent bleeding is not routinely warranted. The inherent risks associated with FFP transfusion such as volume overload or TRALI should be carefully weighed but coagulopathy should be duly corrected.

Strategies to minimise heterologous transfusion should include the use of cell saver. To minimise blood loss maintaining permissive hypotension with controlled hypovolemia can be considered during dissection phase though these strategies are more relevant in chronic liver dis-

ease with portal hypertension and pooling up blood in splanchnic circulation. Additionally, permissive hypotension or hypovolemia can be counterproductive in such cases due to underlying compromised cerebral and renal perfusion.

Presence of minimal or no portal hypertension in ALF associated with absence of abdominal varices helps reduce the risk of surgical bleeding.

Recent studies have demonstrated other potential haemostatic mechanisms- thrombin generation, role of endogenous heparinoids, microparticles and relative role of platelets and fibrinogen in moderating the coagulation disturbances in patients with ALF [57].

Despite having reduced potential to generate thrombin, patients with ALF tend to show accelerated response to thrombin production- once initial amount to activate factors VIII, IX, and XI has been formed, and reduced thrombin inactivation due to activated protein-C resistance, consequently leading to thrombotic potential [58].

A heparin-like effect has also been demonstrated in patients with acute liver failure. Possible mechanism includes release of heparan sulphate from damaged endothelium, release of heparin from damaged liver and reduced renal clearance of heparinoids [59]. Heparinase-modified TEG therefore can be a valuable adjunct in the assessment of coagulopathy related to ALF. This heparin like effect is further enhanced during reperfusion.

Similarly, hyperfibrinolysis has also been observed in the immediate post-reperfusion phase and may be attributed to reduced clearance of t-PA during the anhepatic phase and its release in circulation during reperfusion [60, 61]. Spontaneous recovery from hyperfibrinolysis in the reperfusion phase generally commences 30–60 min but may take up to 2 h to normalise [62].

Viscoelastic tests not only provides information regarding the strength of clot formation but also reflect upon the presence of fibrinolysis. Global assays, thus, have proved to an invaluable tool to help towards a directed therapy and minimising injudicious transfusions and their associated risks.

33.18 Metabolic Derangement

With the failing liver, there is a propensity towards hypoglycaemia, therefore a continuous infusion of dextrose containing fluids with glucose monitoring is essential. Hyperglycaemia, on the other hand may exacerbate cerebral injury and therefore should be avoided.

Infusion of hypertonic saline to maintain S. Na + between 145 and 155 mmol/L in comparison to standard care has resulted in decrease in ICP.

However, liver transplant surgery often warrants large volume fluid administration, transfusion of blood and blood products and use of sodium bicarbonate solution, resulting in gross changes in serum sodium concentration intraoperatively. These changes are often more pronounced in the presence of hyponatremia. Therefore, hypertonic saline solution should be used with caution in these patient population. Due measures including the need for N/2 sodium chloride may be required to prevent rapid changes in sodium levels, ensuring that rate of correction does not exceed 10 mmol/L per 24 h [63].

Ongoing blood boss in the intraoperative period can worsen the underlying acidosis, if left uncorrected, can exacerbate hemodynamic instability. Therefore, metabolic acidosis needs to be addressed with intravascular volume correction or sodium bicarbonate infusion as required.

33.19 Renal Function Management

Intraoperative management of patients with liver failure with underlying renal dysfunction is complex. Conventional anaesthetic techniques such as maintaining "low CVP" and conservative fluid administration to avoid liver congestion and decrease portal pressures- to reduce bleeding and need for transfusion, can cause or worsen kidney injury [64, 65].

It is therefore imperative to maintain adequate blood pressure as well as euvolemia to ensure adequate renal perfusion. Volatile anaesthetics, positive pressure ventilation can further reduce cardiac output, renal blood flow, and conse-

quently glomerular filtration rate. Increased transfusion of blood and blood products can further exacerbate renal injury.

Vasopressors need to be used to treat hypotension was required, with norepinephrine and arginine vasopressin, being most commonly used agents. However, in the background of cerebral oedema, arginine vasopressin analogues should be used with caution.

During the course of surgery, vascular occlusion of portal triad and inferior vena cava clamping, can cause a significant decrease in cardiac output, thereby further compromising renal blood flow. At times, patients with acute liver failure are rendered anhepatic earlier to promote neurological stability, which in turn may significantly alter acid-base balance. Correction of these acid-base derangements is important to prevent hypotension, myocardial depression or life threatening arrhythmias due to underlying hyperkalaemia.

In extreme cases of worsening renal function as reflected by decreased urine output and metabolic derangements (progressive acidosis/hyperkalaemia)—not responding to conventional measures, initiation of renal replacement therapy should be considered.

33.20 Use of Intraoperative CRRT

Continuous renal replacement therapy is often initiated in patients with acute liver failure in preoperative period. Use of CRRT has shown to be beneficial in reducing cerebral oedema, maintaining acid-base balance, maintaining fluid balance, and correcting metabolic derangements esp. in presence of underlying renal dysfunction.

Decision to continue CRRT in the intraoperative period further adds to the intricacy of procedure with need for additional machine, extra circuits, and technical staff to be present in the operating room.

Use of heparin anticoagulation is not recommended due to associated risks of bleeding and citrate anticoagulation can be used instead. Complications of circuit clotting has been reported in patients with ALF.

It is imperative for the anaesthesiologist to be well versed with the functioning of CRRT to avoid/troubleshoot any untoward instances that may arise intraoperatively such as kinking or malfunctioning of CRRT circuits. It is as important to take into account the effect of CRRT on intraoperative drug dosing esp. for drugs that undergo renal excretion, although protein binding and volume of distribution of drugs can also affect their clearance by CRRT. The extra corporeal circulation established with CCRT is prone to induce increased infection risk, hypothermia, thrombocytopenia, and coagulation abnormalities.

Therefore, the decision of continuing CRRT intraoperatively needs to be weighed against the inherent limitations of CRRT in addition to the limited experience of anaesthesiology team with it.

33.21 Postoperative Management

Despite a normal functioning graft, delayed recovery in the postoperative period is expected. Cerebral oedema leading to encephalopathy takes time to recover. Most patients would require postoperative ventilation for at least 24–48 h. Postoperative monitoring of cerebral status in the form of ONSD, Cerebral oximetry, and Pupillometry should continue pending documentation of resolving cerebral oedema. This could be in the form of improving neurological status and if required supported by decreasing cerebral oedema on CT.

After OLT, cerebral oedema resolves slowly and restoration of cerebral autoregulation may take up to 48 h with good allograft function.

> **Key Points**
> 1. Acute liver Failure is acute liver dysfunction characterised by coagulopathy and hepatic encephalopathy.
> 2. Liver transplant continues to remain the only definitive therapy available.

> 3. Conventional coagulation test e.g. PT/INR are poor predictors of bleeding tendencies. Viscoelastic tests are more reliable.
> 4. Different phases of OLT are associated with changes in ICP.
> 5. Mild hypothermia has a neuroprotective effect.
> 6. Hyperventilation should be used as a rescue measure.
> 7. Intracranial pressure monitoring using surrogate markers like ONSD, TCD, $SJvO_2$ and Cerebral oximetry need to be validated.
> 8. Acute liver failure can be frequently complicated by presence of acute kidney injury.
> 9. Intraoperative CRRT, although promising, is not without hazards and should be considered on per case basis.
> 10. Delayed recovery in the postoperative period should be expected.

References

1. Polson J, Lee WM. AASLD position paper: the management of acute liver failure. American Association for the Study of Liver Disease. Hepatology. 2005;41(5):1179–97.
2. Larsen FS, Ejlersen E, Hansen BA, Knudsen GM, Tygstrup N, Secher NH. Functional loss of cerebral blood flow autoregulation in patients with fulminant hepatic failure. J Hepatol. 1995;23:212–7.
3. Larsen FS, Ejlersen E, Clemmesen JO, Kirkegaard P, Hansen BA. Preservation of cerebral oxidative metabolism in fulminant hepatic failure: an autoregulation study. Liver Transpl Surg. 1996b;2:348–53.
4. Larsen FS, Adel Hansen B, Pott F, Ejlersen E, Secher NH, Paulson OB, Knudsen GM. Dissociated cerebral vasoparalysis in acute liver failure. A hypothesis of gradual cerebral hyperaemia. J Hepatol. 1996;25:145–51.
5. Vaquero J, Chung C, Blei AT. Cerebral blood flow in acute liver failure: a finding in search of a mechanism. Metab Brain Dis. 2004;19(3–4):177–94.
6. Ellis A, Wendon J. Circulatory, respiratory, cerebral, and renal derangements in acute liver failure: pathophysiology and management. Semin Liver Dis. 1996;16:379–88.

7. Schneider F, Lutun P, Boudjema K, Wolf P, Tempe JD. In vivo evidence of enhanced guanylyl cyclase activation during the hyperdynamic circulation of acute liver failure. Hepatology. 1994;19:38–44.

8. Stravitz RT. Critical management decisions in patients with acute liver failure. Chest. 2008;134(5):1092–102. https://doi.org/10.1378/chest.08-1071.

9. Lisman T, Stravitz RT. Rebalanced hemostasis in patients with acute liver failure. Semin Thromb Hemost. 2015;41(05):468–73.

10. Pereira SP, Langley PG, Williams R. The management of abnormalities of hemostasis in acute liver failure. Semin Liver Dis. 1996;16:403–14.

11. Lisman T, Leebeek FWG, de Groot PG. Haemostatic abnormalities in patients with liver disease. J Hepatol. 2002;37:280–7.

12. Munoz SJ, Stravitz RT, Gabriel DA. Coagulopathy of acute liver failure. Clin Liver Dis. 2009;13(1):95–107. https://doi.org/10.1016/j.cld.2008.10.001.

13. Ring-Larsen H, Palazzo U. Renal failure in fulminant hepatic failure and terminal cirrhosis: a comparison between incidence, types, and prognosis. Gut. 1981;22:585–59.

14. Tujios SR, Hynan LS, Vazquez MA, Larson AM, Seremba E, Sanders CM, et al. Risk factors and outcomes of acute kidney injury in patients with acute liver failure. Clin Gastroenterol Hepatol. 2015;13:352–9.

15. O'Riordan A, Brummell Z, Sizer E, Auzinger G, Heaton N, O'Grady JG, et al. Acute kidney injury in patients admitted to a liver intensive therapy unit with paracetamol-induced hepatotoxicity. Nephrol Dial Transplant. 2011;26:3501–8.

16. Leithead JA, Ferguson JW, Bates CM, Davidson JS, Lee A, Bathgate AJ, et al. The systemic inflammatory response syndrome is predictive of renal dysfunction in patients with non-paracetamol-induced acute liver failure. Gut. 2009;58:443–9.

17. Wendon J, Panel members, Cordoba J, Dhawan A, Larsen FS, et al. European Association for the Study of the Liver, EASL Clinical Practical Guidelines on the management of acute (fulminant) liver failure. J Hepatol. 2017;66:1047–81.

18. Flood P, Rathmell JP, Shafer S. Stoelting's pharmacology and physiology in anesthetic practice, Chapter 12. 5th ed. Philadelphia: Wolters Kluwer; 2015. p. 323–44.

19. Stephan H, Sonntag H, Schenk HD, Kohlhausen S. Effect of Disoprivan (propofol) on the circulation and oxygen consumption of the brain and CO2 reactivity of brain vessels in the human. Anaesthesist. 1987;36:60–5.

20. Wijdicks EF, Nyberg SL. Propofol to control intracranial pressure in fulminant hepatic failure. Transplant Proc. 2002;34(04):1220–2.

21. Gelman S. General anesthesia and hepatic circulation. Can J Physiol Pharmacol. 1987;65(8):1762–79.

22. Thornton JR, Losowsky MS. Opioid peptides and primary biliary cirrhosis. BMJ. 1988;297:1501–4.

23. Song JC, Sun YM, Zhang MZ, Yang LQ, Tao TZ, Yu WF. The etomidate requirement is decreased in patients with obstructive jaundice. Anesth Analg. 2011;113:1028e32.

24. Baron-Stefaniak J, Götz V, Allhutter A, Schiefer J, Hamp T, Faybik P, Berlakovich G, Baron DM, Plöchl W. Patients undergoing orthotopic liver transplantation require lower concentrations of the volatile anesthetic sevoflurane. Anesth Analg. 2017;125(3):783–9.

25. Kim D, Shin BS, Song I, Han S, Gwak MS, Kim GS, Kim JM, Choi G, Ko JS. Relationship between intraoperative bispectral index and consciousness recovery in patients with hepatic encephalopathy undergoing liver transplant: a retrospective analysis. Transplant Proc. 2019;51(3):798–804.

26. Legrand M, Dupuis C, Simon C, Gayat E, Mateo J, Lukaszewicz AC, et al. Association between systemic hemodynamics and septic acute kidney injury in critically ill patients: a retrospective observational study. Crit Care. 2013;17:R278.

27. Mitchell KH, Carlbom D, Caldwell E, Leary PJ, Himmelfarb J, Hough CL. Volume overload: prevalence, risk factors, and functional outcome in survivors of septic shock. Ann Am Thorac Soc. 2015;12:1837–44.

28. Chen H, Wu B, Gong D, Liu Z. Fluid overload at start of continuous renal replacement therapy is associated with poorer clinical condition and outcome: a prospective observational study on the combined use of bioimpedance vector analysis and serum N-terminal pro-B-type natriuretic peptide measurement. Crit Care. 2015;19:135.

29. Steiner LA, Johnston AJ, Czosnyka M, et al. Direct comparison of cerebrovas-cular effects of norepinephrine and dopamine in head-injured patients. Crit Care Med. 2004;32:1049–54.

30. Eefsen M, Dethloff T, Frederisen JH, et al. Comparison of terlipressin and noradrenalin on cerebral perfusion, intracranial pressure, and cerebral extra- cellular concentrations of lactate and pyruvate in patients with acute liver failure in need of inotropic support. J Hepatol. 2007;47:381–6.

31. Leone M, Asfar P, Radermacher P, Vincent JL, Martin C. Optimizing mean arterial pressure in septic shock: a critical reappraisal of the literature. Crit Care. 2015;19(1):101.

32. Detry O, Arkadopoulos N, Ting P, Kahaku E, Margulies J, Arnaout W, Colquhoun SD, Rozga J, Demetriou AA. Intracranial pressure during liver transplantation for fulminant hepatic failure. Transplantation. 1999;67(5):767–70.

33. Vaquero J, Fontana RJ, Larson AM. Complications and use of intracranial pressure monitoring in patients with acute liver failure and severe encephalopathy. Liver Transpl. 2005;11(12):1581–9.

34. Rajajee V, Vanaman M, Fletcher JJ, Jacobs TL. Optic nerve ultrasound for the detection of raised intracranial pressure. Neurocrit Care. 2011;15:506–15.

35. Klingelhöfer J, Conrad B, Benecke R, Sander D, Markakis E. Evaluation of intracranial pressure from

transcranial Doppler studies in cerebral disease. J Neurol. 1988;235(3):159–62.

36. Bellner J, Romner B, Reinstrup P, Kristiansson KA, Ryding E, Brandt L. Transcranial Doppler sonography pulsatility index (PI) reflects intracranial pressure (ICP). Surg Neurol. 2004;62:45–51.

37. Bhatia V, Batra Y, Acharya SK. Prophylactic phenytoin does not improve cerebral edema or survival in acute liver failure—a controlled clinical trial. J Hepatol. 2004;41:89–96.

38. Trewby PN, Casemore C, Williams R. Continuous bipolar recording of the EEG in patients with fulminant hepatic failure. Electroencephalogr Clin Neurophysiol. 1978;45:107–10.

39. Jalan R. Intracranial hypertension in acute liver failure: pathophysiological basis of rational management. Semin Liver Dis. 2003;23(3):271–82.

40. Privitera GAB, Jalan R. Liver failure: pathophysiological basis and the current and emerging therapies. EMJ Hepatol. 2014;1

41. Jalan R, Olde Damink SW, Deutz NE, Hayes PC, Lee A. Restoration of cerebral blood flow autoregulation and reactivity to carbon dioxide in acute liver failure by moderate hypothermia. Hepatology. 2001;34:50–4.

42. Strauss GI, Møller K, Holm S, Sperling B, Knudsen GM, Larsen FS. Transcranial Doppler sonography and internal jugular bulb saturation during hyperventilation in patients with fulminant hepatic failure. Liver Transpl. 2001;7:352–8.

43. Goldman S, Sutter F, Ferdinand F, Trace C. Optimizing intra-operative cerebral oxygen delivery using noninvasive cerebral oximetry decreases the incidence of stroke for cardiac surgical patients. Heart Surg Forum. 2004;7:E376–81.

44. Taylor WR, Chen JW, Meltzer H, Gennarelli TA, Kelbch C, Knowlton S, et al. Quantitative pupillometry, a new technology: normative data and preliminary observations in patients with acute head injury. J Neurosurg. 2003;98:205–13.

45. Papangelou A, Zink EK, Chang WW, Frattalone A, Gergen D, Gottschalk A, et al. Automated pupillometry and detection of clinical transtentorial brain herniation: a case series. Mil Med. 2018;183:e113–21.

46. Strauss G, Hansen BA, Knudsen GM, Larsen FS. Hyperventilation restores cerebral blood flow autoregulation in patients with acute liver failure. J Hepatol. 1998;28:199–203.

47. Jalan R, Damink SWO, Deutz NE, Lee A, Hayes PC. Moderate hypothermia for uncontrolled intracranial hypertension in acute liver failure. Lancet. 1999;354(9185):1164–8.

48. Karvellas CJ, Todd Stravitz R, Battenhouse H, Lee WM, Schilsky ML, US Acute Liver Failure Study Group. Therapeutic hypother- mia in acute liver failure: a multicenter retrospective cohort analysis. Liver Transpl. 2015;21(01):4–12.

49. Bernal W, Murphy N, Brown S, et al. A multicentre randomized controlled trial of moderate hypothermia to prevent intracranial hypertension in acute liver failure. J Hepatol. 2016;65(02):273–9.

50. Schubert A. Side effects of mild hypothermia. J Neurosurg Anesthesiol. 1995;7:139–47.

51. Bernal W, Wendon J. Acute liver failure. N Engl J Med. 2013;369(26):2525–34.

52. Ringe B, Lubbe N, Kuse E, Frei U, Pichlmayr R. Total hepatectomy and liver transplantation as two-stage procedure. Ann Surg. 1993;218(1):3–9.

53. Ferraz-Neto BH, Moraes-Junior JM, Hidalgo R, Zurstrassen MP, Lima IK, Novais HS, et al. Total hepatectomy and liver transplantation as a two-stage procedure for toxic liver: case reports. Transplant Proc. 2008;40:814–6.

54. Noun R, Zante E, Sauvanet A, Durand F, Bernuau J, Belghiti J. Liver devascularisation improves the hyperkinetic syndrome in patients with fulminant and subfulminant hepatic failure. Transplant Proc. 1995;27(1):1256–7.

55. Pere P, Höckerstedt K, Isoniemi H, Lindgren L. Cerebral blood flow and oxygenation in liver transplantation for acute or chronic hepatic disease without venovenous bypass. Liver Transpl. 2000;6:471–9.

56. Prager MC, Washington DE, Lidofsky SD, Kelley SD, White JD. Intracranial pressure monitoring during liver transplant without venovenous bypass for fulminant hepatic failure. Transpl Proc. 1993;25:1841.

57. Agarwal B, Wright G, Gatt A, et al. Evaluation of coagulation abnormalities in acute liver failure. J Hepatol. 2012;57(4):780–6.

58. Senzolo M, Agarwal S, Zappoli P, Vibhakorn S, Mallett S, Burroughs AK. Heparin-like effect contributes to the coagulopathy in patients with acute liver failure undergoing liver transplantation. Liver Int. 2009;29:54–759.

59. Dzik WH, Arkin CF, Jenkins RL, Stump DC. Fibrinolysis during liver transplantation in humans: role of tissue-type plasminogen activator. Blood. 1988;71(4):1090–5.

60. Porte RJ, Bontempo FA, Knot EA, Lewis JH, Kang YG, Starzl TE. Tissue-type-plasminogen-activator-associated fibrinolysis in orthotopic liver transplantation. Transplant Proc. 1989;21(3):3542.

61. Kang YG, Martin DJ, Marquez J, Lewis JH, Bontempo FA, Shaw BW Jr, et al. Intraoperative changes in blood coagulation and thrombelastographic monitoring in liver transplantation. Anesth Analg. 1985;64(9):888–96.

62. Klinck J, McNeill L, Di Angelantonio E, Menon DK. Predictors and outcome impact of perioperative serum sodium changes in a high-risk population. Br J Anaesth. 2015;114:615–22.

63. Schroeder RA, Kuo PC. Pro: low central venous pressure during liver transplantation–not too low. J Cardiothorac Vasc Anesth. 2008;22(2):311–4.

64. Massicotte L, Beaulieu D, Thibeault L. Con: low central venous pressure during liver transplantation. J Cardiothorac Vasc Anesth. 2008;22(2):315–7.

65. Petroni KC, Cohen NH. Continuous renal replacement therapy: anesthetic implications. Anesth Analg. 2002;94(5):1288–97.

Part VI

Paediatric Liver Transplant

Anesthetic Issues in the Management of Pediatric Liver Transplantation

34

Chitra Chatterji and Vijay Shankar

34.1 Introduction

Liver transplantation remains the only treatment of choice in a patient with end-stage liver disease. Pediatric liver transplant has become a common treatment of choice encouraged by an increasingly successful outcome in end-stage liver disease.

The perioperative management of this population poses unique challenges.

- Different indications according to the age; neonate, infants, and child with their particular characteristics.
- Different comorbidities present in this population.
- Difference in the physiology and size.
- Difference in the surgical techniques.

Through this chapter, we intend to provide an overview of anesthetic management in pediatric patients undergoing living related or cadaveric transplant and an overview also into acute liver failure pediatric patients.

34.2 Indications

The most common etiology for PLT (pediatric liver transplant) is cholestatic disorders like extrahepatic biliary atresia (EHBA) (43%), metabolic disease (13%), and acute hepatic necrosis (11%) [1, 2]. The etiology in 75% of acute liver failure is unknown. The etiologies are given in Table 34.1.

C. Chatterji (✉) · V. Shankar
Department of Anaesthiology and critical care,
Indraprastha Apollo Hospital, New Delhi, India

Table 34.1 Indications for Pediatric Liver Transplantation

Chronic Liver Disease	Metabolic Disorders	Acute Liver Failure	Malignancy	Others
Biliary Atresia	Alpha 1 antitrypsin deficiency	Poisoning	Hepatoblastoma	Budd-Chiari Syndrome
Cryptogenic Cirrhosis	Criggler-Najjar Syndrome	Drug Induced	HCC	Carolis disease
Primary Sclerosing Cholangitis	Cystic Fibrosis	Viral Hepatitis	Sarcoma	Neonatal hemochromatosis
Familial Cholestasis Progressive	Galactossemia		Haemangio-Endothelioma	
Familial Intrahepatic Cholestasis	Gauchers disease			
Autoimmune Hepatitis	Glycogen Storage disorders	Red - **Common in neonates**		
		Violet - **Common in infants**		
Viral Hepatitis	Wilsons Disease	Black - **Common in older children**		
	Niemann-Pick disease			
	Tyrosinemia			

34.3   Basis for Allocation

Earlier waiting list for transplantation was greatly influenced by the disease severity and the duration on the waiting list. The pediatric end-stage liver disease score (PELD) in 2002, predicted the mortality within the next 3 months without transplant. It is valid for children younger than 12 years of age, above which the MELD score is used which incorporates serum bilirubin, INR and serum creatinine. Parameters used in PELD are growth failure, albumin, bilirubin, international normalized ratio (INR), age < 1 year.

$$PELD = 4.80\left[\text{Ln serum bilirubin}\left(\text{mg}/\text{dL}\right)\right] + 18.57\left[\text{Ln INR}\right] - 6.87\left[\text{Ln albumin}\left(\text{g}/\text{dL}\right)\right]$$
$$+ 4.36\left(<1\text{ year old}\right) + 6.67\left(\text{growth failure}\right).$$

PELD exceptions are acute liver failure, hepatopulmonary syndrome, hepatic neoplasms, hepatorenal syndrome, and pulmonary hypertension.

34.4   Timing of Transplantation

This depends on the severity calculated by the PELD score and duration on the waiting list. Age and nutritional status play an important role [3].

In recent times due to better surgical, perioperative management (anesthesia and intensive care), nutritional support, immunosuppressants and elective early living donor liver transplant in this age group has shown improved survival rates similar to older children [4]. The timing of transplantation has been expedited and depends on donor availability, even before the child becomes very sick.

34.5 Pathophysiological Changes, Pre-operative Concerns, and Anesthetic Implications

The complexity of ESLD is enhanced by the multisystem involvement, comorbidities, and social situations. The time period required for work up ranges 1–5 weeks requiring a multidisciplinary team approach. This time period is crucial as it gives a window to assess the severity, presence of congenital anomalies, plan, counsel and make strategies for the specific transplant child. The pathophysiological changes affect all major organ systems.

34.5.1 Pulmonary

- Hypoxemia.
- Hepatopulmonary syndrome (HPS).
- Porto-pulmonary hypertension (POPH).
- Chest infections.

Hypoxemia is multifactorial, most common reason being mechanical restriction due to ascites, hepatosplenomegaly, and pleural effusion. Ascites and pleural effusion can be drained, if massive. Other strategies that can be employed are fluid restriction, diuretics, and albumin infusions.

HPS in acute or chronic liver dysfunction is a syndrome of arterial hypoxemia and right to left shunting due to vasodilation of pulmonary vasculature causing V/Q mismatch and new vessel formation [5]. HPS can be more severe than liver disease and is reversed following transplantation. A fall in arterial oxygen levels on standing from supine, clubbing, and dyspnea with the exclusion of any other cause of hypoxemia is diagnostic. Confirmation is done with Contrast Echocardiography and Technetium 99 labeled micro-aggregated albumin scans.

POPH is rare in pediatric ESLD. Mean PAP (pulmonary artery pressure) >25 mmHg, PCWP (pulmonary capillary wedge pressure) <15 mmHg, PVR (pulmonary vascular resistance) >3 wood units in the presence of portal hypertension. Very little is known about the disease process in pediatric patients. The therapy of POPH in children is challenging and outcomes are dismal.

Chest infections are common due to malnutrition, poor gastric emptying, encephalopathy, mechanical ventilation, recurrent hospitalizations and certain conditions like cystic fibrosis and alpha1 antitrypsin deficiency.

34.5.2 Cardiovascular

- Increased cardiac output (CO).
- Low systemic vascular resistance (SVR).
- Congenital cardiac anomalies (CHD).
- Pulmonary hypertension (PH).
- Cirrhotic cardiomyopathy (CMP).

High CO and low SVR are a result of reduced clearance of vasoactive compounds, e.g., nitric oxide (NO) and also fluid retention due to portal hypertension (PH).

CHD such as atrial septal defect and situs inversus are seen in EHBA children.

PH and pulmonary stenosis have been seen in Alagille syndrome (an autosomal dominant disease characterized by bile duct paucity, cholestasis, and cardiac, musculoskeletal, facial and developmental anomalies).

CMP in pediatrics is an entity evaluated lately especially in biliary atresia (BA). Criteria to diagnose CMP are LVMI (left ventricular mass index) > 95 g/m^2 and relative wall thickness of LV > 0.42 mm. CMP is believed to be more frequent in children especially with BA and is also a predictor of morbidity and mortality [6].

ECG, CXR, ECHO, and cardiac catheterization are required to evaluate.

34.5.3 Central Nervous System

Hepatic encephalopathy is a dangerous complication and is multifactorial. Alterations in cerebral metabolism, accumulation of ammoni and neuroactive peptides have been implicated in the pathophysiology of HE. Precipitating factors are sepsis, nitrogen load from GI bleeding, electrolyte abnormalities, and constipation.

Seizures, airway protection, ventilation, and sedation for procedures would need careful and judicious evaluations.

Non-invasive monitoring of ICP by means of optic nerve sheath diameter and transcranial Doppler are promising monitoring strategies [7].

34.5.4 Renal

- Hepato-renal syndrome (HRS).
- Pre-renal Azotemia.
- Renal failure.

HRS is rare in children and is characterized by impaired RBF, low GFR, elevated serum creatinine, oliguria with low urinary sodium (<20 mmol/L), and high urine/serum creatinine ratio.

Pre-renal azotemia may develop due to fluid restriction and diuretic therapy.

Renal failure due to hyperoxaluria and metabolic disorders are seen.

34.5.5 Gastrointestinal

Gastric emptying is delayed. Intra-abdominal pressure increases due to ascites and organomegaly. Portal hypertension leads to the development of varices. This can present as upper and lower gastrointestinal bleeding. Recurrent hemorrhage with the poor nutritional state can further contribute to anemia.

Impairment of synthetic and metabolic hepatic function leads to impaired drug clearance, glucose hemostasis, and coagulopathy. Glycogen stores are decreased and impaired gluconeogenesis making them prone to hypoglycemia.

Impaired protein synthesis leading to low serum oncotic pressure and high levels of protein-bound drugs. Concentrations of clotting factors due to impaired synthesis or decreased absorption of vitamin K leads to the deficiency of factors II, VII, IX, X, and also antithrombin III, protein C, and protein S.

Splenomegaly also results in the sequestration of platelets and erythrocytes.

Clotting tests and viscoelastic tests show the actual status of the hemostatic condition.

34.6 Pre-operative Workup

Concerns of the systems discussed above should be evaluated in details by a battery of investigations.

Blood tests for complete blood count (Hb, TLC, DLC, platelet count).
Clotting profile with PT, PTT fibrinogen, and FDP.
KFT along with serum electrolytes (Ca, Mg, Na, K) levels. Serum ammonia level when required.
LFT with the bilirubin levels, liver enzymes, albumin, and A/G ratio.
Blood sugar.
Blood grouping and cross-matching.
Serum lactate levels and pH for acidosis.
Baseline cytomegalovirus (CMV) and Epstein–Barr virus (EBV) status.
Blood and urine culture.
Chest X-ray, CT chest.
ECHO or cardiac catheterization (when indicated).

Detailed discussion and history taking with parents/guardian is mandatory. Previous surgeries, hospitalizations (for infections, bleeding, banding, sclerotherapy, dialysis, cardiovascular problems), medications, allergies, vaccination history should be documented.

It is recommended that the vaccination status of the child should be recorded, and the child should be referred for appropriate vaccinations at the time of listing. Many transplant centers will do routine pretransplant serology for vaccine-preventable diseases such as Hepatitis B, Varicella, measles, mumps, and rubella to guide individual vaccine recommendations. Table 34.2 contains recommendations for vaccinations in pediatric patients.

Table 34.2 Immunization s prior to transplantation

Vaccine	Inactivated/live attenuated (I/LA)	Recommended before transplant
Influenza	I	Yes
Hepatitis B	I	Yes
Hepatitis A	I	Yes
Pertussis	I	Yes
Diphtheria	I	Yes
Tetanus	I	Yes
Inactivated polio vaccine	I	Yes
H. influenzae	I	Yes
S. pneumoniae (conjugate vaccine)	I	Yes
S. pneumonia (polysaccharide vaccine)	I	Yes
N. meningitidis	I	Yes
Human papillomavirus	I	Yes
Rabies	I	Yes
Varicella (live-attenuated)	LA	Yes
Rotavirus	LA	Yes
Measles	LA	Yes
Mumps	LA	Yes
Rubella	LA	Yes
BCG	LA	Yes
Smallpox	LA	No
Anthrax	I	No

Explanation of the course of care from presurgical period to the post-surgical and following discharge and long-term care should be done.

Perioperative morbidity, mortality, blood transfusion requirements, ICU stay, mechanical ventilation should be discussed along with consent.

Crucial to the success of the program is an efficient blood bank and a hematology laboratory.

34.7 Pre-operative Medication and Theater Preparation

Antiseptic scrub and bath.

Intravenous dextrose for maintenance fluids.

Antibiotics as per institutional protocol (Usually a board spectrum antibiotic coverage with antifungal. At author's current institute, we use piperacillin—tazobactam, teicoplanin, and fluconazole).

The operating room should be warm prior to induction with the air conditioning preferably turned off. This is especially important as the child will be kept exposed for a while to facilitate placement of intravenous catheters.

Equipment required range from the usual pediatric airway trolley (laryngoscopes, endotracheal tubes, airways, bougies, etc.).

Anesthesia machine capable of delivering low tidal volumes and weaning modes of ventilation.

Suction machine and catheters.

Anesthetic drugs and antibiotics are prepared as per the institutional protocol.

Inotropic drugs as per the table (Table 34.3).

Intravenous lines—2 large bore 22/20/18G as per the age group and venous access available, preferably on either upper limb.

Central venous access in the IJV with a triple lumen 4.5/5.5Fr 8 cm length. Antibiotic impregnated one can be kept for longer especially in children with difficult veins or sick ones.

Sterile lines, water proof, and transparent dressings are mandatory to observe for signs of inflammation at insertion sites.

Arterial lines 24/22/20G for both radial and femoral. Radial line is preferred due to the reliability during the cross-clamping phase. Some anesthesiologists prefer femoral access as in sick children and on high inotropic support, it gives better reliability, as it is more central and larger [8]. Generally, two invasive arterial lines are preferred as one can be used for sampling.

Warming devices for intravenous fluids and blood and blood products.

Bodywarmers such as the temperature control machine (TCM) with water blanket, convection warmers with appropriate blankets.

Nasogastric tube and urinary catheter.

Cotton roll, sponge or head ring to support the head.

Neutral positioning and placement of the child to prevent any pressure sore or positioning-related injury like foot drop and pressure alopecia.

Table 34.3 Dilutions and dosages of commonly used vasoactive drugs

Drug	Dilution	Dosage
Noradrenaline	(0.3 × weight in kg) mg + 50 mL NS 1 mL/h = 0.1 mcg/kg/min	0.05–0.1 mcg/kg/min to a maximum of 1 mcg/kg/min
Adrenaline	(0.3 × weight in kg) mg + 50 mL NS 1 mL/h = 0.1 mcg/kg/min	0.1–1.0 mcg/kg/min
Dopamine	(15 × weight in kg) mg + 50 mL NS 1 mL/h = 5 mcg/kg/min	5–20 mcg/kg/min
Vasopressin	(0.3 × weight in kg) units +50 mL NS 1 mL/h = 0.0001 units/kg/min	0.0003–0.002 units/kg/min
Dobutamine	(15 × weight in kg) mg + 50 mL NS 1 mL/h = 5 mcg/kg/min	5–20 mcg/kg/min

34.8 Intraoperative Management

34.8.1 Induction

Anesthetic induction should be individualized based on the multiple factors evaluated in the preoperative workup. These could be massive ascites, gastrointestinal bleeding, cardiac conditions, pulmonary conditions, and hemodynamic instability.

Since most children would be already having an intravenous (IV) access, IV induction is usually preferred. Pre oxygenation is extremely important as many a times these patients desaturate during layngoscopy. Moreover visualization of larynx might be difficult in certain cases. Its wise to have a smaller size endotracheal tube than the one appropriate for the age of the child. Rapid sequence induction in children with massive ascites is safer.

The choice of induction agent depends on the anesthetic protocol of the institution, usually, they are fentanyl and propofol though ketamine and etomidate can also be used. Succinylcholine and rocuronium are used when rapid sequence induction (RSI) is needed. In most centers atracurium or cisatracurium followed by its infusion is used as muscle relaxants. Higher doses of non-depolarizing muscle relaxants might be required owing to an increased volume of distribution and binding to acute phase reactants. Vecuronium and rocuronium are metabolized in the liver and excreted in bile thus prolonging their action in advanced liver disease. Plasma Pseudocholinesterase level is reduced in liver disease.

Endotracheal intubation is preferably done with a low pressure cuffed endotracheal tube as the variability of pulmonary compliance is an issue due to disease and surgical retraction and manipulation. The cuff pressure should be measured following inflation and just an adequate amount to prevent major leaks is recommended. Newer endotracheal tubes made of polyurethane instead of polyvinyl chloride may help in achieving tracheal sealing at lower pressures. Fixation of the ETT is of utmost importance as it is very common to encounter upper lobe collapse and endobronchial tube migration due to surgical manipulation and retractor application. PEEP of up to 5cmH$_2$O is useful to prevent atelectasis and improve oxygenation.

34.8.2 Intravenous (IV) and Intraarterial (IA) Access

uring of IV and IA access is done after induction of anesthesia. This might take a substantial amount of time and resources depending on the health of the child. Infants and children are particularly prone to inadvertent hypothermia due to their malnourished state, increased cardiac output and peripheral vasodilatation. The OT air conditioning needs to be switched off during securing of lines and placing the child on a warming blanket is very helpful to maintain normothermia. Both active and passive maneuvers should be applied such as conduction warming blanket, convective warming systems such as Bair Hugger, mechanical ventilation with heat and moisture exchanger, and high flow fluid warming devices.

Upper extremities are preferred as IVC cross-clamping is done during the grafting phase. Peripheral IV access with two large bore cannulas in both the upper limbs is ideal. A triple lumen central venous catheter is secured for vasoactive drugs, monitoring the CVP (central venous pressure) and rapid infusion/transfusion during the reperfusion phase or hypovolemic phase. CVP catheter is usually placed using a real-time ultrasound machine to prevent potentially dangerous complications in the already sick, coagulopathic child.

Arterial catheter single or two in number is placed in the radial artery in both the upper limbs. One could be used for sampling or used if the other one gets damped or misplaced. Femoral arterial monitoring is used in certain centers especially in very sick children on high inotropic support or very hemodynamically unstable as they are more central and give a more reliable reading. This could be debatable though as it will be damped during aortic cross-clamping if and when an arterial conduit from the aorta is constructed.

34.8.3 Maintenance of Anesthesia

A mixture of isoflurane/sevoflurane with air and oxygen along with fentanyl and atracurium infusions. Fentanyl does tend to accumulate with repeated boluses or infusion. Remifentanil, which is metabolized by red cell esterases, has a very short half-life and is easily eliminated. Remifentanil is not available in India and we have no experience using it. More important than the technique of anesthesia used are the goals of maintaining hemodynamic stability, temperature, metabolic, and coagulation abnormalities.

34.8.4 Temperature Management

Hypothermia is very common due to numerous reasons like. Exposure of abdomen to room air, infusion of cold fluids, blood and blood products, cold irrigating fluids form the graft and long duration of surgery. The child should be draped

in such a way that ascites and blood should drain away not pool on their bodies. Special drapes are available for the same. Convective warmers and warming mattress should be used. Warm fluids should be used and this can be achieved by using fluid warmers during transfusions or fluid infusions.

34.8.5 Metabolic Management

Hypoglycaemia is common, hence it would be wise to run an infusion of 0.45% normal saline as maintenance during surgical procedure along with monitoring of the blood sugar at regular intervals.

Hypokalemia due to chronic administration of diuretics is common, routine correction is not done unless it is associated with rhythm disturbances and if lower than 3 meq/L. Potassium level usually tends to rise on its own during the course of the operation due to the acidosis, administration of blood products, and reperfusion.

Normal serum ionized calcium levels are very important for preserving myocardial contractility and also for the coagulation pathway. Citrate in the blood products tends to decrease ionized calcium levels, especially during the anhepatic phase. Calcium levels are maintained by administering calcium chloride or calcium gluconate infusions.

34.8.6 Hemodynamic Management

Maintaining hemodynamics is the main focus of anesthetic management in liver transplantation. The reasons for hemodynamics instability are multifactorial. Decreased preload, low systemic vascular resistance, vascular clamping, ongoing fluid, and blood losses are some of the reasons for hypotension.

CVP monitoring is technically unreliable due to changes in intra-abdominal pressures. Massive ascites, when present, can lead to a false elevation of CVP which is followed by a drastic fall on the drainage of ascitic fluid. Maneuvers like retraction of the diaphragm, external compression and pulling of IVC and manipulation of the large-sized liver can lead to erratic reading of CVP. The monitoring of the trend of CVP along with close communication with the surgeon gives an idea of the preload.

Flow trac even though extensively used in adults is not validated for use in children. Most centers do not prefer using pulmonary arterial catheters in children owing to the complications associated with insertion. Minimally invasive cardiac output monitors like PICCO and LIDCO are used in some centers.

TEE is a definitive monitor of the intravascular volume. Small biplanar probes are available for pediatric patients. It provides an excellent assessment of ventricular filling and function along with diagnosing structural abnormalities. However, interpretation of TEE requires significant skill, training and also carries the risk of rupturing esophageal varices.

In addition, constant communication with the surgical team, direct visualization of the IVC and the turgidity of the liver graft is of paramount importance and provides very useful information.

34.8.7 Hematological Management

The degree of coagulopathy present will depend on the severity of liver disease. Blood loss can be significant during the dissection phase especially if the patient has undergone a Kasai procedure. In the past or has had spontaneous bacterial peritonitis. Coagulopathy worsens during the anhepatic phase due to absent synthesis of hepatic clotting factors. Frequent monitoring of coagulation parameters like PT, aPTT, INR, platelets, fibrinogen should be done. Thromboelastogram (Viscoelastic study) will give an idea of the global hemostasis. Observing the surgical field and communication with the surgeon perhaps is the best real-time way to assess coagulation and administer blood products.

In pediatric liver transplant all over the world full correction of the coagulation parameters is not carried out. This is in order to avoid causing vascular thrombosis and early graft occlusion. Correction is done in the presence of an obvious coagulopathic bleed and an abnormal TEG. Depending on the coagulation parameters, decision of the blood product to be used is taken. Preferably cryoprecipitate and platelet transfusion are withheld unless deemed necessary.

In addition to the above, normal calcium level, normothermia, and correction of metabolic acidosis also help in maintaining normal coagulation.

34.9 Stages of Liver Transplantation and the Specific Anesthetic Considerations

34.9.1 Dissection Phase- (Pre-hepatic Stage)

It extends from skin incision to occlusion of hepatic artery and portal vein.

This phase involves mobilization of liver from the inferior vena cava and various adhesions as well as dissection of the porta. There is a potential for significant bleeding from adhesions from previous abdominal surgeries such as Kasai procedure. The aim should be volume replacement to maintain hemodynamic stability, blood glucose levels, and correction of coagulopathy. Excessive ascitic fluid drainage can also lead to hypotension and acidosis and this can be managed by 5% albumin or colloid replacement. Vasopressors such as Nor Adrenaline, dopamine can be started to increase the systemic vascular resistance (SVR).

Application of retractors against the diaphragm reduces the lung compliance and there is an increase in the airway pressure. Ventilatory parameters may need to be readjusted and air entry to both lungs rechecked.

34.9.2 Anhepatic Phase

The characteristic feature is the decrease in venous return due to clamping of the IVC (partial or complete) leading to hypotension though the presence of collaterals may help in better tolerance. There is also compensatory tachycardia to maintain cardiac output.

In children with less developed collaterals especially ones having a relatively normal hepatic function and minimal portal hypertension; acidosis, aggravating hyperkalemia, interruption of gluconeogenesis, and hypoglycemia can be seen.

Care must be taken not to overhydrate the patient during this stage since it may lead to graft edema post-reperfusion.

Acidosis tends to worsen due to decreased clearance of acids and lactate by the liver. Routine administration of soda bicarbonate is not recommended unless the patient is hemodynamically unstable and acidotic.

The anhepatic phase ends with reperfusion of the portal vein. During reperfusion unclamping of the vascular anastomosis is done, the circulatory system of the recipient being exposed to cold fluids, potassium ion, ischemic factors that can lead to hypotension, malignant ventricular dysrhythmia, and unstable hemodynamic states. In anticipation of reperfusion syndrome, all metabolic abnormalities should be corrected prior to reperfusion. The hemoglobin levels are maintained at around 8 g/dL. pH, ionized calcium, and potassium are all kept within the normal range prior to reperfusion.

Temporary administration of 100% oxygen, reduction of volatile agents, stepping up inotropes, a small bolus of calcium chloride, sodium bicarbonate or phenylephrine can mitigate post-reperfusion syndrome. Preparation for necessary cardiopulmonary resuscitation or cardiac defibrillation on occurrence of life-threatening arrhythmias should be always kept in mind.

34.9.3 Neohepatic Phase

This phase is the completion of arterial and biliary anastomosis. Coagulopathy may continue along with oozing from the raw edges of the graft. Volume resuscitation and blood transfusion continues though it has to be judicious to prevent graft congestion and fluid overload. The hematocrit (Hct) is maintained below 30%, the INR and platelet count kept under corrected to decrease blood viscosity in order to decrease chance of arterial and venous thrombosis. As the neohepatic function improves correction of acid base, lactic acidosis, electrolyte abnormalities, and blood sugar levels stabilizes. The production of bile from the graft also gives an idea of the graft function.

On completion of all the anastomosis a Doppler ultrasound is done to confirm vascular patency. Biliary drainage is established by either duct to duct anastomosis or hepatico-jejunostomy.

The risk of hepatic artery thrombosis is higher in pediatric patients especially if there is greater arterial size discrepancy, lower patient weight, reoperation, and longer surgical times. Many institutions take strict initiative to maintain a HCT of <30%. PT, aPTT carefully monitored to prevent over correction. Acetylsalicylic acid, alprostadil (PGE1), and heparin infusions may be started in situations where vascular thrombosis is observed intraoperative. After heparin infusion a close watch on the TEG and aPTT is kept, with a target aPTT being >1.5 times control.

Drains are inserted and abdomen closed. It is important that the anesthesiologist pays attention to the closure of the abdomen to mitigate tight closure leading to respiratory compromise. It can also lead to abdomen compartment syndrome carrying a risk of graft hypoperfusion, and compression. In such cases staged closure of the abdomen is recommended and/or downsizing of the graft prior to anastomosis (Table 34.4).

Table 34.4 Surgical stages and anesthetic considerations

Surgical stage	Anesthetic considerations
Dissection	• Blood loss • Fluid and blood resuscitation • Maintenance of normothermia
Anhepatic	• Fluid management • Correction of hypocalcemia, hyperkalemia, acidosis • Correction of coagulopathy • Prepare for reperfusion with adequate intravascular volume and correction of metabolic abnormalities
Reperfusion	• Management of hypotension • Management of hyperkalemia and hypocalcemia • Fluid and blood replacement • Air embolism
Neohepatic	• Maintain hematocrit around 25% • Preparation for extubation if suitable

34.9.4 Elective Ventilation Vs. on Table Extubation

Traditionally pediatric patients were electively ventilated post-transplantation due to various reasons. Vascular patency was a major problem in the post-operative period with children requiring frequent imaging which was difficult in a restless and agitated child. This coupled with the high rate of re-explorations in children, prolonged use of sedatives and tight abdominal closure meant most of the institutions used to electively ventilate these patients post operatively. However, recently encouraged by positive results of fast tracking in adults many pediatric centers perform on table extubation or early extubation in the ICU which has shown favorable results. At author's current institute, we extubate the patients on table whenever possible at the discretion of the treating anesthetist.

The patient has to fulfill certain criteria to attempt an on table extubation which includes (1) Absence of encephalopathy pre-operatively, (2) Hemodynamic stability, (3) Confirmation of vascular patency by doppler, (4) Absence of tight abdominal closure, (5) Stable blood gases, (6) Absence of massive blood transfusion.

34.9.5 Early Post-operative Course

As mentioned earlier most centers electively ventilate the patients after the transplantation. Opioid infusions are commonly used to sedate the children. An infusion of muscle relaxants can also be added if ventilation becomes difficult due to a diminished lung compliance. Fluid management should be given as per the maintenance requirements and also keeping in mind the loses through the drains which might be quite significant. We usually use a balanced salt solution with dextrose as maintenance and 5% albumin for drain replacement during the first 48 h. Hematocrit is maintained at not more than 25% to reduce the occurrence of vascular thrombosis.

Frequent blood gases are performed to optimize ventilation and also to have an idea about the graft function. It is a good idea to perform a chest X-ray as soon as the patient arrives in the ICU and look for potential problems like misplacement of endotracheal tube and central line, fluid overload, pleural effusions, and position of nasogastric tube. In general, most children undergoing an elective liver transplant and who are having a satisfactory graft function postoperatively can be considered for early extubation. Fast tracking is always preferred if the condition of child permits. This decision should be taken in consultation with the surgeon, hepatologist and the critical care physicians.

34.10 Pediatric Liver Transplantation: Special Circumstances

34.10.1 Acute Liver Failure

Pediatric acute liver failure (PALF) is one of the most challenging critical illnesses which rapidly progresses into a severe multisystem organ failure with unpredictable and potentially devastating complications. The etiology varies according to age. In the neonatal period, neonatal hemochromatosis is the most common cause, whereas in children viral hepatitis, metabolic conditions and drug toxicities are the commonest. The most widely accepted consensus defines PALF as follows [9]:

Biochemical evidence of liver injury in a child without evidence of chronic liver disease.

Coagulopathy not corrected by vitamin K administration.

INR > 1.5 with encephalopathy or INR > 2 without encephalopathy.

There are many criteria which are used worldwide, but the most common criteria used is the Kings college criteria. The Kings college criteria was devised in 1989 to determine if there are any early indices of poor prognosis in patients with acute liver failure. It is important that physicians identify these patients who have less chances of spontaneous recovery and will require liver transplantation (Table 34.5).

34.10.1.1 Management of PAL

F is Management of PALF is complicated and needs a multidisciplinary team in a specialized center. The children should ideally be cared for in an intensive care unit. Intubation and ventilation are carried out pre-emptively if the child presents with encephalopathy in order to prevent aspiration and ensure oxygenation.

Once the airway has been secured the child should be nursed in a calm and quiet room. Propofol is an ideal agent for sedation if the

patient is hemodynamically stable, otherwise, opioid-like fentanyl can also be used. Muscle relaxants like Atracurium can be used to ease ventilation along with high doses of intravenous sedatives.

Once the airway is secured central venous lines and arterial lines are placed to help with regular blood sampling and administration of inotropes. Use of ultrasound while placing these catheters are recommended because of the coagulopathy associated with PALF. As with all other patients with hemodynamic compromise, maintaining adequate intravascular volume status is the first step of management. Once an adequate intravascular volume is achieved and hypotension persists, vasoconstrictor medications should be initiated.

Since raised ICP is the main cause of mortality in ALF measures should be taken to maintain ICP < 20 mm Hg. The child's head should be in a neutral position with 10–15° head up to optimize jugular—venous drainage. Given the association between intracranial hypertension and ammonia, ammonia lowering strategies should be initiated in the form of lactulose, non-absorbable antibiotics, etc. The low molecular weight of ammonia makes it amenable to dialysis, so we employ CRRT in all patients with ammonia more than 100 mmol/L. Fever and shivering must be aggressively controlled as they can lead to surges in ICP. In addition to the above measures, hypertonic saline and mannitol are also administered as part of osmolar therapy to prevent intra cranial hypertension.

Invasive monitoring of intracranial pressures in patients with acute liver failure is controversial as it is associated with bleeding complications with no benefits in overall survival. Ultrasound derived optic nerve sheath diameter and transcranial doppler to measure the pulsatility index of the middle cerebral artery might be useful noninvasive ways to measure intracranial pressure. CT scan can reliably detect the presence of cerebral edema and brain herniation, however, it is associated with the inherent risks of having to transport a critically ill patient.

As it might be expected outcomes post-liver transplantation in acute liver failure is signifi-

Table 34.5 Criteria for Liver Transplantation in Acute Liver failure

Acetaminophen-induced ALF	Non-acetaminophen ALF
1. Arterial pH < 7.3 irrespective of grade of encephalopathy	1. INR > 6.5 (PT > 100 s), irrespective of grade of encephalopathy
OR	OR any 3 of the following:
1. PT > 100 s	1. INR > 3.5 (PT > 50 s)
2. Serum creatinine >3.4 mg/dL	2. Age < 10 or > 40 years
3. Stage 3 or 4 encephalopathy	3. Serum bilirubin >18 mg/dL
	4. Jaundice to encephalopathy interval > 7 days
	5. Non-A, non-B hepatitis, syncratic drug reaction

cantly lower than those with chronic disease. The decision not to proceed for liver transplantation must be made when there are features of irreversible neurological damage like fixed dilated pupils and cerebral herniation on neuroimaging. Patients with cardiovascular instability with escalating inotropes and those with high ventilatory requirements are also unlikely to have favorable outcomes post-liver transplantation.

Intraoperative management of these patients is essentially an extension of the pre-operative ICU management. Additional venous access might have to be secured anticipating the major fluid shifts associated with liver transplantation. If the patient was on CRRT pre-operatively, it should be continued intra operatively as well. Ultrafiltrate of CRRT can be adjusted according to the hemodynamics of the patient. Pupillary reaction and symmetry must be noted at frequent intervals. It is important to know that surges of icp can occur intraoperatively due to the rapid administration of fluid and electrolytes. Continuation of CRRT during the surgery as well as judicious use of fluids, blood, and products will help in tackling this problem.

These patients are sedated and electively ventilated. Neurological monitoring should continue in the early postoperative period. CRRT can be discontinued postoperatively once there is evidence of adequate graft function. Sedation is usually continued for 24–36 h and then subsequently the sedation weaned off. The decision to extubate will depend upon the neurological recovery and adequacy of graft function.

34.10.2 Primary Hyper Oxaluria

Primary hyperoxaluria is a rare autosomal recessive disorder arising from the deficiency of the enzyme alanine glyoxylate aminotransferase located in the liver [10]. This results in the deposition of calcium oxalate crystals in kidney, progressive renal failure, and systemic oxalosis. A combined liver and kidney transplantation is the only solution that results in improved graft and patient survival. These children have varying degrees of cardiac function abnormalities and oxalate osteopathy due to oxalate deposition in the bone marrow. Aggressive renal replacement therapy should be initiated pre-operatively to keep oxalate levels at 30–45 mmol/L. Due to the massive systemic oxalate burden and slow resolubalization of oxalate, it is recommended to continue CRRT intraoperatively and for a few days after the transplantation as well.

34.10.3 Maple Syrup Urine Disease (MSUD)

MSUD is a rare genetic disorder characterized by a unique set of perioperative challenges to the anesthesiologist. It is an autosomal recessive condition caused by a deficiency of the enzyme Branch Chain Alpha Ketoacid Dehydrogenase (BCKDH). This results in excessive accumulation of branch chain amino acids, leucine, and isoleucine. Neurotoxicity is caused by these increased leucine levels with most children presenting in infancy with obtundation and coma leading to cerebral edema. These children are put on a protein-restricted diet and also requires avoidance of catabolic states like prolonged fasting and dehydration [11].

It is important to avoid catabolic states during the pre-operative fasting of these patients. This involves administration of specialized TPN which includes concentrated dextrose solutions. The plasma BCAAs should be normalized prior to surgery and dehydration and acidosis if any should be corrected. Lipid infusion can be used intraoperatively to provide calories avoiding overhydration and hemodilution, thus preventing cerebral edema.

34.11 Conclusion

It has been around 4 decades since the first successful pediatric liver transplantation. In these 4 decades huge advances have been made in the surgical and anesthetic techniques, perioperative care and immunosuppression. Very few children die intraoperatively and in the early postoperative period. However, further studies are required especially for immunosuppression where chronic rejection and lymphoproliferative disorders still cause significant loss of graft. Fast tracking is an exciting concept and is fast catching up with major pediatric transplant centers with significant improvement in outcomes.

Key Points
- Pediatric Liver Transplant necessitates the anesthesiologist to deal with distinct physiology of infants and children.
- Children are more vulnerable to hypothermia and the harmful effects associated with them.
- Managing coagulopathy is extremely important owing to the small calibre of pediatric vessels and the tendency to have thrombosis.
- The success of pediatric liver transplant depends on a multidisciplinary approach including the pediatric hepatologist, transplant surgeon, anesthesiologist, and intensivist.

References

1. Cox KL, Berquist WE, Castillo RO. Pediatric liver transplantation: iLiver transplantation in children. UK Transplant. 2005. www.uktransplant.org.uk.
2. Cox KL, Berquist WE, Castillo RO. Pediatric liver transplantation: indications, timing and medical complications. J Gastroenterol Hepatol. 1999;14(Suppl S):61–6.
3. Chin SE, Shepherd RW, Cleghorn GJ. Survival, growth and quality of life in children after orthotopic liver transplantation: a 5 year experience. J Paediatr Child Health. 1991;22:380–3.
4. Rodeck B, Melter M, Kadorff R, et al. Liver transplantation in children with chronic end stage liver disease: factors influencing survival after transplantation. Transplantation. 1996;62:1071–6.
5. Krowka MJ, Cortese DA. Hepatopulmonary syndrome: current concept in diagnostic and therapeutic considerations. Chest. 1994;105:1528–37.
6. Junge N, et al. Pediatric cirrhotic cardiomyopathy: impact on liver transplant outcomes. Liver Transpl. 2018;24(6):820–30.
7. Kavi T, Gupta A, Hunter K, Schreiber C, Shaikh H, Turtz AR. Optic nerve sheath diameter assessment in patients with intracranial pressure monitoring. Cureus. 2018;10(11):e3546. https://doi.org/10.7759/cureus.3546.
8. Arnal D, Garutti I, Perez-Peña J, Olmedilla L, Tzenkov IG. Radial to femoral arterial blood pressure differences during liver trasplantation. Anaesthesia. 2005;60:766–71. https://doi.org/10.1111/j.1365-2044.2005.04257.
9. Bhatia V, et al. Management of acute liver failure in infants and children: consensus statement of the pediatric gastroenterology chapter, Indian academy of pediatrics. Indian Pediatr. 2013;50:477.
10. Siegal D, Su WS, DaBreo D, Puglia M, Gregor L, Gangji AS. Liver-kidney transplantation in primary hyperoxaluria type-1: case report and literature review. Int J Organ Transplant Med. 2011;2(3):126–32.
11. Díaz VM, Camarena C, de la Vega Á, Martínez-Pardo M, Díaz C, López M, Hernández F, Andrés A, Jara P. Liver transplantation for classical maple syrup urine disease: long-term follow-up. J Pediatr Gastroenterol Nutr. 2014;59(5):636–9.

Challenges in Pediatric Liver Transplant

35

Neelam Mohan and Mohit Vohra

35.1 Introduction

Liver transplantation in pediatrics is a hard-won victory after the contribution from the advanced technologies and the surgical and medical expertise of the transplant team. However, considerable challenges still exist in terms of donor selection, complications following transplant and immunosuppressive barriers based on recipient's immune reactivity and immune tolerance. Creation of further improvised protocols and target-based strategies to deal early and delayed complications and to maintain long-term follow-up is still in a growing phase to meet the challenges of pediatric liver transplant. Besides robust infrastructure, advanced technologies, expertise in medical and surgical field, certain policies, protocols, and decisions need to be strengthened.

35.2 Journey till the Transplant

The child who is being taken as recipient due to an end stage liver disease embarks a unique journey from pre-transplant assessment to the post-transplantation. The first successful pediatric liver transplantation (LT) was done in 1967 by Starzl et al. [1]. Bismuth and Houssin were the first to describe the scope of reduced adult liver in the pediatric population. It was Strong who successfully transplanted the left lobe liver of the mother into her son (recipient). Since then, the science of living donor transplantation (LDLT) is ever growing crossing the obstacles one by one. With the advancement in surgical, anesthetic and medical techniques along with availability of newer immunosuppressive drugs - the outcome of LDLT have been improved worldwide. The most common form of LT performed in Asia, presently is LDLT. The factors which needs a meticulous consideration for this successful journey includes the following.

(a) Detection at the right time and timely referral.
(b) Risk identification and stratification.
(c) Donor Selection.
(d) Co-morbities management in the recipient.
(e) Technical and operational feasibilities.
(f) Successful graft uptake and survival.

35.3 Challenges in Pediatric Liver Transplant

The challenges in the pediatric liver transplant can be understood based on the age and the physiology of pediatric patients, transplanted liver

N. Mohan (✉) · M. Vohra
Department of Pediatric Gastroenterology, Hepatology & Liver Transplantation, Medanta The Medicity, Gurugram, Haryana, India

{rejection, native liver disease, and surgical complications} post-transplant care (sepsis, drug toxicity) and those related to the underlying disease (recurrence of the primary disease in allograft) and many other contributing factors. Sometimes the weight of an adolescent child is more to fulfil the criteria to accept only a single lobe from one donor and hence dual donor are being selected for the two lobes of liver in the recipient to match the required graft recipient body weight ratio (GRWR).

The challenges include timely referral, selection criteria, small for size infant, nutritional status, vaccination status, difference in anatomy and size of vessels as compared to adults (portal vein, hepatic artery and hepatic vein), associated multisystem involvement (renal, brain, cardiac) operational feasibility, medical and surgical expertise, post-transplant intensive unit (ICU) care (including sepsis, immune suppression, post-surgical complications) post-transplant morbidity, longer life expectancy, physiological immaturity, adolescence issues, transition stage to adulthood, and quality of life as compared to the peers (Table 35.1).

1. Selection of pediatric LT candidates: The guidelines or the selection criteria of the pedi-

atric LT candidates varies from center to center across the world. Although the guidelines given by North American Society for Pediatric Gastroenterology Hepatology and Nutrition (NASPGHAN) and American Association for the Study of Liver Diseases (AASLD) have clearly suggested regarding the evaluation and selection of the pediatric LT candidates. The factors such as age at diagnosis, other system involvement, metabolic liver disease, gender bias, distance from their native place to the specialized center, insurance types, and financial dilemmas besides other issues play key role in timely referral.

The commoner indications for LT for which the patient is being referred includes biliary atresia, metabolic liver disease, liver disease associated with other system anomalies like complex congenital heart disease, genetic causes of liver disease, inherited metabolic disease, and complex tumor of liver. The delay in referral not only worsens the ongoing disease but has a substantial impact on the vulnerable organs like brain development and overall growth, development and nutritional status of the child. Besides this pediatric population has lots of specificities which make them more vulnerable to the functional dis-

Table 35.1 Challenges

S. No.	Main challenges	Description
1.	Selection of patient and timely referral	Multiple factors affecting the selection criteria lack of understanding the value of in time referral
2.	Nutritional status	Malnutrition has a deleterious effect on post-transplant status
3.	Vaccination status	Vaccine preventable infections (VPI) are common post-transplant
4.	ABO incompatibility	Increased chances of rejection
5.	Operational feasibility	Advanced technology for assessment
6.	Medical and surgical expertise	Expertise in handling small for size children
7.	Post-transplant ICU care	Well-equipped pediatric ICU
8.	Post-surgical complications	Sepsis, rejection vascular, and biliary complications
9.	Immune suppression	Prolonged and severe side effects
10.	Post-transplant morbidity and mortality	Still higher rates of morbidity and mortality
11.	Physiological immaturity	Effect of metabolic and immune system on growth and development
12.	Adolescence issues	Delicate developmental period
13.	Transition stage to adult	Various psychosocial and socioeconomic issues
14.	Quality of life	Health related quality of life as compared to the peer group

abilities. The prognosis for pediatric LT is also challenging since the list of indications for the pediatric LT is vast but the sample size for the transplant is relatively small. The methods like PELD score to assess the morbidity and mortality of a child or extrapolating adult data to children are not the appropriate way to prognosticate as witnessed in many studies recently.

Despite the advancement in diagnosis and management of acute liver failure (ALF) in children, there is still inability to predict outcome in many cases. In a child presenting with ALF, the challenge is to determine whether the child has potentially treatable condition or LT is necessary and appropriate for the survival of the patient. The prognosis also depends upon the complications such as sepsis, cerebral edema, multiorgan failure, hepatic encephalopathy. Still there is a lack of robust criteria or tools to determine the survival or mortality in ALF. The existing scoring system such as King's College Hospital Criteria (KCHC) and Pediatric End Stage Liver Disease Score (PELDS) has its own limitations. KCHC is relevent only for acute liver failure patient whereas PELDS can be used for chronic liver disease in children. The two criteria KCHC & PELDS are not interchangable [2]. While our capacity to understand and deal with pediatric ALF is constantly improving it still remains a challenging entity. The short-term survival in ALF is good but the long-term survival remains poor as compared to the other indications. The timely referral to an experienced transplant center is the one of the most crucial factors altering the survival rates post-transplant [3]. LDLT with optimization of timing and less cold ischemia time has increased the survival rate.

The timely referral to LT centre is important. The process starts with Identification of patients by the referring unit in a standardized laid down manner. This will result in well timed transplantation and good outcome.

2. Nutritional Status of the child: Children with end stage liver disease offer a more complex challenge regarding the nutritional status,

growth and development, cognition, psychosocial and neuro-development. Nutritional status at liver transplant is an important prognostic factor in outcome and survival. Almost 60% of children undergoing liver transplantation are found to be malnourished. The factors contributing to the poor nutrition list includes frequent admissions, nausea, recurrent vomiting, altered gustatory sensations, ascites, altered mental status, and many more. The metabolic factors responsible are increased metabolic rate, increased resting energy expenditure [4], increased fat oxidation, elevated leptin and TNF-alpha, insulin resistance, decreased insulin like growth factor and reduced glycogen store. A malnourished child undergoing liver transplantation is at increased risk of infections with increase in morbidity and mortality. High calorie diet with protein supplements is given orally. In case of poor oral acceptance occasionally nocturnal nasogastric feeding protocol [5] is followed. High doses of fat-soluble vitamin (A, D, E, K) must be added along with water soluble vitamins in cholestatic liver disease. Increasing the protein calorie malnutrition score (PCM score) pre-transplant increases the survival rates post-transplant.

3. Vaccination and its impact: The incidence of vaccine preventable infections (VPIs) is more in transplant child as compared to general population. In the first 5 years post-transplant the incidence of hospital admission is one in six transplant recipients resulting in significant morbidity, mortality, graft injury, and cost. NASPGHAN (North American Society for Pediatric Gastroenterology, Hepatology and Nutrition) and AASLD (American Association for the Study of Liver Disease) recommend in their joint practice guideline on evaluation of the pediatric patient for transplant that "completion of all age-appropriate vaccinations should occur prior to transplantation and ideally before the development of end stage liver disease [6] and those children who have not completed the necessary vaccine schedule can receive vaccinations on an accel-

erated schedule. Immunizations are a minimally-invasive, cost-effective approach to reducing the incidence of VPIs. The importance of vaccination in pre-transplant phase is crucial because of increased immunogenicity of the vaccines given before the initiation of immunosuppressive drugs. Live vaccines are not indicated due to the risk of acquiring the disseminated vaccine strain disease in an immunocompromised host. Ideally a transplant should not occur until at least 4 weeks [7] following live vaccine administration.

4. ABO incompatible liver transplantation (ABOi LT): It is also one of the challenges which is being optimally managed by breaking the ABO barrier before LT. The recognition of the blood group antigens by recipient immune system can cause complications and graft loss in unmatched liver. As the blood group antigens exist on bile ducts epithelium, the chances of progressive intrahepatic bile duct injury are more [8]. The development of anti--A/B antibody reducing immunosuppressive protocols including plasmapheresis, immunoglobulin, and use of immunomodulators such as rituximab which have made the outcome after living donor (LD) ABO incompatible LT equivalent to that achieved with LD ABO-compatible (ABO-c) [9] (Fig. 35.1).

5. Operational Feasibility: The availability of the latest imaging apparatus using the modern techniques is required to precisely assess the finer anatomical details of the vessels. An effective pre-operative imaging evaluation provides a broad understanding of the vascu-lar size and anatomy of celiac axis, and portal vein, hepatic veins, inferior vena cava besides the parenchymal status and morphology of liver. The ultrasound doppler and CECT with arterial phase sequences provides the information regarding any anatomical variants and accurate vascular measurements. The diameter of portal vein can be measured at the probable anastomosis level which can help us in assessing the chances of portal vein stenosis.

The classification of hepatic artery anatomic variants given by Michel has 10 sub-types, the sub-types II, III, V and IX are most significantly associated [10] with LDLT. In children the multiple arterial feeders in the grafts can cause poor perfusion of the graft. This may require creation of an alternate interposition graft between aorta and hepatic artery for an alternate inflow. Hepatic artery variants usually do not affect liver transplant but only in case the right hepatic artery arises from the superior mesenteric artery which requires for bench reconstruction.

6. Medical and Surgical expertise: The innovative and advanced surgical techniques over the last few years have overcome the hurdles of finding the size matched donors especially in small children. There is tremendous improvement in the graft and patient survival at 1 year after liver transplantation of more than 85%. The long-term survival of these patients is due to fair graft function despite complications. The need for re-transplantation has been decreased significantly. Over the years the surgical skillful techniques of using split, reduced

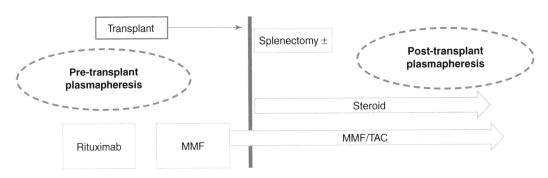

Fig. 35.1 ABO-Incompatible transplant

and living related transplantation have increased the pool and the survival of liver transplantation in children The surgical expertise has managed the technical challenges including vascular anatomy, sufficient volume for metabolic demands of the patient, and biliary drainage. The surgical skills in using the split liver from deceased donors and partial grafts from living donors has resulted in better and prolonged graft viability. The use of a left lateral segment graft (segments II and III) enables to do away the discrepancy of donor to recipient size ratio. For very small babies a further reduction of the left lateral segment is possible to provide a single segment graft (segment II or III). Early surgical interventions for post-operative bleeding, hepatic artery thrombosis or the hepatic or portal vein obstruction often needed for immediate surgical revascularization for salvaging the graft. The uncommon complications like bowel perforation and phrenic nerve injury may also require the surgical expertise for correction-although rarely required [11]. All the above surgical interventions are incomplete without the expert medical management under the guidance of the team headed by pediatric hepatologist.

7. ICU care post-transplantation: The surgery affects almost every system of the body. The patient is shifted to critical care unit immediately after the transplantation with or without tracheal intubation. The intensive critical unit stay is usually directly proportional to the time of extubating after surgery. The early weaning from ventilator is advocated if the patient is hemodynamically active. In patients of long-standing portal hypertension pulmonary vasodilatation results in shunting which leads to desaturation and hence hepatopulmonary syndrome which may require high positive end expiratory pressures keeping the target spo2 > 92% [12]. The other pulmonary complications include pulmonary edema, pleural effusion (right more than left), atelectasis, ventilator associated pneumonia, and very rarely acute respiratory distress syndrome.

Sepsis is the leading cause of morbidity post-transplantation. The infections probably result from donor, post-operative wounds, central venous catheter and intra-arterial catheter and lower respiratory tract from nosocomial sources. Sepsis is frequently encountered and one of the most dreaded complications which can increase the mortality rate. In suspected nosocomial infections hospital culture-based protocol is followed. Central catheters and fungal infection on prolonged antibiotics are also an issue for which vigilant protocols are followed. The feasibility between the immunosuppressant and antibiotics are to be tightly regularized. Serial CRP, procalcitonin, and blood culture plays the pivotal role in upgrading the antibiotics and antifungal drugs accordingly.

Another important parameter in children to be monitored is hemodynamic stability. The volume status of the child depending upon the total intake (oral and intravenous) and output (urine and abdominal drain or aspirates) is an important tool to assess the hemodynamic stability. The hemodynamic status can be measured using invasive to non-invasive methods. The invasive methods include intra-arterial blood pressure monitoring, cardiac output monitoring, and other methods which varies from center to center. The clinical states which may affect the urine output status of the child and indirectly affecting the hemodynamic stability includes hepatorenal syndrome and syndrome of inappropriate antidiuretic secretion (SIADH). To obtain the optimal hemodynamic status of the child requiring fluids, inotropes or vasopressors for optimum cardiac output, the clinical and advance hemodynamic monitoring guides to monitor the actual fluid status.

The electrolytes imbalance is very crucial and need a careful monitoring in post-transplant child. The common electrolyte disturbances seen in post-transplant child are as follows [12].

Electrolyte imbalance needs to be closely monitored and carefully addressed to avoid potential harmful effects like hemolysis, cerebral,

Table 35.2 Electrolyte disturbances

Electrolyte abnormality	Mechanism
Hyponatremia	Common in end staged liver disease. Fluid with high sodium resulting in rapid increase should be avoided
Hyperkalemia	Ischemia -perfusion process during transplant
Hypocalcemia	Citrate in blood products given during surgery chelates calcium
Hypophosphatemia	Increased uptake by regenerating hepatocytes, intracellular shifts
Transient hyperglycemia	Additional insulin infusion may be required

neuromuscular, and myocardial irregularity (Table 35.2).

The neurological complications account for 13–43% in post-transplant children observed in a 1 year follow-up study [13]. The complication usually occurs in first 2 weeks post-transplantation. The commonest manifestation is seizure which is frequently of generalized tonic-clonic variety. The probable causes include hypoglycemia, hypomagnesemia, hyponatremia. Cerebral infarction, hypertension, posterior reversible leukoencephalopathy syndrome (PRES), and adverse effects of immunosuppressive drugs. The modalities of investigations include electroencephalogram (EEG) and brain imaging. The differential diagnosis includes prolonged unconsciousness due to the use of benzodiazepines (Hepatic insufficiency prolongs half-life), intracranial hemorrhage, and meningitis. The antiepileptic of choice is levetiracetam [14] because it does not have liver metabolism and minimum drug interactions.

Another area of pediatric intensive unit care is gastrointestinal (gi) involvement in terms of high gastric aspirates or a paralytic ileus. Such complications sometimes might need re-exploration.

The nutrition of the child even post-transplantation is a big challenge. The aim of 120% of basal energy expenditure and protein supplementation in the range of 1.0–1.3 g/kg/day is fulfilled to promote good wound healing and hepatocyte recovery post-liver transplant [4]. Glucose infusion rate (GIR) should be around 2–3 gm/kg body weight per day of glucose with the frequent sugar monitoring and keeping the blood glucose range between 140 and 180 mg/dl [15]. The role of total parenteral nutrition (TPN) is reserved only in the cases where the cough and swallow reflexes are compromised. The enteral nutrition should be initiated within 12–24 h post-liver transplantation or as soon as possible to prevent the atrophy of intestinal cells and maintain the structural and the functional integrity of the gut. The other advantages of early enteral feeding include prevention of translocation of microorganisms, prevention of bile stasis, and stimulation of portal blood flow.

Late complications. Post-surgical complications:

(a) Early.

- Acute rejection: Acute cellular rejection as a complication usually occurs between 7 days and 6 weeks postoperatively. It is less common in infants (20%) but increases to 40–50% in older children. In majority of cases, it responds with increase in dose of immunosuppression and high dose of steroids.

- Sepsis: It is one of the dreaded complications following transplant. Bacterial infections are common soon after transplant and are related to pretransplant status of the patient, malnutrition and lowered immunity secondary to immunosuppression, malnutrition and pre-transplant status of the patient. In suspected nosocomial infections, hospital-based culture protocols are followed. Fungal infection due to prolonged use of broad spectrum antibiotics and Catheral Related Blood Stream Infection (CRBSI) require stringent protocols.

- Vascular thrombosis and venous outflow obstruction: Portal vein thrombosis occurs in 10–40% in post-Kasai biliary atresia patients usually secondary to narrow fibrotic portal vein. Hepatic artery thrombosis is considered as one of the most devastating complications and it may cause graft loss with increased morbidity and mortality without immediate thrombectomy either by interventional radiology team or surgery [16]. Re-transplant may also be required in these cases. The smaller size of vessels in children make them more prone to this complication as compared to adults. The hepatic artery thrombosis may result in biliary necrosis secondary to ischemia leading to biliary strictures. Hepatic vein stenosis resulting in outflow tract obstruction may present with ascites.

- Biliary Complications Early biliary complications can occur anytime within 12 weeks of transplant. These complications can be biliary leaks, calculi, obstruction or strictures. These complications are commonly observed in reduced size graft recipients. Dysfunction of sphincter of oddi, although rare but is also a documented cause of biliary complications.
- Surgical complications: This includes sudden intra-abdominal hemorrhage due to a surgical cause like slipped ligature which requires re-exploration. Gut perforation may also be seen especially in previously operated patients of biliary atresia with peritonitis.

(b) Late:

- These fall into two categories related to allograft itself sand those related to immunosuppressive drug (IS). These include late biliary stricture, EBV infection, late hepatic artery or portal vein thrombosis, post-transplant lymphoproliferative disease (PTLD), de novo auto immune hepatitis. Nephrotoxicity, hyperlipidemia, obesity, diabetes, hypertension, and hirsutism may occur sequential to immunosuppressive drugs.
- Immunosuppression: This is the critical step in liver transplantation which achieves the balance between allograft rejection and infection. The physiological differences between children and adult makes the use of immunosuppression in children more challenging and more complex. The differences in children as compared to adults includes as follows.

  - Pharmacodynamic and pharmacokinetics of the drugs in children based on their physiology.
  - Lack of clinical trials in children.
  - Incomplete immunization status makes prone towards VPI.
  - Challenges regarding adherence and transition to adulthood.
  - Continuous and close monitoring for the adverse effects and appropriate management of intercurrent infections.
  - Longer exposure period needs continuous assessment of impact on growth and development. The commonly used drugs are steroids, tacrolimus, mycophenolate mofetil, and newer renal protective drugs like sirolimus and everolimus. Under-suppression may lead to rejection which is responsible for graft dysfunction and is being commonly reported in children. It has been observed most commonly within first 6 months of transplant and late acute rejection being observed with non-adherence.

9. A variety of factors contribute to the challenges of immunosuppressive medications in infants and young children. Dispensing medicines as compounded suspension for exact medication concentration, unpalatability of drugs (especially for infants and toddlers) and interaction between supplements, nutrition and immunosuppressive drugs are the most difficult issues to tackle. The common challenges with immunosuppressive drugs are being tabulated (Table 35.3).

Another challenge in children being more prone towards Epstein–Barr Virus (EBV) infection

Table 35.3 Drug dispensing

S. No.	Compounding factor
1.	Dispensing drug as liquid and matching exact concentration
2.	Co-administration of drugs with milk, antacids, and iron may cause chelation of drugs
3.	Presence of food may alter the rate and extent of absorption. Example: Mycophenolate (MMF) to be taken empty stomach for optimal effect
4.	Certain medication needs to be refrigerated and suspension should be shaken before giving like MMF
5.	Children needs 2.7–4.4 times higher dose per kg to reach the same serum concentration
6.	In case of refusal to drug in toddlers nasogastric tube is put to ensure drug delivery
7.	Bone marrow suppression, gastrointestinal disturbances, QTc prolongation, nephrotoxicity, bone disease, and photosensitivity with IS drugs are commoner in children
8.	On-going steroids may lead to short stature, diabetes, hypertension, cosmetic changes (cushingoid facies and striae), mood swings
9.	Gingival and hirsutism are commoner in children with the use of cyclosporine
10.	Neuropsychological deficits and lower cognitive function due to disease and prolonged exposure to immunosuppressive drugs

and more likelihood of PTLD which require alteration in immunosuppressive goals. Immunosuppression following LT is usually high in the initial 3–6 months and gradually tapered thereafter [17]. Development of immune tolerance requiring no immunosuppression is still a subject of understanding in liver transplantation [18].

10. Post-transplant morbidity and mortality: After transplant the currently reported survival rates are more than 95% at 1 year and 85% at 10 years. Children lead a near normal life style including attainment of puberty and development of secondary sexual characteristics and acceptable reproductive life. However, timely and regular follow-up with doctor and frequent blood sampling cannot be ignored. In a series of 200 paediatric transplant from author's center in India, 1-year and 5-year survival rate was 94% and 87% respectively with no statistical difference between the children weighing less or more than 10 kg [19, 20].

11–14. (Physiological Immaturity, Adolescent issues, Transition into adulthood, and Quality of life) The liver transplant recipients who were small children may have challenges once they reach adolescent age. The challenges are not only physical but also psychological, emotional, social, and financial. The main concerns faced in adolescence are mainly the distorted body images, a low feeling for below average academic performance. The mood swings are due to phases of anxiety and depression for the future. In children frequent hospital visits, everyday medication can lead to behavioural issues. This can result in strained parent peer relationship and non adherence to drug regime. Because of the incomplete education, low physical strength makes them seek low profile job which again is an area of disappointment for them.

These challenges are to be tackled by regular counseling of the recipient child and the family by the health care professional. The family including the child may be kept in follow-up of psychologist for timely consult on behavioral and other relevant issues. The government needs to frame policies to provide jobs to liver transplant recipients with a security and a handsome amount to meet the financial challenges of the treatment. Non-government organization should assist such patients in getting the financial support for the long-term medication and daily living. The Ministry of Health needs to take steps to make the non-affording children to complete their studies and create window of opportunities for the kids undergone liver transplant under 18 years. Social isolation due to learning disabilities should be condemned.

References

1. Starzl TE, Hakala TR, Shaw BW Jr, Hardesty RL, Rosenthal TJ, Griffith BP, Iwatsuki S, Bahnson HT. A flexible procedure for multiple cadaveric organ procurement. Surg Gynecol Obstet. 1984;158:223–30.
2. Squires RH, Ng V, Romero R, Ekong U, Hardikar W, Emre S, Mazariego GV. Evaluation of the pediatric patient for liver transplantation: 2014 practice guideline by the American Association for the Study of Liver Diseases, American Society of Transplantation and the North American Society for Pediatric Gastroenterology. Hepatology. 2014;60(1):362–98.
3. Ng VL, Mazariegos GV, Kelly B, Horslen S, McDiarmid SV, Magee JC, et al. Barriers to ideal outcomes after pediatric liver transplantation. Pediatr Transplant. 2019;23(6):e13537. https://doi.org/10.1111/petr.13537.
4. Pawlowska J. The importance of nutrition for pediatric liver transplant patients. Clin Exp Hepatol. 2016;2(3):105–8.
5. Carter-Kent C, Radhakrishnan K, Feldstein AE. Increasing calories, decreasing morbidity and mortanlity: is improved nutrition the answer to better outcomes in patients with biliary atresia? Hepatology. 2007;46(5):1329–31.
6. Feldman AG, Curtis DJ, Moore SL, Kempe A, et al. Under-immunization of pediatric transplant recipients: a call to action for the pediatric community. Pediatr Res. 2020;87(2):277–81.
7. Danzinger-Isakov L, Kumar D, AST Infectious Diseases Community of Practice. Guidelines for vaccination of solid organ transplant candidates and recipients. Am J Transplant. 2009;9 Suppl 4:S258–S62.
8. Honda M, Sugawara Y, Kadohisa M, Shimata K, Sakisaka M, Yoshii D, Uto K, Hayashida S, Ohya Y, Yamamoto H, Yamamoto H, Inomata Y, Hibi T. Long-term outcomes of ABO-incompatible pediatric living donor liver transplantation. Transplantation. 2018;102:1702. https://doi.org/10.1097/TP.0000000000002197.
9. Chaosun N, ma, Chong Dong. The management and outcomes of ABO-incompatible pediatric liver transplantation: experience of a single Chinese center. J Pediatr Surg. 2020;55(12):2647–52.
10. Vohra S, Goyal N, Gupta S. Preoperative CT evaluation of potential donors in living donor liver transplantation. Indian J Radiol Imaging. 2014;24(4):350–9.
11. Goldaracena N, Echeverri J, Kehar M, Deangeis M, Jones N, Ling S, Kamath BM, Avitzur Y, Ng VL, Cattral MS, Grant DR, Ghanekar A. Pediatric living donor liver transplantation with large- for -size left lateral segment grafts. Am J Transplant. 2020;20(2):504–12.
12. Hocky Pudjiadi A. Intensive care management to reduce morbidities following pediatric liver transplantation in Indonesia. J Transpl Reports. 2020;5(4):100064.
13. Nemati H, Kazemi K, Mokarram AT. Neurological complications associated with pediatric liver transplant in Namazi Hospital: one-year follow-up. Int J Organ Transplant Med. 2019;10(1):30–5.
14. Varamphil JJ, Shanmugam N. Post liver transplantation complications: diagnosis and management of seizures. In: Pediatric liver intensive care. Singapore: Springer; 2019. p. 133–136.
15. Cameron R, Kogan-Liberman D. Nutritional considerations in pediatric liver disease. Pediatr Rev. 2014;35(11):493–6.
16. Hackl C, Schlitt HJ, Melter M, Knoppke B, Loss M. Current developments in pediatric liver transplantation. World J Hepatol. 2015;7(11):1509–20.
17. Miloh T, Andrea B, Justin W, Pham T, Hewitt W, Keegan T, Sanchez C, Bulut P, Goss J. Immunosuppression in pediatric liver transplant recipients: unique aspects. Liver Transpl. 2017;23(2):244–56.
18. Tanimine N, Ohira M, Tahara H, Ide K, Tanaka Y, Onoe T, Ohdan H. Strategies for deliberate induction of immune tolerance in liver transplantation: from preclinical models to clinical application. Front Immunol. 2020;11:1615.
19. Mohan N, Karkra S, Rastogi A, Dhaliwal M, et al. Outcome of 200 pediatric living donor liver transplantation in India. Indian Pediatr. 2017;54:913–8.
20. Ueda M, Oike F, Ogura Y, et al. Long term outcome of 600 living donor liver transplants for pediatric patients at a single centre. Liver Transpl. 2006;12:1326–36.

Intensive Care Issues in Post-operative Pediatric Liver Transplantation

36

Maninder Dhaliwal and Veena Raghunathan

36.1 Introduction

Pediatric liver transplantation (LT) has become a standard and definitive treatment for end stage liver disease over last few decades. Advances in pre-transplant care, operative techniques, and post-operative intensive care have led to consistent improved survival and better outcomes. Although the pre-operative condition of patient has an important role in affecting outcome, yet it is not the sole determinant [1]. LT can be successful even in critically ill patients with appropriate supportive care. In more recent years, sicker patients with complicated comorbidities are undergoing LT. Recent addition of certain metabolic diseases as an indication for LT makes the post-operative care even more complex and challenging. This underlines the larger and more crucial role of intensive care management of these children peri-operatively. Pre-existing liver dysfunction associated comorbidities such as hepatopulmonary syndrome, hepatorenal syndrome, etc. along with post-transplant variables such as allograft dysfunction, infection, and surgical issues makes them an unique cohort which requires certain level of expertise to be handled in

intensive care. Careful monitoring, anticipation of problems, and pre-emptive action are essential components to post-LT intensive care management for successful outcomes.

36.2 General Principles

The anesthetist dealing with the child during the liver transplant (LT) operation should accompany the patient to the intensive care unit and a detailed handover should be given to the pediatric intensivist. Handover details should cover all the important intra-operative events such as blood loss, ionotropic requirement, and change in ventilatory requirements when the abdomen is closed, etc. In the liver intensive care unit (ICU) continuous monitoring of vital parameters such as arterial blood pressure (ABP), electrocardiogram (ECG), peripheral oxygen saturation (SpO2), central venous pressure (CVP), and temperature is continued. Some units do additional monitoring with NIRS (near infrared spectroscopy), ScvO2, and SjvO2 monitoring. Bedside ultrasound (USG) and echocardiography are now a routine practice in most of the liver ICU.

Head end elevation, 30–45°, is preferred in normotensive patients. All drains and catheters (nasogastric, bladder, intra-abdominal, biliary, etc.) must be emptied initially and amounts noted. Subsequently hourly output should be measured

M. Dhaliwal (✉) · V. Raghunathan
Department of Pediatric Critical Care, Medanta The Medicity, Gurugram, Haryana, India
e-mail: maninder.dhaliwal@medanta.org

and recorded. Drain output is usually replaced on hourly basis. In addition the colour and consistency of drains is monitored to assess the intra abdominal bleeding. Chest radiograph is performed in all patients to check endotracheal tube position (if intubated) and for assessing lung condition (like collapse, effusion, consolidation etc.). Lung imaging may be repeated if required and regular bedside lung USG (no radiation exposure) can also be performed to assist in diagnosing and decision making. Laboratory investigations include arterial blood gas, complete blood count, coagulation profile (prothrombin time PT/activated partial thromboplastin time PTT, thromboelastogram TEG, fibrinogen), liver and renal function tests, and serum electrolytes (sodium Na, potassium K, magnesium Mg, calcium Ca, chloride Cl, and phosphorous P). Blood investigations are typically repeated 6–12 hourly depending on patient condition. Culture surveillance (blood, urine, endotracheal, and drain fluid) are usually sent depending on institutional protocol. USG Doppler for hepatic vessels and portal vein flow, as a standard should be done daily in children for up to 1 week post-operatively. In infants and small children, some units do twice daily USG Doppler for early detection of vascular issues.

Short-acting, non-hepatotoxic medications are preferred for analgo-sedation during the duration of ventilation (propofol, fentanyl, etc.). Prophylactic antibiotic and antifungal therapy (as per institution protocol) and immunosuppressive therapy are administered. Anticoagulation in the form of either intravenous heparin infusion or low molecular weight subcutaneous heparin may be initiated in high risk patients (small size artery, Budd-Chiari or previous hypercoagulopathy, etc.), with close monitoring of coagulation and clinical parameters to avoid bleeding.

elevate intrathoracic pressures and impair venous return form inferior vena cava and hepatic veins resulting in graft congestion and loss. As a rule extubation is done as early as possible provided biochemical parameters and hemodynamics are stable, with a good liver vessel doppler study. However, the decision to extubate has to be individualized based on pre-operative comorbidities (such as encephalopathy, hepatopulmonary syndrome, etc.) or post-LT complications (such as graft dysfunction, fluid over load, etc.).

Pediatric patients on an average require <48 h of mechanical ventilation post-LT [2]. In selected subgroup of stable patients, tracheal extubation is occasionally feasible immediately at the end of surgical procedure (fast tracking) [3]. Few adult studies have shown that adequate gas exchange can be maintained in cases of early extubation (in O.R or within 3 h of surgery) with no significant difference in the rate of reintubation [3]. However, optimal selection criteria for candidates for early extubation in pediatric LT are not well defined. Also, it is not correct to extrapolate results from a center which advocates fast tracking to any another due to differences in pre-operative condition, surgical skill and duration, graft size and abdominal status, and other factors [4]. Early extubation is generally more feasible in the older children compared to the younger ones and infants [5].

There is an emerging important role for noninvasive ventilation (NIV) and heated humidified high flow nasal cannula (HHHFNC), post-LT. By providing PEEP, NIV is useful to prevent lung atelectasis post-extubation, especially in children with compliant chest walls. This also allows for earlier and safer extubation subsequently leading to lower rates of pneumonia and sepsis post-LT [6].

36.3 Post-op Ventilation and Oxygenation

Lung protective strategy should be generally adopted with tidal volumes 6–8 ml/kg to target a plateau pressure < 30 cm H_2O. High positive end expiratory pressure (PEEP) (>10 cm H_2O) can

36.4 Fluids and Hemodynamics

For the liver graft to function well, it is important to maintain euvolemic state during immediate post-transplant period. Though input–output chart during surgical procedure gives a rough idea on fluid status, it is really difficult to assess the exact status particularly in small infants as insensible and abdominal fluid losses cannot be judged accurately. Several parameters such as heart rate, inferior vena cava (IVC) filling, urine output, post-transplant weight, and CVP are used in combination to access the intravascular volume status. The ultrasonic cardiac output monitors (USCOM) are a more reliable tool in accessing fluid status in such scenario [7].

Hypovolemia can lead to impaired hepatic perfusion, whereas excessive fluids can lead to venous congestion in allograft and can cause graft loss. The pre-existing liver disease induced vasodilatory state, myocardial dysfunction, etc. may resolve slowly over few days post-LT; this may also contribute to hypotension and can explain the need for continued minimal vasopressor/inotrope support in such cases. Dyselectrolytemia, metabolic derangements, reperfusion syndrome, and primary graft dysfunction can all lead to postoperative hemodynamic instability.

In cases of hypovolemia, careful controlled fluid resuscitation should be carried out, with meticulous and continuous reassessment. Synthetic colloids have been demonstrated to be as effective as albumin for fluid resuscitation [8]. Norepinephrine is the usual vasopressor of choice in pediatric post-LT patients. In cases of myocardial dysfunction, dobutamine is conventionally used. Hypertension has also been described in 20–70% patients of pediatric patients undergoing LT [9, 10]. This occurs due to interplay of multiple variables: high volume status, steroid, calcineurin inhibitor, and high renin levels. Medications used to treat hypertensive crisis include sodium nitroprusside infusion or calcium channel blockers initially. Angiotensin converting enzyme inhibitors and beta blockers are subsequently added as needed. Hypertension must be well controlled in the post-LT patient as there is higher risk of bleeding due to the presence of coagulopathy/thrombocytopenia in these patients.

36.5 Electrolytes and Metabolic Issues

Lactate in post-LT patient have a special role. In addition to diagnosing and treating shock, lactate is a good surrogate marker of good graft function during immediate post-transplant period. The lactate reaches peak during anhepatic phase of surgery and once the new allograft is implanted the lactate should start showing a declining trend. Persistent hyperlactatemia or progressive increase after surgery is a marker for graft dysfunction. Usual maintenance fluid in children is 5% or 10% dextrose with additives. This is to provide at least 4–6 mg of glucose/min. In case of hyperglycemia, rather than decreasing the dextrose concentration, providing adequate glucose along with insulin infusion should be carried out. This hyperglycemia can be due to transient insulin resistance during postoperative period. On the other hand, persistent hypoglycemia should alert the possibility of graft dysfunction.

Most of the children with chronic liver disease (CLD) would be having long standing hyponatremia before surgery. This may require low sodium fluids during post-LT period, to avoid rapid increase in serum sodium levels. Regular electrolyte monitoring is essential. Hypocalcemia may be present, especially if a patient has received massive amounts of blood products (citrate-induced). This needs to be corrected. Hypokalemia and hypomagnesemia may also occur and have to monitored regularly and should be appropriately supplemented.

36.6 Pulmonary Issues

1. Pleural effusion: Pleural effusions are very common post-LT (around 30%) and seen most often on the right side [4]. This pleural fluid collection is usually reactionary, and is due to movement of ascitic fluid across the diaphragm. Fluid collection also occurs due to surgical

handling and placement of a foreign graft tissue below the diaphragm. Most of these effusions resolve spontaneously with careful restriction of volume intake and/or cautious diuretic therapy. Chest tube insertion is rarely needed; only if respiratory compromise occurs.

2. Atelectasis: This is a unique concern, especially in the smaller children, which can delay extubation or lead to respiratory distress post-extubation. Patients who are malnourished or have abdominal distension have added risk. Regular chest physiotherapy post-LT plays both a preventive as well as therapeutic role to achieve lung expansion.

3. Pulmonary edema: This can occur due to fluid overload and/or myocardial dysfunction. Careful attention to volume status and fluid restriction is the key to prevent this.

4. Ventilator induced pneumonia (VAP): prolonged post-op ventilation could predispose to VAP. Strict asepsis, implementation of VAP bundle, early extubation, non-invasive ventilation, and regular physiotherapy helps in reducing the risk.

5. Acute respiratory distress syndrome (ARDS): The mechanism for development of ARDS post-LT are manifold. These include transfusion related acute lung injury (TRALI), severe reperfusion injury, and infection induced ARDS. Low tidal volume with high PEEP strategy is the dictum for ventilator strategy in ARDS, the same is applicable to the post-LT scenario. Inhaled nitric oxide may be used in cases of refractory hypoxemia. Role of HFOV and prone ventilation is unclear, but if indicated it is used.

6. Right hemidiaphragm paralysis due to phrenic nerve injury is a rare complication which may hamper weaning process [11].

36.7 Post-operative Hematological Issues: Bleeding and Coagulopathy

Most of the children who undergoes LT are coagulopathic. Due to the usage of various blood products during the surgery, PT/International normalized ratio (INR) measured at 4–6 h after surgery would reflect the true coagulation profile. Coagulation is also used as marker of graft functionality. During immediate post-operative period PT/INR is monitored on regular interval to check that it is improving. In case of progressive worsening of INR, fibrinogen and platelets are to be checked and are usually corrected before giving fresh frozen plasma (FFP). While correcting coagulopathy risk of bleeding must be carefully balanced against risk of thrombosis of hepatic vessels. Overcorrection of coagulopathy and thrombocytopenia should be avoided. Thromboelastography (TEG) is useful to guide the type and amount of blood component transfusion needed along with PT/PTT, fibrinogen, and platelet counts [12]. The usual target levels are INR 1.5–2, fibrinogen >100 mg/dl and platelet >50,000/mcL [13]. But these target parameters are not the rule always, clinical examination and surgical team inputs are necessary before giving blood products.

Thrombocytopenia is commonly seen post-LT and may persist for about 2 weeks: it occurs due to platelet activation and consumption following reperfusion and hypersplenism. Some centers advocate target threshold of <20,000/mcL along with active bleeding to transfuse platelets [14]. Monitoring of serial blood Hb levels along with drain Hb level and drain amount will help to identify active ongoing bleeding. Imperfectly achieved surgical hemostasis (e.g.: slippage of surgical knot), hypocalcemia, and thrombocytopenia can cause postsurgical bleed. In cases of persistent or increasing bleeding, re-exploration is indicated. Intra-operative use of recombinant factor VII has been shown to control profuse bleeding without increasing rate of thrombotic events. Restrictive transfusion strategy is advocated as it has been shown to improve patient outcomes [15].

36.8 Gastrointestinal (GI) Concerns

1. Ileus: Post-operative ileus may occur due to the use of analgesia, intra-operative gut handling, dyselectrolytemia (e.g.: hypokalemia),

and occasionally sepsis. In patients with biliary atresia with kasai portoenterostomy, LT procedure is complicated by bowel adhesions, thereby increased risk of perforation in such patients. Bowel perforation during post-LT period may be silent with absence of classical signs such as rigidity, fever, etc. due to immunosuppressive drugs. In cases of clinical suspicion (persistent abdominal pain, increasing gastric aspirates, and abdominal distension) further evaluation with imaging (abdominal CT) is essential and abdominal re-exploration would be required in some cases. Elevated abdominal drain amylases and visibly dirty abdominal drain could give clue towards intestinal perforation.

2. Gastrointestinal (GI) bleeding: Stress-induced and steroid induced gastroduodenal ulceration can lead to upper GI bleeding post-LT. Massive upper GI bleed is usually from esophageal varix secondary to portal vein (PV) thrombosis, hence urgent evaluation by endoscopy and ultrasound doppler must be done. Any lower GI bleed or hematochezia requires CT angiography to look at bleeding site in small and large bowel. The management consists of cessation of antiplatelet drugs and anticoagulants. PT/aPTT, platelet count, fibrinogen need to be evaluated and blood product support needs to be given according to laboratory and clinical parameters. Upper GI endoscopy is essential in cases of significant bleeding; it has both diagnostic and therapeutic value.

3. Intra-abdominal hypertension: Intra-abdominal hypertension can occur occasionally in the smaller babies, where graft size is large, leading to a tight closure. This is detrimental to liver perfusion and may also lead to progressive shock and organ dysfunction, particularly kidneys. There must a high alert for this complication whenever large grafts are used, and occasionally the abdomen is left open and temporary closure devices are used in order to prevent this complication.

36.9 Neurological Issues

Children who were ventilated due to encephalopathy prior to LT, neurological recovery might be slow as the cerebral oedema takes time to resolve. Seizures during post-LT period is not uncommon and could occur in around 30% cases [15]. Etiology for seizures during post-LT would include dyselectrolytemia, hypertension, calcineurin inhibitor toxicity, posterior reversible encephalopathy syndrome (PRES), acute cerebral infarctions, hemorrhages, continue myelinolysis (CPM), [9, 16] etc. Though serum electrolytes levels might be normal, rapid fluctuations in serum electrolytes due to multiple colloids and crystalloids are also implicated as important risk factor. Screening CT of brain to be performed in all children with seizure to rule out any bleed or vascular event. Self-limiting brief seizures usually does not require treatment. For recurrent seizures or a single seizure with potentially epileptogenic abnormalities on brain imaging or EEG, antiepileptic drug (AED) therapy should be initiated. Levetiracetam is the drug of choice for post-LT seizures due to lack of significant hepatic metabolism or drug interactions. AEDs can usually be discontinued after 1–3 months, provided the child is seizure-free and EEG is normal. Other neurological disturbances such as headache, confusion, hallucinations, tremor, and speech apraxia can be seen due to adverse effects of immunosuppressive drugs.

36.10 Acute Kidney Injury (AKI)

AKI during post-LT is multi-factorial. Pre-transplant status (severe liver dysfunction, shock, hepatorenal syndrome), intra-operative hemodynamic instability, prolonged use of vasoconstrictors, massive blood transfusions, post-op use of immunosuppressive agents (tacrolimus, cyclosporine), antibiotics (aminoglycosides, colistin), and antifungals (amphotericin B) with nephrotoxic side effects could all contribute towards AKI. Hemodynamic-mediated AKI generally resolves spontaneously. Several renoprotective agents (dopamine, prostaglandins) have been studied but none have been proven to be effective to prevent post-LT (AKI) [17]. In case of worsening AKI: reducing/withholding tacrolimus should be considered. Alternative agents like sirolimus, and/or mycophenolate mofetil can be given for immunosuppression [18]. Whenever feasible nephrotoxic drugs like aminoglycosides, colistin, and amphoterin B must be avoided. When AKI is advanced causing fluid and metabolic issues in critically sick children, continuous renal replacement therapy (CRRT) is the preferred modality of management.

36.11 Immunosuppression

Calcineurin inhibitors (CNIs) particularly tacrolimus forms the mainstay of immunosuppression after LT. It is a potentially nephrotoxic agent and has many undesirable side effects. Tacrolimus doses are adjusted by drug level monitoring. Of particular note is the drug interaction between fluconazole and tacrolimus. Azole antifungals inhibit the metabolism of tacrolimus mediated by CYP3A4. Steroid are used as adjutants during immediate post-transplant period and gradually weaned in 3–6 months. Different institutes have their own policy/protocol on steroid weaning. Other drugs which are used include mycophenolate mofetil (B & T cell proliferation inhibitor, renal sparing, no drug level monitoring needed), cyclosporine (T helper cell inhibitor), sirolimus (IL-2 transduction inhibitor), and IL2 receptor blocking antibodies (Daclizumab, basiliximab). Detailed discussion of immunosuppression is beyond the scope of this article. Table 36.1 enlists the side effect profile of the commonly used agents. Research is ongoing to develop new immunosuppressive protocols which are renal sparing and steroid free.

Table 36.1 Common drugs used in liver transplant and their side effect profile

Drug	Side effects
Glucocorticoids	Hypertension Dyselectrolytemia Gastroduodenal ulceration Mood disturbances Fluid retention Hyperglycemia Pancreatitis
Tacrolimus	Hypertension Nephrotoxicity Hyperglycemia Seizures and neurological symptoms (tremor, headache, etc.)
Cyclosporine	Hypertension Neurological symptoms (seizure, headache, confusion) Nephrotoxicity Dyselectrolytemia Gingival hyperplasia
Mycophenolate mofetil	Anemia, thrombocytopenia, leukopenia Hypertension Dyselectrolytemia Myopathy Tachycardia
Sirolimus	Anemia, thrombocytopenia, leukopenia Hyperlipidemia Poor wound healing

36.12 Infections

Post-LT patients are at high risk for infection. Pre-operative liver dysfunction and malnutrition along with the use of post-operative immunosuppression and presence of multiple devices (central lines, drains, etc.) in situ make them prone for acquiring infections. Post-transplant prophylactic antibiotics are given for 5 days and are usually stopped. Antifungal prophylaxis (oral fluconazole) is given as a institutes protocol for 2–3 weeks or until patient is discharged from hospital. If the recipient is cytomegalovirus (CMV) negative and the donor is CMV positive, treatment with intravenous ganciclovir is given for at least 2 weeks. Clinical signs of sepsis may be subtle due to steroids/immunosuppression. Laboratory septic parameters must be closely followed for development of leukocytosis/leukopenia and positive cultures; and focus of infection must be sought. Prompt treatment with appropriate broad spectrum or specific antibiotics/antifungal is an essential component.

36.13 Nutrition

Nutritional support is an important part of post-LT care. Pre-operative malnutrition, surgical stress, and steroid administration all contribute to increased nutritional demand post-op. Pre-operative malnutrition is associated with higher risk of post-LT infections and longer ICU stay. Caloric intake should be aimed at 120–130% of calculated basal energy expenditure and protein intake of 1.5–2 g/kg must be provided [19]. Early enteral nutrition has been shown to be beneficial and causes lesser metabolic issues and decreased infection rates [20]. Since most of the infants with LT would have hepaticojejunostomy immediate enteral nutrition might not be practically possible. In such children with malnutrition, total or partial parenteral nutrition is recommended from post-op day one until 50–70% enteral feeds are achieved. Replacing abdominal drain loss with intravenous 5% albumin is another strategy to prevent protein loss.

36.14 Early Post-operative Complications Specific to Liver Graft

36.14.1 Primary Graft Failure

This is a dreaded complication of LT where the new liver graft fails to function. Though the exact reason is unclear, many factors such as advanced donor age, prolonged ischemic time (>18 h), >30% macrosteatosis, and reperfusion injury have been implicated [21]. Liver dysfunction is severe (transaminases usually >5000 U/L) and hypoglycaemia and coagulopathy occur. Management is mainly supportive: high concentration dextrose infusion, regular FFP transfu-

sion, and appropriate neuroprotective measures and renal support are given. Prostaglandin E1 and N-acetyl cysteine infusion have been used across various centers, however, results have not been consistent. If there is no graft recovery in 24–36 h, emergency re-transplantation is indicated, without which progressive multiorgan dysfunction and eventually death results.

36.14.2 Size Discrepancy of Graft

The ideal graft should be 0.8–2% of recipient body weight. Size discrepancy is problematic in both ways—both large and small sized grafts have their own set of issues. When Graft to recipient weight ratio (GRWR) < 0.8% (small for size) congestion of the graft may occur due to high portal flow resulting in delayed synthetic liver function, cholestasis and increased susceptibility for infections. However, this is not common in the small-sized pediatric patient. Large for size transplants (GRWR > 4) even with use of split/reduced grafts can occur especially in patients <10 kg [22]. Abdominal closure in these cases may be tight or not completely possible. Higher intrabdominal pressures may lead to abdominal compartment syndrome and compromised blood perfusion to the new liver graft. In some cases full abdominal closure is not possible; and temporary abdominal mesh/bogota bag need to be placed followed by closure after 2 weeks [22].

36.14.3 Rejection

Acute rejection can occur at any time after LT but is common in first 5–10 days post-LT. Clinical manifestations may be absent or subtle in mild to moderate rejection, while in severe rejection non-specific symptoms such as fever, abdominal pain, etc. can be present. Any rise in transaminases above base line should raise the possibility of rejection. Liver biopsy is essential for confirmation and will show lymphocytic infiltrate in the portal space. Duct and endothelial damage can be seen and in severe cases hepatocyte destruction occurs. Adjustment in baseline immunosuppressive drug doses along with pulse dose steroids usually suffices as treatment [20]. Rejection must be recognized and managed early, as it is detrimental for graft survival. A close differential is a sepsis, differentiating this needs careful interpretation of clinical and laboratory parameters.

36.14.4 Vascular Issues

Hepatic artery thrombosis (HAT): This is a potentially fatal complication with an incidence of 1.5–25% in children [23]. It is more common in children compared to adults and more so in living donor transplants as the anastomosis is between smaller sized vessels. Sensitivity of doppler ultrasound to detect HAT can be 100% and should be performed daily for the first week post-LT. CT arteriography is confirmatory when vessel cannot be identified on ultrasound. After detection, urgent thrombectomy is indicated either by surgical or radiological interventional technique [24]. Failure to detect or intervene in cases of HAT leads to rapid graft necrosis and death. Urgent retransplantation is indicated if revascularization of hepatic artery is not achieved. Prophylactic low molecular weight heparin, antiplatelet drugs (aspirin), systemic anticoagulation (in high risk cases) are used based on institution-specific protocols. HAT and biliary complications are interlinked as the biliary tract is almost exclusively supplied by hepatic artery.

Portal vein thrombosis (PVT): Clinical manifestations include worsening signs of portal hypertension (GI bleeding due to varices, increasing ascites, encephalopathy) and worsening liver function tests. The diagnosis is by doppler ultrasound. Early thrombosis is usually successfully relieved by surgical/radiological interventional procedure or by emergency shunt surgery to relieve the portal hypertension. Late thrombosis are usually persistent and tend to get compensated over time.

36.14.5 Biliary Issues

These are known as the "Achilles heel" of LT and are more frequent in living donor transplantation [25]. Bile leak can occur due to faulty surgical anastomosis, necrosis or biliary tract ischemia.

Cut surface leak can also occur especially in case of split/partial grafts. Bile leaks usually occur towards the end of the first week post-LT. They can present as fever, bilious abdominal drain, increased gamma-glutamyl transferase (GGT), and leukocytosis. Biliary leak increases the risk of fungal sepsis. While in older children who had duct to duct anastomosis; ERCP and stenting can help while in small children with hepaticojejunostomy, usually surgical intervention is required to detect and repair site of leak. Biliary strictures may occur late in the post-LT course which are treated by percutaneous/endoscopic dilatation or surgical re-exploration.

36.15 Conclusion

Post-LT intensive care management involves anticipation of problems and pre-emptive intervention. Essential components of PICU care include hemodynamic stabilization, early extubation, appropriate fluid-electrolyte therapy, strict asepsis, early recognition, and appropriate management of sepsis, AKI, and organ dysfunction. Unique aspects of monitoring in post-LT children include monitoring graft function and flow in hepatic vasculature. Prompt identification and treatment of complications is the key to reduce mortality and morbidity post-LT.

Key Points

- Post-operative intensive care in pediatric liver transplantation is complex and challenging.
- Optimal fluid management and hemodynamics are essential for liver graft functioning and successful outcomes.
- Early extubation must be targeted; NIV is an emerging useful adjunct to prevent pulmonary complications and allow early extubation.
- Thorough knowledge of graft and vascular issues are essential for anticipation and timely management of complications which are unique to liver transplantation.

References

1. Chologitas E, Betrosian A, Senzolo M, Shaw S, Patch D, Manousou P, et al. Prognostic models in cirrhotics admitted to intensive care units better predict outcome when assessed at 48 h after admission. J Gastroenterol Hepatol. 2008;23:1223–7.

2. Tannuri U, Tannuri AC. Postoperative care in pediatric liver transplantation. Clinics. 2014;69(S1):42–6.

3. Biancofiore G, Bindi ML, Romanelli AM, Boldrini A, Bisà M, Esposito M, Urbani L, Catalano G, Mosca F, Filipponi F. Fast track in liver transplantation: 5 years' experience. Eur J Anaesthesiol. 2005;22:584–90.

4. Kukreti V, Daound H, Bola SS, Singh RN, Atkinson P, Kornecki A. Early critical care course in children after liver transplant. Crit Care Res Pract. 2014;2014:725748.

5. Ulukaya S, Ayanoglu HO, Acar L, Tokat Y, Kilic M. Immediate tracheal extubation of the liver transplant recipients in the operating room. Transplant Proc. 2002;34(8):3334–5.

6. Antonelli M, Conti G, Bufi M, Costa MG, Lappa A, Rocco M, Gasparetto A, Meduri GU. Noninvasive ventilation for treatment of acute respiratory failure in patients undergoing solid organ transplantation: a randomized trial. JAMA. 2000;283:235–24.

7. Su B-C, Lin C-C, Su C-W, Hui Y-L, Tsai Y-F, Yang M-W, Lui P-W. Ultrasonic cardiac output monitor provides accurate measurement of cardiac output in recipients after liver transplantation. Acta Anesthesiol Taiwan. 2008;46:171–7.

8. Boldt J, Priebe HJ. Intravascular volume replacement therapy with syntetic colloids: is there an influence on renal function? Anesth Analg. 2003;96:376–82.

9. Mohan N, Karkra S, Rastogi A, Dhaliwal M, Raghunathan V, Goyal D, et al. Outcome of 200 pediatric living donor liver transplantation in India. Indian Pediatr. 2017;54:913–8.

10. Ganschow R, Nolkemper D, Helmker K, Harps E, Commentz JC, Broering DC, et al. Intensive care management after pediatric liver transplantation: a single-center experience. Pediatr Transplant. 2000;4(4):273–9.

11. Garcia S, Ruza F, Gonzalez M, et al. Evolution and complications in the immediate postoperative period after pediatric liver transplantation: our experience with 176 transplantations. Transplant Proc. 1999;31(3):1691–5.

12. Wang SC, Shieh JF, Chang KY, Chu YC, Liu CS, Loong CC, Chan KH, Mandell S, Tsou MY. Thromboelastography-guided transfusion decreases intraoperative blood transfusion during orthotopic liver transplantation: randomized clinical trial. Transplant Proc. 2010;42:2590–3.

13. Gopal BP, Kapoor D, Raya R, Subrahmanyam M, Juneja D, Sukanya B. Critical care issues in adult liver transplantation. Indian J Crit Care Med. 2009;13:113–9.

14. Kim J, Yi NJ, Shin WY, Kim T, Lee KU, Suh KS. Platelet transfusion can be related to liver regeneration after living donor liver transplantation. World J Surg. 2010;34:1052–8.

15. Lacroix J, Hebert PC, Hutchison JS, et al. Transfusion strategies for patients in pediatric intensive care units. N Engl J Med. 2007;356:1609–19.

16. Beresford TP. Neuropsychiatric complications of liver and other solid organ transplantation. Liver Transpl. 2001;7:S36–4.

17. Cabezuelo JB, Ramírez P, Ríos A, Acosta F, Torres D, Sansano T, et al. Risk factors of acute renal failure after liver transplantation. Kidney Int. 2006;69:1073–80.

18. Tannuri U, Gibelli NE, Maksoud-Filho JG, Santos MM, Pinho-Apezzato ML, Velhote MC, et al. Mycophenolate mofetil promotes prolonged improvement of renal dysfunction after pediatric liver transplantation: experience of a single center. Pediatr Transplant. 2007;11(1):82–6.

19. Plauth M, Cabré E, Riggio O, Assis-Camilo M, Pirlich M, Kondrup J, DGEM (German Society for Nutritional Medicine), Ferenci P, Holm E, Vom Dahl S, Müller MJ, Nolte W, ESPEN (European Society for Parenteral and Enteral Nutrition). ESPEN guidelines on enteral nutrition: liver disease. Clin Nutr. 2006;25:285–94.

20. Hasse JM. Nutrition in clinical practice. Gastrointestinal disorders and their connections to nutrition. Nutr Clin Pract. 2008;23:259.

21. Uemura T, Randall HB, Sanchez EQ, Ikegami T, Narasimhan G, McKenna GJ, et al. Liver retransplantation for primary nonfunction: analysis of a 20-year single-center experience. Liver Transpl. 2007;13(2):227–33.

22. Akdur A, Kirnap M, Ozcay F, Sezgin A, Ayvazoglu Soy HE, Karakayali YF, et al. Large-for-size liver transplant: a single center experience. Exp Clin Transplant. 2015;13(Suppl 1):108–10.

23. Crippin J. Pathogenesis/pathology of organ dysfunction. In: Norman DJ, Suki WN, editors. Primer on transplantation. Mt Laurel, NJ: American Society of Transplantation Physicians; 1998. p. 321–7.

24. Gibelli NE, Tannuri U, Velhote MC, Santos MM, Gibelli NE. Hepatic artery thrombosis after pediatric liver transplantation: graft salvage after thrombectomy and reanastomosis. In: IV Congresso Brasileiro de Transplante de Fígado, Pâncreas e Intestino Delgado [Brazilian congress of liver, pancreas and small bowel transplantation] and III Encontro de Transplantadores de Pâncreas e Pâncreas-rim [Meeting of pancreas and kidney-pancreas transplant surgeons], Belo Horizonte, 2004.

25. Duailibi DF, Ribeiro MAF. Biliary complications following deceased and living donor liver transplantation: a review. Transplant Proc. 2010;42:517–20.

Part VII

Post-operative Issues

Fast Tracking in Liver Transplantation

37

Pooja Bhangui and Prachi Gokula

37.1 Introduction

Liver transplantation (LT) since its inception has undergone a paradigm shift not only in terms of technique and perioperative patient management, but also in terms of recipient outcomes following transplant. While deceased donor liver transplantation (DDLT) is the predominant form of LT performed in the West, lack of adequate number of deceased donations, fueled the need for living donor liver transplantation (LDLT) in the East [1]. Today, Asia leads the world in terms of numbers of LDLTs, technical innovations, and success with LDLT, with some centers performing more than 200 LTs annually [2].

With the increasing feasibility and acceptable outcomes with LT in patients with end-stage liver disease (ESLD), the focus has now shifted from just "good" postoperative recovery to "rapid" recovery, and early discharge from hospital. The concept of "fast tracking" liver transplant recipients has thus emerged.

Traditionally, all liver transplant recipients have been subjected to a certain mandatory period of mechanical ventilation in ICU, with gradual weaning off. This practice of mandatory mechanical ventilation in patients after a major surgery was first challenged in cardiac anesthesia by Prakash et al. [3], and then expanded to other surgical disciplines, and major surgical procedures including LT.

The multisystem effect of ESLD, associated comorbidities typically seen in these patients like diabetes mellitus, obesity, cirrhotic cardiomyopathy, and sometimes a poor performance status makes immediate extubation difficult after LT. However, with evolution of the surgical and anesthetic practices successful early extubation and fast tracking in liver transplantation has indeed become a reality, and its implementation can be further expanded, especially in experienced and high volume centers.

37.2 Definition and Evolution of Fast Tracking in LT

"Fast tracking (FT)" aims at rapid progress from preoperative preparation to surgery and early discharge. There are varying definitions of FT in LT. While some authors have restricted it to on-table (in the operating room) extubation [4], others have broadened the use of the term to include tracheal extubation within 3 h of surgery [5]. Recently, complete avoidance of ICU has also been incorporated in the concept of fast tracking [6].

Prakash et al. [3] first demonstrated that early extubation either immediately or within 3 h of a

P. Bhangui (✉) · P. Gokula
GI and Liver Transplant Anesthesia, Institute of Anesthesia and Critical Care, Medanta-The Medicity, Gurgaon, India
e-mail: pooja.bhangui@medanta.org; Prachi.Gokula@Medanta.org

© The Author(s), under exclusive license to Springer Nature Singapore Pte Ltd. 2023
V. Vohra et al. (eds.), *Peri-operative Anesthetic Management in Liver Transplantation*,
https://doi.org/10.1007/978-981-19-6045-1_37

major surgical procedure was possible. His team successfully extubated 123 out of 142 adult patients within 3 h of open heart surgery.

The concept of early extubation with its attendant benefits was then further extrapolated to other major surgeries including liver transplant recipients [4]. Rossaint et al. [7] reported that they were successful in extubating 5 out of 36 recipients immediately after LT, and the rest was extubated within an average of 6 h after LT. There were no pre-defined selection criteria in their study for immediate extubation. Based on their findings, they proposed that use of minimal fluids during the surgery was one of the keys to early extubation. Fluid management in their patients was based upon fall in cardiac index and ventricular filling pressures.

Mandell et al. [4] further evaluated the feasibility and cost effectiveness of fast tracking in liver transplant recipients in two institutions, University of Colorado (UC) and University of California at San Francisco (UCSF). At UC, pre- and intraoperative criteria, derived from retrospective analysis of patients who were successfully extubated within 8 h of surgery, were established. UNOS status 3/4, absence of comorbidities, age <50 years, and no hepatic encephalopathy were preoperative criteria; whereas, good donor liver function, <10 units of packed RBC transfusion during surgery, no vasoactive support at the end of surgery and alveolar-arterial oxygen gradient <150 mmHg were the intra operative criteria, which could predict planned extubation in the OR and FT. At UCSF, patients were given trial of extubation without any pre-structured criteria, based on clinical judgment of the attending anesthesiologist. Sixteen of 67 patients at UC, and 25 of 106 patients at UCSF, were immediately extubated. Retrospective comparison of the results between two universities also proved the cost effectiveness and feasibility of successful immediate extubation.

These initial studies were then followed by attempts at early extubation in other LT centers around the world. Two of the largest published series included those reported by Baincofiore et al. (211/365 recipients extubated on table) and

Skurzak et al. (575/652 recipients extubated on table) [8, 9]. In their experience over 5 years, Biancofiore et al. [8] noted a progressive increase in the fraction of patients who were immediately extubated in OR as the study period progressed, and towards the end of the study period, 82.5% of recipients were extubated on table. Only 2 of the 211 immediately extubated patients needed re-intubation. Their study showed that the MELD score of 11 had the best predictive value for rapid extubation. Skurzak et al. [9] generated a prognostic score for safe operating room extubation after liver transplantation (SORELT) score (Table 37.1) based upon the data from 597/652 patients extubated on table.

Table 37.1 Proposed clinical criteria for operating room extubation after liver transplantation

Mandell et al. [8]	
Preoperative criteria	UNOS status 3 or 4
	Age <50 years
	No comorbidities
	No encephalopathy
Intraoperative criteria	Good donor liver function
	Administered RBCs <10
	No vasoactive support at the end of surgery
	Alveolar- arterial O₂ gradient <150 mmHg
Mandell et al. [6]	
Encephalopathy and BMI index >34 predicted extubation failure	
Biancofiore et al. [9]	
MELD score of less 11 correlated positively with successful extubation in OR	
Cammu et al. [10]	
Preoperative criteria	No acute liver failure or encephalopathy
Intraoperative factors	Good donor liver function
	Less than 10 U of packed red blood cells
	Hemodynamic stability
	Alveolar-arterial oxygen gradient of less than 200 mmHg

Table 37.1 (continued)

Skurzak et al. [11]
• SORELT score—safe operating room extubation after liver transplantation
Major criteria
• 7 units packed red blood cells transfused intraoperatively
• Lactate ≥3.4 mmol/L at end of surgery
Minor criteria
• Patient not at home
• Duration of surgery ≥5 h
• Vasopressors at end of surgery—dopamine >5 µg/kg/min or norepinephrine >0.05 µg/kg/min)
SORELT score-derived criteria (fewer than two major/ one major plus two minor/ three minor criteria) were considered for OR extubation
Bhangui et al. [12]
Pre-operative criteria
• Age <50 years
• Patient BMI <22–26 kg/m²
• METS >4
• Admission from home
• Well-controlled co-morbid condition (diabetes mellitus, hypertension, thyroid disease)
• MELD score <20, CTP class A, B (only selected CTP Class C patients)
Intraoperative criteria
• Use of <5 units of packed red blood cells during surgery
• Low inotropic requirement at the end of surgery (single inotrope, noradrenaline dose <0.05 mcg/kg/min)
• Decreasing trend of lactates on arterial blood gas post reperfusion
• Short duration of surgery (<12 h)
• Actual GRWR ratio >0.7
• Low-risk vascular anastomoses (especially hepatic artery anastomosis, no multiple arterial anastomoses, no size mismatch)
Patients with hepatic encephalopathy/renal replacement therapy (SLED, CRRT)/fulminant hepatic failure/morbid obesity/co-existing HPS or POPH were excluded
Chae et al. [13]
• Preoperative psoas muscle index positively correlates with successful immediate extubation
• Intraoperative factors—CRRT, development of significant PRS and FFP transfusion requirements negatively influence the proposition of early extubation

With the success of early extubation in the OR, the concept of fast tracking was given a further impetus by Mandell et al. [11] publishing

their successful attempt to directly shift the extubated patients to surgical ward, thereby completely bypassing the ICU. Out of 147 patients enrolled in the study, 111 were extubated immediately post-surgery. 83 patients /111(74.7%) and 28/111 (25.3%) were successfully transferred to surgical ward and IMCU respectively, without intervening ICU care.

37.3 To Fast Track or Not? That's the Question

37.3.1 Be Careful Before You Fast Track

Historically, LT recipients have been electively ventilated for 48 h with the rationale that positive pressure ventilation with sedation may decrease surgical stress, improve hemodynamic stability, and facilitate early recovery [14]. Although there is evidence in favor of early extubation protocols, still a section of clinicians prefer the traditional approach of a certain mandatory period of postoperative mechanical ventilation followed by gradual weaning off.

Liver transplant being a complex procedure is associated with extreme hemodynamic alterations often putting the recipients and their cardiopulmonary system under varying degrees of stress, and the practice of early extubation may not provide the required time for the patient to recuperate.

A period of mechanical ventilation and gradual weaning off allows optimization of the cardiopulmonary system and promotes recovery from the stress of surgery. The possible need for re-explorations also adds to the reluctance in early extubation.

37.3.2 Benefits of the Fast Track Approach

Proponents of early extubation often argue in favor of avoiding the complications associated with mechanical ventilation. Kaiser et al. [15] reported the negative impact of PEEP on liver graft hemodynamics. This was, however, challenged by Saner et al. [16] who proposed that a PEEP of up to 10 mbar did not influence hepatic arterial and venous flow. Although controversial, positive pressure ventilation can alter the liver hemodynamics adversely, thereby early extubation helps in preventing graft dysfunction from impaired hepatic hemodynamics. Apart from decreasing the complications of positive pressure ventilation, early extubation is definitely associated with increased patient comfort and compliance.

Immunosuppressed post-LT recipients may also be particularly vulnerable to ventilator-associated pneumonia with prolonged ventilation. Prolonged mechanical ventilation may also increase right ventricular afterload and even induce venous congestion of the liver graft, especially in those with pre-existing tricuspid regurgitation and raised pulmonary artery pressures (which is not uncommon in end-stage liver disease patients). Furthermore, hepatic venous drainage is better in spontaneously breathing patients as it reduces intrapleural pressure, thereby increasing cardiac end-diastolic volume, which in turn increases cardiac output and hepatic blood flow. Improved donor graft circulation could aid in early liver graft recovery and regeneration.

In terms of cost effective practices, early extubation definitely scores higher as it decreases the cost incurred during the ICU stay, and also a reduced cost due to the shorter length of hospital stay. This improved utilization of resources is especially pertinent in developing nations with limited resources at their disposal. In a systematic review by Rando et al. [17] in 2011, practice of early extubation was shown to be associated with decreased ICU stay and overall shorter hospital stay, thereby decreasing the overall economic burden. It was therefore recommended that early extubation could be carefully applied in new programs, as it helps in reducing cost of ICU stay without subjecting the patients to increased risks. Similarly, Loh et al. [18] found a decrease in 2.5–3 days in the length of hospital stay following a fast tracking protocol post-LT, with significant savings in health care cost.

37.4 Anesthesia For Fast Tracking

Advances in balanced anesthesia techniques and monitoring systems allowing rapid arousal from anesthesia, like use of remifentanil (due to its rapid elimination), may aid in FT [19].

Some of the principles to guide anesthesia for FT include the following:

(a) Balanced anesthesia using barbiturates/propofol combined with opioids at induction, followed by maintenance with inhalational agents along with narcotic infusion. Anesthesia is typically maintained with continuous infusion of rocuronium/cis-atracurium and fentanyl infusion with Isoflurane in air/O_2 gas mixture.

(b) Monitoring includes electrocardiography, pulse oximetry, invasive arterial pressure, central venous and advanced venous access, and continuous cardiac output monitoring.

(c) Dose regulation of inhalational agents: requirements of various drugs, including inhalational agents decrease significantly during anhepatic phase. Similarly, higher MELD score is also associated with decreased requirement of inhalational agents.

(d) Careful titration of anesthetic agents to prevent over dosage and delayed emergence. Bispectral index monitoring thereby plays a significant role in patients planned for early extubation.

(e) Neuromuscular blockade using different NMDAs ranging from vecuronium and rocuronium to atracurium and cis-atracurium. Since, different NMDAs undergo variable hepatic metabolism, neuromuscular monitoring becomes an essential tool to monitor the degree of muscle strength prior to trial of extubation.

(f) Adequate titration of the total dosage of *opioids* used in the perioperative period to ensure adequate analgesia and anesthetic depth, without causing excessive sedation and respiratory depression. Liver transplant recipients have reported to have reduced opioid requirement in the perioperative period when compared with patients undergoing other major abdominal surgeries. Another option is to use fentanyl-free periods intermittently during the surgery, instead of continuous fentanyl since it has a long context-sensitive time.

(g) In possible candidates of immediate extubation, muscle relaxant and opioid infusion can be discontinued upon ensuring good flow on Doppler ultrasound on completion of all vascular anastomoses and adequate graft function. Prior to extubation, adequate hemostasis by the surgeon should be confirmed and required correction of abnormal TEG values, if any, should be ensured. Patients, thereafter, meeting the extubation criteria can be safely given a trial of immediate extubation.

37.5   Fast Tracking in the LDLT Setting

Most of the studies that have reported on feasibility and safety of fast tracking have been in the DDLT setting. There is a difference though between the DDLT and LDLT recipients. In adult-to-adult LDLT, the partial graft (right or left lobe) usually takes time to regenerate and attain optimal function. Higher incidence of vascular complications leading to re-exploration is a possibility owing to small size and stumps of vessels in the harvested graft. In addition, surgical duration, and consequently total anesthesia time for the recipient, is also more in LDLT compared to DDLT. Hence, experience with only a few cases of FT LDLT recipients has been published so far [10, 20, 21]. Bhangui et al. [21] reported successful extubation in OR in 15 LDLT recipients, which comprised only 2% of LDLTs performed during the study period, this confirms the difficulty in fast tracking LDLT recipients even in high volume, and experienced LDLT center. Fast-tracked patients were young, had a low BMI, most were CTP class A or B, had a low MELD score, METs' score of 4–6, and no significant comorbidities. Also, most fast-tracked patients had no need for major BT. None of the patients in this subgroup required immediate re-intubation, all recovered well with short ICU and hospital

stay and there were no major complications. Chae et al. [13] based upon a relatively large number of subset of LDLT recipients proposed preoperative psoas muscle index to positively correlate with successful immediate extubation.

LDLT is an opportunity for an "elective" procedure, hence adequate patient and donor preparation, as well as planning for immediate postoperative care is possible in the LDLT setting. Thus, experienced anesthesia teams in high volume LDLT centers should try and fast track more recipients in the near future.

37.6   Criteria For Fast Tracking

The search for ideal criteria for planned on table extubation, and fast tracking in the recipients is still on. Predetermined criteria could help streamline the perioperative course of the patients and increase the number of patients who can be given the trial of early extubation. Each institution has indeed defined criteria for patient selection based upon their unique patient profile, often influenced by their national selection policy for organ allocation.

However, in general, extubation criteria employed in various studies till date have broadly remained similar. Parameters used to assess the adequacy of neuromuscular reversal are - patient breathing spontaneously, awake, able to follow simple commands, respiratory rate ≤35 breaths/min, tidal volume ≥5 mL/kg and heart rate ≤20% above baseline.

Table 37.1 summarizes the various clinical criteria for operating room extubation after liver transplantation, as proposed by several authors.

37.7   Future Prospects

An optimal utilization of resources by reducing ICU and overall hospital stay, without any apparent increase in adverse effects as a direct consequence, should encourage more anesthetists to attempt fast tracking in a well selected group of recipients.

One of the arguments often stated for reluctance in adopting the concept fast tracking is the lack of evidence based on comparable patient data with different national policies in selection criteria of patients. As a consequence, results of these studies cannot be extrapolated to local institutions dealing with sicker or a different profile of patients.

Fast tracking can be viewed as a component of an enhanced recovery program after surgery (ERAS) but it lacks the definite end goals as described in different stages of ERAS program [12]. Thereby, the lack of required multimodal and multidisciplinary approach towards a common goal has been a hurdle in the wider acceptance of FT in LT. Incorporation of multidisciplinary team approach in the care of liver transplant recipients can be a step in the required direction. Different multispecialty teams should be involved in preoperative optimization of the patients with effective plan of care tailored to meet and address the uniqueness of each patient and their disease process. With the commitment on part of surgeons, anesthesiologists, and other disciplines, in conjunction with dynamic interactions between them at various stages of perioperative care can help us achieve the desired results.

Key Points

- Fast tracking in liver transplantation is feasible and is cost effective.
- Early extubation is one of the ingredients of fast tracking.
- Possible fast tracking patients should be identified before transplantation.
- There is a difference between DDLT and LDLT recipient for fast tracking as surgical duration much longer in LDLT.
- There should be pre-defined criteria for extubating patient in operating theater.
- Acute liver failure patient are ineligible for on table extubation.

References

1. Lee SG. Asian contribution to living donor liver transplantation. J Gastroenterol Hepatol. 2006;21:572–4.
2. Bhangui P, Sah J, Choudhary N, et al. Safe use of right lobe live donor livers with up to 20% macrovesicular steatosis without compromising donor safety and recipient outcome. Transplantation. 2020;104:308–16.
3. Prakash O, Jonson B, Meij S, et al. Criteria for early extubation after intracardiac surgery in adults. Anesth Analg. 1977;56:703–8.
4. Mandell MS, Lockrem J, Kelley SD. Immediate tracheal extubation after liver transplantation: experience of two transplant centers. Anesth Analg. 1997;84:249–53.
5. Biancofiore G, Romanelli AM, Bindi ML, et al. Very early tracheal extubation without predetermined criteria in a liver transplant recipient population. Liver Transpl. 2001;7:777–82.
6. Aniskevich S, Pai SL. Fast track anesthesia for liver transplantation: review of the current practice. World J Hepatol. 2015;7:2303–8.
7. Rossaint R, Slama K, Jaeger M, et al. Fluid restriction and early extubation for successful liver transplantation. Transplant Proc. 1990;22:1533–4.
8. Biancofiore G, Bindi ML, Romanelli AM, et al. Fast track in liver transplantation: 5 years' experience. Eur J Anaesthesiol. 2005;22:584–90.
9. Skurzak S, Stratta C, Schellino MM, et al. Extubation score in the operating room after liver transplantation. Acta Anaesthesiol Scand. 2010;54:970–8.
10. Aneja S, Raina R. Immediate postoperative extubation after liver transplantation at our centre: a report of two cases. Indian J Anaesth. 2011;55:392–4.
11. Mandell MS, Lezotte D, Kam I, Zamudio S. Reduced use of intensive care after liver transplantation: influence of early extubation. Liver Transpl. 2002;8:676–81.
12. Brustia R, Slim K, Scatton O. Enhanced recovery after liver surgery. J Visc Surg. 2019;156(2):127–37.
13. Chae MS, Kim JW, Jung JY, et al. Analysis of pre- and intraoperative clinical for successful operating room extubation after living donor liver transplantation: a retrospective observational cohort study. BMC Anesthesiol. 2019;19:112.
14. Stock PG, Payne WD. Liver transplantation. Crit Care Clin. 1990;6:911–26.
15. Kaisers U, Langrehr JM, Haack M, Mohnhaupt A, Neuhaus P, Rossaint R. Hepatic venous catheterization in patients undergoing positive end-expiratory pressure ventilation after OLT: technique and clinical impact. Clin Transpl. 1995;9:301–6.

16. Saner FH, Olde Damink SW, Pavlaković G, et al. Is positive end-expiratory pressure suitable for liver recipients with a rescue organ offer? J Crit Care. 2010;25:477–82.

17. Rando K, Niemann CU, Taura P, Klinck J. Optimizing cost- effectiveness in perioperative care for liver transplantation: a model for low- to medium-income countries. Liver Transpl. 2011;17:1247–78.

18. Loh CA, Croome KP, Burcin Taner C, Keaveny AP. Bias-corrected estimates of reduction of post-surgery length of stay and corresponding cost savings through the widespread national implementation of fast-tracking after liver transplantation: a quasi-experimental study. J Med Econ. 2019;22:684–90.

19. Nöst R, Thiel-Ritter A, Scholz S, Hempelmann G, Müller M. Balanced anesthesia with remifentanil and desflurane: clinical considerations for dose adjustment in adults. J Opioid Manag. 2008;4:305–9.

20. Cammu G, Decruyenaere J, Troisi R, et al. Criteria for immediate postoperative extubation in adult recipients following living-related liver transplantation with total intravenous anesthesia. J Clin Anesth. 2003;15:515–9.

21. Bhangui P, Bhangui P, Gupta N, et al. Fast tracking in adult living donor liver transplantation: a case series of 15 patients. Indian J Anaesth. 2018;62:127–30.

Early Post-operative Care of Liver Transplant Recipient

38

Sachin Gupta and Deeksha Singh Tomar

38.1 Introduction

Liver transplant (LT) has become a very viable and successful option for patients with both acute and chronic liver disease with advances in the management technique. It is a multidisciplinary collaboration which leads to higher graft survival rates. As the experience and acceptability of LT is increasing, sicker population are being considered for this definitive treatment. High quality and dedicated critical care management is required for increasing the graft survival and also to prevent any complications arising due to other distant organ dysfunctions in these sicker population in the immediate post-operative period.

The early post-operative period is a very critical phase and it involves very stringent monitoring of various organ functions such as cardiorespiratory function, the graft performance, renal functions, and any other unexpected complications arising due to non-hepatic issues. The intensive care unit (ICU) management revolves around optimal hemodynamic stabilization, judicious fluid management to avoid fluid overload, assessing and preserving kidney function, pre-

vention of graft rejection, and very strict infection control practices.

38.2 General Considerations

The immediate post-operative period is an extension of the intra-operative period and the entire focus should be on optimal ventilation to avoid hypoxemia and hypercarbia, optimization of fluid administration to avoid both hypo-and hypervolemia, and assessment of graft function. The ICU team should be made aware of the pre-LT status of the patient like the model-for end stage-liver-disease (MELD) score; intra-operative clinical course like the need for transfusion, total fluid administered, vasopressors needed, acid-base status; and the graft quality like graft-to-recipient weight ratio (GRWR), graft steatosis if any [1]. The ICU should also be aware of any incidence of reperfusion syndrome in the intra-operative period.

The LT recipient after shifting to ICU should undergo certain physiological and laboratory parameter monitoring as given in Table 38.1.

S. Gupta (✉) · D. S. Tomar
Narayana Superspeciality Hospital, Gurgaon, India

Table 38.1 Monitoring in the immediate post-operative period (within first 24 h)

Physiological monitoring	Laboratory parameters
Mandatory	Arterial blood gas with
Electrocardiogram (ECG)	lactate levels (frequency depends on criticality)
Central venous pressure (CVP)	Complete hemogram
Invasive arterial pressure	Renal function test
	Liver function test
Rectal temperature	Blood sugar
Ventilatory parameters	Electrolytes
Conscious level off sedation	Coagulation parameters
	Chest X-ray
Total intake output including drain output	Drain bilirubin
Optional or if present	Drain hemoglobin
Cardiac output	
Extravascular lung water	
Pulmonary artery wedge pressure	
Jugular venous oxygen saturation (SjVO$_2$)	

38.3 Cardiovascular and Hemodynamics

All efforts should be done to prevent hypotension in the immediate postoperative period as it is the most common complication. If hypotension persists, then it leads to graft ischaemia and compromises graft recovery [2, 3]. The hemodynamic behavior of immediate post-LT patient is a continuum of the pre-operative status i.e. high cardiac output with low systemic vascular resistance (SVR). *Due to this vasodilated state, there is always a propensity for central hypovolemia leading to hypotension* [4]. Hypotension can also be due to ongoing bleeding due to coagulopathy, major fluid losses due to high drain output or even sustained reperfusion syndrome.

One should always keep a high index of suspicion for cardiovascular complications as LT patients are at high risk to develop these complications. The incidence of pulmonary edema, arrhythmias, dilated cardiomyopathy (also known as Takotsubo Cardiomyopathy or stress cardiomyopathy or apical ballooning syndrome or broken heart syndrome), myocardial ischaemia or shock is up to 70% in patients post-LT [5, 6].

Pulmonary edema is probably the most common complication after LT with an incidence as high as 47% [5, 7]. The possible reasons are fluid shifts that happen in the immediate post-operative period due to increase in SVR and high cardiac afterload. The fluid therapy should be very judicious and if possible one should take use of invasive hemodynamic monitoring tools like VolumeView if present. The conventional static indices like central venous pressure (CVP) monitoring is erratic and should not be relied upon to judge the preload status of the patient. *The fluids administered for optimization of hemodynamics should be a combination of both crystalloid and colloids like albumin.* As these patients have a tendency for fluid sequestration, albumin should form a major component of fluid therapy in the immediate post-operative period. Non-invasive techniques like bedside use of ultrasound (Fig. 38.1) to perform inferior vena cava measurement, lung ultrasound to look for B-Lines indicative of wet lungs and calculate velocity time integral by 2D echocardiogram should be done to optimize fluid management.

Patients can have subtle signs like tachycardia and hypotension which are early features of cardiomyopathy or even myocardial ischaemia. Electrocardiogram, 2D ECHO and if needed coronary angiogram should be performed for definitive diagnosis and management.

The drain losses should be replenished around two-thirds volume with 5% albumin so as to maintain adequate intravascular volume [8]. Vasopressor like norepinephrine should be used whenever hypotension persists after adequate volume resuscitation. The presence of systemic hypertension is as high as 50% [9] in the postoperative period and should be managed initially with intravenous labetalol and then later on converted to oral drugs like calcium channel blockers or beta blockers.

Fig. 38.1 Lung ultrasound

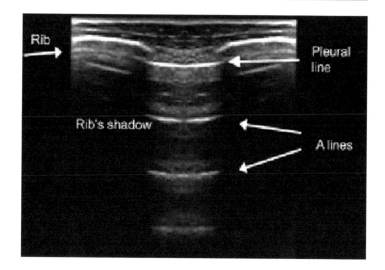

38.4   Respiratory System

Majority of the patients are shifted to ICU on mechanical ventilation and they should be planned for fast tracking weaning process and extubation. This has become possible due to better surgical skills and better anesthetic techniques along-with use of modern anesthetic agents which are cleared from the body very rapidly. *Early extubation is the preferred ventilator strategy for LT recipients as it is associated with low incidence of ventilator associated pneumonia (VAP) and better mobilization* [10]. The extubation time depends upon many factors as given in Table 38.2.

Patients with lung pathology are the ones who require prolonged mechanical ventilation. Glanemann et al. [18] showed that recipients who require more than 24 h of mechanical ventilation in the post-operative period have a high incidence of VAP. Acute respiratory distress syndrome (ARDS) is one of the most common complications after transplant. Intra-operative reperfusion syndrome, massive blood transfusion, prolonged surgery are some of the risk factors which may lead to ARDS. Low tidal volume ventilator strategy should be followed so as to prevent ventilator inflicted lung injury (VILI). *The target should be to keep the plateau pressure below 30 cm H_2O.* Other ventilator modes apart from assist control

Table 38.2 Factors affecting early extubation

Pre-operative	Intra-operative	Post-operative
Obesity [11] with BMI > 34 kg/m²	Emergency transplant [15]	Graft dysfunction [12, 14, 16]
Acute liver failure [12]	Massive blood transfusion [12, 16]	Hemodynamic instability
On mechanical ventilation [13]	Prolonged surgery [17]	
Neurological impairment [14]	Hemodynamic instability	
MELD [12–14] > 11	Re-transplant	

have not been studied in LT patients and so their use is limited. Recruitment maneuvers are generally avoided in LT patients as they cause affect graft function due to congestion and can also increase intracranial pressure especially in patients operated for acute liver failure. Similarly, prone ventilation is generally avoided due to recent abdominal surgery. The target of ventilation should be to avoid hypoxemia and hypercapnia. The use of non-invasive ventilation (NIV) post-extubation can be attempted in patients who experience respiratory failure [19] as it has been shown in few studies to be associated with decrease incidence of VAP and sepsis.

Patients who are difficult to wean should be given spontaneous breathing trials on a daily basis and if they fail this for at least 7 days, then they should undergo tracheostomy, preferably percutaneous to liberate from mechanical ventilation.

38.5 Renal and Electrolyte Balance

Renal insufficiency in the post-transplant period has an incidence varying from 5 to 50% [20] depending upon the definition used to define acute kidney injury (AKI). There are number of causative factors for renal dysfunction like use of massive blood transfusion, pre-existing hepatorenal syndrome, prolonged duration of cross clamping of vena cava intra-operatively, high vasopressor requirement, and use of nephrotoxic medications [21].

The immediate post-operative period should focus on optimization of intravascular volume and avoidance of use of any nephrotoxic medications. Hypotension should be avoided and if need arises, then vasopressors should be instituted. Antibiotics should be administered based on creatinine clearance. The use of diuretics should be restricted as it has been shown to be associated with increased incidence of AKI. *Help of Risk, Injury, Failure, Loss of function and End stage (RIFLE) score can be taken to stage the patient for AKI.* Monitoring AKI in LT patients is difficult as serum creatinine rises very late due to poor muscle mass ratio in liver disease patients [22]. Oliguria is generally the first clinical sign.

If acute kidney injury develops in the immediate post-transplant period, then renal replacement therapy (RRT) in the form of hemodialysis should be initiated. Dialysis is associated with poor outcome in transplant patients. Continuous assessment of intravascular volume by dynamic indices of hemodynamic monitoring should be instituted so as to avoid intravascular hypo-or hypervolemia and renal vasoconstriction by overuse of vasoconstrictive agents. Immunosuppressive agents should be changed from calcineurin inhibitors to less nephrotoxic agents like cyclosporine or sirolimus. *Continuous renal replacement therapy (CRRT) should be used when patient is hemody-namically unstable and there is fluid retention and severe acid base disturbance.* Preferably, regional citrate anticoagulation (RCA) technique should be used for CRRT so as to avoid use of heparin and the risk for bleeding.

Electrolyte imbalance like hypernatremia, hyperkalemia, hypomagnesemia, and hypophosphatemia are very common in the immediate postoperative period. Sodium imbalance occurs due to overzealous use of saline based fluid resuscitation and albumin. One should be very watchful for this as it affects the sensorium of the patient and also results in fluid retention. Hyperkalemia can be due to new onset AKI or also due to use of calcineurin inhibitor immunosuppressive agent. As these patients are very prone for arrhythmias, hyperkalemia should be managed very aggressively by glucose insulin drip, salbutamol nebulization, calcium chloride. Hypomagnesemia is associated with delayed graft function and so supplementation of magnesium sulfate to keep the levels in normal range should start in the immediate postoperative period. Hypophosphatemia is associated with poor reflexes and it may affect the weaning of patients from mechanical ventilation.

38.6 Graft Function Assessment

Graft function should be constantly assessed as it not only reflects as coagulopathy but it also affects other organ functions as well. All patients in the immediate post-transplant period are coagulopathic as it takes time for the newly implanted liver to pick its synthetic function [7]. *The improvement in graft function is seen by normalization of International normalized ratio (INR).* Failure to see such a correction should prompt to do a workup for graft dysfunction and sepsis as these two are the two most important causes of persisting coagulopathy.

Routine transfusion of blood products to normalize the numbers should not be practiced as it increases the load on the heart and also can be detrimental to the graft by increasing the risk of thrombosis in the newly anastomosed vessels [23].

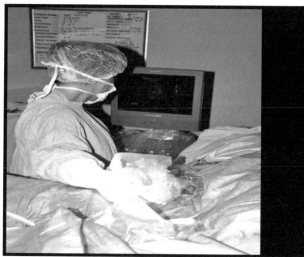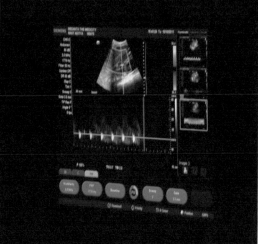

Fig. 38.2 Vascular flows—Doppler

Transfusion should be reserved only for patients who are bleeding. If possible, one should take help of thromboelastrogram (TEG) to decide on the type of blood product required to be transfused.

Improving bilirubin, correction of acidosis, normalization of glucose, improvement in the conscious level of the patient, adequate urine output, recovery from hypothermia are indicators of normal graft function. In the initial phase, liver enzymes may be elevated but they start declining over the next few days. Use of N-Acetylcysteine (NAC) in the first 48 h after transplant has been shown to fasten the process of graft recovery as it avoids further reperfusion injury. Constant monitoring of blood lactate levels in the first few days also helps in diagnosing graft dysfunction as rising lactates is a strong indicator of either primary non-function or sepsis.

Daily liver Doppler (Fig. 38.2) should be done in the first few days to look for vascular performance of the newly implanted liver. It also helps in diagnosing intra-abdominal collections and pleural effusions. Inability to visualize portal vein or hepatic artery flow should prompt to do a angiography to look for any vascular complication like hepatic artery thrombosis (HAT) as it is a life threatening complication. If the liver func-

tion is worsening with normal vascular flows, then liver biopsy can be performed by experienced intervention radiologist to look for rejection.

38.7 Neurological Management

The patients operated for acute liver failure (ALF) are at higher risk of developing neurological complications in the immediate post-operative period. *Seizures, altered sensorium due to continuation of encephalopathy from pre-LT period and intracranial bleeding are the most common neurological complications* [24]. Poor sensorium can be due to graft dysfunction, intracranial bleeding or even new onset intracranial infections. Seizures can arise as a complication of immunosuppressive drug like the calcineurin inhibitors [25]. One should look for sudden onset quadriparesis as cerebral pontine myelinolysis is a known complication more so after ALF transplant.

These patients should undergo rapid awakening after transplant so that any change in sensorium is picked up early. ALF patients take a longer duration to wake up due to resolution in cerebral edema post-LT and also due to higher grade of encephalopathy pre LT. Any sudden change in sensorium should be immediately investigated by performing a non-contrast CT brain.

38.8 Pain Management

Although liver transplant is one of the most extensive abdominal surgeries but still the postoperative pain is not severe in nature [26]. As most of the analgesics are metabolized and cleared by the hepatobiliary system, drug accumulation is possible in the poorly functioning graft. The reduced need for analgesics in LT patients can be due to increased levels of endogenous neuropeptides which are involved in pain modulation [27]. As the risk of drug accumulation is there, a constant watch on sensorium and respiratory efforts should be made.

Opioids like Fentanyl is generally the most preferred analgesic as it has minimal effect on liver and hemodynamics [28]. Certain other drugs like Tramadol can be tried with a watch for vomiting. Drugs like paracetamol should be avoided as it can cause liver injury.

38.9 Infection Prophylaxis

Liver transplant patients are at a very high risk of infections and it is one of the most common causes of mortality in the post-operative period [29]. There are many risk factors but the major ones are prolonged hospital stay pre-transplant and immunosuppression post-transplant. *The early infections are related to hospitalization and include pneumonia, urinary tract infection, blood stream infections, and surgical site infections* [30]. The most common organisms suspected should be Coagulase-negative and Coagulase-positive *Staphylococci, Enterococcus* species, *Klebsiella* species, *Pseudomonas aeruginosa, Escherichia coli*, and *Candida albicans* [31].

The antibiotics and antifungal prophylaxis should be based on the local microbiota.

Generally, these patients receive a third generation cephalosporin along with a glycopeptide for prophylaxis against methicillin resistant staphylococcus aureus (MRSA) and an azole based antifungal. Selective gut decontamination has not shown any clear benefit and rather can lead to increase in hospitalization days as per the Cochrane Database analysis [32]. Cytomegalovirus (CMV) prophylaxis should be given only to high risk patients who have received massive blood transfusion intra-operatively, requiring bolus doses of immunosuppression for early graft dysfunction or re-transplant patients. *Routine surveillance cultures like blood, urine, and drain sites should be sent to diagnose infections early.* Measurement of procalcitonin may add some clinical benefit in management of the patients although the cut-offs may not be the same as for non-transplant population as the levels of procalcitonin rise transiently after transplant and then settles over next few days even in the absence of infections [33]. However, the trend of procalcitonin should guide the clinician about a new onset infection.

Transplant patients may not mount the same response to sepsis as seen in other patients and so a high index of suspicion is required. Tachycardia, decrease in urine output, increase in liver enzymes, change in sensorium, rise in lactates and even low grade fever are subtle signs of infections. The threshold to upgrade antibiotics to Cabapenems or Colistin and Echinocandin or Liposomal Amphotericin B should be very low as the mortality is high once infection sets in. The need for vascular catheters like central venous line and arterial line should be judged on a daily basis and if possible should be removed as soon as possible. Same principle should be followed with urinary catheter. Presence of intra-abdominal collection which is not being drained by the existing drains should warrant an insertion of percutaneous pigtail insertion either under ultrasound or CT guidance. The use of adjuvant therapies like endotoxin or cytokine haemadsorption system has not shown any clear benefit and should not be a part of the standard care regimen.

38.10 Nutrition Management

Cirrhotic patients have abnormalities in metabolism of various nutritional elements and are generally malnourished in the pre-transplant phase. Malnutrition is associated with an increase in post-operative infectious complications, weaning difficulty from ventilator and prolongation of hospital stay [34].

In the immediate post-LT period, patients are kept nil per oral for first 24 h and then are initiated on clear liquids orally if the gastric aspirate was minimal. This is to stimulate the bowel for peristalsis and once they start tolerating the liquids, the oral diet is escalated. *The energy requirement is generally 120–130% of the basal requirement* [35] *and should comprise of high quality protein, carbohydrate, and fat components.* There should be no reduction of protein component even if there is encephalopathy in the post-operative period and the patients should receive almost 1.5–2 g protein/kg of weight [35]. If the patient is not able to consume oral feed due to decrease in sensorium, then enteral feeding should be initiated through nasogastric tube. Parenteral nutrition should only be used if all attempts to use gastrointestinal tract have failed. Both tube and oral feeding can be given simultaneously till the time patients starts consuming almost 80% of the daily requirement through oral feeding.

38.11 Physiotherapy

As these patients undergo prolonged surgery and are lying down for the first few post-operative days, physiotherapy plays a very vital role. Chest physiotherapy involves both passive and active exercises like vibration therapy to mobilize secretions from the peripheral to central bronchioles from where the patient can cough and remove them, incentive spirometry where the patient blows in to improve the functional residual capacity and prevent atelectasis (Fig. 38.3). On the third post-operative day, if other organ functions are improving, then the patient should be made to mobilize out of bed. This also helps in

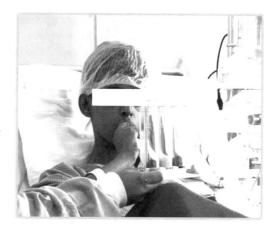

Fig. 38.3 Spirometry

bowel functioning and improving peristalsis. All attempts should be made to keep the patient busy with some or the other form of physiotherapy for most part of the day.

38.12 Psychosocial Management

The patients undergoing transplant may be in some grade of encephalopathy and so they may not be aware of the time and place. *In the post-operative period, once their encephalopathy settles, they may become delirious due to new surroundings, surgical stress, pain, and frequent monitoring* [36]. It is characterized by confusion, agitation, change in sensorium, disorientation. Once diagnosed, it should be managed with low dose of antipsychotics and non-pharmacological measures like family meeting and behavioral interventions. Apart from delirium, depression is the another psychiatric disorder observed. The incidence varies from 5 to 46% [37]. Counseling and making them aware of the present times generally helps these patients.

38.13 Conclusion

With the advancement in surgical and anesthetic technique, liver transplant has become a successful procedure for end-stage liver disease patients. The immediate post-operative management revolves around optimization of hemodynamic, respiratory, renal, and gastrointestinal functions. Graft recovery monitoring plays a very significant role in the outcome of the patient. The trend of the early post-operative period determines the outcome of the patient.

Key Points
- Fluid overload should be avoided as it leads to cardiac complications and graft dysfunction.
- Fast tracking weaning protocols should be followed in the post-LT period.
- Oliguria is the first indicator of renal dysfunction.
- Graft monitoring like sensorium, correction in acidosis, resolution of hypothermia, normalization of glucose determines the outcome of the patient.
- Antibiotics and antifungals should be given as per the local policy to prevent any infectious complications.
- Upgradation of antibiotics should have a low threshold.
- Coagulation abnormalities should not be corrected unless the patient is bleeding.
- Analgesia should be patient centric. Opioids are generally the choice of drug.
- Feeding should be attempted in all patients either through oral or enteral route.

References

1. Keegan MT, Kramer DJ. Perioperative care of the liver transplant patient. Crit Care Clin. 2016;32(3):453–73. https://doi.org/10.1016/j.ccc.2016.02.005.
2. Moreno R, Berenguer M. Post-liver transplantation medical complications. Ann Hepatol. 2006;5(2):77–85.
3. Fabbroni BM. Anaesthesia for hepatic transplantation. Contin Educ Anaesth Crit Care Pain. 2006;6(5):171–5.
4. Al-Hamoudi WK. Cardiovascular changes in cirrhosis: pathogenesis and clinical implications. Saudi J Gastroenterol. 2010;16(3):145–53.
5. Wray CL. Liver transplantation in patients with cardiac disease. Semin Cardiothorac Vasc Anesth. 2018;22(2):111–21.
6. Dec GW, Kondo N, Farrell ML, Dienstag J, Cosimi AB, Semigran MJ. Cardiovascular complications following liver transplantation. Clin Transpl. 1995;9(06):463–71.
7. Therapondos G, Flapan AD, Plevris JN, Hayes PC. Cardiac morbidity and mortality related to orthotopic liver transplantation. Liver Transpl. 2004;10(12):1441–53.
8. Feltracco P, Barbieri S, Galligioni H, Michieletto E, Carollo C, Ori C. Intensive care management of liver transplanted patients. World J Hepatol. 2011;3(03):61–71.
9. Najeed SA, Saghir S, Hein B, et al. Management of hypertension in liver transplant patients. Int J Cardiol. 2011;152(1):4–6.
10. Błaszczyk B, Wrońska B, Klukowski M, et al. Factors affecting breathing capacity and early tracheal extubation after liver transplantation: analysis of 506 cases. Transplant Proc. 2016;48(5):1692–6.
11. Mandell MS, Lezotte D, Kam I, Zamudio S. Reduced use of intensive care after liver transplantation: patient attributes that determine early transfer to surgical wards. Liver Transpl. 2002;8(8):682–7.
12. Glanemann M, Hoffmeister R, Neumann U, et al. Fast tracking in liver transplantation: which patient benefits from this approach? Transplant Proc. 2007;39(2):535–6.
13. Huang CT, Lin HC, Chang SC, Lee WC. Pre-operative risk factors predict post-operative respiratory failure after liver transplantation. PLoS One. 2011;6(08):e22689.
14. Biancofiore G, Romanelli AM, Bindi ML, et al. Very early tracheal extubation without predetermined criteria in a liver transplant recipient population. Liver Transpl. 2001;7(09):777–82.
15. Zeyneloglu P, Pirat A, Guner M, Torgay A, Karakayali H, Arslan G. Predictors of immediate tracheal extubation in the operating room after liver transplantation. Transplant Proc. 2007;39(4):1187–9.
16. Glanemann M, Langrehr J, Kaisers U, et al. Postoperative tracheal extubation after orthotopic liver transplantation. Acta Anaesthesiol Scand. 2001;45(3):333–9.
17. Skurzak S, Stratta C, Schellino MM, et al. Extubation score in the operating room after liver transplantation. Acta Anaesthesiol Scand. 2010;54(8):970–8.
18. Glanemann M, Busch T, Neuhaus P, Kaisers U. Fast tracking in liver transplantation. Immediate postoperative tracheal extubation: feasibility and clinical impact. Swiss Med Wkly. 2007;137:187–91.
19. Antonelli M, Conti G, Bufi M, Costa MG, Lappa A, Rocco M, Gasparetto A, Meduri GU. Noninvasive

ventilation for treatment of acute respiratory failure in patients undergoing solid organ transplantation: a randomized trial. JAMA. 2000;283:235–41.

20. Paramesh AS, Roayaie S, Doan Y, Schwartz ME, Emre S, Fishbein T, Florman S, Gondolesi GE, Krieger N, Ames S, Bromberg JS, Akalin E. Post-liver transplant acute renal failure: factors predicting development of end-stage renal disease. Clin Transpl. 2004;18:94–9.

21. Kundakci A, Pirat A, Komurcu O, Torgay A, Karakayali H, Arslan G, et al. Rifle criteria for acute kidney dysfunction following liver transplantation: incidence and risk factors. Transplant Proc. 2010;42:4171–4.

22. Lucey MR, Terrault N, Ojo L, Hay JE, Neuberger J, Blumberg E, et al. Long-term management of the successful adult liver transplant: 2012 practice guideline by the American Association for the Study of Liver Diseases and the American Society of Transplantation. Liver Transpl. 2013;19:3–26.

23. Massicotte L, Beaulieu D, Thibeault L, Roy JD, Marleau D, Lapointe R, et al. Coagulation defects do not predict blood product requirements during liver transplantation. Transplantation. 2008;85:956–62.

24. Živković SA. Neurologic complications after liver transplantation. World J Hepatol. 2013;5(8):409–16.

25. Campagna F, Biancardi A, Cillo U, Gatta A, Amodio P. Neurocognitive- neurological complications of liver transplantation: a review. Metab Brain Dis. 2010;25(1):115–24.

26. Feltracco P, Carollo C, Barbieri S, Milevoj M, Pettenuzzo T, Gringeri E, et al. Pain control after liver transplantation surgery. Transplant Proc. 2014;46(7):2300–7.

27. Pai SL, Aniskevich S, Rodrigues ES, Shine TS. Analgesic considerations for liver transplantation patients. Curr Clin Pharmacol. 2015;10(1):54–65.

28. Milan Z. Analgesia after liver transplantation. World J Gastroenterol. 2015;7(21):2331–5.

29. Laici C, Gamberini L, Bardi T, Siniscalchi A, Reggiani ML, Faenza S. Early infections in the intensive care unit after liver transplantation-etiology and risk factors: a single-center experience. Transpl Infect Dis. 2018;20(2):e12834.

30. Romero FA, Razonable RR. Infections in liver transplant recipients. World J Hepatol. 2011;3:83–92.

31. Blair JE, Kusne S. Bacterial, mycobacterial, and protozoal infections after liver transplantation–part I. Liver Transpl. 2005;11:1452–9.

32. Gurusamy KS, Kumar Y, Davidson BR. Methods of preventing bacterial sepsis and wound complications for liver transplantation. Cochrane Database Syst Rev. 2008;3:CD006660.

33. Zazula R, Prucha M, Tyll T, Kieslichova E. Induction of pro-calcitonin in liver transplant patients treated with anti-thymocyte globulin. Crit Care. 2007;11:R131.

34. Figueiredo F, Dickson ER, Pasha T, Kasparova P, Therneau T, Malinchoc M, DiCecco S, Francisco-Ziller N, Charlton M. Impact of nutritional status on outcomes after liver transplantation. Transplantation. 2000;70:1347–52.

35. Sanchez AJ, Aranda MJ. Nutrition in hepatic failure and liver transplantation. Rev Gastroenterol Mex. 2007;72:365–70.

36. Guarino M, Stracciari A, Pazzaglia P. Neurological complications of liver transplantation. J Neurol. 1996;243:137–42.

37. Russell RT, Feurer ID, Wisawatapnimit P, Salomon RM, Pinson CW. The effects of physical quality of life, time, and gender on change in symptoms of anxiety and depression after liver transplantation. J Gastrointest Surg. 2008;12:138–44.

Assessment of Early Graft Function and Management of Early Graft Failure

39

Akila Rajakumar, Premchandar Velusamy, and Ilankumaran Kaliamoorthy

Abbreviations

ALF	acute liver failure
ALT	Alanine aminotransferases
AST	Aspartate aminotransferases
CIT	cold ischemia time
CRRT	continuous renal replacement therapy
DCD	donation after cardiac death
DDLT	Deceased donor liver transplantation
EAD	early allograft dysfunction
ECLS	extracorporeal liver support systems
HVP	high volume plasmapheresis
ICG-PDR	Indocyanine green-plasma disappearance rate
IPGF	initial poor graft function
IRI	ischemia reperfusion injury
LDLT	Living donor liver transplantation
LiMax	Liver maximal function capacity
LT	Liver transplantation
MARS	Molecular adsorbent recirculating system
MEAF	Model for early allograft function
NAC	N-acetyl cysteine
PEEP	positive end expiratory pressure
PGD	primary graft dysfunction
PLP	Plasmapheresis
PNF	primary non function
PRS	reperfusion syndrome
RRT	renal replacement therapy
SIRS	systemic inflammatory response

Liver transplantation (LT) has now been universally accepted as the standard of care for patients with decompensated end-stage liver disease, acute liver failure (ALF), and a few other metabolic disorders. Resumption of graft function during and immediately after surgery is very crucial in determining patient outcomes. Graft survival approximates patient survival in most circumstances. Although the rates of cadaveric donation have increased, there seems to be a disproportionate increase in the number of recipients on waitlist. Living donor liver transplantation (LDLT) was developed with the main purpose of reducing waitlist mortality which, unfortunately, has not been able to provide a complete solution for the problem. To overcome this, the transplant community has increased the margins for acceptance of a donor in deceased donor liver transplantation (DDLT) and a smaller volume graft in LDLT to prioritize donor safety [1, 2]. This has led to increasing use of marginal grafts which increase the likelihood of primary graft dysfunction (PGD). It has been well demonstrated that recipients who develop PGD have a higher risk of

A. Rajakumar (✉) · P. Velusamy · I. Kaliamoorthy
Department of Liver Intensive Care and Anaesthesia,
Dr. Rela Institute and Medical Centre, Chennai, India

morbidity and mortality, but the benefits might outweigh the risks of dying in the waitlist without a suitable organ.

Primary graft dysfunction (PGD) is a sequalae of the ischemia reperfusion injury (IRI) in the liver graft [3]. The spectrum of PGD ranges from primary non function (PNF) which results in death or retransplantation to early allograft dysfunction (EAD) which is also referred to as initial poor graft function (IPGF) by some authors. Presumably the severity of IRI is a major determinant of graft outcomes. PNF is a severe form of IRI resulting in irreversible graft failure without other technical or immunological factors [4, 5]. Sinusoidal endothelial cell damage seems to be central to the pathophysiology of PGD [6]. Closure biopsies also referred to as time zero biopsy has shown to be a significant predictor of graft and patient outcomes. Acute inflammatory infiltration of the graft and hepatocellular damage ranging from ballooning degeneration to coagulative necrosis has been observed immediately post-reperfusion in the closure graft biopsies studied [7]. Severe IRI shown in these biopsies help in predicting PGD earlier and initiate aggressive management strategies including decision on retransplantation [8].

39.1 Incidence, Predictors, and Outcome of PGD

Incidence of EAD has shown to be between 15 and 27% and PNF has a reported incidence of 4–8% [9–12]. EAD incidence has increased over the recent years because of more prevalent use of marginal and extended criteria donors [13].

Donor age, fatty liver on donor biopsy, prolonged cold ischemia time (CIT), prolonged ICU stay of the donor, retransplantation and renal insufficiency, preop recipient ICU stay, and intraoperative transfusions have been shown as predictors of PGD [11, 12, 14–18]. A higher incidence of PGD has been observed in donation after cardiac death (DCD) donors [16, 17]. Larger graft in a smaller recipient is also shown to be a risk factor for EAD [19, 20]. In the Adult to Adult Living Liver (A2ALL) group, left lobe grafts,

lower GRWR grafts, higher preop bilirubin, higher portal reperfusion pressure, and donor factors including advanced age and higher BMI were found to be risk factors for EAD. Recipients with EAD had a 5.2 times higher risk of graft loss than those without EAD and the incidence of graft loss was found to be 24% in their EAD cohort [21]. EAD is associated with increased susceptibility to sepsis, prolonged ICU and hospital stay, which has huge implications on resources [11, 14, 15, 22]. EAD has been shown to be an independent risk factor for graft loss and mortality [11, 13, 22–25]. In the Olthoff study, [11] among the 23.2% of recipients with EAD, 18.8% died, whereas 1.8% of recipients without EAD died. The rate of graft loss was 26.1% for patients with EAD and 3.5% for patients without EAD.

With this huge burden of adverse outcomes in PGD, the liver transplant community is presented with the ever increasing challenges to plan and implement strategies to decrease complications related to marginal grafts. Factors predictive of PGD should be well understood to enable donor–recipient matching. During donor–recipient matching, it has been strongly recommended to avoid a combination of risk factors like the combination of donor steatosis (30–60%) and prolonged CIT as advised by Busuttil and Tanaka [26]. In recipients who have a higher probability of PGD, all intraoperative and postoperative factors which could add on to the risk should be optimized as much as possible. Aggressive and defined perioperative strategies should be in place to handle these patients to avoid graft loss and mortality.

There are several scores developed to predict outcome of a transplant, which can predict graft loss to a great extent, based on donor and recipient factors like donor risk index, [27] survival outcomes following liver transplantation score, [28] Donor Model for End-Stage Liver Disease (D-MELD) score [29]. These scores can be used to make informed decisions regarding donor–recipient matching and also help to explain to patients what their post-transplant survival would be. This would be more helpful in recipients who receive marginal grafts.

39.2 Assessment of Early Graft Function

Early graft failure in the form of PNF is an uncommon but very challenging and stressful scenario for the transplant team and patient's family. Early recognition of the problem, incorporation of multidisciplinary inputs, excellent communication among team members and family and reassessments at frequent intervals followed by execution of planned strategies in anticipation of impending complications are all keys to success in managing this cohort of patients. Multiorgan dysfunction sets in at the late stages of graft failure both in PNF and EAD, when recovery of graft function becomes impossible. It is, therefore, imperative to identify signs of early graft failure to decide if urgent retransplantation is required and also to identify grafts with potential to recover with meticulous postoperative care. In patients with EAD, a milieu ideal for regeneration will help avoid graft loss.

Graft function is determined by multiple factors—quality of donor graft, ischemia times, graft reperfusion, technical factors at anastomosis, intraoperative course, and pre-existing status of the recipient. Identifying potentially modifiable risk factors could help in the initiation of early interventions that could mitigate the course of PGD.

Of all the solid organ transplants, biomarkers are readily and easily available to assess dynamic graft function in LT. These should be used with clinical parameters to assess and evaluate graft function and early graft failure. Graft function is usually assessed by a combination of assessment of operating field and bile production, clinical parameters, requirement for multiorgan support, laboratory parameters, and the need for blood products, specifically for clotting support. But the clinical and laboratory derangements are not entirely specific for graft function and can be deranged due to pre-existing medical status of the patient and other new onset perioperative factors.

Assessment of graft function should begin, as early as, immediately after reperfusion and continued onto the postoperative period. PNF is usu-

ally evident on table after reperfusion. EAD can be picked up on table but usually manifests in the postoperative period. A good functioning graft usually presents itself, at reperfusion, as a uniform well perfused liver which becomes soft in consistency as noted by the surgeons, along with other factors like, start of bile production, improving coagulopathy, stabilization of hemodynamics, improvement in urine output, and stabilization with falling trends in lactate levels and acidosis. PNF usually presents with a stiff liver at reperfusion, reperfusion syndrome, worsening hemodynamics, worsening coagulopathy with massive bleeding and massive transfusion requirements, no improvements or fall in urine output, worsening lactate levels, and acidosis.

The superurgent listing criteria for PNF as accepted by Organ Procurement and Transplantation Network (OPTN) is the PNF of a transplanted liver within 7 days of implantation; as defined by (a) or (b):

(a) AST ≥ 3000 and one or both of the following:
   - INR ≥ 2.5.
   - Acidosis, defined as having an arterial pH ≤ 7.30 or venous pH of 7.25 and/or lactate ≥ 4 mmol/L.
(b) Anhepatic candidate.
   https://optn.transplant.hrsa.gov/media/1200/optn_policies.pdf

Various definitions for EAD has been proposed by several authors [11, 14, 18, 30–34]. Table 39.1 lists out the commonly used definitions and some have included criteria for PNF also.

Several functional tests which depend on the presence of active liver function have been studied to assess postoperative graft function. Despite several limitations, Indocyanine Green - Plasma Disappearance Rate (ICG-PDR) and Liver Maximal Function Capacity (LiMax) tests have been well studied for detection of early allograft failure. Daily determination of ICG PDR [35, 36] in the postoperative period has been shown to determine graft function with values showing an improving trend with as the graft function recov-

Table 39.1 Definitions of EAD

Study authors	Primary graft dysfunction
Ploeg RJ [18]	IPGF was defined as a form of PDF with AST >2000 U/L, PT > 16 s and ammonia >50micromol/L on post-transplant day 2–7 PNF—Non-sustaining function of liver after liver transplant leading to death or retransplant within 7 days
Deschênes M [14]	EAD was defined by the presence of at least one of the following between 2 and 7 days after liver transplantation: Serum bilirubin >10 mg/dL, prothrombin time (PT) ≥17 s, and hepatic encephalopathy
Nanashima et al. [34]	EAD—two consecutive measurements of ALT or AST > 1500 IU/L within first 72 h after transplant
Broering et al. [30]	Primary poor graft function as one of the transaminases (alanine transaminase, aspartate transaminase, and glutamate dehydrogenase) more than 2000 U/L or requirement of fresh frozen plasma for more than 5 days postoperatively PNF—Re-transplant within 10 days of implantation or death from a non-functioning graft
Olthoff et al. [11]	EAD—presence of one or more of the following variables: Bilirubin >10 mg/dL, INR > 1.6 on day 7, AST or ALT >2000 U/L within the first 7 postoperative days
Dhillon et al. [32]	Graft function assessed as average liver enzymes [(AST + ALT)/2)] on day 2 <285 IU/L: Good function285–986 IU/L: Average function>986 IU/L: IPGF PNF—death or re transplant within 7 days of liver transplant
Mathe et al. [33]	IPGF—AST or ALT levels >1500 U/L on two consecutive measurements within the first 72 h after LT PNF—Poor graft function of the allograft culminating into death or re-transplant
Chen X. et al. [31]	EAD—Presence of one or more of the following variables bilirubin ≥10 mg/dL, INR ≥ 1.6 on day 7 with AST or ALT >2000 U/L within the first 7 postoperative days

ers. ICG PDR is a safe bedside test but multiple confounders affecting PDR is the limitation resulting in poor specificity. LiMax is a real time breath test performed using ^{13}C methacetin. When administered intravenously, it is selectively metabolized by cytochrome P450 1A2 (CYP1A2), an enzyme exclusively expressed by hepatocytes and is excreted by ventilation. An estimate of this enzyme kinetics can be obtained with the $^{13}CO_2/^{12}CO_2$ ratio. Non-EAD patients showed significantly higher LiMax within 6 h after LT than EAD patients [37, 38]. Various external factors and genetic variability influence cytochrome activity and hence this test has poor specificity in determining liver function post LT.

Bedside determination of serum lactate levels is a well-established excellent predictor of graft function post-LT. The rate of fall of serum lactate levels is used to predict survival in ICUs for patients admitted with varying causes within the first 6 h of admission [39]. The same was demonstrated in a study from China [40] with post-LT patients. Non-EAD patients showed a significantly higher lactate clearance compared to patients who developed EAD subsequently.

Persistent thrombocytopenia, [41, 42] low factor V levels [43], have all been shown to be significantly associated with EAD. But it is not clear if thrombocytopenia is a cause or consequence of EAD.

39.3 Scoring Systems for Assessment of Graft Function Post-LT

In an effort to identify predictors for PGD, Wagener and colleagues [44] demonstrated that MELD on day 5 was found to be the best predictor of 90-day survival. They demonstrated that the best cut-off of MELD score on day 5 for predicting 90-day mortality or graft loss was 18.9 and a MELD score > 18.9 on postoperative day 5 was a better predictor than any other laboratory value or definition of EAD. In a study from Spain, Pareja et al. [12]developed a model scoring system for continuous grading of early allograft function following liver transplantation—Model for early allograft function (MEAF) score using easily available parameters—ALT, bilirubin, and

INR in the first three postoperative days. For easy use, the model's range of score points has been set between 0 and 10.

and increasing score points reflect increasing severity of EAD. With the use of a nomogram, each recipient's score can be calculated at the bedside. They demonstrated significant association between MEAF scores and patient survival at 3, 6, and 12 months. In another study from Belgium, MEAF score was shown to be superior to EAD in predicting 1-year survival [10].

In a study from UCLA, another model called Liver Graft Assessment Following Transplantation (L-GrAFT) was developed as a dynamic assessment of graft function using 10 days post-transplant values of AST, bilirubin, INR, and platelet counts and analyzing their trends and the rates of normalization. A score of 1–5 was given and the authors demonstrated that this score model was superior to other binary EAD classifications and MEAF score in predicting 3-month graft survival [45].

39.4 Management of a Failing Graft

Whenever PGD is anticipated or suspected based on intraoperative course, strict strategies need to be implemented. In addition to the failing allograft, the clinical course becomes quite stormy due to additional factors like preoperative recipient physiology which deteriorates further, the physiological stress of surgery, ischemia reperfusion injury, immune activation, and multiorgan dysfunction. Multidisciplinary team input and collaborative working is essential.

In the LDLT setting, it has been observed that if the early period after transplantation is well supported, majority of PGD would recover without much consequences [46].

39.4.1 Deteriorating Recipient Physiology in PGD

Due to PGD, all other organ systems of the recipient suffer and extra hepatic organ failure sets in

very rapidly. Worsening coagulopathy necessitates coagulation correction and transfusion of large amounts of blood and blood products. The lungs can suffer because of transfusion associated lung injury (TRALI), transfusion associated circulatory overload (TACO) or acute lung injury due to systemic inflammatory response (SIRS) triggered by struggling graft. SIRS results in increased vasopressor requirement which can lead to peripheral circulatory failure which perse can add to the burden of lactate load. Acidosis resulting from PGD and renal dysfunction further increases refractoriness to vasopressors. The magnitude of these changes varies from patient to patient and also depends on the preoperative status of the recipient.

39.4.2 General Principles of Management

All efforts should be made to extract maximal function of the failing graft and enhance liver regeneration. Optimizing and preventing extra hepatic organ system dysfunction is the most important goal which facilitates an appropriate milieu conducive for liver regeneration or to stabilize the patient for retransplantation. All efforts should be made to prevent iatrogenic injury at any stage.

39.4.3 Meticulous Surgical Care

As much as possible, thorough hemostasis should be ensured. Venous drainage should be good to avoid any further congestion. In centers, where routine use of intraoperative ultrasound doppler is not practiced, it is advisable to use in suspected cases of PGD to ensure patency of venous and arterial anastomosis and adequate outflow. When in the ICU, it is prudent to exclude all reversible causes of PGD by imaging, either by a bedside Doppler or Contrast enhanced CT scan. Immediate re-exploration, in cases of vascular thrombosis, can avoid retransplantation or death.

39.4.4 ICU Management

In the postoperative period, supportive therapy should be aggressive and pre-emptive. ICU care can be divided to (a) general supportive care for each of the organ systems and (b) specific interventions for PGD.

39.5   General Supportive Care

39.5.1 Neurological Support

PGD is occasionally evident by failure to wake up at the end of surgery in fast track centers and inappropriate sensorium in other recipients. Sensorium changes can range from subtle delays in awakening to rapidly developing coma. Recent evidence shows glial edema and increased serum levels of γ-amino butyric acid and inhibitory neural receptor activity are associated with hepatic encephalopathy [47]. Hyperammonemia has paradoxical central nervous system effects; increasing inhibitory γ-amino butyric acid receptor sensitivity and independently causing neuronal excitation and seizure activity [48, 49].

Patient evaluation should be directed towards excluding and eliminating neurological diseases which can have a similar presentation as EAD. Electroencephalography can detect status epilepticus without motor manifestations, which has an increased incidence in advanced hepatic encephalopathy [50]. A triphasic wave pattern on the encephalogram suggests hepatic coma but cannot be distinguished from other causes of neuroinhibition such as calcineurin inhibitor neurotoxicity. Therefore, serum immunosuppressant levels are part of the standard evaluation of recipients with impaired level of consciousness [51].

Neuroimaging using high-resolution computed tomography or magnetic resonance can help in the identification of posterior reversible leukoencephalopathy syndrome (PRES) and intracerebral bleeding, conditions that occur with greater frequency in critically ill transplant recipients due to immune suppression and a reduction

in blood clotting, respectively and also the rare complication of osmotic demyelination. The most common clinical manifestation of PRES is seizures and 30% seem to have an intracranial bleed, thus suggesting vascular dysregulation/damage as contributing factors [52]. Because imaging can lag behind clinical findings, serial studies may be necessary [53, 54]. Other monitors such as transcranial Doppler, continuous electroencephalography, and cerebral oximetry have not been systematically evaluated for neurological outcome in PGD and there is no agreement on when to initiate monitoring.

The clinical management of these patients is neuroprotection as in ALF for patients with PNF and careful neuromonitoring and delaying extubation in patients who develop EAD. All principles for neuroprotection applied in ALF brain should be used in PNF [55].

There is still disagreement about the benefits and risks of invasive intracranial pressure monitoring. Although there are often marked abnormalities in the standard coagulation tests, very few hemorrhagic complications have been reported with invasive intracranial pressure monitoring devices [56]. Yet, the use of subdural and subarachnoid catheters has not been associated with better outcomes in patients with acute liver failure [57–61].

Treatment aims to reduce cerebral edema if present. It is recommended to maintain a serum sodium of 145–155 mmol/L and use of hypertonic saline when indicated has shown to improve outcome in ALF [62, 63]. Routine monitoring of serum sodium and osmolality helps control the risk of developing neurological injury due to myelinosis. Bolus therapy with mannitol/hypertonic saline is recommended when there is clinical evidence of raised intracranial pressure. Administration of nonabsorbable disaccharides like lactulose/lactitol, antibiotics like oral rifaximin, and other drugs like L-ornithine-L-aspartate improves outcome in chronic liver disease by reverting hepatic encephalopathy, although no benefit is achieved in ALF [55]. Their role in EAD is yet to be studied.

39.5.2 Mechanical Ventilation

It has been shown that these patients are at increased risk of ALI due to graft failure and the mediators [64]. Indirect injury affecting lung endothelium is seen more frequently in patients with liver disease and is probably attributable liver failure than the direct epithelial injury seen in other forms of critical illness [65]. Ongoing requirement for blood products further increase the risk of transfusion associated lung injury and circulatory overload. Prolonged ventilator requirement puts them at an increased risk of ventilator associated pneumonia and the requirement of tracheostomy.

Preemptive lung protective ventilation strategies are the most effective way of reducing the incidence and severity of ALI from any underlying cause [66]. The recent international expert panel based consensus recommendations for perioperative ventilation [67] recommends protective strategies and to initiate ventilation with tidal volume of 6–8 mL/kg predicted body weight and positive end expiratory pressure (PEEP) 5 cm H_2O. PEEP could then be individualized as per status of oxygenation. Whenever recruitment maneuvers are required, the lowest effective pressure and shortest effective time or fewest number of breaths to be used. Positive end expiratory pressure up to 15 cm H_2O is associated with preserved hepatic venous outflow and can be used in patients following liver transplantation [68].

39.5.3 Cardiovascular Support

The systemic inflammatory response in these patients results from the IRI and the mediators cause marked vasodilation and vasoplegia. The clinical picture is indistinguishable from septic shock. Relative endogenous vasopressin deficiency has been demonstrated in patients with liver disease and this could be the reason for vasodilatory shock seen in liver failure similar to septic shock [69].

Goal directed fluid therapy is recommended [70]. A thorough insight into all fluid therapy trials recommend that clinicians should focus on the precision for using invasive or non-invasive approaches at the initial presentation of high risk patients [71]. Intravenous fluids should be meticulously titrated keeping in mind the risks of graft congestion and cerebral edema vs. inadequate perfusion. In this cohort of patients, fluids and vasopressor use should be guided by cardiac output monitoring.

When vasopressors are needed, norepinephrine is recommended as first choice followed by vasopressin. This combination is supported by few studies in ALF because of favorable effects on intracranial pressure and preservation of cerebral perfusion [72]. A reduction in portal flow helps control symptoms of portal hypertension, including hepatorenal syndrome [73].

Norepinephrine is recommended as a first line treatment with the addition of vasopressin if the mean arterial blood pressure is less than 65 mm Hg in patients with septic shock as per surviving sepsis guidelines. It has been shown that these patients respond by a 20% increase in MAP with exogenous vasopressin [69]. When ionotropes are required, dobutamine should be used. It has not been possible to identify a target blood pressure associated with better survival. Complications such as atrial fibrillation were more common with higher vasopressor induced blood pressures [74].

Crystalloids can contribute to dilutional coagulopathy and can increase risk of bleeding. Colloids are recommended in protein rich drain losses including ascites. A common ratio for replacement is 8 g of 20% albumin per liter ascites drained when no other fluids are administered [75]. The indications for use of fresh frozen plasma are primarily for coagulation correction in profound coagulopathy or for invasive procedures. Factor concentrates like prothrombin complex concentrates, fibrinogen concentrates, and recombinant activated factor VII in some instances, are preferred whenever possible, for the advantage of avoiding fluid overload, immunological issues, and lung injury caused by blood products [76, 77].

When used with guidance from point of care coagulation tests, these concentrates have been found to be safe [78, 79]. The use of vitamin K is currently not supported by clinical trials [80].

39.5.4 Renal Support

PGD affects renal function, severity of which depends on the severity of IRI, hemodynamic instability and the presence or pre-existing renal disease. Conditions such as immune-mediated glomerular and interstitial injury was noted in 42% of cirrhotic patients on renal biopsy [81]. It has also been observed that even under normal circumstances, there is a significant decline in renal function accompanied by impaired renal oxygenation directly after liver transplantation [82]. This happens despite hyperdynamic systemic circulation. It is obvious that these changes will be exaggerated during PGD.

Renal dysfunction occurring due to graft failure had a very high mortality and the risk is further increased with requirement of renal replacement therapy [83]. Associated manifestations require attention—fluid overload, acidosis, and other electrolyte disturbances necessitating renal replacement therapy (RRT). These patients with EAD also tend to have higher rates of progression of renal dysfunction and non-recovery compared to others without EAD [84].

In the data from US acute liver failure study group, continuous renal replacement therapy (CRRT) was shown to cause significant reduction in serum ammonia and improve transplant free survival [85] and the same has been demonstrated in children with acute liver failure [86]. Observations from patients with acute liver failure show that early renal replacement therapy in patients with associated renal dysfunction increases graft and patient survival [87]. It has also been well established that CRRT is better than intermittent RRT in acute liver failure because of the slower changes in serum osmolality and a smaller effect on arterial pressure which is thought to preserve cerebral perfusion and avoid fluctuations in hemodynamics and intracranial pressure [88, 89]. Ammonia clearance is closely correlated with ultrafiltration rate and increasing ultrafiltration rates have shown rapid decline in ammonia levels [90].

39.5.5 Infection Prevention and Control

This cohort of patients are extremely susceptible to infections because of impaired acute phase cellular and protein response, reduced portal filtering capacity, and gut translocation [91], in addition to immunosuppressive therapy, longer duration of ventilation, invasive lines and drains, and frequent use of extracorporeal circuits increase the risk of infection. Periodic surveillance cultures and screening, broad spectrum antibacterials and antifungals as per the local hospital antibiogram, and very stringent infection control measures should be instituted.

39.5.6 Nutritional Support

In patients with acute liver failure, nutritional goals would be to ensure adequate provision of energy by exogenous administration of glucose, lipid, proteins/amino acids, vitamins, and trace elements. In patients with hyperacute disease, it is preferred to defer nutritional protein support for 24–48 h until hyperammonemia is controlled. Protein supplementation should be done with monitoring of serum ammonia levels [92]. Otherwise, nutritional therapy principles should be similar to other critically ill patients and we should aim to initiate and establish enteral feeding within 5–7 days of the onset of any acute illness [92]. As in all critically ill patients, this improves gut mucosal integrity and bacterial flora. While parenteral nutrition is an option if enteral feeding is not possible, the risk of infection and cholestasis is increased.

In those patients with hypermetabolism, peak metabolic requirements was noticed on tenth day post-transplant [93]. By the end of 12 months post-transplant, the metabolic state was comparable to other healthy individuals [93, 94]. It is important to supply the extra energy requirements in this group of patients.

39.5.7 Immunosuppression

Despite severity of illness, these patients require immunosuppression to prevent the added complication of graft rejection. Serum levels of immunosuppressants should be carefully monitored because graft dysfunction interferes with drug metabolism and makes these patients more prone to the drug side effects. The risk of infection and renal dysfunction has to be balanced against graft rejection [95].

39.6 Specific Interventions

39.6.1 Use of *N*-Acetyl Cysteine

N-Acetyl cysteine (NAC) is a rich source of sulfydryl groups which help in replenishing glutathione stores [96]. Glutathione acts as a free radical scavenger and contributes to the antioxidant effect of NAC. The anti-inflammatory properties are well proven [97–100]. Free radicals are believed to play a major role in the pathogenesis of ischemia reperfusion injury resulting in primary graft dysfunction manifesting as PNF or EAD [101]. The role of NAC in acetaminophen induced fulminant liver failure has been well established [55, 102]. Beneficial effects have also been demonstrated in non-acetaminophen ALF [103–106]. NAC has, therefore, been widely used in ALF of all etiologies and in liver resections because of the fact that it is cheap, easily available and devoid of major adverse effects, hence its use in PNF can be justified.

In an experimental model with rats, NAC was shown to reduce the effects of ischemia reperfusion injury after warm ischemia or liver transplantation by an improvement of microcirculation and reduction of leukocyte endothelium interaction [107]. In a study on intraoperative use of NAC, in doses recommended for fulminant liver failure, modest improvement in oxygen transport was observed, but no difference noted on the reperfusion syndrome (PRS), postoperative graft function, rejection, infection or other complications [108].

In another RCT, there was no difference in incidence of PRS, immediate graft function, acute kidney injury or long-term graft, and patient survival in patients receiving NAC. The authors proposed further studies to evaluate its efficiency by continuing NAC for a longer duration and use in donor as well as recipient [109]. In a RCT in LDLT, use of NAC in live donors until graft harvest and in recipients during implantation and continued for 96 h did not show any difference in incidence of early graft function, postoperative AKI, hospital stay, and mortality [110]. Therefore, routine intraoperative use of NAC is not supported by existing literature.

In a RCT on deceased donors by D'Amico et al. [111], NAC infusion at a dose of 300 mg/kg commenced an hour before beginning of liver procurement and a locoregional NAC infusion given through portal vein) was shown to significantly improve 3-month and 12-month graft survival. This effect on early graft function and survival was more pronounced in the cohort of patients who received marginal grafts.

39.6.2 Role of Plasma Exchange in Graft Failure

Plasmapheresis (PLP) has been used for a long time in acute liver failure due to various etiologies including PNF and in EAD [112]. It helps in removal of free and protein-bound toxic substrates with supply of fresh plasma with clotting factors and albumin. PLP also helps in removal of inflammatory mediators and attenuates activation of innate immune pathway and can thus prevent multi organ dysfunction in ALF [113].

Improvement in biochemical parameters and coagulopathy has been demonstrated in all studies evaluating PLP in PGD [114, 115]. Clinical improvement evidenced by reduction in systemic inflammatory response syndrome (SIRS) and sequential organ failure assessment (SOFA) scores has been observed in ALF patients treated with high volume plasmapheresis(HVP) [113]. Although used widely, there has been only one RCT performed till date to evaluate plasma exchange in ALF and this has demonstrated improved outcome in patients with ALF by significantly increasing liver transplant-free survival [113]. HVP has now been included in the European guidelines as level 1, grade 1 recommendation in the management of ALF [55]. As per the available literature, most of the studies have continued PLP until retransplantation or clinical improvement or death of the patient.

PLP has been used widely for EAD also but no proper RCT has been performed. Studies have shown beneficial effects of PLP in EAD in the LDLT setting [116–118] as well as in DDLT setting [114, 119, 120]. In a study of 107 EAD recipients from Korea, it was observed that PLP improved biochemical parameters and coagulation profile and survival was significantly better compared to those who did not undergo PLP [116].

PLP has the advantage of being simple and easy to use, readily available, and economical liver support system. It is, therefore, an excellent tool in the management of PGD, in countries where retransplantation is not always feasible, due to scarcity of donor organs and the financial burden. Apart from all other known problems with extracorporeal circuit, PLP non-selectively removes substances from blood. Essential medications like antibiotics and immunosuppressants can be removed and the degree of removal is not yet very clearly understood [121, 122].

39.6.3 Other Artificial Liver Support Systems in PGD

A variety of artificial liver support systems have emerged for the treatment of liver failure but none except HVP has shown survival benefit till date [123]. Molecular adsorbent recirculating system (MARS) has shown the most benefit so far and has been extensively studied, has shown temporary improvement in systemic hemodynamics and encephalopathy [123]. Recent meta-analysis [124] suggests that extracorporeal liver support systems (ECLS) may reduce mortality and improve hepatic encephalopathy in patients with liver failure. It has been strongly recommended that well designed RCTs are needed to

determine the magnitude of that effect and to see which modality is better and which cohort of patients will benefit from ECLS [125].

39.7 Use of Prostaglandins

Prostaglandins with their anti-inflammatory properties, platelet inhibition, and vasodilation are presumed to improve hepatic microcirculatory flow. However, a systematic analysis of randomized controlled studies did not show improvement in all-cause mortality for cadaveric primary nonfunction [126]. A pilot study on the use of the PGI_2 analogue iloprost showed improvement in early postoperative graft function [127]. Further to this, a German multicenter study termed the PRAISE study is underway to evaluate the effect of intravenous iloprost on graft function after liver transplantation [128]. In a study on LDLT recipients, perioperative PGE1 infusion was shown to reduce the incidence of post-transplant renal dysfunction but no difference in incidence of PGD was observed [129]. In a setting of small for size grafts, continuous portal infusion of PGE1 was shown to attenuate portal hypertension, suppress antidonor immune responses, improved graft function resulting in better survival [130].

39.8 Other Experimental Strategies

IRI is the predominant contributor for PGD and is a complex process whose understanding is gradually evolving. On the basis of this understanding, drugs targeted at relevant pathways to ameliorate IRI are being developed and tested in animal models with promising outcomes with respect to EAD [131]. For instance, dexmedetomidine (DEX) treatment seems to protect liver against IRI in rodents by decreasing inflammation through suppressed TLR4/NF-κB pathway [132, 133]. DAS-OLT trial has been designed to prospectively evaluate the effect of DEX in cadaveric LT [134].

To conclude, early graft failure in the form of PNF or EAD has serious adverse outcomes for the patient as well as the transplant unit. Identifying and understanding the predictors of PGD, proper donor–recipient matching and other relevant perioperative strategies along with regular assessment of graft function for early recognition of PGD can help in stabilizing the postoperative course of the patient and mitigating adverse outcomes. Meticulous ICU care with focused multi-system organ support can help in stabilizing the patient until graft regeneration and recovery or retransplantation.

Key Points

- Ischemia reperfusion injury is the most important cause of early graft dysfunction.
- Early graft dysfunction is identified within the first 7 days of transplantation and all supportive measures need to be instituted to facilitate graft regeneration and recovery.
- EAD patients require additional neurological, respiratory, cardiovascular, and renal support in the postoperative period.
- EAD patients are susceptible to infections and therefore require close monitoring.
- NAC, plasmapheresis, and artificial liver support have a role in improving outcome.
- Prostaglandins improve hepatic microcirculatory blood flow and are shown to be valuable in EAD.

References

1. Lai JC, Feng S, Roberts JP. An examination of liver offers to candidates on the liver transplant wait-list. Gastroenterology. 2012;143(5):1261–5.
2. Barshes NR, Horwitz IB, Franzini L, Vierling JM, Goss JA. Waitlist mortality decreases with increased use of extended criteria donor liver grafts at adult liver transplant centers. Am J Transplant. 2007;7(5):1265–70.
3. Zhai Y, Petrowsky H, Hong JC, Busuttil RW, Kupiec-Weglinski JW. Ischaemia-reperfusion injury in liver transplantation--from bench to bedside. Nat Rev Gastroenterol Hepatol. 2013;10(2):79–89.
4. Clavien PA, Harvey PR, Strasberg SM. Preservation and reperfusion injuries in liver allografts. An overview and synthesis of current studies. Transplantation. 1992;53(5):957–78.
5. Burton JR Jr, Rosen HR. Diagnosis and management of allograft failure. Clin Liver Dis. 2006;10(2):407–35.
6. Clavien PA. Sinusoidal endothelial cell injury during hepatic preservation and reperfusion. Hepatology. 1998;28(2):281–5.
7. Deschenes M, Forbes C, Tchervenkov J, Barkun J, Metrakos P, Tector J, et al. Use of older donor livers is associated with more extensive ischemic damage on intraoperative biopsies during liver transplantation. Liver Transpl Surg. 1999;5(5):357–61.
8. Ali JM, Davies SE, Brais RJ, Randle LV, Klinck JR, Allison ME, et al. Analysis of ischemia/reperfusion injury in time-zero biopsies predicts liver allograft outcomes. Liver Transpl. 2015;21(4):487–99.
9. Bolondi G, Mocchegiani F, Montalti R, Nicolini D, Vivarelli M, De Pietri L. Predictive factors of short term outcome after liver transplantation: a review. World J Gastroenterol. 2016;22(26):5936–49.
10. Jochmans I, Fieuws S, Monbaliu D, Pirenne J. "Model for early allograft function" outperforms "early allograft dysfunction" as a predictor of transplant survival. Transplantation. 2017;101(8):e258–e64.
11. Olthoff KM, Kulik L, Samstein B, Kaminski M, Abecassis M, Emond J, et al. Validation of a current definition of early allograft dysfunction in liver transplant recipients and analysis of risk factors. Liver Transpl. 2010;16(8):943–9.
12. Pareja E, Cortes M, Hervas D, Mir J, Valdivieso A, Castell JV, et al. A score model for the continuous grading of early allograft dysfunction severity. Liver Transpl. 2015;21(1):38–46.
13. Briceno J, Ciria R, de la Mata M, Rufian S, Lopez-Cillero P. Prediction of graft dysfunction based on extended criteria donors in the model for end-stage liver disease score era. Transplantation. 2010;90(5):530–9.
14. Deschenes M, Belle SH, Krom RA, Zetterman RK, Lake JR. Early allograft dysfunction after liver transplantation: a definition and predictors of outcome. National Institute of Diabetes and Digestive and Kidney Diseases liver transplantation database. Transplantation. 1998;66(3):302–10.
15. Howard TK, Klintmalm GB, Cofer JB, Husberg BS, Goldstein RM, Gonwa TA. The influence of preservation injury on rejection in the hepatic transplant recipient. Transplantation. 1990;49(1):103–7.
16. Lee DD, Croome KP, Shalev JA, Musto KR, Sharma M, Keaveny AP, et al. Early allograft dysfunction after liver transplantation: an intermediate outcome measure for targeted improvements. Ann Hepatol. 2016;15(1):53–60.
17. Lee DD, Singh A, Burns JM, Perry DK, Nguyen JH, Taner CB. Early allograft dysfunction in liver

transplantation with donation after cardiac death donors results in inferior survival. Liver Transpl. 2014;20(12):1447–53.

18. Ploeg RJ, D'Alessandro AM, Knechtle SJ, Stegall MD, Pirsch JD, Hoffmann RM, et al. Risk factors for primary dysfunction after liver transplantation--a multivariate analysis. Transplantation. 1993;55(4):807–13.

19. Biancofiore G, Bindi ML, Romanelli AM, Bisa M, Boldrini A, Consani G, et al. Postoperative intra-abdominal pressure and renal function after liver transplantation. Arch Surg. 2003;138(7):703–6.

20. Taner CB, Bulatao IG, Willingham DL, Perry DK, Sibulesky L, Pungpapong S, et al. Events in procurement as risk factors for ischemic cholangiopathy in liver transplantation using donation after cardiac death donors. Liver Transpl. 2012;18(1):100–11.

21. Pomposelli JJ, Goodrich NP, Emond JC, Humar A, Baker TB, Grant DR, et al. Patterns of early allograft dysfunction in adult live donor liver transplantation: the A2ALL experience. Transplantation. 2016;100(7):1490–9.

22. Croome KP, Hernandez-Alejandro R, Chandok N. Early allograft dysfunction is associated with excess resource utilization after liver transplantation. Transplant Proc. 2013;45(1):259–64.

23. Croome KP, Wall W, Quan D, Vangala S, McAlister V, Marotta P, et al. Evaluation of the updated definition of early allograft dysfunction in donation after brain death and donation after cardiac death liver allografts. Hepatobiliary Pancreat Dis Int. 2012;11(4):372–6.

24. Pokorny H, Gruenberger T, Soliman T, Rockenschaub S, Langle F, Steininger R. Organ survival after primary dysfunction of liver grafts in clinical orthotopic liver transplantation. Transpl Int. 2000;13(Suppl 1):S154–7.

25. Salvalaggio P, Afonso RC, Felga G, Ferraz-Neto BH. A proposal to grade the severity of early allograft dysfunction after liver transplantation. Einstein (Sao Paulo). 2013;11(1):23–31.

26. Busuttil RW, Tanaka K. The utility of marginal donors in liver transplantation. Liver Transpl. 2003;9(7):651–63.

27. Feng S, Goodrich NP, Bragg-Gresham JL, Dykstra DM, Punch JD, DebRoy MA, et al. Characteristics associated with liver graft failure: the concept of a donor risk index. Am J Transplant. 2006;6(4):783–90.

28. Rana A, Hardy MA, Halazun KJ, Woodland DC, Ratner LE, Samstein B, et al. Survival outcomes following liver transplantation (SOFT) score: a novel method to predict patient survival following liver transplantation. Am J Transplant. 2008;8(12):2537–46.

29. Halldorson JB, Bakthavatsalam R, Fix O, Reyes JD, Perkins JD. D-MELD, a simple predictor of post liver transplant mortality for optimization of donor/recipient matching. Am J Transplant. 2009;9(2):318–26.

30. Broering DC, Topp S, Schaefer U, Fischer L, Gundlach M, Sterneck M, et al. Split liver transplantation and risk to the adult recipient: analysis using matched pairs. J Am Coll Surg. 2002;195(5):648–57.

31. Chen XB, Xu MQ. Primary graft dysfunction after liver transplantation. Hepatobiliary Pancreat Dis Int. 2014;13(2):125–37.

32. Dhillon N, Walsh L, Kruger B, Ward SC, Godbold JH, Radwan M, et al. A single nucleotide polymorphism of toll-like receptor 4 identifies the risk of developing graft failure after liver transplantation. J Hepatol. 2010;53(1):67–72.

33. Mathe Z, Paul A, Molmenti EP, Vernadakis S, Klein CG, Beckebaum S, et al. Liver transplantation with donors over the expected lifespan in the model for end-staged liver disease era: is mother nature punishing us? Liver Int. 2011;31(7):1054–61.

34. Nanashima A, Pillay P, Verran DJ, Painter D, Nakasuji M, Crawford M, et al. Analysis of initial poor graft function after orthotopic liver transplantation: experience of an australian single liver transplantation center. Transplant Proc. 2002;34(4):1231–5.

35. Levesque E, Saliba F, Benhamida S, Ichai P, Azoulay D, Adam R, et al. Plasma disappearance rate of indocyanine green: a tool to evaluate early graft outcome after liver transplantation. Liver Transpl. 2009;15(10):1358–64.

36. Olmedilla L, Lisbona CJ, Perez-Pena JM, Lopez-Baena JA, Garutti I, Salcedo M, et al. Early measurement of indocyanine green clearance accurately predicts short-term outcomes after liver transplantation. Transplantation. 2016;100(3):613–20.

37. Lock JF, Schwabauer E, Martus P, Videv N, Pratschke J, Malinowski M, et al. Early diagnosis of primary nonfunction and indication for reoperation after liver transplantation. Liver Transpl. 2010;16(2):172–80.

38. Stockmann M, Lock JF, Malinowski M, Niehues SM, Seehofer D, Neuhaus P. The LiMAx test: a new liver function test for predicting postoperative outcome in liver surgery. HPB (Oxford). 2010;12(2):139–46.

39. Nguyen HB, Rivers EP, Knoblich BP, Jacobsen G, Muzzin A, Ressler JA, et al. Early lactate clearance is associated with improved outcome in severe sepsis and septic shock. Crit Care Med. 2004;32(8):1637–42.

40. Wu JF, Wu RY, Chen J, Ou-Yang B, Chen MY, Guan XD. Early lactate clearance as a reliable predictor of initial poor graft function after orthotopic liver transplantation. Hepatobiliary Pancreat Dis Int. 2011;10(6):587–92.

41. Lesurtel M, Raptis DA, Melloul E, Schlegel A, Oberkofler C, El-Badry AM, et al. Low platelet counts after liver transplantation predict early posttransplant survival: the 60-5 criterion. Liver Transpl. 2014;20(2):147–55.

42. Li L, Wang H, Yang J, Jiang L, Yang J, Wang W, et al. Immediate postoperative low platelet counts after living donor liver transplantation predict early allograft dysfunction. Medicine (Baltimore). 2015;94(34):e1373.

43. Zulian MC, Chedid MF, Chedid AD, Grezzana Filho TJ, Leipnitz I, de Araujo A, et al. Low serum factor

V level: early predictor of allograft failure and death following liver transplantation. Langenbeck's Arch Surg. 2015;400(5):589–97.

44. Wagener G, Raffel B, Young AT, Minhaz M, Emond J. Predicting early allograft failure and mortality after liver transplantation: the role of the postoperative model for end-stage liver disease score. Liver Transpl. 2013;19(5):534–42.

45. Agopian VG, Harlander-Locke MP, Markovic D, Dumronggittigule W, Xia V, Kaldas FM, et al. Evaluation of early allograft function using the liver graft assessment following transplantation risk score model. JAMA Surg. 2018;153(5):436–44.

46. Chae MS, Kim Y, Lee N, Chung HS, Park CS, Lee J, et al. Graft regeneration and functional recovery in patients with early allograft dysfunction after living-donor liver transplantation. Ann Transplant. 2018;23:481–90.

47. Ellul MA, Gholkar SA, Cross TJ. Hepatic encephalopathy due to liver cirrhosis. BMJ. 2015;351:h4187.

48. Shawcross DL, Wendon JA. The neurological manifestations of acute liver failure. Neurochem Int. 2012;60(7):662–71.

49. Ferenci P, Lockwood A, Mullen K, Tarter R, Weissenborn K, Blei AT. Hepatic encephalopathy-definition, nomenclature, diagnosis, and quantification: final report of the working party at the 11th World Congresses of Gastroenterology, Vienna, 1998. Hepatology. 2002;35(3):716–21.

50. Brenner RP. The interpretation of the EEG in stupor and coma. Neurologist. 2005;11(5):271–84.

51. Zivkovic SA. Neurologic complications after liver transplantation. World J Hepatol. 2013;5(8):409–16.

52. Cruz RJ Jr, DiMartini A, Akhavanheidari M, Iacovoni N, Boardman JF, Donaldson J, et al. Posterior reversible encephalopathy syndrome in liver transplant patients: clinical presentation, risk factors and initial management. Am J Transplant. 2012;12(8):2228–36.

53. Lidofsky SD, Bass NM, Prager MC, Washington DE, Read AE, Wright TL, et al. Intracranial pressure monitoring and liver transplantation for fulminant hepatic failure. Hepatology. 1992;16(1):1–7.

54. Munoz SJ, Robinson M, Northrup B, Bell R, Moritz M, Jarrell B, et al. Elevated intracranial pressure and computed tomography of the brain in fulminant hepatocellular failure. Hepatology. 1991;13(2):209–12.

55. European Association for the Study of the Liver. Electronic address eee, Clinical practice guidelines p, Wendon J, Panel m, Cordoba J, Dhawan A, et al. EASL clinical practical guidelines on the management of acute (fulminant) liver failure. J Hepatol. 2017;66(5):1047–81.

56. Stravitz RT, Lisman T, Luketic VA, Sterling RK, Puri P, Fuchs M, et al. Minimal effects of acute liver injury/acute liver failure on hemostasis as assessed by thromboelastography. J Hepatol. 2012;56(1):129–36.

57. Blei AT, Olafsson S, Webster S, Levy R. Complications of intracranial pressure monitoring in fulminant hepatic failure. Lancet. 1993;341(8838):157–8.

58. Karvellas CJ, Fix OK, Battenhouse H, Durkalski V, Sanders C, Lee WM, et al. Outcomes and complications of intracranial pressure monitoring in acute liver failure: a retrospective cohort study. Crit Care Med. 2014;42(5):1157–67.

59. Keays RT, Alexander GJ, Williams R. The safety and value of extradural intracranial pressure monitors in fulminant hepatic failure. J Hepatol. 1993;18(2):205–9.

60. Vaquero J, Fontana RJ, Larson AM, Bass NM, Davern TJ, Shakil AO, et al. Complications and use of intracranial pressure monitoring in patients with acute liver failure and severe encephalopathy. Liver Transpl. 2005;11(12):1581–9.

61. Peck M, Wendon J, Sizer E, Auzinger G, Bernal W. Intracranial pressure monitoring in acute liver failure: a review of 10 years experience. Crit Care. 2010;14(S1):P542.

62. Murphy N, Auzinger G, Bernel W, Wendon J. The effect of hypertonic sodium chloride on intracranial pressure in patients with acute liver failure. Hepatology. 2004;39(2):464–70.

63. Stravitz RT, Kramer AH, Davern T, Shaikh AO, Caldwell SH, Mehta RL, et al. Intensive care of patients with acute liver failure: recommendations of the U.S. Acute Liver Failure Study Group. Crit Care Med. 2007;35(11):2498–508.

64. Audimoolam VK, McPhail MJ, Wendon JA, Willars C, Bernal W, Desai SR, et al. Lung injury and its prognostic significance in acute liver failure. Crit Care Med. 2014;42(3):592–600.

65. Luo L, Shaver CM, Zhao Z, Koyama T, Calfee CS, Bastarache JA, et al. Clinical predictors of hospital mortality differ between direct and indirect ARDS. Chest. 2017;151(4):755–63.

66. Sadowitz B, Jain S, Kollisch-Singule M, Satalin J, Andrews P, Habashi N, et al. Preemptive mechanical ventilation can block progressive acute lung injury. World J Crit Care Med. 2016;5(1):74–82.

67. Young CC, Harris EM, Vacchiano C, Bodnar S, Bukowy B, Elliott RRD, et al. Lung-protective ventilation for the surgical patient: international expert panel-based consensus recommendations. Br J Anaesth. 2019;123(6):898–913.

68. Saner FH, Olde Damink SW, Pavlakovic G, Sotiropoulos GC, Radtke A, Treckmann J, et al. How far can we go with positive end-expiratory pressure (PEEP) in liver transplant patients? J Clin Anesth. 2010;22(2):104–9.

69. Wagener G, Kovalevskaya G, Minhaz M, Mattis F, Emond JC, Landry DW. Vasopressin deficiency and vasodilatory state in end-stage liver disease. J Cardiothorac Vasc Anesth. 2011;25(4):665–70.

70. Kendrick JB, Kaye AD, Tong Y, Belani K, Urman RD, Hoffman C, et al. Goal-directed fluid therapy in the perioperative setting. J Anaesthesiol Clin Pharmacol. 2019;35(Suppl 1):S29–34.

71. Nguyen HB, Jaehne AK, Jayaprakash N, Semler MW, Hegab S, Yataco AC, et al. Early goal-directed therapy in severe sepsis and septic shock: insights and comparisons to ProCESS, ProMISe, and ARISE. Crit Care. 2016;20(1):160.

72. Bjerring PN, Eefsen M, Hansen BA, Larsen FS. The brain in acute liver failure. A tortuous path from hyperammonemia to cerebral edema. Metab Brain Dis. 2009;24(1):5–14.

73. Bari K, Garcia-Tsao G. Treatment of portal hypertension. World J Gastroenterol. 2012;18(11):1166–75.

74. D'Aragon F, Belley-Cote EP, Meade MO, Lauzier F, Adhikari NK, Briel M, et al. Blood pressure targets for vasopressor therapy: a systematic review. Shock. 2015;43(6):530–9.

75. Cardenas A, Gines P, Runyon BA. Is albumin infusion necessary after large volume paracentesis? Liver Int. 2009;29(5):636–40; discussion 40–1.

76. Tanaka KA, Esper S, Bolliger D. Perioperative factor concentrate therapy. Br J Anaesth. 2013;111(Suppl 1):i35–49.

77. McDowell Torres D, Stevens RD, Gurakar A. Acute liver failure: a management challenge for the practicing gastroenterologist. Gastroenterol Hepatol (N Y). 2010;6(7):444–50.

78. Kirchner C, Dirkmann D, Treckmann JW, Paul A, Hartmann M, Saner FH, et al. Coagulation management with factor concentrates in liver transplantation: a single-center experience. Transfusion. 2014;54(10 Pt 2):2760–8.

79. Hartmann M, Walde C, Dirkmann D, Saner FH. Safety of coagulation factor concentrates guided by ROTEM-analyses in liver transplantation: results from 372 procedures. BMC Anesthesiol. 2019;19(1):97.

80. Polson J, Lee WM. American Association for the Study of liver D. AASLD position paper: the management of acute liver failure. Hepatology. 2005;41(5):1179–97.

81. Pichler RH, Huskey J, Kowalewska J, Moiz A, Perkins J, Davis CL, et al. Kidney biopsies may help predict renal function after liver transplantation. Transplantation. 2016;100(10):2122–8.

82. Skytte Larsson J, Bragadottir G, Redfors B, Ricksten SE. Renal function and oxygenation are impaired early after liver transplantation despite hyperdynamic systemic circulation. Crit Care. 2017;21(1):87.

83. Thongprayoon C, Kaewput W, Thamcharoen N, Bathini T, Watthanasuntorn K, Lertjitbanjong P, et al. Incidence and impact of acute kidney injury after liver transplantation: a meta-analysis. J Clin Med. 2019;8(3):372.

84. Wadei HM, Lee DD, Croome KP, Mai L, Leonard D, Mai ML, et al. Early allograft dysfunction is associated with higher risk of renal nonrecovery after liver transplantation. Transplant Direct. 2018;4(4):e352.

85. Cardoso FS, Gottfried M, Tujios S, Olson JC, Karvellas CJ, Group USALFS. Continuous renal replacement therapy is associated with reduced serum ammonia levels and mortality in acute liver failure. Hepatology. 2018;67(2):711–20.

86. Deep A, Stewart CE, Dhawan A, Douiri A. Effect of continuous renal replacement therapy on outcome in pediatric acute liver failure. Crit Care Med. 2016;44(10):1910–9.

87. Knight SR, Oniscu GC, Devey L, Simpson KJ, Wigmore SJ, Harrison EM. Use of renal replacement therapy may influence graft outcomes following liver transplantation for acute liver failure: a propensity-score matched population-based retrospective cohort study. PLoS One. 2016;11(3):e0148782.

88. Davenport A, Will EJ, Davidson AM. Improved cardiovascular stability during continuous modes of renal replacement therapy in critically ill patients with acute hepatic and renal failure. Crit Care Med. 1993;21(3):328–38.

89. Davenport A, Will EJ, Davison AM. Effect of renal replacement therapy on patients with combined acute renal and fulminant hepatic failure. Kidney Int Suppl. 1993;41:S245–51.

90. Slack AJ, Auzinger G, Willars C, Dew T, Musto R, Corsilli D, et al. Ammonia clearance with haemofiltration in adults with liver disease. Liver Int. 2014;34(1):42–8.

91. Donnelly MC, Hayes PC, Simpson KJ. Role of inflammation and infection in the pathogenesis of human acute liver failure: clinical implications for monitoring and therapy. World J Gastroenterol. 2016;22(26):5958–70.

92. Plauth M, Bernal W, Dasarathy S, Merli M, Plank LD, Schutz T, et al. ESPEN guideline on clinical nutrition in liver disease. Clin Nutr. 2019;38(2):485–521.

93. Perseghin G, Mazzaferro V, Benedini S, Pulvirenti A, Coppa J, Regalia E, et al. Resting energy expenditure in diabetic and nondiabetic patients with liver cirrhosis: relation with insulin sensitivity and effect of liver transplantation and immunosuppressive therapy. Am J Clin Nutr. 2002;76(3):541–8.

94. Plank LD, Metzger DJ, McCall JL, Barclay KL, Gane EJ, Streat SJ, et al. Sequential changes in the metabolic response to orthotopic liver transplantation during the first year after surgery. Ann Surg. 2001;234(2):245–55.

95. Pillai AA, Levitsky J. Overview of immunosuppression in liver transplantation. World J Gastroenterol. 2009;15(34):4225–33.

96. Meister A. Glutathione deficiency produced by inhibition of its synthesis, and its reversal; applications in research and therapy. Pharmacol Ther. 1991;51(2):155–94.

97. Fukuzawa K, Emre S, Senyuz O, Acarli K, Schwartz ME, Miller CM. N-acetylcysteine ameliorates reperfusion injury after warm hepatic ischemia. Transplantation. 1995;59(1):6–9.

98. Harrison P, Wendon J, Williams R. Evidence of increased guanylate cyclase activation by acetylcysteine in fulminant hepatic failure. Hepatology. 1996;23(5):1067–72.

99. Kharazmi A, Nielsen H, Schiotz PO. N-acetylcysteine inhibits human neutrophil and monocyte chemotaxis and oxidative metabolism. Int J Immunopharmacol. 1988;10(1):39–46.

100. Kim DY, Jun JH, Lee HL, Woo KM, Ryoo HM, Kim GS, et al. N-acetylcysteine prevents LPS-induced pro-inflammatory cytokines and MMP2 production in gingival fibroblasts. Arch Pharm Res. 2007;30(10):1283–92.

101. Montalvo-Jave EE, Escalante-Tattersfield T, Ortega-Salgado JA, Pina E, Geller DA. Factors in the pathophysiology of the liver ischemia-reperfusion injury. J Surg Res. 2008;147(1):153–9.

102. Harrison PM, Wendon JA, Gimson AE, Alexander GJ, Williams R. Improvement by acetylcysteine of hemodynamics and oxygen transport in fulminant hepatic failure. N Engl J Med. 1991;324(26):1852–7.

103. Hu J, Zhang Q, Ren X, Sun Z, Quan Q. Efficacy and safety of acetylcysteine in "non-acetaminophen" acute liver failure: a meta-analysis of prospective clinical trials. Clin Res Hepatol Gastroenterol. 2015;39(5):594–9.

104. Lee WM, Hynan LS, Rossaro L, Fontana RJ, Stravitz RT, Larson AM, et al. Intravenous N-acetylcysteine improves transplant-free survival in early stage non-acetaminophen acute liver failure. Gastroenterology. 2009;137(3):856–64 e1.

105. Squires RH, Dhawan A, Alonso E, Narkewicz MR, Shneider BL, Rodriguez-Baez N, et al. Intravenous N-acetylcysteine in pediatric patients with nonacetaminophen acute liver failure: a placebo-controlled clinical trial. Hepatology. 2013;57(4):1542–9.

106. Stravitz RT, Sanyal AJ, Reisch J, Bajaj JS, Mirshahi F, Cheng J, et al. Effects of N-acetylcysteine on cytokines in non-acetaminophen acute liver failure: potential mechanism of improvement in transplant-free survival. Liver Int. 2013;33(9):1324–31.

107. Thies JC, Koeppel TA, Lehmann T, Schemmer P, Otto G, Post S. Efficacy of N-acetylcysteine as a hepatoprotective agent in liver transplantation: an experimental study. Transplant Proc. 1997;29(1–2):1326–7.

108. Bromley PN, Cottam SJ, Hilmi I, Tan KC, Heaton N, Ginsburg R, et al. Effects of intraoperative N-acetylcysteine in orthotopic liver transplantation. Br J Anaesth. 1995;75(3):352–4.

109. Hilmi IA, Peng Z, Planinsic RM, Damian D, Dai F, Tyurina YY, et al. N-acetylcysteine does not prevent hepatorenal ischaemia-reperfusion injury in patients undergoing orthotopic liver transplantation. Nephrol Dial Transplant. 2010;25(7):2328–33.

110. Bavikatte A, Sudhindran S. Perioperative influence of N-acetylcysteine (NAC) on early post transplant outcome of recepient in live donor liver transplantation (LDLT): a double blind randomized controlled trial. HPB. 2016;18:e160.

111. D'Amico F, Vitale A, Piovan D, Bertacco A, Ramirez Morales R, Chiara Frigo A, et al. Use of N-acetylcysteine during liver procurement: a prospective randomized controlled study. Liver Transpl. 2013;19(2):135–44.

112. Tan EX, Wang MX, Pang J, Lee GH. Plasma exchange in patients with acute and acute-on-chronic liver failure: a systematic review. World J Gastroenterol. 2020;26(2):219–45.

113. Larsen FS, Schmidt LE, Bernsmeier C, Rasmussen A, Isoniemi H, Patel VC, et al. High-volume plasma exchange in patients with acute liver failure: an open randomised controlled trial. J Hepatol. 2016;64(1):69–78.

114. Camci C, Akdogan M, Gurakar A, Gilcher R, Rose J, Monlux R, et al. The impact of total plasma exchange on early allograft dysfunction. Transplant Proc. 2004;36(9):2567–9.

115. Akdogan M, Camci C, Gurakar A, Gilcher R, Alamian S, Wright H, et al. The effect of total plasma exchange on fulminant hepatic failure. J Clin Apher. 2006;21(2):96–9.

116. Choe W, Kwon SW, Kim SS, Hwang S, Song GW, Lee SG. Effects of therapeutic plasma exchange on early allograft dysfunction after liver transplantation. J Clin Apher. 2017;32(3):147–53.

117. Yamamoto R, Nagasawa Y, Marubashi S, Furumatsu Y, Iwatani H, Iio K, et al. Early plasma exchange for progressive liver failure in recipients of adult-to-adult living-related liver transplants. Blood Purif. 2009;28(1):40–6.

118. Park CS, Hwang S, Park HW, Park YH, Lee HJ, Namgoong JM, et al. Role of plasmapheresis as liver support for early graft dysfunction following adult living donor liver transplantation. Transplant Proc. 2012;44(3):749–51.

119. Lee JY, Kim SB, Chang JW, Park SK, Kwon SW, Song KW, et al. Comparison of the molecular adsorbent recirculating system and plasmapheresis for patients with graft dysfunction after liver transplantation. Transplant Proc. 2010;42(7):2625–30.

120. Rammohan A, Sachan D, Logidasan S, Sathyanesan J, Palaniappan R, Rela M. World J Hematol 2017;6(1):24–7.

121. Cheng CW, Hendrickson JE, Tormey CA, Sidhu D. Therapeutic plasma exchange and its impact on drug levels: an ACLPS critical review. Am J Clin Pathol. 2017;148(3):190–8.

122. Ibrahim RB, Liu C, Cronin SM, Murphy BC, Cha R, Swerdlow P, et al. Drug removal by plasmapheresis: an evidence-based review. Pharmacotherapy. 2007;27(11):1529–49.

123. Larsen FS. Artificial liver support in acute and acute-on-chronic liver failure. Curr Opin Crit Care. 2019;25(2):187–91.

124. Alshamsi F, Alshammari K, Belley-Cote E, Dionne J, Albrahim T, Albudoor B, et al. Extracorporeal liver support in patients with liver failure: a systematic review and meta-analysis of randomized trials. Intensive Care Med. 2020;46(1):1–16.

125. Fuhrmann V, Bauer M, Wilmer A. The persistent potential of extracorporeal therapies in liver failure. Intensive Care Med. 2020;46(3):528–30.

126. Cavalcanti AB, De Vasconcelos CP, Perroni de Oliveira M, Rother ET, Ferraz L Jr. Prostaglandins for adult liver transplanted patients. Cochrane Database Syst Rev. 2011;11:CD006006.

127. Barthel E, Rauchfuss F, Hoyer H, Habrecht O, Jandt K, Gotz M, et al. Impact of stable PGI(2) analog iloprost on early graft viability after liver transplantation: a pilot study. Clin Transpl. 2012;26(1):E38–47.

128. Barthel E, Rauchfuss F, Hoyer H, Breternitz M, Jandt K, Settmacher U. The PRAISE study: a prospective, multi-center, randomized, double blinded, placebo-controlled study for the evaluation of iloprost in the early postoperative period after liver transplantation (ISRCTN12622749). BMC Surg. 2013;13:1.

129. Bharathan VK, Chandran B, Gopalakrishnan U, Varghese CT, Menon RN, Balakrishnan D, et al. Perioperative prostaglandin e1 infusion in living donor liver transplantation: a double-blind, placebo-controlled randomized trial. Liver Transpl. 2016;22(8):1067–74.

130. Onoe T, Tanaka Y, Ide K, Ishiyama K, Oshita A, Kobayashi T, et al. Attenuation of portal hypertension by continuous portal infusion of PGE1 and immunologic impact in adult-to-adult living-donor liver transplantation. Transplantation. 2013;95(12):1521–7.

131. Zhou J, Chen J, Wei Q, Saeb-Parsy K, Xu X. The role of ischemia/reperfusion injury in early hepatic allograft dysfunction. Liver Transpl. 2020;26(8):1034–48.

132. Wang Y, Wu S, Yu X, Zhou S, Ge M, Chi X, et al. Dexmedetomidine protects rat liver against ischemia-reperfusion injury partly by the alpha2A-adrenoceptor subtype and the mechanism is associated with the TLR4/NF-kappaB pathway. Int J Mol Sci. 2016;17(7):995.

133. Chen Z, Ding T, Ma C-G. Dexmedetomidine (DEX) protects against hepatic ischemia/reperfusion (I/R) injury by suppressing inflammation and oxidative stress in NLRC5 deficient mice. Biochem Biophys Res Commun. 2017;493(2):1143–50.

134. Ni C, Masters J, Zhu L, Yu W, Jiao Y, Yang Y, et al. Study design of the DAS-OLT trial: a randomized controlled trial to evaluate the impact of dexmedetomidine on early allograft dysfunction following liver transplantation. Trials. 2020;21(1):582.

Postoperative Renal Dysfunction in Recipient

40

Piyush Srivastava, Anil Agrawal, and Amit Jha

Abbreviations

ADQI	Acute disease quality initiative
AKI	Acute kidney injury
ATN	Acute tubular necrosis
CKD	Chronic kidney disease
CKD-EPI	Chronic kidney disease epidemiology
CNI	Calcineurin inhibitor
Cys C	Cystatin C
DCD	Donation after circulatory death
DDLT	Deceased donor liver transplantation
ESRD	End-stage renal disease
EVR	Everolimus
GFR	Glomerular filtration rate
GRWR	Graft-recipient body weight ratio
HCV	Hepatitis C virus
HRS	Hepatorenal syndrome
ICA	International club of ascites
IL-18	Interleukin-18
KDIGO	Kidney disease: improving global outcomes
LDLT	Live donor liver transplantation
LT	Liver transplantation
MDRD	Modification of diet in renal disease
MELD	Model of end-stage liver disease
MMF	Mycophenolate mofetil
mTOR	Mammalian target of rapamycin
NASH	nonalcoholic steatohepatitis
NGAL	Neutrophil gelatinase-associated lipocalin
PRS	Post reperfusion syndrome
RBC	Red blood cell
RRT	Renal replacement therapy
SBP	Spontaneous bacterial peritonitis
SCr	Serum creatinine
SLKT	Simultaneous liver kidney transplantation

40.1 Objective

This chapter will:
1. Asses renal function before and after liver transplantation
2. Present the risk factors for early postoperative acute kidney injury after liver transplantation, including pre-LT, intraoperative factors, and post-LT factors.
3. Present the factors affecting renal dysfunction in long-term survivors.
4. Suggest strategies to reduce risk factors.

P. Srivastava (✉) · A. Agrawal · A. Jha
Liver Transplant Anesthesia and Critical Care,
Fortis Hospitals, Noida, India

40.2   Preamble

AKI is a common and significant complication after liver transplantation (LT), and is associated with increased acute rejection, infection, hospital length of stay, utilization of resources, and health care costs and poor long-term survival [1, 2]. Although the survival of LT recipients has improved substantially over the past few decades, mortality rates related to post-LT, AKI, and subsequent progressive CKD remain high and are of increasing concern [1–5]. Sometimes these patients require transient renal replacement therapy (RRT) immediately following LT.

Recent studies have demonstrated a wide variety of risk factors for the development of post-LT AKI and its aetiology is therefore considered multifactorial. Presence of AKI in pre-transplant set up is a predisposing factor for post-transplant chronic kidney disease (CKD), both which may lead to higher morbidity and mortality especially in patients with acute tubular necrosis (ATN) prior to LT as compared to patients with hepatorenal syndrome. The cumulative risk of developing chronic renal failure post-LT has been described to be approximately 8–18% at 1–5 years after LT. Therefore identifying the risk factors for AKI or progressive CKD after LT and developing strategies to either minimize the risks for AKI or retard the progression of CKD should be an integral part in the management of LT recipients. Assessment of renal function pre- and post-LT and an overview of the literature on the risk factors for early postoperative AKI and those affecting progressive CKD in long-term survivors are presented. Suggested therapeutic approaches to prevent, halt, or ameliorate renal dysfunction are also discussed.

40.3   Definition of AKI

Our understanding of the scope of renal dysfunction at the time of liver transplantation is often clouded due to paucity of accepted definitions, as evidenced by the many studies that do not differentiate between AKI, CKD, and AKI superimposed on CKD. Although it is often clinically obvious when renal dysfunction occurs, there is currently no consensus on the definition of AKI in the setting of liver transplantation, and this makes the existing literature difficult to compare. Several definitions based on different criteria have been used to define AKI. Many of them were complex, it became crucial to establish a consensual and accurate definition of AKI that could ideally be used globally.

40.3.1   RIFLE Criteria

In May 2002, the acute dialysis quality initiative (ADQI) group for the study of AKI, composed of nephrologists and intensivists, came together reached to a consensus with the purpose of defining AKI. They introduced the consensual RIFLE (risk, injury, failure, loss of kidney function, and end-stage kidney disease) classification for AKI definition which was published in May 2004 in critical care [6].

The RIFLE criteria consider three stages of severity of AKI (risk, injury, and loss) based on changes in serum creatinine levels and urine output. The temporal pattern of the SCr and/or UO variation is also relevant for defining AKI: the deterioration of renal function must be sudden (1–7 days) and sustained (persisting >24 h).

The RIFLE-criteria were subsequently evaluated in a large multicentre intensive care population and shown to be a sensitive definition of AKI and associated with increased hospital mortality. Similarly, in a retrospective cohort of 300 liver transplant recipients, O'Riordan et al. [7], used RIFLE-criteria to classify post-LT AKI and found that AKI-Injury (AKI-I) occurred in 11% and AKI-Failure (AKI-F) in 26% patients; AKI-F was also associated with inferior short-term patient survival. Similar results were found by Kundacki et al. in his smaller study cohort (n = 112) [8]. Another author demonstrated that the 23% of recipients had AKI-R, 21% AKI-I, and 16% AKI-F in a cohort of 440 Living-Donor Liver Transplantations [9].

Despite its clinical use, the RIFLE criteria has important shortcomings. First, baseline SCr is necessary to define and classify AKI; and several studies have found out that determination of AKI based on SCr has number of limitation [10]. Second, decreased UO is sensitive and frequent in AKI; however, it also has some important limitations in defining and staging AKI [11].

It must also be highlighted that the RIFLE criteria has only evaluated in a minority (<2%) of patients included in prospective studies. This major concern definitely did limit the analysis of other clinical or laboratory variables with prognostic impact on the epidemiology of AKI.

40.3.2 Acute Kidney Injury Network (AKIN) Classification

In 2007 the Acute Kidney Injury Network (AKIN) group, a multidisciplinary consensus workgroup of nephrologists and critical care physicians, proposed a more sensitive and strict definition of AKI and it is a later version of the RIFLE classification with some modifications [12].

In these AKIN criteria a smaller change in SCr was used as threshold for diagnosis of AKI. To ensure that the renal insult is acute and representative of events within a clinically relevant time period, a time constraint of 48 hours for diagnosis of AKI was defined. Furthermore, patients on renal replacement therapy (RRT) were also considered to have met the criteria for stage 3 AKI. The "Loss" and "End-stage" categories of RIFLE were omitted since they were considered to be outcomes instead of stages of AKI (Table 40.1). Later two studies with larger cohort among intensive care patients validated these modified criteria [14, 15]. Similarly, in even a small rise of serum creatinine seem to be associated with higher short-term mortality among the cirrhotic and liver transplant recipients. In a cohort of 193 consecutive liver transplantations, AKI according to AKIN criteria was reported in 60% of recipients and 28-day and 1- year mortality were 15% and 26% in patients with AKI compared to 0% and 4% in patients without AKI [16]. Furthermore, in a study of 70 liver transplant recipients AKIN criteria identified AKI in an additional 13% of recipients compared to the RIFLE-criteria [17]. A large European validation study of the AKIN criteria also emphasized that despite the lower diagnostic threshold for AKI, the AKIN criteria performed similarly as the RIFLE-criteria in terms of defining outcome [14].

Table 40.1 Current diagnostic criteria for acute kidney injury (AKI) in the general population and in patients with cirrhosis

	RIFLE criteria	AKIN criteria	KDIGO criteria	Conventional criteria
Diagnostic criteria	Increase in SCR to ≥1.5 times baseline, within 7 days, or GFR decreases>25% or U/O <0.05 ml/kg/h for 6 h	Increase in SCr by ≥0.3 mg/dl (26.5 μmol/L) within 48 h; or Increase in SCr ≥1.5 times baseline within 48 h; or urine volume <0.5 ml/kg/h for 6 h	Increase in SCr by ≥0.3 mg/dl (26.5 μmol/L) within 48 h; or increase in SCr to ≥1.5 times baseline, which is known or presumed to have occurred within the prior 7 days; or Urine volume <0.5 ml/kg/h for 6 h	A percentage increase in SCr of 50% or more to a final value of SCr >1.5 mg/dl (133 μmol/L)
Staging	Risk SCr increase 1.5–1.9 times baseline; or GFR decrease 25–50%; or Urine output <0.5 ml/kg/h for 6 h	Stage 1 SCr increase 1.5–1.9 times baseline; or SCr increase ≥0.3 mg/dl (26.5 μmol/L); or Urine output <0.5 ml/kg/h for 6 h	Stage 1 SCr increase 1.5–1.9 times baseline; or Cr increase ≥0.3 mg/dl (26.5 μmol/L); or Urine output <0.5 ml/kg/h for 6–12 h	None

(continued)

Table 40.1 (continued)

	RIFLE criteria	AKIN criteria	KDIGO criteria	Conventional criteria
	Injury SCr increase 2.0–2.9 times baseline; or GFR decrease 50–75%; or Urine output <0.5 ml/kg/h for 12 h	Stage 2 SCr increase 2.0–2.9 times baseline; or Urine output <0.5 ml/kg/h for 12 h	Stage 2 SCr increase 2.0–2.9 times baseline; or Urine output <0.5 ml/kg/h for ≥12 h	
	Failure SCr increase ≥3.0 times baseline; or GFR decrease 50–75%; or sCr increase ≥4.0 mg/dl (353.6 μmol/L) with an acute increase of at least 0.5 mg/dl (44 μmol/L); or Urine output <0.3 ml/kg/h for ≥24 h; or Anuria for ≥12 h	Stage 3 SCr increase 3.0 times baseline; or SCr increase ≥4.0 mg/dl (353.6 μmol/L) with an acute increase of at least 0.5 mg/dl (44 μmol/L); or Urine output <0.3 ml/kg/h for ≥24 h; or Anuria for ≥12 h	Stage 3 SCr increase 3.0 times baseline; or SCr increase to ≥4.0 mg/dl (353.6 μmol/L); or Initiation of renal replacement therapy; or Urine output <0.3 ml/kg/h for ≥24 h; or Anuria for ≥12 h	

AKIN acute kidney injury network, *GFR* glomerular filtration rate, *KDIGO* kidney disease improving global outcome, *RIFLE* risk, injury, failure, loss, end-stage renal disease, *SCr* serum creatinine

40.3.3 KIDGO Revision of RIFLE and AKIN Criteria

In 2012, the Kidney Disease Improving Global Outcomes (KDIGO) released their clinical practice guidelines for acute kidney injury (AKI), which build off of the RIFLE criteria and the AKIN criteria [18]. This revised AKI classification merged the AKIN and RIFLE-criteria by including both an increase of serum creatinine by ≥26 μmol/L within 48 h as well as an increase to ≥1.5 times baseline within 7 days as threshold for diagnosis of AKI. The further details of KDIGO criteria have been described in Table 40.1. Till now few studies have used the revised KDIGO criteria to evaluate post-LT AKI. Trinh et al. [19] identified KDIGO-AKI in 57% of 491 liver transplant recipients, of whom 33% had stage I, 14% stage II, and 10% stage III. A single-centre cohort of 1152 patients observed KDIGO-AKI ≥ stage II in 33% recipients, but did not report AKI stage I [20]. In both studies post-LT AKI was associated with higher incidence of CKD and reduced short- and long-term patient survival [19, 20].

40.4 Why Do We Need to Change the Conventional Diagnostic Criteria for AKI?

This should be borne in mind when interpreting current definition and diagnostic criteria of renal failure in cirrhosis?" Currently, studies on AKI in patients with cirrhosis showed that AKI defined by an absolute increase in SCr P0.3 mg/dl (26.5 lmol/L) and/or P50% from baseline is associated with a higher probability of the patients being transferred to the intensive care unit, a longer hospital stay, and an increased in-hospital as well as 90-day and mid-term mortality [21–24]. On the basis of this evidence, all the experts at International Consensus Conference and the ICA has agreed to change the current definition of renal failure by introducing a modified version of the KDIGO criteria for the diagnosis of AKI in patients with cirrhosis (Table 40.2). In the new ICA criteria for the diagnosis of AKI, the use of urine output as one of the criteria has been removed since it does not apply to patients with cirrhosis (i.e., many patients are oliguric but have preserved kidney function). Staging system of

Table 40.2 International club of ascites (ICA-AKI) new definitions for the diagnosis and management of AKI in patients with cirrhosis

Subject	Definition
Baseline SCr	A value of SCr obtained in the previous 3 months, when available, can be used as baseline SCr. In patients with more than one value within the previous 3 months, the value closest to the admission time to the hospital should be used. In patients without a previous SCr value, the SCr on admission should be used as baseline
Definition of AKI	Increase in SCr $\geq$0.3 mg/dl ($\geq$26.5 µmol/L) within 48 h; or A percentage increase SCr $\geq$50% from baseline which is known, or presumed, to have occurred within the prior 7 days
Staging of AKI	Stage 1: increase in SCr $\geq$0.3 mg/dl (26.5 µmol/L) or an increase in SCr $\geq$1.5-fold to 2-fold from baseline Stage 2: increase in SCr >2-fold to 3-fold from baseline Stage 3: increase of SCr >3-fold from baseline or SCr $\geq$4.0 mg/dl (353.6 µmol/L) with an acute increase $\geq$0.3 mg/dl (26.5 µmol/L) or initiation of renal replacement therapy
Progression of AKI	Progression Progression of AKI to a higher stage and/or need for RR Regression Regression of AKI to a lower stage

AKI acute kidney injury, *RRT* renal replacement therapy, *SCr* serum creatinine

the AKI helps in defining severity of renal dysfunction once it sets in and also allows to identify the patients at high risk and to manage different stages of AKI.

40.5 Assessment of Renal Function Before and After Liver Transplantation

Exogenous markers (inulin or iohexol) or endogenous markers like SCr or CysC is readily accessible in routine clinical practice [25, 26]. Although measured GFR remains the gold standard in assessment of renal function, SCr or creatinine-based equations overestimates true GFR, particularly in the setting of severe renal dysfunction or more severe liver disease. In recent years, Cys C has been studied extensively as an alternative endogenous marker of kidney function in cirrhotic patients. Cys C is a nonglycosylated low molecular weight basic protein produced at a constant rate by nucleated cells and less influenced by factors that may influence SCr, such as muscle mass and gender. In a study comparing the performance of various creatinine SCr and Cys C-based GFR-predicting equations in LT candidates (including CKD-EPI (creat), CKD-EPI (Cys C), and CKD-EPI (creat-Cys C) and the 4- and 6-variable Modification of Diet in Renal Disease (MDRD) and Hoek formulas), De Souza et al. [27] demonstrated that Cys C-based had a better performance than creatinine-based equations, with CKD-EPI (Cys C) equation showing the best performance regardless of the severity of ascites and in the presence of significant renal dysfunction defined as GFR less than 60 mL/min. In a small Japanese study of 14 cirrhotic patients, Adachi et al. [28] similarly demonstrated that Cys C-based GFR-estimating equations had better performances compared with creatinine-based equations in terms of bias, precision, and accuracy. However, the superior performance of Cys C above creatinine in cirrhotic patients with GFR less than 80 mL/min has not been demonstrated consistently [29].

Similar to the cirrhotic population, Cys C also has been suggested to be a more accurate filtration marker than creatinine among LT recipients. In a study to evaluate whether the addition of Cys C improves GFR estimation compared with various GFR estimating equations, Allen et al. [30] demonstrated that Cys C based equations had superior performance in GFR estimation compared with creatinine-based equations, whereas CKD-EPI (creat-Cys C) outperformed those with either marker alone. A total of 586 iothalamate-measured GFR in 401 LT recipients were available for analysis. Of the five GFR estimation equations examined, CKD-EPI (creat-Cys C) was shown to have the highest coefficient of determination (R^2 of 0.83), followed by CKD-EPI (Cys C) (R^2 of 0.78), MDRD-6 (R^2 of 0.77), and MDRD-4 and CKD-EPI (creat) (R^2 of 0.76

for both). Nonetheless, the CKD-EPI (creat-Cys C) formula still underestimated measured GFR by approximately 12%, particularly in low GFR groups.

Although not yet readily available in many centres, Cys C-based equations may enable clinicians to more accurately assess renal function in LT candidates and recipients. However, Cys C levels may be increased in high cell turnover states (such as hyperthyroidism, steroid use, and malignancy), advanced age, gender and ethnicity, fat mass, and diabetes, among others. Although, more costly and complicated, traditional studies evaluating the renal clearance of inulin or radioisotopes such as iothalamate remain the gold standard for evaluating renal function in patients with liver cirrhosis and in LT recipients.

Post-LT, several factors like inflammation and immunosuppression may affect Cys C level, thus hampering the accurate estimation of GFR, though higher discrepancy has been seen in the lowest GFR group. Serum Cys C itself or as part of the equation to measure GFR was the strongest independent predictor of mortality, an observation also noted in other populations [31, 32].

40.6   Biomarkers of AKI

Though, SCr, blood urea, fraction excretion of sodium or urine output itself are used worldwide to diagnose and determine the aetiology of AKI, but they are still considered as poor marker to ascertain presence of AKI. These limitations further go up in the patients with concurrent cirrhosis. In candidates for LT, it has been shown that there is a poor correlation between conventional markers and biopsy findings [33, 34].

These biomarkers should ideally be able to identify early stages of AKI to allow interventions aimed at preventing progression and facilitating recovery. Biomarkers could also provide information about the aetiology of AKI and help distinguishing functional changes from structural renal damage thus helping in prediction of outcome. Up to now several biomarkers for AKI have been identified. Although these novel AKI biomarkers have primarily been evaluated in general intensive care populations, they are also being studied in liver transplant recipients primarily in pre-transplant setting [35]. The most studied biomarkers associated with tubular damage are neutrophil gelatinase-associated lipocalin (NGAL), kidney injury molecule-1 (KIM-1), liver fatty acid-binding protein (L-FABP), and interleukin 18 (IL-18) [36].

Markers of acute tubular injury has been found to be more predictable as it shows the ischemia related events but unfortunately not always specific thus yet to be validated. NGAL, a small secreted polypeptide, is markedly upregulated in response to tubular injury and subsequently detectable in plasma and urine. Nickolas et al. have shown that measurement of NGAL in plasma or urine helps in detecting early AKI pre-transplant [37]. Studies had found that measurement of NGAL at ICU admission has high positive predictive value for the development of severe AKI in a large prospective mixed ICU population [38]. In one of the studies among liver transplantation recipients, a single measurement of plasma NGAL within 24 h predicted AKI and severe AKI with a high degree of accuracy and was superior to SCr at determining which patients were at risk of post-LT AKI [39]. Recently a small study highlighted a significant observation by showing that urinary NGAL was a sensitive biomarker for the development of CNI-induced AKI early after liver transplantation [40]. Despite these evidence, there are also increasing concerns regarding specificity of NGAL for renal damage as it has been found to have inconsistent association. NGAL is produced at a low level in many different tissues and both acute and chronic systemic inflammation contributes to the release of NGAL thus posing a challenge in identification of AKI and spectrum of kidney dysfunction as well. In a study of 107 liver transplant recipients, author found that plasma and urinary NGAL were not only associated with postoperative renal function, but also with white blood cell count and other inflammation parameters [41].

Renal biomarkers predictive of recovery from AKI after LT could enhance decision algorithms regarding the need for simultaneous liver-kidney transplant (SLKT) or renal sparing regimens [12, 35]. In a single-centre study, Levitsky et al. found that levels of TIMP-1 and osteopontin along with patient characteristics (age, diabetes) were able to differentiate between recipients that developed reversible versus irreversible AKI post LT [12].

Recent advances in molecular biology have resulted in promising biomarkers for AKI and CKD diagnoses; concerns remain that hamper broad clinical application. Thus more research studies are necessary to implement them successfully into clinical practice in order to facilitate early diagnosis, guide interventions, and monitor disease progression.

40.7 Burden of Renal Dysfunction After Liver Transplantation

The detrimental effect of AKI after LT was recognized several decades ago, with 1-year CKD incidence of 52% and hospital mortality as high as 90% in recipients requiring RRT [42]. Since, several blooming, particularly in surgery, perioperative care and immunosuppression have significantly improved outcomes in liver transplant recipients. However, AKI still remains an important risk factor for morbidity and mortality after liver transplantation. United Network for Organ Sharing data show 1-, 5-, and 10-year liver transplant recipient survival rates of 88%, 74%, and 60%, respectively [43]. In NIDDK long-term follow-up study by Watt et al. looked at risk factors for mortality in liver transplant recipients [44] and found that recipient survival rates 1, 3, 5, and 10 years after transplantation were 87.0%, 78.6%, 74.9%, and 59.4%, respectively. As for the cause of death, 6.8% were directly attributed to kidney failure. Renal dysfunction before or after liver transplantation modified the risk for overall death more than 1 year after transplantation [hazard ratio (HR) 1/4 3.59] and for hepatic failure-associated death (HR 1/4 5.1). Renal dysfunction before or after liver transplantation conveyed an HR for death of 2.66. Furthermore, the timing of renal dysfunction predicted the risk of

mortality more than 1 year after liver transplantation. In comparison with normal pre- transplant renal function, renal dysfunction developing less than 1 year after transplantation resulted in an HR for death of 2.41; renal dysfunction 1–5 years after transplantation resulted in an HR of 6.58; and the development of renal dysfunction more than 5 years after transplantation afforded an HR for death of 7.49. Zhu et al. [16] evaluated consequences of post–liver transplant AKI for mortality and found 28-day and 1-year mortality rates for liver transplant recipients who did not develop AKI were 0% and 3.9%, respectively. However, in those who developed AKI, the mortality rates were markedly increased to 15.5% and 25.9%, respectively.

Several studies confirmed previous observations that the occurrence of mild AKI is associated with decreased patient survival after liver transplantation. The development of renal dysfunction (both AKI and CKD) after liver transplantation appears to be associated with a profound mortality risk. It is unclear whether AKI after liver transplantation is the primary driver of worse mortality outcomes or is merely associative. There is a strong association between the development of CKD and increased mortality after liver transplantation, but as with AKI, causality is unclear. Regardless, renal dysfunction after liver transplantation is a marker of increased LOS, nonrenal complications, poor outcomes, and prevention should be a major focus of post-transplant care.

40.8 Risk Factors for Postoperative Acute Kidney Injury After Orthotopic Liver Transplantat

Patients with cirrhosis have an higher risk of developing renal dysfunction, both short and long term, and is associated with several complications, additional organ failure, and marked decrease in short-term survival [45]. AKI has been reported to develop in 17–95% of LT recipients, whereas severe AKI requiring perioperative RRT occurred in 5–35% of patients [46, 47]. The broad range in the incidence reported may be attributed to, in part, the poor standardization of criteria, defining AKI among studies. In one study consisting of 424 LT recipients, AKI within the first 3 days after transplantation occurred in 52% of patients [48]. The former was defined as "50% increase in serum creatinine from preoperative baseline value or a 26.5 μmol/L increase from baseline within 48 h without urine output" [48]. Although the development of AKI after LT are often multifactorial and difficult to establish, they can be linked to three distinct time frames in relation to the LT: the pre-LT, intraoperative, and post-LT periods (immediate and long term) and summarize suggested risk factors for early postoperative AKI and strategies to reduce risk factors.

40.8.1 Pre-transplantation Risk Factors

Pre-transplantation renal dysfunction and HRS are well-established risk factors for post transplantation AKI. Other suggested risk factors include higher serum bilirubin levels, hypoproteinemia, hypoalbuminemia, hyponatremia, viral hepatitis, high serum lactate levels, and severity of liver disease as reflected by the Child-Pugh or MELD scores. The Organ Procurement and Transplantation Network recently has incorporated sodium into the MELD score. As of January 2016, the MELD-Na score is employed in the liver allocation system in the United States. Selected studies evaluating potential pretransplant risk factors for postoperative AKI and suggested pathogenic mechanisms and their preventive measures are discussed.

40.8.2 Hyponatremia

The presence of hyponatremia, defined as a serum sodium level below 130 mEq/L at the time of transplantation, has been suggested to be associated with a high rate of complications after LT,

including neurologic disorders, infectious complications, and AKI during the first month after transplantation [49]. It is well established that the presence of hyponatremia identifies a group of patients with cirrhosis who have severe impairment in circulatory function. The latter may act in concert with the intraoperative and perioperative hemodynamic changes to increase the risk of postoperative AKI.

In a single-centre retrospective study consisting of 134 LT recipients, AKI occurred in nearly half of patients (46.7%) in the postoperative period. Serum sodium was lower in the AKI compared with the non-AKI groups ($p = 0.02$). Viral hepatitis, longer warm ischemia time, and high levels of serum lactate were found to be risk factors for AKI, whereas a high MELD-Na score is a predictor for HD need [50]. A greater than eightfold increase in post-transplant HD need was observed among patients with a MELD-Na score of at least 22 (OR 8.4, 95% CI = 1.5–46.5). Among LT recipients with viral liver disease, it is speculated that undiagnosed viral glomerulonephritis and superimposed hemodynamic instability may play a causative role in the development of AKI after LT. In a small series of 30 LT recipients with hepatitis C who underwent intraoperative kidney biopsy, membranoproliferative glomerulonephritis was found in 12, IgA nephropathy in 7, and mesangial glomerulonephritis in 6 [51].

40.8.3 Hypoalbuminemia

A meta-analysis of observational clinical studies showed that lower serum albumin was an independent predictor of AKI and death after AKI development [52]. The odds of development of AKI in association with low serum albumin were more than doubled among the six studies of surgical or intensive care unit patients and nearly tripled among studies in other hospital settings. For every 10 g/L decrement in serum albumin, the odds of developing AKI increased by 134% (CI 1.74–3.14) [52].

The mechanisms how low serum albumin increases the risk of postoperative AKI remain unclear. Nonetheless, it has been suggested that hypoalbuminemia modifies Starling's forces in the systemic capillaries and results in the reduction of GFR [53]. Hypoalbuminemia also has been suggested to alter the pharmacokinetics of potentially nephrotoxic drugs, thereby increasing the risk of AKI. In a prospective study consisting of 104 patients treated with intravenous amikacin for at least 36 h, low serum albumin was found to be associated with amikacin accumulation in the plasma and an increased risk of nephrotoxicity [54]. It is speculated that specific ligand-binding properties of albumin may mediate renoprotection in patients treated with nephrotoxic drugs. In his propensity score analysis of 998 consecutive patients Sang et al. found that hypoalbuminemia within two postoperative days is an independent risk factor for acute kidney injury following living donor liver transplantation. Prevalence of AKI based on RIFLE and mortality after LTx was higher in patients with hypoalbunemeia [55].

40.8.4 Hyperbilirubinemia

The association between high serum bilirubin level and postoperative AKI has long been recognized. The spectrum of cholaemic nephrosis ranges from proximal tubulopathy to bile cast nephropathy and it is usually seen in prolong cholestasis or ACLF. In a clinicopathologic study of 44 jaundiced subjects (41 autopsies and 3 kidney biopsies), 18 had bile casts involving distal nephron segments and 6 had extension to proximal tubules. Eleven of 13 patients with HRS and all 10 with alcohol-related cirrhosis had tubular bile casts. A significant correlation was found between these casts and higher serum total and direct bilirubin levels ($p = 0.0001$ and $p = 0.003$, respectively). Furthermore, a trend toward higher serum creatinine, aspartate transaminase, and alanine transaminase levels were observed among patients with bile casts compared with those without. It is suggested that bile cast-associated AKI is due to direct bile and bilirubin toxicity and tubular obstruction analogous to that observed with myeloma or myoglobin casts [56].

40.8.5 Liver Disease Severity

Post-LT AKI occurs much more commonly than postoperative AKI in the rest of the surgical population with normal preoperative renal function [57–59]. Several studies have shown an association between pre-LT MELD score and post-LT AKI [2, 3, 15, 59]. In a retrospective study consisting of more than 600 recipients of liver-only transplants, Sanchez et al. [60] demonstrated that MELD scores greater than 21 were significant predictive indicators of the need for renal replacement therapy after LT. The association between MELD score and severe AKI also was demonstrated by others too. In a retrospective study consisting of 153 LT recipients, hepatic encephalopathy, deceased donor liver transplant (compared with living donor transplant), MELD score, and intraoperative blood loss were found to be independent predictive factors for postoperative continuous renal replacement therapy [61]. A more favourable renal outcome was observed among LT recipients with hepatocellular carcinoma (HCC) as the indication for LT. The study findings suggest that liver disease severity as reflected by high MELD score portends a worse renal prognosis. LT recipients with HCC generally had preserved liver function and a lower MELD score than LT recipients with end-stage liver disease. However, the impact of pre-LT AKI on prevalence of post-LT AKI stills needs to be made clear. Of note, Hilmi et al. found that neither age, baseline renal function, nor the majority of intraoperative variables were associated with the development of early post-LT AKI. She further clarified that female sex, high Child–Pugh score high MELD without renal dysfunction and other factors were associated with higher incidence of post-LT AKI [48].

40.9 Strategies to Reduce Pre-transplantation Risk Factors

Every effort should be made to prevent or minimize the risk of developing pre-transplantation AKI or HRS. Suggested predictive and precipitating factors for the development of HRS and proposed preventive measures are given in Table 40.3. The potential benefits of diuretics, lactulose, contrast dye exposure, nephrotoxic medications, and nonsteroidal anti-inflammatory drugs must be balanced carefully against the risk of precipitating HRS. Large-volume paracentesis in patients with severe hypoalbuminemia or ascites without peripheral oedema has been suggested to increase the risk for the development of acute volume depletion and potential HRS. In such cases, the use of albumin has been strongly advocated. In general, albumin has been suggested to be more effective and safer than artificial plasma expanders in the prevention of

Table 40.3 Predictive and precipitating factors for the development of hepatorenal syndrome and proposed preventive measures

Predictive and precipitating factors	Management of HRS

Predictive factors
• Hyponatremia <133 mEq/L
• High MELD score
• Arterial hypotension (mean arterial pressure <85 mmHg)
• Elevated neurohormones
  – Plasma renin activity
  – Aldosterone
  – Norepinephrine levels
Precipitating factors
• Poor cardiac output (<6.0 L/ min)
• Elevated intrarenal resistive index
• Infections (bacterial infection, predominantly SBP)
• Large volume paracentesis without albumin support
• Acute alcoholic hepatitis
• +/− Gastrointestinal (GI) bleed
	Avoid further renal damage
	• Discontinue nephrotoxic medication
	Reverse hypovolemia
	• Discontinue diuresis
	• Volume resuscitation
	Albumin 1 g/kg on day 1 followed by 20–40 g/day þ splanchnic vasoconstrictors
	• Norepinephrine infusion to increase mean arterial pressure >10 mmHg or
	• Midodrine: up to 15 mg orally/8 hours þ octreotide 200 mg SQ/8 h or
	• Vasopressin or
	• Terlipressin: 1–2 mg/4–6 h for maximum of 14 days
	Renal replacement therapy
	Transjugular intrahepatic portosystemic shunt (TIPS)
	Liver transplantation

circulatory dysfunction [62]. Albumin administration is also recommended in patients with spontaneous bacterial peritonitis along with antibiotics to reduce the mortality and risk of HRS. Infections other than SBP should be treated with antibiotics as infections notorious as to jeopardize the renal function in cirrhosis. Another drug frequently used to prevent renal dysfunction in cirrhosis is N-acetylcysteine. Though several studies has found no role in improving renal function, but one of studies has demonstrated that death due to HRS was lower in patients who received N-acetylcysteine.

40.9.1 Studies Evaluating the Effect of Terlipressin in HRS

Terlipressin is a vasopressin analogue that can improve hemodynamic and GFRs in patients with HRS when given with albumin. In early studies, it demonstrated utility when used as a bridge to maintain renal function until liver transplantation [63]. Maximum dose of terlipressin can be up to 2 mg/4 h and continuous infusion is preferred over boluses to avoid dose related complications. Results of the REVERSE study demonstrated that terlipressin plus albumin was more effective than albumin alone in improving renal function in patients with cirrhosis and type 1 HRS. A significant decrease in SCr from baseline to end of treatment was observed among terlipressin versus placebo treated patients. SCr decreased by 1.1 mg/dL in the terlipressin compared with 0.6 mg/dL in the placebo-treated groups, respectively ($p < 0.001$) [64]. In a prospective, randomized, open-label study of 200 cirrhotic patients with SBP and bilirubin exceeding 4 mg/dL or creatinine exceeding 1 mg/dL, Salman et al. [65] demonstrated no significant difference in renal impairment or mortality among patients randomized to receive albumin (n = 50), terlipressin (n = 50), low-dose albumin + terlipressin (n = 50), or midodrine (n = 50). Terlipressin alone or terlipressin in combination with low-dose albumin was associated with improvement in systemic, renal, and splanchnic haemodynamics. Terlipressin and albumin + terlipressin were associated with decreased cardiac output and portal flow, and increased systemic vascular resistance compared with albumin after 3 and 10 days. It was concluded that terlipressin and low-dose albumin + terlipressin may be a reasonable therapeutic alternative to standard-dose albumin in high-risk SBP patients. Reversal of HRS can be achieved in more than 60% of patients with the use of terlipressin and albumin [66, 67]. However, relapse after discontinuation of therapy is not uncommon and even significant proportion of responders develop post-transplant AKI and CKD [66]. Further studies are needed to validate the utility of terlipressin in AKI among cirrhosis.

40.9.2 Role of Nonpharmacological Therapies

The provision of RRT is not straight forward in the context of ESLD and decision should be made on clinical grounds. There is paucity of prospective randomized trials demonstrating a survival benefit with RRT. The decision to initiate RRT in this population must include consideration of the reversibility of the renal failure and the likelihood of LT, in addition to the degree of severity of AKI. Though optimal timing of RRT initiation remains a topic of much debate, meta-analyses examining the timing of initiation of RRT [68–70], have suggested that earlier initiation of RRT in patients with AKI may have a beneficial impact on survival. In patients deemed appropriate for the initiation of RRT, several modalities can be considered, specifically, continuous RRT (CRRT) and conventional HD. Although there is no prospective evidence to demonstrate the advantage of one modality over the other, CRRT carries the advantage of improved cardiovascular tolerance, which is particularly relevant in patients with ESLD due to vulnerability to hemodynamic decompensation.

The use of trans-jugular intrahepatic portosystemic shunt (TIPS) and extracorporeal liver support therapy in the treatment of HRS is not well established. One uncontrolled study that looked at the long-term effects of a TIPS in non-transplantable patients with HRS suggested an improvement in renal function and a possible survival advantage [71]. Using a TIPS in addition to pharmacotherapy has been found to enhances the improvement in renal function, reduces ascites, and helps in cases in which patients relapsed after medical therapy [72–74]. The TIPS carries risk of post-procedure hepatic encephalopathy and other complications therefore, the balance between risks and benefits should be taken into consideration. The TIPS is absolutely contraindicated in patients with severe pulmonary hypertension and congestive heart failure [75]. The use of MARS may play some role in improving renal function in patients with HRS; however, evidences are not convincing [76].

40.9.3 Role of Simultaneous Liver and Kidney Transplant

SLK transplantation may be needed among patients with ESRD with cirrhosis and symptomatic portal hypertension, but more often required for patients who are listed for LT and have concomitant renal dysfunction or injury. Guidelines and policies towards SLK transplantation are described in Table 40.4.

Patients with ESLD receiving kidney transplant have higher 10-year survival rates than those maintained on dialysis [77]. The frequency of SLKT has increased dramatically in the MELD era, with changes in organ allocation policies. There has been increase in absolute numbers of donor kidneys diverted to the SLK pool from 138 in 2000 to 738 in 2016 as analysed using the latest UNOS dataset. The benefits of simultaneous liver and kidney transplant must be weighed against the potential for longer wait times [78]. Overall, liver transplant alone is likely sufficient for patients with type 1 HRS for less than 4 weeks, and SLKT is recommended for those with HRS at risk of nonrecovery of renal function [79]. Presently, there is a lack of hard evidence to guide us, so it is important to approach this issue in a thoughtful and systematic way (Table 40.5).

Table 40.4 Published guidelines and policies towards simultaneous liver and kidney transplantation

OPTN Policy 3.5.10 2009	• CKD with dialysis need • CKD (GFR less than 30 mL/min and proteinuria >3 g/day) • Sustained AKI with dialysis need for 6 weeks or longer (dialysis at least twice per week) • Sustained AKI with GFR less than 25 mL/min for 6 weeks or more but not on dialysis • Metabolic disease

Nadim et al. [79]	• Persistent AKI more than 4 weeks with one of the following
	  – Increase in serum creatinine more than threefold from baseline or on dialysis
	  – GFR less than 35 mL/min (MDRD-6) or less than 25 mL/min (iothalamate)
	• CKD more than 3 months with one of the following
	  – Estimated GFR less than 40 mL/min (MDRD-6) or less than 30 mL/min (iothalamate)
	  – Proteinuria more than 2 g/day
	  – Kidney biopsy showing >30% glomerulosclerosis or >30% interstitial fibrosis

Formica et al. [80]	• CKD: estimated GFR of <60 mL/min for >90 days prior to listing and an estimated GFR of <35 mL/min at the time of listing • Sustained AKI: a combination of dialysis and estimated GFR <25 mL/min for 6 consecutive weeks' duration • Metabolic disease • Safety net for kidney after liver transplantation • Regional sharing of kidney for SLK with high MELD score

Table 40.5 Summary of postoperative risk factors for renal dysfunction in LT recipients and treatment strategies

Time period post-OLT	Risk factors for renal dysfunction	Treatment strategies
AKI in the immediate postoperative period	Sepsis	• Maintenance of MAP >65 mmHg • Optimal antimicrobial therapy with renal dose adjustment, avoiding nephrotoxic drugs • Need for postoperative RRT
	Graft dysfunction	• Perioperative strategies to reduce IR injury • Role of machine perfusion in marginal grafts • Postoperative plasmapheresis
	Acute CNI nephrotoxicity	• Induction immunosuppression with Basiliximab/ATG and delayed introduction (POD 4–6) of CNI • Reduced dose Tacrolimus (target trough levels <8 ng/ml)
	Postoperative blood transfusion	• Point of care haemostasis testing and guided judicious blood component therapy, avoiding overtransfusion
Persistent AKI and progress to CKD (first 6 months)	Chronic CNI nephrotoxicity	• Reduced dose Tacrolimus with MMF • Tacrolimus minimization and switch to Everolimus (1–3 months post-LT)
	Hypertension	• Target BP <140/90 mmHg • Target BP <130/80 mmHg in those with DM and/or proteinuria • ACE inhibitors/ARBs preferred for long-term renoprotection
CKD (> 6 months to years after OLT)	CNI toxicity	• CNI minimization (levels <5 ng/ml) plus MMF • CNI withdrawal and switch to mTOR inhibitors (results variable if switched >2 years post-LT)
	DM	• Target HBA1c <7% • Insulin/oral hypoglycaemic agents • Dietary and lifestyle modifications • Early reduction in steroid dosing
	HCV recurrence	• Target: achieving SVR with DAAs (e.g., sofosbuvir), interferon-free regimens preferred
	Dyslipidemia	• Target LDL <100 mg/dl, Triglyceride <250 mg/dl • Hydrophilic statins (Pravastatin/Fluvastatin) preferred
		• Early referral to Nephrology team in recipients with progressive CKD • Renal biopsy to find the aetiology and directed therapy instead of empiric changes in immunosuppression

40.10 Intraoperative Risk Factors

Liver transplantation is high-risk surgery with a significant risk of hypotension, tissue hypoperfusion and blood loss, which are known risk factors for postoperative AKI [81]. Blood loss is not uncommon during liver transplant especially during dissection phase. Several studies have shown strong relationship between post-LT AKI and the amount of blood loss or perioperative red blood cell (RBC) transfusions, which is frequently used as surrogate marker of blood loss [82, 83]. Intraoperative hemodynamic instability largely represented by blood loss, vascular clamping, ischemia–reperfusion injury, and the use of vasopressors is an important complication during LT that contributes to the development of AKI after LT and has a negative impact on patient outcomes [61, 84, 85]. The duration of intraoperative hypotension and the length of anhepatic time are key predictors for immediate post-LT AKI [86]. Clamping of the portal vein and cross clamping of inferior vena cava (IVC) during the anhepatic phase compromises the venous return from the lower extremities and splanchnic bed and may result in decreased cardiac output and blood pressure, increased systemic vascular resistance, and reduced perfusion to vital organs. The latter may lead to renal hypoperfusion and potential ischemic kidney injury. Although venovenous bypass (VVB) has been shown to improve or restore normal hemodynamic physiology during the anhepatic phase, the use of VVB has not been shown consistently to decrease the incidence of perioperative or early postoperative AKI [87, 88]. In one single-centre study, the degree of renal dysfunction (assessed by inulin clearance) measured at various perioperative periods (anaesthesia induction, hepatectomy, anhepatic phase, biliary anastomosis, and 24 h after surgery) was not significantly different between LT recipients randomized to receive VVB support or no VVB support at any time point, with the exception of the anhepatic phase, which demonstrated a more marked renal function impairment in patients without VVB support. Nevertheless, renal function on postoperative day 7 and the need for HD/hemofiltration during the first week were similar in both groups. Multivariate analysis revealed that low mean arterial pressure at anaesthesia induction was an independent risk factor for early postoperative severe AKI [88]. Vena cava-sparing technique (piggy back technique) avoids complete IVC clamping for caval anastomosis, hence preservation of caval flow during the entire procedure maintains venous return thus reduces the risk of hemodynamic instability and prevents congestion of the kidneys [89]. Cabezuelo et al. [90], showed that, compared with the standard surgical technique (with or without VVB), the piggyback technique significantly reduces the probability of AKI after liver transplantation. It is speculated that this is partly due to the reduction in retroperitoneal blood loss, because the piggyback technique. In addition, it permits venous return to the heart during the anhepatic phase and avoids hemodynamic variation during inferior vena cava clamping. In a retrospective study conducted to evaluate the clinical outcome of three different surgical techniques, including retrohepatic caval resection (RCV) with VVB (RCV + VVB; $n = 104$), piggyback without VVB (PB-only; $n = 174$), Sakai et al. [91] similarly demonstrated a lower incidence of AKI ($p = 0.0001$) and better patient and graft survival in the PB-only group.

The ischemia-reperfusion injury during reperfusion phase of liver transplantation is known for its risk of severe hemodynamic instability. Following reperfusion of the graft, most patients develops some degree of hypotension which can last for more than minutes, but usually resolves within 30–60 min. This phenomenon has been termed the postreperfusion syndrome (PRS) [92, 93]. Several studies have demonstrated that PRS is an independent risk factor for post-LT AKI. Moreover, in a large retrospective cohort of DBD LT and LDLT, the decrease in blood pressure after reperfusion correlated well with both post-LT AKI severity.

Perioperative fluid management during LT has been linked to high prevalence of post-LT AKI. Use of the colloid solution hydroxyethyl starch (HES) [94, 95] in fluid resuscitation in sepsis and critically ill patients, was associated with an increased need for RRT compared to the use of crystalloids. In a smaller retrospective study of LT recipients the use of HES was also an independent risk factor for post-LT AKI. However, there is an increasing concern that high-chloride-containing crystalloids fluids, like normal saline, can cause hyperchloremic acidosis, which subsequently may impair renal blood flow and provoke AKI [96].

In his observational study among 158 LT patients Nadeem et al. concluded the same. After stepwise multivariate regression, administration of greater than 3200 ml of chloride-liberal fluids (HR 6.25, 95% CI 2.69–14.5, $P <0.000$) remained significant predictors for post-LT AKI [97]. Another small study indeed showed that both the infusion of large amounts of colloid fluids and high-chloride containing crystalloid fluids was associated with post-LT AKI [98].

Although large, prospective clinical trials are lacking, it is conceivable that intraoperative risk factors for the development of perioperative and early postoperative AKI in LT are similar to those in other surgical settings. These may include an anaesthesia induced decrease in effective blood volume, pre-existing cardiovascular disease or severe cardiomyopathy, prolonged episode of hypotension, severe intravascular volume depletion, and uses of drugs that can adversely affect intrarenal haemodynamic. In this respect, hemodynamic instability associated with a prolonged anhepatic phase and major bleeding during hepatectomy potentially can predispose patients undergoing LT to postoperative AKI.

40.11 Strategies to Reduce Intraoperative Risk Factors

Evidence-based intraoperative interventions to prevent or ameliorate AKI post-LT are not much. Nonetheless, management of coagulopathy, control of bleeding during surgery, judicious use of blood and blood product, careful attention to management of fluid and electrolytes, and avoidance of hypotensive episodes remain mainstay towards protection the kidneys from intraoperative injury.

Whether the use of the piggyback technique, as opposed to the standard surgical technique (with or without VVB), significantly reduces the probability of AKI after liver transplantation remains speculative. In recent years, most centres advocate the use of piggyback alone without VVB with favourable results.

The 2013 Cochrane review showed a lack of a reno-protective effect of various pharmacologic agents and surgical techniques. The pharmacologic measures include dopamine and its analogues, diuretics, calcium channel blockers, ACE inhibitors, N-acetylcysteine, atrial natriuretic peptide, sodium bicarbonate, antioxidants, and erythropoietin. It was also noticed that there is no reliable evidence from the available literature to suggest that interventions during surgery can protect the kidneys from damage [99].

40.12 Postoperative Risk Factors

Factors that have been shown to cause or predispose LT recipients to postoperative AKI, particularly ATN, include ischemic or toxic insult to the kidneys, prolonged hypotension, sepsis, sustained prerenal AKI, the use of nephrotoxic drugs, contrast nephropathy, delayed liver graft function or primary graft nonfunction or small for size syndrome, and postreperfusion syndrome or ischemia-reperfusion injury. It is suggested that reactive oxygen species such as superoxide anion, hydrogen peroxide, and hydroxyl radical released by donor livers with prolonged warm ischemia time play a contributory role in the development of AKI [100]. It has been shown that hypoalbuminemia, a common finding in liver transplant patients with severe cirrhosis, has been associated with the development of AKI [101]. However, the administration of albumin failed to show any benefit on the outcome of AKI. Other suggested predictive factors include prolonged treatment with dopamine or vasopressors, repeat laparotomy, intraabdominal hypertension, and perioperative volume of transfused blood products. The introduction of cyclosporine or tacrolimus in the post-transplantation period may exacerbate further renal dysfunction. Finally, polypharmacy, and specifically the use of multiple antibiotics, may contribute to postoperative AKI because of drug-induced tubulointerstitial nephritis.

40.12.1 Strategies to Reduce Postoperative Risk Factors

Bleeding and infectious complications in the perioperative period should be sought and treated aggressively. The use of contrast studies or nephrotoxic drugs should be minimized or avoided.

Therapeutic approaches in the postoperative period should be modified in patients with pre-existing HRS or pre-transplantation renal dysfunction. The cornerstone of postoperative immunosuppression in LT involves the use of CNI. The nephrotoxicity associated with CNI therapy has both acute and chronic effects. The following section presents an overview of the literature on the use of various immunosuppressive strategies to prevent postoperative AKI.

40.13 Early Renal Protection Strategies Post-OLT (0–6 Months)

Calcineurin inhibitors (tacrolimus, cyclosporine) are the cornerstone of immunosuppression following OLT and have resulted in improved graft survival over the last few decades. The standard immunosuppression regimens followed in most transplant centres include methylprednisolone (started on POD 0), mycophenolate mofetil (MMF), and tacrolimus (started on POD 1–2). However, acute CNI nephrotoxicity, superimposed on other risk factors for postoperative AKI, can lead to significant renal dysfunction in the first month after OLT. CNI-sparing immunosuppression strategies are the key to renal protection in the early weeks to months after transplant.

40.13.1 Induction Therapy to Delay CNI Initiation

Recipients at high risk of post-OLT AKI and subsequent progression to CKD are candidates for induction therapy with polyclonal or monoclonal antibodies so as to facilitate delayed initiation of CNIs. The International Liver Transplantation Society (ILTS) Consensus Statement on immunosuppression (2018), formulated by an eminent global panel of transplant surgeons, hepatologists, nephrologists, and pharmacologists, also strongly recommend antibody induction regimens to delay CNI initiation in patients with renal insufficiency [102].

40.13.2 Polyclonal Induction Therapy with Antithymocyte Globulin (ATG)

Induction immunosuppression with ATG to allow delayed tacrolimus initiation after OLT has been investigated by few researchers. Iglesias et al. analysed the UNOS database of 1720 LT recipients with pre-transplant renal dysfunction and identified the predictors of renal recovery post-LT in these patients [103]. ATG induction with delayed introduction of tacrolimus in the first week after OLT was associated with 2.2-fold increase in recovery of renal function compared to patients not receiving ATG. Similarly, ATG induction (short-term) along with steroids and MMF followed by delayed tacrolimus initiation till postoperative day 4 or 5 was associated not only with fewer rejection episodes but also improved renal parameters at discharge and at 1-year post-OLT [104, 105]. The safety issues that need to be addressed with induction immunosuppression include risk of infections and post-transplant malignancies. ATG induction therapy was not found to be associated with overall increased infections including cytomegalovirus infections and risk of malignancy. However, the Asian Liver Transplant Network guidelines (2019) on immunosuppression in LT recipients recommend that ATG induction is associated with more leukopenia and worse adverse effect profile compared to induction with IL-2 receptor antibodies [106].

40.13.3   Monoclonal Antibody Induction Therapy (Daclizumab, Basiliximab)

Monoclonal antibodies targeting IL-2 receptor (e.g., Daclizumab) have also been utilized as induction immunosuppression in OLT recipients in order to allow delayed introduction of tacrolimus. Renal functional improvement with this regimen (daclizumab induction, steroids, MMF, and delayed low-dose tacrolimus starting from POD4-6) was validated for 1, 6, and 12 months post-transplant in Canadian as well as European (ReSpECT Study) multicentric prospective randomized trials [107, 108]. However, owing to unfavourable adverse effect profile, Daclizumab has been withdrawn from both US and European markets in the last 2–3 years.

Basiliximab (anti IL-2 receptor antibody) has been utilized as steroid-sparing induction immunosuppressant agent in paediatric OLT recipients. It is now also being used in adult OLT recipients with renal dysfunction to allow delayed introduction of tacrolimus so as to minimize acute CNI nephrotoxicity [109]. It has been associated with better renal function and less need for renal replacement therapy in the early postoperative period [102].

40.14   Reduced CNI Exposure

40.14.1   MMF Plus Reduced Dose Tacrolimus

MMF (1–2 g/day) has been utilized in the early postoperative period with reduced tacrolimus

dose (target trough levels <10 ng/ml for the first 4 weeks followed by trough levels <8 ng/ml for the next few months) in patients with pre-OLT renal dysfunction so as to minimize the acute nephrotoxic effects of CNIs. This strategy has led to lesser decline of the renal function not only in the immediate postoperative period but also till the first year after OLT without increased rejection episodes [110, 111]. Leucopenia, thrombocytopenia, GI disturbances occur more frequently in patients receiving higher doses of MMF.

40.14.2   Use of mTOR Inhibitors (Sirolimus/Everolimus)

The inclusion of mammalian target of rapamycin (mTOR) inhibitors in the immunosuppression regimen to reduce CNI exposure has been found to be beneficial in terms of renal function post-OLT. De novo use of Sirolimus immediately after OLT, as a substitute to tacrolimus, however, is not recommended because of a high incidence of graft loss and hepatic artery thrombosis [112].

Early switch from CNI based therapy to sirolimus plus MMF (1–3 months after OLT), instead of de novo use, may lead to significant improvement in renal function in long-term survivors. This has been validated in many prospective trials including the multicentric Spare-the-Nephron Liver trial with no differences in patient and graft survival [113, 114]. The limitation of this renal sparing strategy is the increased risk of acute rejection in the early months after transplant.

EVR is a hydroxyethyl derivative of sirolimus with faster absorption, shorter half-life and a twice daily dosing schedule. Early introduction of everolimus 1 month after OLT in combination with low-dose tacrolimus to minimize irreversible CNI nephrotoxicity has been found to improve renal function up to 3 years after transplant [115]. However, complete withdrawal of tacrolimus in early months after OLT is not recommended in view of increased episodes of rejection and graft loss.

40.15 Factors Affecting Renal Function in Long-Term Survivors

Chronic kidney disease progressing to ESRD in LT recipients is second most common among other nonrenal solid organ transplant recipients (commonest in intestinal transplant recipients) [116]. The incidence of CKD following OLT varies from 10% to 45% depending on the cut-off chosen by the different investigators and varied duration of follow-up [116–118]. Creatinine-based equations, used by most of these researchers, tend to overestimate the GFR in post-OLT patients. Allen et al. used measured GFR by iothalamate clearance to determine the prevalence of renal dysfunction after OLT [117]. At 25 years after OLT, 9% required renal transplant while 7%, 21%, and 18% had measured GFR >60, 59–30, and <30 ml/min/1.73m² respectively. The mortality risk increased exponentially in patients with mGFR <30 ml/min (Hazard ratio 2.67).

Sharma et al. proposed a three-hit model for the development of CKD after LT [119]. The preoperative renal dysfunction in cirrhotics (e.g., HRS) constitute the first hit while the intraoperative risk factors (donor factors and surgical factors, as mentioned already) render the second hit to the renal function. The third hit to the kidneys leading to postoperative AKI and eventually CKD is due to the calcineurin inhibitor (CNI) nephrotoxicity and other risk factors like diabetes, dyslipidemia, hypertension, etc. The decline in renal function post-OLT is biphasic. The first phase, seen in the first 3–6 months, is characterized by a sharp decline in GFR and is attributed predominantly to the acute nephrotoxicity of the immunosuppressants, particularly the CNIs. The second phase is more gradual but persistent leading to the development of CKD over 1–5 years following transplant. The renal protection strategies post-OLT, therefore, can be stratified according to the risk factors prevalent in the early and the late post-transplant periods.

40.16 Renal-Sparing Strategies (Long Term, >6 Months Post-OLT)

40.16.1 CNI Minimization/ Withdrawal

Chronic CNI nephrotoxicity is the most common cause of CKD in LT recipients. It is related to dose as well as duration of therapy post-transplant. It is characterized pathologically by striped interstitial fibrosis, tubular damage and arteriolar hyalinosis [120].

The American Society of Transplant (Liver and Intestine) expert panel recommended that tacrolimus, in reduced dose, is essential for the immunological graft protection in the first year after transplant [121]. In patients with CKD post-OLT attributable to CNI toxicity, early initiation of everolimus (<1 year) in combination with reduction and subsequent withdrawal of CNI may be beneficial [122]. Adverse effects like impaired wound healing, dyslipidemia, proteinuria should be kept in mind while initiating mTOR inhibitors. Withdrawal of CNIs should be done in selected patients with no episodes of recent rejection in last 4–8 weeks. Late switch (>1 year post-OLT) from CNIs to MMF/mTOR inhibitors should be done in an individualized manner based on the benefit in terms of improvement in GFR and risk of increased rejection episodes.

40.16.2 Role of Renal Biopsy

CNI nephrotoxicity is not the only risk factor for CKD in long-term survivors post-OLT. Many patients progress to CKD despite reduced dose CNI within few months after transplant. Hence further reduction of CNI or switch to everolimus might not lead to halting the progression of CKD and, rather, might as well be associated with increased rejection episodes. Patients with deteriorating renal function or developing proteinuria after OLT should undergo a renal biopsy to confirm the aetiology [123]. It has been found to be a safe procedure (ultrasound guided percutaneous/transjugular route) and provides an array of information pertinent to management of CKD. Apart from the characteristic histologic findings of CNI toxicity, the renal biopsy may point towards other causes such as hypertension, diabetic nephropathy, HCV-associated membranoproliferative nephritis, amyloidosis, IgA nephropathy, etc. Management strategies targeted towards the specific aetiology might be better individualized according to the biopsy findings thereby avoiding empiric changes in immunosuppression.

40.16.3 Modification of Risk-Factors Other Than CNIs

Hypertension, diabetes mellitus, HCV recurrence, and dyslipidemia have been demonstrated to be independent risk factors for CKD in liver transplant recipients. Proper management of these modifiable risk factors may be useful to the progression of CKD in these patients [124].

40.16.3.1 Hypertension
Hypertension is a common long-term postoperative complication in OLT recipients owing to the use of steroids and CNIs. Dihydropyridine calcium channel blockers (Amlodipine, nifedipine) are the first line antihypertensive in the immediate postoperative period because of induced renal vasodilation. ACE inhibitors and ARBs (angiotensin receptor blockers) are the preferred agents for long-term management of hypertension in CKD post-LT and diabetic patients because of their renoprotective properties [102]. They are usually avoided in the first month after OLT and in patients with AKI.

40.16.3.2 Diabetes Mellitus
New onset diabetes after transplant (NODAT) and pre-existing DM are strong predictors of CKD in LT recipients. HbA1c screening should

be done at 3, 6, and 12 months post-transplant in all patients and annually thereafter. Lifestyle modification, diabetic diet, minimization of corticosteroids, and CNIs are critical to optimum glycaemic control along with pharmacotherapy (insulin and oral hypoglycaemics). There is not enough evidence in favour of or against newer oral hypoglycaemic agents in post-LT setting.

40.16.3.3 Dyslipidemia
Dyslipidemia is common after LT, as an adverse effect of immunosuppressant medications (steroids, CNIs and mTOR inhibitors). Fluvastatin and Pravastatin are preferred treatment options because of fewer drug interactions with CNIs [102]. Lipid profile should be advised at 3 and 6 months post-transplant in all patients and annually thereafter. Fish oil, fibric acid derivatives, and avoidance of sirolimus are recommended for the management of hypertriglyceridemia in these patients.

40.16.3.4 Management of HCV Recurrence
Recurrence of HCV infection is common post-OLT and is an established risk factor for renal function impairment and progression to CKD. The mechanism of HCV induced renal injury includes predominantly cryoglobulinemia related immune complex deposition and membranoproliferative glomerulonephritis. Sustained virological response using DAA (direct acting antivirals) like sofosbuvir has been demonstrated to prevent worsening of renal function in post-transplant patients compared to interferon-based regimens [125, 126].

40.16.3.5 Referral to Nephrology
Liver transplant recipients should receive nephrology consultation in the following circumstances: (1) acute decline in GFR detected on follow-up (20 GFR <30 ml/min), (2) Urine albumin >300 mg/24 h, (3) CKD with refractory hypertension or hyperkalaemia, and (4) RBCs > 20/high power field on urine microscopy.

40.17 Conclusion

This chapter emphasizes current knowledge as well as knowledge gaps, including the need for efforts to more optimally evaluate and improve renal function in LT recipients. AKI is common after LT, whereas CKD increase in incidence in long-term survivors who often have excellent function of their allograft. Identifying the risk factors for renal dysfunction and developing strategies to prevent, halt, or ameliorate renal function should be an integral part of management of LT candidates and recipients. Perioperative and immediate postoperative nephroprotective strategies are not well developed and need to move beyond delaying CNI therapy for a few days post-LT. Preventing intraoperative AKI and eliminating CNI therapy with novel immunosuppressive agents would likely improve post-LT GFR the greatest; however, prospective randomized trials are needed. However, manipulation of immunosuppressive therapy such as CNI minimization or withdrawal in the face of severe acute kidney injury may be futile. The added risks of acute rejection should be weighed carefully against the benefits. Furthermore, once CKD has set in >1 year post-LT, there are no known immunosuppressive modifications that reliably improve GFR. Recipients of SLKT may not be fully protected from renal dysfunction and can experience chronic immunologic injury and other renal injury events. Given the increasing SLKT population, novel immunosuppressive strategies and approaches more similar to those of kidney transplant only recipients need to be evaluated. There are promising biomarkers of renal injury available for study to detect early AKI, which may ultimately lead to targeted strategies to avert significant postoperative renal injury and CKD.

Keynotes

1. Pretransplant renal dysfunction and pre-existing HRS are well-established risk factors for post-transplant AKI. The potential benefits of diuretics, lactulose, contrast dye exposure, or nephrotoxic medications must be used judiciously against the risk of precipitating AKI.

2. In large volume paracentesis, albumin infusion is recommended. In the setting of SBP, albumin infusion is recommended as a treatment modality.

3. Intraoperative risk factors for the development of perioperative AKI are likely similar to those in nontransplant settings. Aggressive control of intraoperative bleeding, management of fluid and electrolyte abnormalities, minimizing IR injury, and avoidance of hypotensive episodes are imperative in the perioperative period.

4. Post-transplant AKI is likely multifactorial and may include ischemic or toxic insult to the kidneys, prolonged hypotension, sepsis, sustained prerenal AKI, and the use of CNI or other nephrotoxic drugs. Bleeding and infectious complications should be treated promptly and aggressively.

5. Monoclonal or polyclonal antibody induction and delayed and reduced CNI exposure in a regimen may improve renal function without increased rejection risk or graft loss. The use of CNI sparing protocols in patients with pre-existing HRS or pre-transplant renal dysfunction should be individually tailored

6. The use of CNI sparing protocols in patients with pre-existing hepatorenal syndrome or pre-transplant renal dysfunction should be individually tailored but need to balance against unacceptable acute rejection rates and graft loss.

7. Preventing intraoperative AKI and eliminating CNI therapy with novel immunosuppressive agents would likely improve post-LT GFR the greatest No known immunosuppressive modifications that reliably improve GFR.

References

1. Bilbao I, Charco R, Balsells J, et al. Risk factors for acute renal failure requiring dialysis after liver transplantation. Clin Transpl. 1998;12:123–9.
2. Kim WH, Lee HC, Lim L, et al. Intraoperative oliguria with decreased SvO predicts acute kidney injury after living donor liver transplantation. J Clin Med. 2018;8:29.
3. Hamada M, Matsukawa S, Shimizu S, et al. Acute kidney injury after paediatric liver transplantation: incidence, risk factors, and association with outcome. J Anesth. 2017;31:758–63.
4. Yoo S, Lee HJ, Lee H, et al. Association between perioperative hyperglycemia or glucose variability and postoperative acute kidney injury after liver transplantation: a retrospective observational study. Anesth Analg. 2017;124:35–41.
5. Jochmans I, Meurisse N, Neyrinck A, et al. Hepatic ischemia/reperfusion injury associates with acute kidney injury in liver transplantation: prospective cohort study. Liver Transpl. 2017;23:634–44.
6. Manjunath G, Sarnak MJ, Levey AS, et al. Prediction equations to estimate glomerular filtration rate: an update. Curr Opin Nephrol Hypertens. 2001;10:785–92.
7. O'Riordan A, Wong V, McQuillan R, et al. Acute renal disease, as defined by the RIFLE criteria, post-liver transplantation. Am J Transplant. 2007;7:168–76.
8. Kundakci A, Pirat A, Komurcu O, et al. Rifle criteria for acute kidney dysfunction following liver transplantation: incidence and risk factors. Transplant Proc. 2010;42:4171–4.
9. Utsumi M, Umeda Y, Sadamori H, et al. Risk factors for acute renal injury in living donor liver transplantation: evaluation of the RIFLE criteria. Transpl Int. 2013;26:842–52.
10. Macedo E, Bouchard J, Soroko SH, et al. Fluid accumulation, recognition and staging of acute kidney injury in critically-ill patients. Crit Care. 2010;14:R82.
11. Hoste EA, Kellum JA. Acute kidney injury: epidemiology and diagnostic criteria. Curr Opin Crit Care. 2006;12:531–7.
12. Levitsky J, Baker TB, Jie C, et al. Plasma protein biomarkers enhance the clinical prediction of kidney injury recovery in patients undergoing liver transplantation. Hepatology. 2014;60:2017–26.
13. Mehta RL, Kellum JA, Shah SV, et al. Acute kidney injury network: report of an initiative to improve outcomes in acute kidney injury. Crit Care. 2007;11:R31.
14. Joannidis M, Metnitz B, Bauer P, et al. Acute kidney injury in critically ill patients classified by AKIN versus RIFLE using the SAPS 3 database. Intensive Care Med. 2009;35:1692–702.
15. Thakar CV, Christianson A, Freyberg R, et al. Incidence and outcomes of acute kidney injury in intensive care units: a Veterans Administration study. Crit Care Med. 2009;37:2552–8.
16. Zhu M, Li Y, Xia Q, et al. Strong impact of acute kidney injury on survival after liver transplantation. Transplant Proc. 2010;42:3634–8.
17. Karapanagiotou A, Dimitriadis C, Papadopoulos S, et al. Comparison of RIFLE and AKIN criteria in the evaluation of the frequency of acute kidney injury in post-liver transplantation patients. Transplant Proc. 2014;46:3222–7.
18. Work Group Membership. Kidney Int Suppl. 2012;2:2.
19. Trinh E, Alam A, Tchervenkov J, et al. Impact of acute kidney injury following liver transplantation on long-term outcomes. Clin Transpl. 2017;31:1.
20. Leithead JA, Rajoriya N, Gunson BK, et al. The evolving use of higher risk grafts is associated with an increased incidence of acute kidney injury after liver transplantation. J Hepatol. 2014;60:1180–6.
21. Belcher JM, Garcia-Tsao G, Sanyal AJ, et al. Association of AKI with mortality and complications in hospitalized patients with cirrhosis. Hepatology. 2013;57:753–62.
22. Piano S, Rosi S, Maresio G, et al. Evaluation of the Acute Kidney Injury Network criteria in hospitalized patients with cirrhosis and ascites. J Hepatol. 2013;59:482–9.
23. Fagundes C, Barreto R, Guevara M, et al. A modified acute kidney injury classification for diagnosis and risk stratification of impairment of kidney function in cirrhosis. J Hepatol. 2013;59:474–81.
24. Tsien CD, Rabie R, Wong F, et al. Acute kidney injury in decompensated cirrhosis. Gut. 2013;62:131–7.
25. Levitsky J, Baker T, Ahya SN, et al. Outcomes and native renal recovery following simultaneous liver-kidney transplantation. Am J Transplant. 2012;12:2949–57.
26. Vagefi PA, Qian JJ, Carlson DM, et al. Native renal function after combined liver-kidney transplant for type 1 hepatorenal syndrome: initial report on the use of postoperative Technetium-99 m-mercaptoacetyltriglycine scans. Transpl Int. 2013;26:471–6.
27. De Souza V, Hadj-Aissa A, Dolomanova O, et al. Creatinine-versus cystatine C-based equations in assessing the renal function of candidates for liver transplantation with cirrhosis. Hepatology. 2014;59:1522–31.
28. Adachi M, Tanaka A, Aiso M, et al. Benefit of cystatin C in evaluation of renal function and prediction of survival in patients with cirrhosis. Hepatol Res. 2015;45(13):1299–306.
29. Beben T, Rifkin DE. GFR estimating equations and liver disease. Adv Chronic Kidney Dis. 2015;22(5):337–42.
30. Allen AM, Kim WR, Larson JJ, et al. Serum cystatin C as an indicator of renal function and mortality in liver transplant recipients. Transplantation. 2015;99(7):1431–5.

31. Shlipak MG, Matsushita K, Arnlov J, et al. Cystatin C versus creatinine in determining risk based on kidney function. N Engl J Med. 2013;369:932–43.

32. Gowrishankar M, VanderPluym C, Robert C, et al. Value of serum cystatin C in estimating renal function in children with non-renal solid organ transplantation. Pediatr Transplant. 2015;19:27–34.

33. Wadei HM, Geiger XJ, Cortese C, et al. Kidney allocation to liver transplant candidates with renal failure of undetermined etiology: role of percutaneous renal biopsy. Am J Transplant. 2008;8:2618–26.

34. Trawale JM, Paradis V, Rautou PE, et al. The spectrum of renal lesions in patients with cirrhosis: a clinicopathological study. Liver Int. 2010;30:725–32.

35. Francoz C, Nadim MK, Durand F, et al. Kidney biomarkers in cirrhosis. J Hepatol. 2016;65:809–24.

36. Tanriover B, Mejia A, Weinstein J, et al. Analysis of kidney function and biopsy results in liver failure patients with renal dysfunction: a new look to combined liver kidney allocation in the post-MELD era. Transplantation. 2008;86:1548–53.

37. Nickolas TL, O'Rourke MJ, Yang J, et al. Sensitivity and specificity of a single emergency department measurement of urinary neutrophil gelatinase-associated lipocalin for diagnosing acute kidney injury. Ann Intern Med. 2008;148:810–9.

38. de Geus HR, Bakker J, Lesaffre EM, et al. Neutrophil gelatinase-associated lipocalin at ICU admission predicts for acute kidney injury in adult patients. Am J Respir Crit Care Med. 2011;183:907–14.

39. Portal AJ, McPhail MJ, Bruce M, et al. Neutrophil gelatinase–associated lipocalin predicts acute kidney injury in patients undergoing liver transplantation. Liver Transpl. 2010;16:1257–66.

40. Tsuchimoto A, Shinke H, Uesugi M, et al. Urinary neutrophil gelatinase-associated lipocalin: a useful biomarker for tacrolimus-induced acute kidney injury in liver transplant patients. PLoS One. 2014;9:e110527.

41. Hryniewiecka E, Gala K, Krawczyk M, et al. Is neutrophil gelatinase-associated lipocalin an optimal marker of renal function and injury in liver transplant recipients? Transplant Proc. 2014;46:2782–5.

42. Jerry McCauley DHVT, Starzl TE, Puschett JB. Acute and chronic renal failure in liver transplantation. Nephron. 1990;55:121–8.

43. Thuluvath PJ, Guidinger MK, Fung JJ, et al. Liver transplantation in the United States, 1999-2008. Am J Transplant. 2010;10(2):1003–19.

44. Watt KD, Pedersen RA, Kremers WK, et al. Evolution of causes and risk factors for mortality post-liver transplant: results of the NIDDK long-term follow-up study. Am J Transplant. 2010;10:1420–7.

45. Wong F, O'Leary JG, Reddy KR, et al. New consensus definition of acute kidney injury accurately predicts 30-day mortality in patients with cirrhosis and infection. Gastroenterology. 2013;145:1280–8.

46. Pham PT, Pham PC, Wilkisnon AH, et al. Renal function outcomes following liver transplantation and combined liver-kidney transplantation. Nat Clin Pract Nephrol. 2007;3(9):507–14.

47. Contreras G, Garces G, Quartin AA, et al. An epidemiology study of early renal replacement therapy after orthotopic liver transplantation. J Am Soc Nephrol. 2002;13:228–33.

48. Hilmi IA, Damian D, Al-Khafaji A, et al. Acute kidney injury following orthotopic liver transplantation: incidence, risk factors, and effects on patient and graft outcomes. Br J Anaesth. 2015;114(6):919–26.

49. Londono MC, Guevara M, Rimola A, et al. Hyponatremia impairs early posttransplant outcome in patients with cirrhosis undergoing liver transplantation. Gastroenterology. 2006;130:1135–43.

50. Barreto AGC, Daher EF, Silva GB, et al. Risk factors for acute kidney injury and 30-day mortality after liver transplantation. Ann Hepatol. 2015;14(5):688–94.

51. McGuire BM, Julian BA, Bynon JS Jr, et al. Glomerulonephritis in patients with hepatitis cirrhosis undergoing liver transplantation. Ann Intern Med. 2006;144:735–41.

52. Wiederman CJ, Wiederman W, Joannidis M. Hypoalbuminemia and acute kidney injury: a meta-analysis of observational studies. Intensive Care Med. 2010;36(10):1657–65.

53. Cabezuelo JB, Ramirez P, Rios A, et al. Risk factors of acute renal failure after liver transplantation. Kidney Int. 2006;69:1073–80.

54. Contreras AM, Ramirez M, Cueva L, et al. Low serum albumin and the increased risk of amikacin nephrotoxicity. Rev Investig Clin. 1994;46:37–43.

55. Sang BH, Bang JY, Jun-Gol Song JG, et al. Hypoalbuminemia within two postoperative days is an independent risk factor for acute kidney injury following living donor liver transplantation: a propensity score analysis of 998 consecutive patients. Crit Care Med. 2015;43(12):2552–61.

56. Van Slambrouck CM, Salem F, Meehan SM, et al. Bile cast nephropathy is a common pathologic finding for kidney injury associated with severe liver dysfunction. Kidney Int. 2013;84(1):192–7.

57. Barri YM, Sanchaz EQ, Jennings LW, et al. Acute kidney injury after liver transplantation: definition and outcome. Liver Transpl. 2009;15:475–83.

58. Abelha FJ, Botelho M, Fernandes V, Barros H. Determinations of postoperative acute kidney injury. Crit Care. 2009;13:R79.

59. Thakar CV. Perioperative acute kidney injury. Adv Chronic Kidney Dis. 2013;20:67–75.

60. Sanchez EQ, Gonwa TA, Levy MF, et al. Preoperative and perioperative predictors of the need for renal replacement therapy after orthotopic liver transplantation. Transplantation. 2004;78:1048–54.

61. Kim JM, Jo YY, Na SW, et al. The predictors for continuous renal replacement therapy in liver transplant recipients. Transplant Proc. 2014;46:184–91.

62. Cardenas A, Gines P, Runyon BA, et al. Is albumin infusion necessary after large volume paracentesis? Liver Int. 2009;29(5):636–40.

63. Rajekar H, Chawla Y. Terlipressin in hepatorenal syndrome: evidence for present indications. J Gastroenterol Hepatol. 2011;26(1):109–14.

64. Boyer TD, Sanyal AJ, Wong F, et al. Terlipressin plus albumin is more effective than albumin alone in improving renal function in patients with cirrhosis and hepatorenal syndrome type 1. Gastroenterology. 2016;1550(7):1579–89.

65. Salman TA, Edrees AM, El-Said HH, et al. Effect of different therapeutic modalities on systemic, renal, and hepatic hemodynamics and short-term outcomes in cirrhotic patients with spontaneous bacterial peritonitis. Eur J Gastroenterol Hepatol. 2016;28(7):777–85.

66. Rodriguez E, Henrique Pereira G, Sola E, et al. Treatment of type 2 hepatorenal syndrome in patients awaiting transplantation: effects on kidney function and transplantation outcomes. Liver Int. 2015;21:1347–54.

67. Ghosh S, Choudhary NS, Sharma AK, et al. Noradrenaline vs terlipressin in the treatment of type 2 hepatorenal syndrome: a randomized pilot study. Liver Int. 2013;33:1187–93.

68. Wierstra BT, Kadri S, Alomar S, et al. The impact of "early" versus "late" initiation of renal replacement therapy in critical care patients with acute kidney injury: a systematic review and evidence synthesis. Crit Care. 2016;122:1291–8.

69. Zou H, Hong Q, Xu G, et al. Early versus late initiation of renal replacement therapy impacts mortality in patients with acute kidney injury post cardiac surgery: a meta-analysis. Crit Care. 2017;21:150.

70. Karvellas CJ, Farhat MR, Sajjad I, et al. A comparison of early versus late initiation of renal replacement therapy in critically ill patients with acute kidney injury: a systematic review and meta-analysis. Crit Care. 2011;15:R72.

71. Brensing KA, Textor J, Perz J, et al. Long term outcome after transjugular intrahepatic portosystemic stent-shunt in non-transplant cirrhotics with hepatorenal syndrome: a phase II study. Gut. 2000;47(2):288–95.

72. Wong F, Pantea L, Sniderman K, et al. Midodrine, octreotide, albumin, and TIPS in selected patients with cirrhosis and type 1 hepatorenal syndrome. Hepatology. 2004;40(1):55–64.

73. Alessandria C, Venon WD, Marzano A, et al. Renal failure in cirrhotic patients: role of terlipressin in clinical approach to hepatorenal syndrome type 2. Eur J Gastroenterol Hepatol. 2002;14(12):1363–8.

74. Boyer TD, Haskal ZJ, American Association for the Study of Liver Diseases. The role of transjugular intrahepatic portosystemic shunt in the management of portal hypertension. Hepatology. 2005;41:386–400.

75. Boyer TD, Haskal ZJ, American Association for the Study of Liver Diseases. The role of transjugular intrahepatic portosystemic shunt (TIPS) in the management of portal hypertension: update 2009. Hepatology. 2010;51(1):306.

76. Mitzner SR, Stange J, Klammt S, et al. Improvement of hepatorenal syndrome with extracorporeal albumin dialysis MARS: results of a prospective, randomized, controlled clinical trial. Liver Transpl. 2000;6(3):277–86.

77. Paramesh AS, Roayaie S, Doan Y, et al. Post-liver transplant acute renal failure: factors predicting development of end-stage renal disease. Clin Transpl. 2004;18(1):94–9.

78. Hmoud B, Kuo YF, Wiesner RH, et al. Outcomes of liver transplantation alone after listing for simultaneous kidney: comparison to simultaneous liver kidney transplantation. Transplantation. 2015;99(4):823–8.

79. Nadim MK, Kellum JA, Davenport A, et al. Hepatorenal syndrome: the 8th international consensus conference of the Acute Dialysis Quality Initiative (ADQI) Group. Crit Care. 2012;16(1):R23.

80. Formica RN, Aeder M, Boyle G, et al. Simultaneous liver-kidney allocation policy: a proposal to optimize appropriate utilization of scarce resources. Am J Transplant. 2016;16:758–66.

81. Goren O, Matot I. Update on perioperative acute kidney injury. Curr Opin Crit Care. 2016;22:370–8.

82. Chen J, Singhapricha T, Hu K-Q, et al. Postliver transplant acute renal injury and failure by the RIFLE criteria in patients with normal pretransplant serum creatinine concentrations: a matched study. Transplantation. 2011;91:348–53.

83. Smoter P, Nyckowski P, Grat M, et al. Risk factors of acute renal failure after orthotopic liver transplantation: single-center experience. Transplant Proc. 2014;46:2786–9.

84. Rahman S, Davidson BR, Mallett SV. Early acute kidney injury after liver transplantation: predisposing factors and clinical implications. World J Hepatol. 2017;9(18):823–32.

85. Rueggeberg A, Boehm S, Napieralski F, et al. Development of a risk stratification model for predicting acute renal failure in orthotopic liver transplantation recipients. Anaesthesia. 2008;63(11):1174–80.

86. Chen X, Ding X, Shen B, et al. Incidence and outcomes of acute kidney injury in patients with hepatocellular carcinoma after liver transplantation. J Cancer Res Clin Oncol. 2017;143(7):1337–46.

87. Shaw BW Jr, Martin DJ, Marquez JM, et al. Advantages of venous bypass during orthotopic transplantation of the liver. Semin Liver Dis. 1985;5:344.

88. Grande L, Rimola A, Cugat E, et al. Effect of venous bypass on postoperative renal function in liver transplantation: results of a randomized, controlled trial. Hepatology. 1996;23:1418–28.

89. Belghiti J, Panis Y, Sauvanet A, et al. A new technique of side to side caval anastomosis during orthotopic hepatic transplantation without inferior vena caval occlusion. Surg Gynecol Obstet. 1992;175:270–2.

90. Cabazuelo JB, Ramirez P, Acosta F, et al. Does the standard vs. piggyback surgical technique affect the development of acute renal failure after

orthotopic liver transplantation? Transplant Proc. 2003;35:1913–24.

91. Sakai T, Matsusaki T, Marsh JW, et al. Comparison of surgical methods in liver transplantation: retrohepatic caval resection with venovenous bypass (VVB) versus piggyback (PB) with VVB versus PB without VVB. Transpl Int. 2010;23(12):12447–58.

92. Paugam-Burtz C, Kavafyan J, Merckx P, et al. Postreperfusion syndrome during liver transplantation for cirrhosis: outcome and predictors. Liver Transpl. 2009;15:522–9.

93. Kalisvaart M, de Haan JE, Hesselink DA, et al. The postreperfusion syndrome is associated with acute kidney injury following donation after brain death liver transplantation. Transpl Int. 2017;30(7):660–9.

94. Myburgh JA, Finfer S, Bellomo R, et al. Hydroxyethyl starch or saline for fluid resuscitation in intensive care. N Engl J Med. 2012;367:1901–11.

95. Perner A, Haase N, Guttormsen AB, et al. Hydroxyethyl starch 130/0.42 versus Ringer's acetate in severe sepsis. N Engl J Med. 2012;367:124–34.

96. Hoorn EJ. Intravenous fluids: balancing solutions. J Nephrol. 2017;30(4):485–92.

97. Nadeem, et al. Chloride-liberal fluids are associated with acute kidney injury after liver transplantation. Crit Care. 2014;18:625.

98. Salahuddin N, Sammani M, Hamdan A, Joseph M, Al-Nemary Y, Alquaiz R, et al. Fluid overload is an independent risk factor for acute kidney injury in critically Ill patients: results of a cohort study. BMC Nephrol. 2017;18:45.

99. Zacharias M, Mugawar M, Herbison GP, et al. Interventions for protecting renal function in the perioperative period. Cochrane Database Syst Rev. 2013;9:CD003590. https://doi.org/10.1002/14651858.

100. Barreto AG, Daher EF, Silva Junior GB, et al. Risk factors for acute kidney injury and 30-day mortality after liver transplantation. Ann Hepatol. 2015;14(5):688–94.

101. Wiedermann CJ, Wiedermann W, Joannidis M, et al. Hypoalbuminemia and acute kidney injury: a meta-analysis of observational clinical studies. Intensive Care Med. 2010;36:1657–65.

102. Charlton M, Levitsky J, Aqel B, O'Grady J, Hemibach J, Rinella M, et al. International Liver Transplantation Society consensus statement on immunosuppression in liver transplant recipients. Transplantation. 2018;102(5):727–43.

103. Iglesias J, Frank E, Mahendru S, et al. Predictors of renal recovery in patients with pre-orthotopic liver transplant (OLT) renal dysfunction. BMC Nephrol. 2013;14:147–58.

104. Bajjoka I, Hsaiky L, Brown K, et al. Preserving renal function in liver transplant recipients with rabbit anti-thymocyte globulin and delayed initiation of calcineurin inhibitors. Liver Transpl. 2008;14:66–72.

105. Soliman T, Hetz H, Burghuber C, et al. Short term induction therapy with anti-thymocyte globulin and delayed use of calcineurin inhibitors in orthotopic liver transplantation. Liver Transpl. 2007;13:1039–44.

106. Tan PS, Muthiah MD, Koh T, Teoh YL, Chan A, Kow A, et al. Asian Liver Transplant Network clinical guidelines on immunosuppression in liver transplantation. Transplantation. 2019;103(3):470–80.

107. Yoshida EM, Marotta PJ, Greig PD, Kneteman NM, Marleau D, Cantarovich M, et al. Evaluation of renal function in liver transplant recipients receiving daclizumab (zenapax), mycophenolate mofetil, and a delayed, low-dose tacrolimus regimen vs. a standard dose tacrolimus and mycophenolate regimen: a multicenter randomized clinical trial. Liver Transpl. 2005;11:1064–72.

108. Neuberger JM, Mamelok RD, Neuhaus P, Pirenne J, Samuel D, Isoniemi H, et al. Delayed introduction of reduced-dose tacrolimus, and renal function in liver transplantation: the ReSpECT study. Am J Transplant. 2009;9:327–36.

109. Turner AP, Knechtle SJ. Induction immunosuppression in liver transplantation: a review. Transpl Int. 2013;26:673–83.

110. Boudjema K, Camus C, Saliba F, Calmus Y, Salame E, Pageaux G, et al. Reduced dose tacrolimus with mycophenolate mofetil vs. standard dose tacrolimus in liver transplantation: a randomized study. Am J Transplant. 2011;11:965–76.

111. Durand F. How to improve long term outcome after liver transplantation? Liver Int. 2018;S1:134–8.

112. Asrani SK, Wiesner RH, Trotter JF, Klintmalm G, Katz E, Maller E, et al. De novo sirolimus and reduced-dose tacrolimus versus standard-dose tacrolimus after liver transplantation: the 2000-2003 phase II prospective randomized trial. Am J Transplant. 2014;14(2):356–66.

113. Lebranchu Y, Thierry A, Toupance O, Westeel PF, Etienne I, Thervet E, et al. Efficacy on renal function of early conversion from cyclosporine to sirolimus 3 months after renal transplantation: concept study. Am J Transplant. 2009;9(5):1115–23.

114. Teperman L, Moonka D, Sebastian A, et al. Calcineurin inhibitor-free mycophenolate mofetil/sirolimus maintenance in liver transplantation: the randomized Spare-the-Nephron trial. Liver Transpl. 2013;19(7):675–89.

115. Fischer L, Saliba F, Kaiser GM, et al. Three-year outcomes in de novo liver transplant patients receiving everolimus with reduced tacrolimus: follow-up results from a randomized, multicenter study. Transplantation. 2015;99(7):1455–62.

116. Ojo AO, Held PJ, Port FK, et al. Chronic renal failure after transplantation of a nonrenal organ. N Engl J Med. 2003;349:931–40.

117. Allen AM, Kim WR, Therneau TM, et al. Chronic kidney disease and associated mortality after liver transplantation – a time-dependent analysis using measured glomerular filtration rate. J Hepatol. 2014;61:286–92.

118. Meraz-Munoz A, Garcia-Juarez I, et al. Chronic kidney disease in liver transplantation. Evaluation of kidney function. Rev Gastroenterol Mex. 2019;84:57–68.

119. Sharma P, Bari K. Chronic kidney disease and related long-term complications following liver transplantation. Adv Chronic Kidney Dis. 2015;22(5):404–11.

120. Chapman JR. Chronic calcineurin inhibitor nephrotoxicity – lest we forget. Am J Transplant. 2011;11:693–7.

121. Levitsky J, O'Leary JG, Asrani S, et al. Protecting the kidney in liver transplant recipients. Practice-based recommendations from the American Society of Transplantation Liver and Intestine Community of Practice. Am J Transplant. 2016;16(9):2532–44.

122. Zhang W, Fung J. Limitations of current liver transplant immunosuppressive regimens: renal considerations. Hepatobiliary Pancreat Dis Int. 2017;16:27–32.

123. Welker MW, Weiler N, Bechstein WO, et al. Key role of renal biopsy in management of progressive chronic kidney disease in liver graft recipients. J Nephrol. 2019;32:129–37.

124. Aberg F, Mäkisalo H, Nordin A, et al. Long-term renal function deteriorates at a similar rate among liver transplant patients with preserved renal function at 1 year and in the general population: Is chronic calcineurin inhibitor nephrotoxicity overrated? Transplant Proc. 2013;45(3):1182–7.

125. Satapathy SK, Joglekar K, Molnar MZ, et al. Achieving sustained virological response in liver transplant recipients with hepatitis C decreases risk of decline in renal function. Liver Transpl. 2018;24:1040–9.

126. Beig J, Orr D, Harrison B, Gane E, et al. Hepatitis C virus eradication with new interferon-free treatment improves metabolic profile in hepatitis C virus–related liver transplant recipients. Liver Transpl. 2018;24:1031–9.

Immunosuppression

41

Jayshri A. Shah

41.1 Introduction

Liver transplantation (LT) is the main treatment option for patients with end stage liver disease. When a solid organ such as liver is transplanted from donor to recipient, the recipient identifies the organ as foreign body and mounts an immune response against it causing graft rejection and subsequently loss of graft function in the recipient. Since the inception of liver transplantation in 1963, numerous immunosuppressive agents have become available to help improve outcomes of liver transplant recipients [1]. New agents have evolved over last few decades with better side-effect profiles, but calcineurin inhibitors (CNI) continue to remain the backbone for immunosuppression. Despite all advances, the challenges remain to maintain optimal level of immunosuppression thereby preventing rejection and adverse effects associated with the medication.

This review will help understand the journey of immunosuppression in liver transplantation. It outlines the current choice of immunosuppressive agents in adults, paediatric recipients, management of complications acute cellular rejection (ACR), chronic rejection, complications associated with immunosuppressive therapy, choice of drug in special situations such as pregnancy, hepatitis C virus (HCV), hepatocellular cancer, and chronic kidney disease. Finally, this review will briefly discuss the concept of immunological tolerance - and answer the question, can immunosuppression be withdrawn post transplant?

41.2 Immunosuppressive Agents

Immunosuppressive agents are required in all stages post-LT, the optimal drug, dose may differ depending on the phase. The phases of immunosuppression are classified as follows: [2–4].

1. Induction (in early stage): initial immunosuppressive regimen used in the first 30 days after transplantation when the alloreactivity is very high.
2. Maintenance (in the late phase): is the period after 30 days of transplantation and used indefinitely thereafter.
3. Treatment of ACR: is addition of immunosuppressive agents when histological diagnosis of acute rejection is made (Table 41.1).

J. A. Shah (✉)
East Kent University Hospitals NHS Foundation
Trust, Kings College Hospital, London, UK
e-mail: jayshri.shah@nhs.net

© The Author(s), under exclusive license to Springer Nature Singapore Pte Ltd. 2023
V. Vohra et al. (eds.), *Peri-operative Anesthetic Management in Liver Transplantation*,
https://doi.org/10.1007/978-981-19-6045-1_41

Table 41.1 Shows the timeline with the advances in immunosuppressive medication used post-LT for induction of immunosuppression or maintenance of remission

Immunosuppressive Agent	Timeline	Indication
Pharmacological/non-biological agents	1963 to 1976	Induction/maintenance of immunosuppression, treatment of ACR
(1) Corticosteroids	1963 to 1976	
Methylprednisolone	1995	Maintenance of Immunosuppression
Prednisolone	2004	Treatment of rejection
(2) Antimetabolites	1973	Maintenance of immunosuppression
Azathioprine	1984	Maintenance of immunosuppression, treatment of rejection, special use in malignancy
Mycophenolate (MMF)	2000	
Mycophenolic Acid (MPA)	2010	
	1985 (withdrawn from market due to reduced use since 2010)	Induction of immunosuppression
(3) Calcineurin Inhibitors	2000	Treatment of steroid resistant rejection
Cyclosporin (CyA)	2000	
Tacrolimus		
(4) mTOR inhibitors		
Sirolimus (Rapamycin)		
Everolimus		
Biological agents		
(1) T cell depleting		
Monoclonal Anti CD3(OKT3)		
Antithymocyte Globulin (Horse and Rabbit derived)		
(2) Non-T cell depleting		
Basiliximab		
Daclizumab		
Belatacept		

41.3 Classification of Immunosuppressive Agents Based on Mechanism of Action

Early immunosuppression was suboptimal. Last few decades have seen an array of novel immunosuppressive agents due to recent advances in molecular and cellular immunology [5, 6]. Specific agents are discussed individually below.

41.3.1 Corticosteroids: Methylprednisolone/Prednisolone

Mechanism of Action: Inhibit T cell derived and Antigen Presenting cell (APC) cytokine expression of IL-1, IL-2, IL-3, and IL-6.

Dose: It is variable across LT centres. Bolus of 500–1000 mg iv of Methylprednisolone administered in the first few post-operative days followed by rapid taper and switched to oral Prednisolone over few days. Prednisolone 40–60 mg/day is gradually tapered off over 3–6 months. By 1 year after transplant, only 38% remain on the drug. In some patients such as those with recurrent ACR, autoimmune liver disease, corticosteroids cannot be stopped completely and need to be continued at a lower dose [7].

The side-effects are summarized in Table 41.2.

41.3.2 Calcineurin Inhibitors (CNI):Cyclosporin(CyA), Tacrolimus (Tac)

Mechanism of Action: Both CyA and Tac bind to cytoplasmic receptors(cyclophilin and

Table 41.2 Side-effects seen with corticosteroids

- Hypertension
- Fluid retention
- Hyperglycaemia
- Impaired wound healing
- Cataract
- Mental status changes
- Myopathy
- Osteoporosis

Table 41.3 Side-effects of Calcineurin inhibitors

(a) **Side-effects of tacrolimus**
• Diabetes
• Hyperkalaemia
• Gastrointestinal, nausea, vomiting
• Hypertension
• Tremor
• Headache
• Hypomagnesemia
• Renal dysfunction
(b) **Side-effects of cyclosporin**
• Hypertension
• Hirsutism
• Gingival hyperplasia
• Hyperkalaemia
• Renal dysfunction
• Hypomagnesemia

KF-binding protein 12 respectively, the resulting complexes Inhibit calcineurin which plays a vital role in cytokine activation CNIs are the most common choice for immunosuppression across LT centres worldwide.

1. *Cyclosporin*: Two formulations are available. The standard formulation (Sandimmune) came first but requires emulsification step and therefore has unpredictable bioavailabilty. The newer formulation are microemulsion preconcentrates(Neoral), lipophilic solvent with consistent bioavailability.

   CyA initial dose ranges from 10 to 15 mg / kg/day in two divided doses.

   Dose adjustment based on trough level(C0) within 24 hours of commencing CyA.

   Target Range post-LT.

   Week 1–2: 250–350 ng/mL

   Week 3–4: 200–300 ng/mL

   Week 5–24: 150–250 ng/mL

   Week 25–52: 100–200 ng/mL

   Recently dose adjustments based on blood concentration at 2 h after dose (C2) target level 850–1400 ng/mL) appears to correlate with C0 monitoring [8].

2. *Tacrolimus(Tac)* It is the drug of choice in approximately 90% cases of LT, its use has been increasing progressively since 1998. Tac is 100 times more potent than CyA. Tac Absorption occurs in duodenum but not influenced by the presence of bile unlike CyA.

   Dose guidelines - 0.1 to 0.15 mg/kg/day orally in divided doses every 12 hourly. It can be given sublingual, if patient is unable to take orally. Intravenous formulation is available but seizures remain a significant risk and therefore best avoided. Doses are adjusted based on trough level. Therapeutic goals for Tac level in the first 4–6 weeks after transplant range from 10 to 15 ng/mL and thereafter 5–10 ng/mL is acceptable.

A meta-analysis including 3813 patients showed immunosuppression with Tac reduces mortality at 1 and 3 years post-transplant, reduced graft loss, reduced rejection, and steroid resistant rejection [9, 10]. Comparison of side-effects between the two CNIs are given in Table 41.3.

A prolonged release formulation of Tac is now available as once daily dosing. The efficacy and safety profile is similar to twice daily formulation. This has shown a favourable impact on patients who inadvertently forget to take medicines, improving compliance and adherence to immunosuppression [11–13].

41.3.3 Antimetabolites

Azathioprine (AZA), Mycophenolate mofetil (MMF) Mycophenolic acid (MPA) Mechanism of action: AZA is a prodrug of 6-mercaptopurine(6-MP) inhibits inosine monophosphate dehydrogenase(IMPDH), thereby reducing purine synthesis, affecting T and B lymphocyte proliferation. MMF is rapidly absorbed and hydrolysed to form MPA, which is the active metabolite.

1. *Azathioprine*:

AZA was one of the first immunosuppressive agents to be used in LT. Thiopurine methyl transferase (TPMT) enzyme is responsible for metabolizing 6-MP leading to over accumulation of 6-thioguanine nucleotides (TGN). Small number of patients who have deficiency of TPMT may not be able to tolerate AZA due to severe bone marrow suppression. Accumulation of 6-methyl mercaptopurine (6-MMP) can result in hepatotoxicity. TGN level monitoring during treatment and ratio of 6-MMP/TGN may be useful but the tests are expensive, complex, and not easily available [14].

Dose: 1–2 mg/kg per day.

AZA was used initially as the only immunomodulatory agent for maintenance of immunosuppression but later has been administered as an adjunct to CNI. With advent of novel immunosuppressive agents, the role of AZA has reduced and been replaced with MMF/MPA. However, the evidence of a significant benefit in terms of preventing ACR using MMF instead of AZA is very poor [15].

2. *Mycophenolate mofetil and Mycophenolic Acid*:

Dose of MMF: 1 g every 12 h. Taken orally (also available as iv formulation).

Dose of MPA: 720–1440 mg daily divided into two doses. MPA is also available as an enteric coated, delayed release agent (EC-MPA) this has been developed to reduce the gastrointestinal side-effects by delaying MPA release until small intestine [16].

It is usually commenced at lower doses and gradually increased to dose that can be tolerated. The toxicity is poorly correlated with blood level. It is therefore commenced at lower doses and gradually increased to a dose that can be tolerated. It has high bioavailability and monitoring drug level is not usually recommended. Although can be used in some cases.

MMF is used for both treatment and prevention of rejection in combination with CNI. It is the second most common immunosuppressant used at the time of discharge from transplantation. As it does not have any renal

Table 41.4 Side-effects with antimetabolites (AZA MMF)

Gastrointestinal: Nausea, Vomiting, Diarrhoea
• Anaemia
• Leucopenia
• Thrombocytopenia

toxicity, numerous studies have demonstrated the benefit of using MMF in patients with chronic renal insufficiency which allows lowering the dose of nephrotoxic CNI [15, 17, 18]. Approximately, 45% patients discontinue the drug due to side-effects which are outlined in Table 41.4.

41.3.4 mTOR inhibitors: Sirolimus/ Rapamycin (SRL) Everolimus (EVR)

Mechanism of action: Sirolimus is a macrolide antibiotic structurally similar to tac, binding to FK binding protein but inhibits the mammalian target of rapamycin inhibitors (mTORI). Both SRL and EVR block signal 3 of cell activation from IL-2 receptors in T cells and B cells.

SRL is available as 0.5 mg, 1mg and 2 mg tablet.

Loading dose of 6 mg for 1 day is recommended, but most programmes will initiate therapy at 1–2 mg daily.

Target concentration 4–12 ng/mL ranges depending on the use of other immunosuppressants and time of transplant.

EVR dose guidelines: taken orally 1 mg twice daily. It is started at lower dose and gradually increased as tolerated.

Blood trough level 3–8 ng/mL.

Sirolimus was approved for use in renal transplant in 1999. Due to its non-nephrotoxic property, it has been used along with CNIs (allowing to lower the dose of CNI) in liver transplant recipients with renal dysfunction. However, studies have not shown a significant improvement in renal function after 1 year in these patients [19–21]. A black box warning was placed on its use after multicentre trials showed that SRL was associated with an increase in risk of graft loss, hepatic artery thrombosis (HAT), and death. Most cases of HAT were reported in patients who received sirolimus early within 30 days of LT. However, the incidence of HAT related to sirolimus use varies in different reports [22–24].

Everolimus is another mTOR inhibitor, which was not available for clinical use until 2010. Several studies have shown beneficial effects on renal function after 2 years when EVR is combined with low dose tacrolimus early post-LT, without adverse effects on rejection rates. However, rejection rates are higher when EVR is used as a single agent without CNI. Concomitant use of CNI and mTORIs is recommended to reduce the risk of rejection which is increased when mTORIs are used alone. Also avoid mTOR I introduction for the first 30 days post-LT to avoid the risk of HAT and allow time for wound healing. The side-effects and drug interactions are summarized in the below table.

However, further studies are needed to assess the value of mTORIs as primary immunosuppressor post-LT either as a single agent or when combined with other immunosuppressants [25–27].

The side-effects are summarized in Table 41.5.

Antitumour effect of mTORI: mTOR signalling plays a role in tumour angiogenesis and proliferation in patients with hepatocellular cancer (HCC). In patients with HCC, SRL based immunosuppression has been shown to be associated with lower tumour recurrence rate and longer overall survival compared to patients on CNI. Similarly the protective effect due to antip-

roliferative effect, showing reduced recurrence rate on post-LT HCC has been reported. However, EVR has not been sufficiently investigated in clinical trials in this group of patients [28, 29].

41.3.5 Antibodies/Biological Immunosuppressive Agents

The overall use of biological immunosuppressive agents for induction of immunosuppression was approximately 26%, the rate has gradually increased over the years. Biological agents provide an opportunity to reduce the dose of other concomitant immunosuppressive agents (CNI and corticosteroids) with the aim to reduce the side-effects associated with steroids and CNI use (Table 41.6).

(i) In patients with renal dysfunction to avoid CNI in the immediate post-transplant period and help with delayed CNI introduction to preserve renal function.

(ii) To reduce the need for early corticosteroid use (as compared to corticosteroid induction, these agents cause less hyperglycaemia, hypertension, and CMV infection). Steroid free strategy has been found to be beneficial in patients with HCV.

Table 41.6 Side-effects of Biological Induction Agents

Basiliximab/dacluzimab
• Hypersensitivity reaction
• Mild side-effects
Antithymocyte globulin
• Cytokine release syndrome (fever, chills, hypotension)
• Thrombocytopenia, leukopenia
• Serum sickness
Muromonab
• Severe cytokine release syndrome
• Pulmonary oedema
• Acute renal failure
• Gastrointestinal disturbances
• Changes in central nervous
Alemtuzumab
• Mild CK-release syndrome
• Neutropenia, anaemia, idiosyncratic pancytopenia, autoimmune thrombocytopenia
• Thyroid disease

Table 41.5 Side-effects of mTOR inhibitors

(a) **Side-effects of sirolimus**
• Anaemia, leucopenia, thrombocytopenia
• Dyslipidemia
• Hepatic artery thrombosis
• Interferes with wound healing
• Interstitial lung disease
• Mouth ulcers, skin rash
• Albuminuria
(b) **Side-effects of Everolimus**
• Gastrointestinal: Diarrhoea
• Proteinuria
• Urinary tract infections
• Peripheral oedema

There are two types of biological agents in this group [2, 3].

(a) *T cell depleting antibodies*: further divided into.

    Polyclonal: Antithymocyte globulin(ATG).

    Monoclonal: Anti-CD52(Alemtuzumab) OKT3 (muromonab) [30, 31].

    Mechanism of Action: These antibodies destroy T cells, B cells, or both. This results in cytokine release responsible for number of systemic symptoms after the first dose. The risk of infections with cytomegalovirus (CMV), fungi and development of post-transplant lymphoproliferative disease (PTLD) is high with use of these agents. Recovery from its effect can take months to even years.

    Polyclonal antibodies:

    ATG: Two preparations are available.

    Equine ATG (eATG, ATGAM).

    Rabbit origin (rATG, Thymoglobulin).

    ATG has been predominantly used for steroid resistant rejection and for induction of immunosuppression.

    Dose: 3 day induction protocol 2.5 mg/kg, when the first dose id delayed up to 48 h post-LT.

    Intermittent dosing based on CD3, whereby second dose of ATG only given if CD3 count is above 20 cells/mm [30–32].

    Monoclonal antibodies:

    OKT3 monoclonal antibody directed to CD3 receptors, has been discontinued since 2010 due to significant side-effects and newer agents available.

    Alemtuzumab: Several side-effects including risk of recurrence of Hepatitis C virus(HCV) have limited its use as an induction agent for immunosuppression. Further studies are required to address risk versus benefit [33, 34].

(b) *Non-T cell depleting antibodies*

    Anti IL2 receptors: Basiliximab, Dacluzimab.

Mechanism of Action: These are humanized monoclonal antibodies or fusion proteins that bind to IL-2 receptors on T cells, thereby suppressing the proliferative response of T cells to IL-2. These are less immunogenic and therefore trigger less cytokine release, reducing the risk of complications such as diabetes, CMV infections, higher glomerular filtration rate, lower risk of PTLD, and HCV recurrence. Also the rate of ACR was reduced and rejection free survival increased .

IL2 antagonists - Daclizumab, Basilixiamb have shown the above mentioned benefits in various studies. However, daclizumab has been withdrawn from market since 2010 due to diminished demand [35–38].

41.4 Choice of Immunosuppressive Agents in Specific LT Population

Since the first liver transplant, a wide variety of immunosuppressive agents are available, each with a risk benefit profile. Newer drugs are available with better potency and reduced toxicity. To avoid long term toxicity and help improve outcomes post LT it is important to tailor the immunosuppression for special patient population such as:

- Renal impairment.
- Hepatitis C (HCV).
- Hepatocellular cancer (HCC).
- Paediatric patients.
- Pregnancy.

Tailoring immunosuppression to various patient population as a concept has evolved over the years. This helps to assign patients to immunosuppression protocols that best fit their needs.

41.4.1 Immunosuppression in Patients with Renal Impairment

Approximately, 18% patients will develop chronic renal dysfunction post-LT defined as GFR </= 29 mL/min. Pretransplant renal dysfunction is the most important determinant of post-transplant CKD. Sicker patients usually have high MELD (Model for End stage Liver disease) scores which is partly driven by creatinine. Multiple studies have suggested that duration of pretransplant renal dysfunction affects post-transplant renal outcomes. There is a suggestion that in the absence of parenchymal renal disease, patients with renal dysfunction of <12 weeks are likely to have recovery of renal function after LT. The other important factors which contribute include the presence of diabetes, hypertension, acute kidney injury (AKI) pretransplant and post-LT and finally the use of CNIs based immunosuppression which is the most common cause of end stage renal disease(ESRD) post-LT [39]. Some of the additional risk factors leading to renal injury include the following.

HCV infection: The risk of CKD is also found to be higher in LT patients with HCV infection due to glomerulonephritis [40].

Prolonged exposure to nephrotoxic drugs.

Prolonged ischemia and hemodynamic instability.

It is very important to identify pre-liver transplant patients who are at risk for evolution of ESRD post LT, so that patients can be identified appropriately for combined liver/kidney transplantation [41].

41.4.1.1 Recommendations of Immunosuppressive Agents in Patients with Renal Dysfunction

The administration of induction agents in particular IL-2R antibody can be used to delay introduction of CNI.

Also MMF can be continued to allow lower doses of CNI in patients with renal dysfunction. This approach is associated with significant improvement in renal function without increase in rejection rate. Some studies have also shown that AZA with low dose CNI can improve renal function, however, there is an increased risk of rejection seen in some cases. There are no RCT's performed directly comparing AZA and MMF with respect to renal function [15, 17, 18, 42].

Conversion to SRL can be done safely in LT recipients with renal dysfunction without increased risk of infection and graft loss [21].

Early EVR-based, CNI-free immunosuppression is feasible and has shown to improve renal function but this benefit comes with increased risk of rejection [26, 43].

41.4.2 Immunosuppression in HCV Liver Transplant Patients

Post-transplant HCV recurrence is almost universal if HCV viral load is detectable at the time of transplant. Also in approximately 10% LT recipients, fibrosis progression can be very rapid resulting in early graft loss. In approximately 30% patients HCV recurrence results in progressive fibrosis leading to cirrhosis in 5 years [44–46].

Besides various studies showing the role of immunosuppression regimen, several factors influence the complications associated with HCV recurrence

- Viral load in host and donor.
- Recipients' immune response.
- Donor age.
- Pretransplant viral load and genotype.

41.4.2.1 Role of Immunosuppression in HCV Recurrence

A meta-analysis including five RCTs has not shown significant difference in terms of mortality, graft survival, biopsy proven acute rejection, fibrosing cholestatic hepatitis between Tac based vs. CyA based immunosuppression [47].

There is evidence of association of increase in HCV viral loads due to steroid boluses used to treat ACR, however, the effect of steroid maintenance is controversial. The link between steroid therapy and HCV replication after LT in these patients prompted many centres to try the approach of rapid steroid withdrawal. Robust data on this approach is lacking and there is some evidence to suggest that rapid reduction in steroid dosage may be harmful for HCV recurrence. There are some studies available where steroid maintenance was compared to steroid free regimen in HCV transplanted patients, and these studies failed to show a significant difference with regard to liver fibrosis and viral loads. The protective role of steroid withdrawal still requires further investigation [48].

There remains a controversy regarding the best antiproliferative agent for HCV recipients. Some of the studies do suggest that maintenance with AZA is associated with less fibrosis progression compared to MMF. With the current data available, the evidence to support use of MMF over AZA is lacking [49].

Among mTORI, SRL has certainly raised some interest due to its potential benefit of reducing HCV replication and risk of significant fibrosis in post-LF HCV recipients. However, studies have also shown increased risk of mortality and graft loss with the use of SRL in both HCV and non-HCV LT recipients. Data on role of EVR and HCV recurrence after LT is limited [50, 51].

OKT3 and alemtuzumab use have been associated with severe HCV recurrence. There was no significant difference with regard to liver fibrosis and HCV replication in HCV LT recipients treated with IL-2R antagonists, with some studies showing no harm and others showing increased recurrence [52, 53].

To summarize, tailoring immunosuppression in HCV patients remains challenging due to conflicting evidence from various studies. However, the newer directly acting antiviral agents (DAAs) are available for treatment of HCV pretransplant and post-LT with promising results. The new DAAs have helped to obviate the need to focus on immunosuppression regimen and concerns of HCV recurrence and fibrosis progression in this group of patients.

41.4.3 Immunosuppression in Patients with HCC

The incidence of HCC continues to rise, therefore number of patients receiving LT for HCC is high. Recurrence of HCC post-LT remains a great concern. Many factors influence the risk of HCC recurrence, related to tumour, the patient and type of immunosuppression [54]. Although the biological behaviour of the tumour, waiting time, alpha-fetoprotein level (AFP) are very important, immunosuppression does play a central role in risk of HCC recurrence post-LT.

CNIs have shown properties of promoting tumour growth in experimental models. The blood levels of CNI appear to play a role in HCC recurrence rather than the type of CNI, suggesting a dose-dependent relationship. The association between the serum level of tacrolimus in the first month after LT with the risk of HCC recurrence has been studied and it was observed that patients with a level above 10 ng/mL presented a 2.8-fold higher risk of HCC recurrence.

MMF, although has antiproliferative effect, has not shown to play a role in the prevention of HCC recurrence. There are no data on influence of AZA and HCC recurrence available.

mTORI have been shown to have antitumorigenic effect as they inhibit cell proliferation and angiogenesis. SRL has shown its beneficial effect in several studies A meta-analysis including 42 studies showed a lower frequency of HCC recurrence among patients treated with an mTOR inhibitor, if the HCC was within the Milan criteria. The benefit of SRL is evident in 3–5 years in these patients. There is no evidence that SRL improves the long-term recurrence free survival beyond 5 years. Very limited data is available on role of EVR in these patients [28, 55–57].

41.4.4 Immunosuppression in Paediatric Patients

LT has evolved over several decades revolutionizing the outcomes of children with ESLD or liver based metabolic defects. LT in children is usually curative, recurrence of underlying disease is less common. In children, both pharmacokinetics and dynamics of immunosuppressive agents are different from adults, which affects absorption, distribution, metabolism, and drug excretion. The paediatric population may require higher doses to achieve appropriate medication trough levels due to developmental changes that occur with increasing age. The expected period of exposure of immunosuppressive agents is longer in children, this can have an impact on compliance, risk of infections, and carcinogenesis. Children are at increased risk of developing PTLD due to higher risk of exposure to Epstein–Barr Virus (EBV). In children, medications often must be available in liquid form which may not be easily available in the recommended concentrations. Suspensions can be unpalatable resulting in non-adherence to medication. It is also important to focus on age appropriate immunization in order to avoid vaccine-preventable diseases.

Although same immunosuppressive agents are used in adults and paediatric population, lack of clinical trials remains an issue for newer agents available and the management of immunosuppression in children challenging [58, 59].

41.4.5 Immunosuppression in Pregnant Patients

More female patients in child bearing age group receive LT. Concerns remain with regard to maternal outcome, including graft risk, choice of immunosuppression, and foetal outcomes.

Some studies have shown that pregnancies post-LT are high risk due to increased risk of complications including pre-eclampsia and pre-term delivery. These vary depending on timing of pregnancy after LT. The time of conception is advised to be at least 1 year after LT, for better outcome waiting longer (>2 years) has been suggested.

As regards immunosuppression regimens, steroids use is associated with gestational diabetes and hypertension, requiring additional monitoring. Both Tac and CyA based regimens can be safely used during pregnancy with not much difference in the complication rate such as hypertension, diabetes, renal insufficiency, and neurotoxicity. The complications can be minimized by careful drug level monitoring. Azathioprine can be used during pregnancy, however, MMF is teratogenic and this medication must be stopped for 6–12 weeks before conception. Data on safety of mTORIs in pregnancy is limited [60–62].

41.5 Can Immunosuppression Be Withdrawn After LT?

Outcomes following LT have improved due to advances in immunosuppression protocols and availability of newer agents. A careful balance to prevent rejection and avoid complications associated with the medication has been the approach over several years. With the current immunosuppression, there is still a risk of acute rejection of 10–40% and risk of chronic rejection is approximately below 5%.

However, liver has been shown to be more tolerogenic than other organs, whereby donor and recipients are matched only with ABO compatibility. Limited evidence has shown that approximately 20–25% liver transplant patients may develop operational tolerance maintaining their allografts after withdrawal of immunosuppression. Attempts at withdrawal is done late after LT (many months/years). Majority of patients will suffer rejection after immunosuppression withdrawal and have severe complications. Currently, there are no assays or data available on how to identify patients who have the immunological milieu which is favourable for immunosuppression withdrawal. Also, there is no evidence that immunosuppression withdrawal decreases patient morbidity. The goal should be to maintain adequate graft function and avoid complications associated with long-term use of immunosuppression. This can be achieved by minimizing the dose, although an ideal minimized protocol has yet to be established [63, 64].

References

1. Van Thiel DH, Makowa L, Starzl TE. Liver transplantation: where it's been and where it's going. Gastroentetol Clin North Am. 1988;17:1–18.
2. Weisner RH, Fung JJ. Present state of immunosuppressive therapy in liver transplant recipients. Liver Transpl. 2011;17:ppS1–9.
3. Moini M, Schilsky ML, Tichy EM. Review on immunosuppression in liver transplantation. World J Hepatol. 2015;7(10):1355–68.
4. Encke J, Uhl W, Stremmel W, Sauer P. Immunosuppression and modulation in liver transplantation. Nephro Dial Transplant. 2004;19(Suppl 4):iv22–5.
5. Trotter JF. Rejection and immunosuppression trends in liver transplantation. In Medical Care of Liver Transplant Patient, 4th ed. Hoboken, New Jersey: Wiley. p 297–310.
6. EASL Clinical Practice Guidelines. Liver Transplantation. J Hepatol. 2015:26–30.
7. Trouillot TE, Shrestha R, Kam I, Wachs M, Everson GT. Successful withdrawal of prednisolone after adult liver transplantation for autoimmune hepatitis. Liver Transpl Surg. 1999;5:375–80.
8. Villamil F, Pollard S. C2 monitoring of cyclosporine in de novo liver transplant recipients: the clinicians perspective. Liver Transpl. 2004;10:577–83.
9. McAlister VC, Haddad E, Renouf E, Malthaner RA, Kjaer MS, Gludd LL. Cyclosporin versus tacrolimus as primary immunosuppressant after liver transplantation:a meta-analysis. Am J Transplant. 2006;6:1578–85.
10. O'Grady JG, Hardy P, Burroughs AK, Elbourne D. Randomized controlled trial of tacrolimus versus microemulsified cyclosporine (TMC)in liver transplantation:post study surveillance to 3 years. Am J Transplant. 2007;7:137–41.
11. Dumortier J, Guillaud O, Boillot O. Conversion from twice daily tacrolimus to once daily tacrolimus in long term stable liver transplant recipients: A single Centre experience with 394 patients. Liver Transpl. 2013;19:529–33.
12. Trunecka P, Boillot O, Seehofer D, Pinna AD, Fischer L, Ericzon BG, et al. Once daily prolonged-release tacrolimus (ADVAGRAF) versus twice daily tacrolimus(PROGRAF)in liver transplantation. Am J Transplant. 2010;10:2313–23.
13. Beckebaum S, Iacob S, Sweid D, Sotiropoulos GC, Saner F, Kaiser G, et al. Efficacy, safety and immunosuppressant adherence in stable liver transplant patients converted from a twice –daily tacrolimus –based regimen to once-daily tacrolimus extended release formulation. Transpl Int. 2011;24:666–75.
14. Ford LT, Berg JD. Thiopurine S-methyltransferase(TPMT) assessment prior to starting thiopurine drug treatment; a pharmacogenomics test whose time has come. J Clin Pathol. 2010;63:288–95.
15. Wiesner R, Rabkin J, Klintmalm G, McDiarmid S, Langnas A, Punch J, et al. A randomized double – blind comparative study of mycophenolate mofetil and azathioprine combination with cyclosporine and corticosteroids in primary liver transplant recipients. Liver Transpl. 2001;7:442–50.
16. Miras M, Carballo F, Egea J, Martinez C, Alvarez-Lopez MR, Sanchez-Bueno F, et al. Clinical evolution in the first 3 months of patients after liver transplantation in maintenance phase converted from mycophenolate mofetil to mycophenolate sodium due to gastrointestinal complications. Transplant Proc. 2007;39:2314–7.
17. Schlitt HJ, Barkmann A, Boker KH, et al. Replacement of calcineurin inhibitors with mycophenolate mofetil in liver transplant patients with renal dysfunction: a randomized controlled study. Lancet. 2001;357:587–91.
18. Nashan B, Saliba F, DurandF,et al. Pharmacokinetics, efficacy and safety of mycophenolate mofetil in combination with standard–dose or reduced–dose tacrolimus in liver transplant recipients. Liver Transpl 2009;15:136–147.
19. Shenoy S, Hardinger KL, Crippin J, Desai N, Korenblat K, Lisker-Melman M, et al. Sirolimus conversion in liver transplant recipients with renal dysfunction: a prospective, randomized, single Centre trial. Transplantation. 2007;83:1389–92.
20. Fairbanks KD, EustaceJA FD, Thuluvath PJ. Renal function improves in liver transplant recipients when switched from a calcineurin inhibitor to sirolimus. Liver Transpl. 2003;9:1079–85.
21. Asrani SK, Leise MD, West CP. Use of sirolimus in liver transplant recipients with renal insufficiency:A systemic review and meta-analysis. Hepatology 2010;52:1360–1370.
22. Molinari M, Berman K, Meeberg G, Shapiro JA, Bigam D, Trotter JF, et al. Multicentric outcome analysis of sirolimus-based immunosuppression in 252 liver transplant recipients. Transpl Int. 2010;23:155–68.
23. Dunkleberg JC, Trotter JF, Wachs M, Bak T, Kugelmas M, Steinberg T, et al. Sirolimus as primary immunosuppression in liver transplant is not associated with hepatic artery or wound complications. Liver Transpl. 2003;9:463–8.

24. McKenna GJ, Trotter JF. Sirolimus-it doesn't deserve its bad Rap(a). J Hepatol. 2012;56:285–7.

25. Yee M-L, Tan H-H. Use of everolimus in liver transplant. World J of Hepatol. 2017;9(23):990–1000.

26. Saliba F, De Simone P, Nevens F, De Carlis L, Metselaar HJ, Beckebaum S, et al. Renal function at two years in liver transplant patients receiving everolimus: results of a randomized, multicenter study. Am J Transplant. 2013;13:1734–45.

27. Rainer G, Jorg-Matthias P, Martin J, Guido J. The role of everolimus in liver transplantation. Clin Exp Gastroenterol. 2014;7:329–43.

28. Menon KV, Hakeem AR, Heaton ND. Meta-analysis:recurrence and survival following use of sirolimus in liver transplantation for hepatocellular carcinoma. Aliment Pharmacol Ther. 2013;37:411–9.

29. Jeng LB, Thorat A, Hsieh TW, Yang HR, Yeh CC, Chen TH, et al. Experience of using everolimus in the early stage of living donor liver transplantation. Transplant Proc. 2014;46:744–8.

30. Eason JD, LossGE BJ, Nair S, Mason AL. Steroid free liver transplantation using rabbit antithymocyte globulin induction: results of a prospective randomized trial. Liver Transpl. 2001;7:693–7.

31. Eghtesad B, Forrest T, Fijiki M, Diago T, Hodgkinson P, Hashimoto K, et al. A pilot randomized controlled clinical trial of thymoglobulin (r-ATG) induction with extended delay of calcineurin inhibitor therapy in liver transplantation-interim analysis(abstract). Liver Transpl. 2011;17(suppl 1):S85.

32. Marks WH, IIsley JN, Dharnidharka VR. Post transplantation lymphoproliferative disorder in kidney and heart transplant recipients receiving thymoglobulin: a systematic review. Transplant Proc. 2005;37:2607–8.

33. Magliocca JF, Knechtle SJ. The evolving role of alemtuzumab (Campath-1H) for immunosuppressive therapy in organ transplantation. Transpl Int. 2006;19:705–14.

34. Marcos A, Eghtesad B, Fung JJ, Fonts P, Patel K, Devera M, et al. Use of alemtuzumab and tacrolimus monotherapy for cadaveric liver transplantation:with particular reference to hepatitis C virus. Transplantation. 2004;78:966–71.

35. Neuberger JM, Mamelok RD, Neuhaus P, Pirenne J, Samuel D, Isoniemi H, et al. For ReSpECT study group. Delayed introduction of reduced-dose tacrolimus and renal function in liver transplantation: the ReSpECT study. Am J Transplant. 2009;9:327–36.

36. Goralczyk AD, Hauke N, Bari N, Tsui TY, Lorf T, Obed A. Interleukin 2 receptor antagonists for liver transplant recipients: a systematic review and meta-analysis of controlled studies. Hepatology. 2011;54:541–54.

37. Penninga L, Wettergren A, Wilson CH, Chan AW, Steinbruchel DA, Gluud C. Antibody induction versus corticosteroid induction for liver transplant recipients. Cochrane Database Syt Rev. 2014;5:CD010252.

38. Ramirez CB, Doria C, di Francesco F, Iaria M, Kang Y, Marino IR. Basiliximab induction in adult liver transplant recipients with 93% rejection –free patient

39. Bahirwani R, Reddy RK. Outcomes after liver transplantation: chronic kidney disease. Liver Transpl. 2009;15:S70–4.

40. McGuire BM, Julian BA, Bynon JS Jr, Cook WJ, King SJ, Curtis JJ, et al. Brief communication: glomerulonephritis in patients with hepatitis C cirrhosis undergoing liver transplantation. Ann Intern Med. 2006;144:735–41.

41. Davis CL, Gonwa TA, Wilkinson AH. Identification of patients best suited for combined liver-kidney transplantation:Part II. Liver Transpl. 2002;8:193–211.

42. Hong M, Angus PW, Jones RM, Vaughan RB, Gow PJ. Predictors of improvement in renal function after calcineurin inhibitor withdrawal for post-liver transplant renal dysfunction. Clin Transpl. 2005;19:193–8.

43. Sterneck M, Kaiser GM, Heyne N, Richter N, Rauchfuss F, Pascher A, et al. Everolimus and early calcineurin inhibitor withdrawal: 3 year results from a randomized trial in liver transplantation. Am J Transplant. 2014;14:701–10.

44. Gee I, Alexander G. Review: liver transplantation for hepatitis C virus related liver disease. Post Grad Med J. 2005;81:765–71.

45. Joshi D, Pinzani M, Carey I, Agarwal K. Recurrent HCV after liver transplantation-mechanisms, assessment and therapy. Nat Rev Gastroenterol Hepatol. 2014;11:710–21.

46. Samonakis DN, Triantos CK, Thalheimer U, Quaglia A, Leandro G, Teixeira R, et al. Immunosuppression and donor age with respect to severity of HCV recurrence after liver transplantation. Liver Transpl. 2005;11:386–95.

47. Duvoux C, Firpi R, Grazi GL, Levy G, Renner E, Villamil F. Recurrent hepatitis C virus infection post liver transplantation:impact of choice of calcineurin inhibitor. Transpl Int. 2013;26:358–72.

48. Berenguer M, Aguilera V, Prieto M, San Juan F, Rayon JM, Benlloch S, et al. Significant improvement in the outcome of HCV-infected transplant recipients by avoiding rapid steroid tapering and potent induction immunosuppression. J Hepatol. 2006;44:717–22.

49. Germani G, Pleguezuelo M, Villamil F, Vaghjiani S, Tsochatzis E, Andreana L, et al. Azathioprine in liver transplantation: a reevaluation of its use and a comparison with mycophenolate mofetil. Am J Transplant. 2009;9:1725–31.

50. Kelly MA, Kaplan M, Nydam T, Wachs M, Bak T, Kam I, Zimmerman MA. Sirolimus reduces the risk of significant hepatic fibrosis after liver transplantation for hepatitis C virus: a single –Centre experience. Transpl Proc. 2013;45:3325–8.

51. De Simone P, Metselaar HJ, Fischer L, Dumortier J, Boudjema K, Hardwigsen J, et al. Conversion from a calcineurin inhibitor to everolimus therapy in maintenance liver transplant recipients: a prospective, randomized multicenter trial. Liver Trasnpl. 2009;15:1262–9.

52. Fillipponi F, Callea F, Salizzoni M, Grazi GL, Fassati LR, Rossi M, et al. Double blind comparison of hepatitis C histological recurrencve rate in HCV + liver transplant recipients given basiliximab+steroids or basiliximab+placebo in addition to cyclosporine and azathioprine. Transplantation. 2004;78:1488–95.

53. Marcos A, Eghtesad B, Fung JJ, Fontes P, Patel K, Devera M, et al. Use of alemtuzumab and tacrolimus monotherapy for cadaveric liver transplantation: with particular reference to hepatitis C virus. Transplantation. 2004;78:966–71.

54. Filgueira NA. Hepatocellular carcinoma recurrence after liver transplantation: risk factors, screening and clinical presentation. World J Hepatol. 2019;11(3):261–72.

55. Rodríguez-Perálvarez M, Tsochatzis E, Naveas MC, Pieri G, García-Caparrós C, O'Beirne J, Poyato-González A, Ferrín-Sánchez G, Montero-Álvarez JL, Patch D, Thorburn D, Briceño J, De la Mata M, Burroughs AK. Reduced exposure to calcineurin inhibitors early after liver transplantation prevents recurrence of hepatocellular carcinoma. J Hepatol. 2013;59:1193–9.

56. Rodríguez-Perálvarez M, Guerrero M, Barrera L, Ferrín G, Álamo JM, Ayllón MD, Artacho GS, Montero JL, Briceño J, Bernal C, Padillo J, Marín-Gómez LM, Pascasio JM, Poyato A, Gómez-Bravo MA, De la Mata M. Impact of early initiated Everolimus on the recurrence of hepatocellular carcinoma after liver transplantation. Transplantation. 2018;102:2056–64.

57. Zimmerman MA, Trotter JF, Wachs M, Bak T, Campsen J, Skibba A, et al. Sirolimus –based ImmunosuppressionFollowing liver transplantation for hepatocellular carcinoma. Liver Transpl. 2008;14:633–8.

58. Miloh T, Barton A, Wheeler J, Pham Y, Hewitt W, Keegan T, et al. Review article: immunosuppression in pediatric liver transplant recipients: unique aspects. Liver Transpl. 2017;23:244–56.

59. Dhawan A. Immunosuppression in pediatric liver transplantation: are little people different? Liver Transpl. 2011:S13–9.

60. Westbrook RH, Yeoman AD, Agarwal K, Aluvihare V, O'Grady J, Heaton N, et al. Outcomes of pregnancy following liver transplantation: the King's college hospital experience. Liver Transpl. 2015;21:1153–9.

61. Baskiran A, Karakas S, Ince V, Kement M, Ozdemir F, Ozsav O, et al. Pregnancy after liver transplantation: risks and outcomes. Transplant Proc. 2017;49(8):1875–8.

62. Sifontis NM, Coscia LA, Constantinescu S, Lavelanet AF, Moritz MJ, Armenti VT. Pregnancy outcomes in solid organ transplant recipients with exposure to mycophenolate mofetil or sirolimus. Transplantation. 2006;82:1698–702.

63. Porrett P, Shaked A. The failure of immunosuppression withdrawal: patient benefit is not detectable, inducible or reproducible. Liver Transpl. 2011;17:S66–8.

64. Adams DH, Sanchez-Fueyo A, Samuel D. Review: from immunosuppression to tolerance. J Hepatol. 2015;62:S170–85.

Part VIII

Special Situations

Anesthesia for Interventional Radiology in CLD and Transplanted Patient

42

Sumit Goyal

42.1 Introduction

Interventional radiology (IR) is the key component of every multidisciplinary liver transplantation program. Advances in the field of IR have proved to be useful in managing both pre- and post-liver transplant patients. For pre-transplant candidates, IR helps in treating complications of portal hypertension and liver tumors [1]. The interventional radiologist helps in reducing morbidity and mortality of post-liver transplant recipients by treating vascular and biliary anastomotic complications. They also have role in monitoring of graft rejection with the help of liver biopsies [1].

With an increased range of complex IR procedures and medically challenging patients, demand for anesthesiologist's services has increased. Anesthesiologists working in IR must be comfortable with providing well tolerated care to ill patients in a non-operating environment [2]. Two way effective communication with a dedicated team is crucial.

Anesthetic management of patients in interventional radiology requires knowledge of the procedure to be performed, its duration, intraoperative requirements with regard to fluid management/apnea/positioning, complications, and postoperative management of this unique patient population

[2]. The patient factors like medical condition and preference also need to be considered when planning type of anesthesia. The choice of anesthesia can range from monitored anesthesia care (MAC) to general/regional/local anesthesia.

42.2 Basic Considerations for Providing Anesthesia for IR

The American Society of Anaesthesiologist (ASA) guidelines for providing non-operating room anesthesia (NORA) should be followed [3].

- The standard of care for pre- and post-anesthesia in non-operating room should be the same as that of operating room. Monitoring equipment, anesthesia machine, location of cardiopulmonary resuscitation equipment, anesthesia, and emergency drugs should be checked. Adequately trained staff to support anesthesiologist must be there.
- Induction is usually done in radiology suite, on anesthetic trolley as procedure table has no provision of tilting. Then patient should be shifted to procedure table.
- Radiological equipment restricts mobility and access to the patient's head. Facilities for invasive monitoring and cardiopulmonary resuscitation should be available in the radiology suite.

S. Goyal (✉)
Liver Transplant Anaesthesia and Critical Care, Max Centre for Liver and Biliary Sciences, Max Super Speciality Hospital, New Delhi, India

Fig. 42.1 Portoveno-
gram showing TIPS
stent in situ

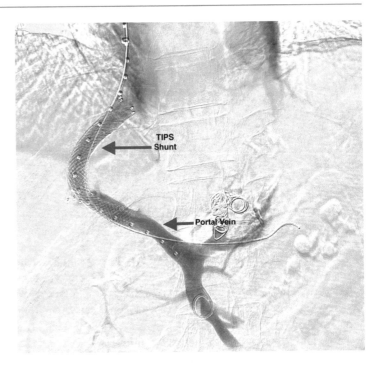

TIPS
Shunt

Portal Vein

- Radiation exposure must be considered, and contrast reactions must be anticipated.
- Following procedure, the patient should be shifted to an appropriate post-anesthesia care unit, accompanied and monitored by anesthesia trained personnel.

42.2.1 Anesthesia for Interventional Radiology for the Pre-Transplant Patients

42.2.1.1 Transjugular Intrahepatic Portosystemic Shunt (TIPS)

The transjugular intrahepatic portosystemic shunt (TIPS) is a minimally invasive procedure, preferred for the management of portal hypertension [4]. The stent creates the intrahepatic shunt between hepatic and portal vein and thus decompresses the portal venous system.

42.2.1.2 TIPS Procedure

TIPS is usually performed by interventional radiologists in angiography suite. A needle catheter is passed via the right internal jugular vein in to the hepatic vein and then track is made into the intra-

hepatic portion of the portal vein. This hepatic track is then dilated and kept patent through deployment of metallic stent [5] (Fig. 42.1).

42.2.1.3 Indication and Contraindications

The two indications with the strongest clinical evidence of TIPS efficacy are secondary prevention of esophageal variceal bleeding and treatment of refractory ascites [6, 7]. Other indications with limited evidence are portal hypertensive gastropathy, gastric antral vascular ectasia, refractory hepatic hydrothorax, hepatorenal syndrome, Budd-Chiari syndrome, and hepatopulmonary syndrome [6, 7].

Absolute contraindications to TIPS placement include severe pulmonary hypertension (mean pulmonary pressure > 45 mmHg), severe tricuspid regurgitation, congestive heart failure, severe liver failure, and polycystic liver disease [6, 7]. Relative contraindications include recurrent HE, hepatocellular carcinoma, severe coagulopathy (International Normalized Ratio more than 5), thrombocytopenia of less than 20,000/mm^3, moderate pulmonary hypertension, portal vein thrombosis, and obstruction of all hepatic veins [6, 7].

42.2.1.4 Complications

The cannulation of right IJV can cause carotid artery puncture, tension pneumothorax or hemothorax, thoracic duct injury or brachial plexus injury [8]. Cardiac arrhythmias can occur during advancement of catheter from right IJV to inferior vena cava [5, 8]. Although transient but sometimes may require cardioversion in case associated with hypotension [5]. Cardiac perforation and tamponade have been also reported [5]. Other fatal complications can be portal vein rupture, liver capsule rupture, injury to hepatic artery and biliary tracts [8]. Stent thrombosis, occlusion or migration can occur in the later course [8].

42.2.1.5 Anesthesia

Detailed preoperative assessment is required since hepatic dysfunction is associated with a wide range of co-morbidities.

42.2.1.6 Preoperative

Patient presenting for TIPS may have large amount of ascites or other complications of chronic liver diseases such as hepatic hydrothorax, cirrhotic cardiomyopathy, hepatorenal syndrome, encephalopathy, and coagulopathy.

If TIPS is indicated for refractory ascites or hepatic hydrothorax, large volume paracentesis or thoracentesis should precede the procedure [6, 8]. For assessment of cardiovascular system, transthoracic echocardiography is mandatory to exclude left ventricular dysfunction and pulmonary artery hypertension [5, 8]. The post-TIPS elevation in preload can precipitate heart failure in patients with pre-existing overt heart failure or severe tricuspid regurgitation or worsen portopulmonary hypertension. Chest radiograph may reveal pleural effusion. The laboratory test required are complete blood counts, coagulation parameters, blood group, kidney and liver function tests.

Significant thrombocytopenia (platelets count less than 50,000/mm) or coagulopathy (Internationalized Normal Ratio more than 1.5) should be corrected [8].

Neurological evaluation for the presence of hepatic encephalopathy and its severity should be done as it can worsen after the procedure due to shunting of ammonia and other neurotoxins.

42.2.1.7 Anesthesia Technique

The procedure can be performed under monitored anesthesia care (MAC) sedation or general anesthesia depending on patients physical and mental status and practitioner's experience.

As per literature, general anesthesia with endotracheal intubation is safe and the recommended technique [5, 8–10]. The points in favor of general anesthesia are as follows:

- The presence of ascites and pleural effusion by reducing functional residual capacity can cause respiratory embarrassment [8]. Therefore, controlled mechanical ventilation is helpful in providing motionless patient with breath hold during stent dilatation [8].
- Ascites can also raise intragastric pressure increasing the risk of gastric contents aspiration [5, 8].
- Intraoperative hemodynamic instability can occur due to injury to portal vein, hepatic artery or liver capsule.
- Balloon dilatation of intrahepatic track may cause severe pain, discomfort, sympathetic stimulation, and hemodynamic changes [5, 8].
- The duration can be long, uncomfortable to lie in supine position [5, 8, 9].

Rapid sequence induction of anesthesia should not be done on angiography table as it lacks provision of tilting. So separate table with tilting facility should be used for induction [8].

Large bore intravenous access should be established on the side most accessible to the anesthetist [8]. Invasive arterial pressure monitoring is required in case of hemodynamic instability.

Urinary catheterization and patient warming are also required. A board spectrum antibiotic coverage should be given and continued for 24 h [8].

Altered pharmacokinetics and pharmacodynamics seen in liver disease should be taken in consideration while choosing anesthesia drugs.

Fig. 42.2 Fluoroscopic image showing microwave ablation of a previously embolized hepatocellular carcinoma

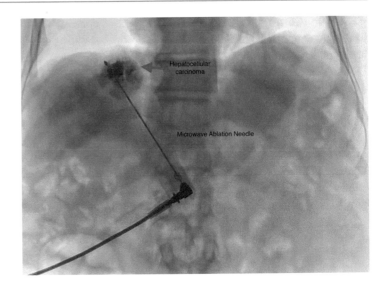

Propofol in titrated dose can be used as induction agent. Succinylcholine, atracurium or cis-atracurium are muscle relaxants of choice. Opioids with shorter duration of action like fentanyl or remifentanil are safe. The maintenance of anesthesia can be done with any inhalational agent or total intravenous anesthesia [8].

Post-procedure, patient should be shifted to high dependency unit or intensive care unit for close monitoring for complications such as pulmonary edema, hepatic encephalopathy, sepsis, contrast induced nephropathy, and acute hepatic failure. The use of prophylactic diuretics has been mentioned to reduce the fluid load on systemic circulation after TIPS and preventing cardiopulmonary complications [1].

42.2.1.8   Radiofrequency Ablation

Radiofrequency ablation has been accepted as minimally invasive technique for treating small hepatocellular carcinomas (HCC). Radiofrequency is a localized thermal treatment technique in which a high frequency alternating current increases the temperature of tissues beyond 60 °C causing coagulative necrosis near by the electrode [11, 12]. Typically under ultrasound or computed tomography guidance, one or more applicators (needles, electrodes, or antennae) are advanced from the skin into or adjacent to the targeted hepatic tumor [1]. It can be performed using percutaneous, laparoscopy, or lapa-

rotomy technique. It helps in controlling tumor progression while awaiting transplant (Fig. 42.2).

42.2.1.9   Anesthesia

The role of the anesthesiologist in hepatocellular carcinoma ablation therapy is to facilitate patient safety and satisfaction as well as to ensure that the patient have minimal pain during the procedure [12]. Several anesthesia methods including local anesthesia, epidural anesthesia, paravertebral block, and general anesthesia have been reported for percutaneous radio frequency ablation (PRFA) of hepatic malignancy [13]. The choice of anesthesia will depend on both patient factors and site, size, and location of the tumor [14].

42.2.1.10   Monitored Anesthesia Care

Local anesthesia with intravenous sedation is most commonly used for PRFA of small HCC. However, rarely some patients may experience severe pain and anxiety resulting in termination of procedure and insufficient tumor ablation area [13, 15].

42.2.1.11   General Anesthesia

The location of tumor adjacent to the parietal peritoneum is an independent risk factor of higher pain level during PRFA of HCC [16]. It may be due to stimulation of thermal or multimodal nociceptors in the parietal peritoneum. Large tumor, history of multiple ablations and longer duration of ablation are other risk factors related to intra-procedural pain [16]. Therefore, general anesthesia (GA) should be preferred in these situations. Another advantage of GA is that by reducing hepatic blood flow, can increase the ablation diameter [15, 17].

For PRFA of small HCC, Lai et al. reported that the patients who opted for GA were at reduced risk of recurrence but no effect on overall survival compared to epidural anesthesia [17]. In another retrospective study, Kuo et al. demonstrated that PRFA under GA did not alter recurrence and overall survival rate as compared to non-GA group [15]. However, the patients undergoing RFA with GA required fewer sessions to obtain an equivalent complete response than non-GA group and shorter hospital stay [15]. In GA group, controlled ventilation allowed operator to place needle more precisely due to longer time interval between the breaths [15]. One limitation of GA is inability to provide post procedural analgesia.

42.2.1.12 Epidural Anesthesia

Literature about the role of epidural anesthesia for PRFA is very limited. Recently in a retrospective study, Choi et al. reported that thoracic epidural anesthesia was associated with shorter procedure time, lower post procedural pain and lower opioid consumption during and after the procedure as compared to MAC group [13]. However, epidural may have limited role in case of coagulopathy because of hepatic cirrhosis. The advantage of epidural anesthesia is ability to provide post procedural analgesia.

42.2.1.13 Thoracic Paravertebral Block

Thoracic paravertebral block (TPVB) represents another method of providing anesthesia for PRFA. TPVB is an anesthetic technique of depositing local anesthesia at the emergence of the spinal nerves from the thoracic intervertebral foramina [18]. Ning et al. used the right TPVB for anesthesia during PRFA of hepatic tumors in 20 patients and concluded as a safe and effective technique for the anesthetic management of

PRFA of hepatic tumors [19]. Piccioni et al. evaluated the efficacy and safety of TPVB (without sedation) in 12 patients with hepatic tumors undergoing PRFA and concluded that TPVB produced satisfactory unilateral anesthesia with minor side effects [20]. Gazzera et al. evaluated the efficacy of ultrasound-guided TPVB for PRFA in 30 patients with liver tumors. Significantly, ten patients (33.3%) experienced moderate-to-severe pain that required IV sedation [18]. Recently, Elyazed et al. assessed and compared the efficacy of TPVB with that of local anesthetic (LA) infiltration with sedation, for the anesthetic management of PRFA of liver tumors. VAS was significantly lower in TPVB group than LA group during and after the procedure. Number of patients requiring GA was significantly higher in LA group. Thus, concluded TPVB as safe and more effective than LA with sedation in relieving pain during PRFA procedure of hepatic tumors [21].

The failure to achieve total visceral anesthesia as a result of the inability to block the ipsilateral parasympathetic as well as left sided sympathetic fibers may be considered a major drawback of a unilateral TPVB [18, 21]. The average complication rate reported in the literature varies between 2.6 and 5%: the most common reported complications are hypotension (4.6%), hematoma due to the accidental puncture of vessels (3.8%), pleural lesions (1.1%) and pneumothorax (0.5%) [18].

42.2.2 Anesthesia for Interventional Radiology for Post-Liver Transplant Patients

Liver transplant recipients have benefited from major technological advances in the field of IR. The role of IR in post-transplant period is to provide treatment for vascular and biliary complications. Thus, improving graft and patient survival and avoiding surgical revision and re-transplantation [22].

For IR interventions in immediate post-transplant period, patient may be hemodynamically unstable, may be intubated, on mechanical ventilation and acidotic. The role of anesthesiologist is to transport these sick recipients from intensive care unit to the radiology suite safely and maintain hemodynamics and hemostasis during the procedure. Coagulation monitoring should be done using whole blood viscoelastic tests.

Patients with late complications may have graft dysfunction in form of deranged liver tests, coagulation defects. The clinical presentation of vascular complications is often indistinguishable from other post transplantation complications (biliary complications, rejection, graft dysfunction, infections) [22]. The type of immunosuppressive regime and their side effects, its interaction with anesthesia and other drugs also need to be considered [23]. These issues are discussed extensively elsewhere in this book.

42.2.2.1 Hepatic Artery Complications

Hepatic artery thrombosis (HAT) is a potentially life-threatening complication of liver transplant. Graft dysfunction is more commonly seen in early HAT (less than 1 month after transplant), whereas biliary complications are more common in late HAT [24]. For HAT, preferred endovascular intervention for revascularization is catheter directed thrombolytic therapy [22, 24]. Thrombolytic therapy in the very early post-transplant period is associated with a high risk of bleeding complications [24]. For hepatic artery stenosis, endovascular management includes percutaneous transluminal angioplasty and stent placement [22, 24]. Regarding anesthesia of choice, there is no published data but author feel it should be done under monitored anesthesia care. GA is rarely required.

42.2.2.2 Portal Vein Complications

Endovascular management for portal vein stenosis is usually performed through percutaneous transhepatic angioplasty [22, 24]. Patients with portal vein stenosis may be asymptomatic or may have clinical symptoms of portal hypertension, such as ascites, splenomegaly, gastrointestinal tract bleeding, and thrombocytopenia. This transhepatic approach can cause bleeding, so MAC is the preferred choice of anesthesia [22]. Periprocedural anticoagulation may be required.

42.2.2.3 Biliary Complications

Complications include biliary stricture, bile leakage, biliary stones, and bilomas [22]. Biliary obstructions and leaks usually require interventions. Endoscopic retrograde cholangiopancreatography (ERCP) is used to treat biliary complications in patients with duct to duct anastomosis [22]. In case of choledochojejunostomy or failure of ERCP, percutaneous transhepatic cholangiography (PTC) is preformed to manage biliary complications followed by biliary drain placement [22]. Possible complications of PTC are hemobilia, intra or extrahepatic hematoma, and fever with bacteremia. Multiple sessions of PCT are required. PTC should be performed under monitored anesthesia care [22]. Intravenous antibiotic prophylaxis should be administered before all procedures.

42.3 Conclusion

The ability of interventional radiology to treat the lesions or complications noninvasively with minimal morbidity helps in avoiding the need of surgical explorations and retransplant. Coordination of care between surgeons, interventional radiologist, and anesthesiologist in transplant team is crucial for the successful treatment of transplant patients. The anesthesiologist must focus on providing anesthetic and perioperative care by ensuring familiarity with the expanding range of IR procedures.

Key Points
- IR is a key component of liver transplantation program.
- TIPS procedure though minimally invasive can results in vast changing in portal hemodynamics.
- Post-TIPS procedure neurological evaluation is necessary to rule out hepatic encephalopathy.
- Biliary complications are more common in living donor liver transplantation.
- MAC may need to be converted to general anesthesia during the IR procedure.

Acknowledgments None.

References

1. Shamimi-Noori S. Interventional radiology for the pre-transplant patient. In: Doria C, editor. Contemporary liver transplantation: the successful liver transplant program. Cham: Springer; 2016. p. 1–2.

2. Landrigan-Ossar M. Common procedures and strategies for anaesthesia in interventional radiology. Curr Opin Anesthesiol. 2015;28(4):458–63.

3. American Society of Anesthesiologists. Statement on non-operating room anesthetizing locations, last amended. 2013. http://www.asahq.or.

4. Bhogal HK, Sanyal AJ. Transjugular intrahepatic portosystemic shunt: an overview. Clin Liver Dis. 2012;1(5):173.

5. DeGasperi A, Corti A, Corso R, Rampoldi A, Roselli E, Mazza E, Fantini G, Prosperi M. Transjugular intrahepatic portosystemic shunt (TIPS): the anesthesiological point of view after 150 procedures managed under total intravenous anesthesia. J Clin Monit Comput. 2009;23(6):341–6.

6. Copelan A, Kapoor B, Sands M. Transjugular intrahepatic portosystemic shunt: indications, contraindications, and patient work-up. Semin Interv Radiol. 2014;31(3):235–42.

7. Fidelman N, Kwan SW, LaBerge JM, Gordon RL, Ring EJ, Kerlan RK Jr. The transjugular intrahepatic portosystemic shunt: an update. Am J Roentgenol. 2012;199(4):746–55.

8. Chana A, James M, Veale P. Anaesthesia for transjugular intrahepatic portosystemic shunt insertion. BJA Educ. 2016;16(12):405–9.

9. Kam PC, Tay TM. The role of the anaesthetist during the transjugular intrahepatic porto-systemic stent shunt procedure (TIPPS). Anaesth Intensive Care. 1997;25(4):385–9.

10. Scher C. Anesthesia for transjugular intrahepatic portosystemic shunt. Int Anesthesiol Clin. 2009;47(2):21–8.

11. Minami Y, Kudo M. Radiofrequency ablation of hepatocellular carcinoma: a literature review. Int J Hepatol. 2011;2011:104685.

12. Amornyotin S, Jirachaipitak S, Wangnatip S. Anesthetic management for radiofrequency ablation in patients with hepatocellular carcinoma in a developing country. J Anesth Crit Care. 2015;3(1):00086.

13. Choi EJ, Choi YM, Kim HJ, Ok HG, Chang EJ, Kim HY, Yoon JU, Kim KH, Byeon GJ. The effects of thoracic epidural analgesia during percutaneous radiofrequency ablation for hepatocellular carcinoma. Pain Res Manag. 2018;2018:4354912.

14. Chakravorty N, Jaiswal S, Chakravarty D, Jain RK, Agarwal RC. Anaesthetic management of radiofrequency tumor ablation: our experience. Indian J Anaesth. 2006;50:123–7.

15. Kuo YH, Chung KC, Hung CH, Lu SN, Wang JH. The impact of general anesthesia on radiofrequency ablation of hepatocellular carcinoma. Kaohsiung J Med Sci. 2014;30(11):559–65.

16. Lee S, Rhim H, Kim YS, Choi D, Lee WJ, Lim HK, Shin B. Percutaneous radiofrequency ablation of hepatocellular carcinomas: factors related to intraprocedural and postprocedural pain. Am J Roentgenol. 2009;192(4):1064–70.

17. Lai R, Peng Z, Chen D, Wang X, Xing W, Zeng W, Chen M. The effects of anesthetic technique on cancer recurrence in percutaneous radiofrequency ablation of small hepatocellular carcinoma. Anesth Analg. 2012;114(2):290–6.

18. Gazzera C, Fonio P, Faletti R, Dotto MC, Gobbi F, Donadio P, Gandini G. Role of paravertebral block anaesthesia during percutaneous transhepatic thermoablation. Radiol Med. 2014;119(8):549–57.

19. Cheung Ning M, Karmakar MK. Right thoracic paravertebral anaesthesia for percutaneous radiofrequency ablation of liver tumours. Br J Radiol. 2011;84(1005):785–9.

20. Piccioni F, Fumagalli L, Garbagnati F, Di Tolla G, Mazzaferro V, Langer M. Thoracic paravertebral anesthesia for percutaneous radiofrequency ablation of hepatic tumors. J Clin Anesth. 2014;26(4):271–5.

21. Elyazed MM, Abdullah MA. Thoracic paravertebral block for the anesthetic management of percutaneous radiofrequency ablation of liver tumors. J Anaesthesiol Clin Pharmacol. 2018;34(2):166.

22. Miraglia R, Maruzzelli L, Caruso S, Milazzo M, Marrone G, Mamone G, Carollo V, Gruttadauria S, Luca A, Gridelli B. Interventional radiology procedures in adult patients who underwent liver transplantation. World J Gastroenterol: WJG. 2009;15(6):684.

23. Brusich KT, Acan I. Anesthetic considerations in transplant recipients for nontransplant surgery. In: Organ donation and transplantation: current status and future challenges. London: IntechOpen; 2018. p. 229.

24. Thornburg B, Katariya N, Riaz A, Desai K, Hickey R, Lewandowski R, Salem R. Interventional radiology in the management of the liver transplant patient. Liver Transpl. 2017;23(10):1328–41.

Acute on Chronic Liver Failure: An Update

43

Manasvi Gupta and Rakhi Maiwall

Abbreviations

ACLF	Acute on chronic liver failure
AKI	Acute kidney injury
AKIN	Acute kidney injury network
ALF	Acute liver failure
AOPP	Advanced oxidative protein products
APASL	Asian Pacific Association for the study of liver
ATN	Acute tubular necrosis
ATP	Adenosine triphosphate
CAM	Complementary and alternative medicines
CK18	Caspase-cleaved keratin18
CLD	Chronic liver disease
CLIF	Chronic liver failure
CRP	C-reactive protein
CRRT	Continuous renal replacement therapy
CysC	Cystatin C
DAMP	Damage associated molecular patterns
DDLT	Deceased donor liver transplant
EASL	European Association for the study of liver
eGFR	Estimated glomerular filtration rate
FPSA	Fractionated plasma separation and adsorption
G-CSF	Granulocyte colony stimulating factor
HBV	Hepatitis-B virus
HCC	Hepatocellular carcinoma
HE	Hepatic encephalopathy
HIV	Human immunodeficiency virus
HMGB1	High mobility group protein B1
HRS	Hepatorenal syndrome
iACLF	Infection related
ICA	International club of ascites
ICU	Intensive care unit
IL	Interleukin
IL-1RA	IL-1 receptor antagonist
INR	International normalized ratio
K18	Keratin 18
KCH	King's College Hospital criteria
KIM-1	Kidney-Injury molecule
LDLT	Living donor liver transplant
L-FABP	Liver fatty acid binding protein
LPS	Lipopolysaccharide
LT	Liver transplant
MAP	Mean arterial pressure
MARS	Molecular adsorbents recirculatory system
MELD	Model for end-stage liver disease
MERTK	Mer tyrosine-protein kinase
MHE	Minimal hepatic encephalopathy
NAC	N-acetyl cysteine

M. Gupta
Department of Internal Medicine, University of Connecticut, Farmington, CT, USA

R. Maiwall (✉)
Department of Hepatology, Institute of Liver and Biliary Sciences, New Delhi, India

NACSELD	North American consortium for the study of end-stage liver disease
NASH	Non alcoholic steatohepatitis
NGAL	Neutrophil gelatinase-associated lipocalin
OLT	Orthotopic liver transplantation
PAMPs	Pathogen-associated molecular patterns
PICD	Paracentesis induced circulatory dysfunction
PIRO	Predisposition, injury, response, organ failure
RAAS	Rennin–Angiotensin aldosterone
ROTEM	Rotational thromboelastometry
SBP	Spontaneous bacterial peritonitis
SIRS	Systemic inflammatory response syndrome
SOFA	Sequential organ failure assessment
SPAD	Single-pass albumin dialysis
TEG	Thromboelastography
TNF-α	Tumor necrosis factor alpha

43.1 Introduction

The incidence of acute on chronic liver failure (ACLF) has been steadily increasing secondary to excessive alcohol use, usage of over-the-counter hepatotoxic drugs, complementary and alternative medicines, and the rising epidemic of non-alcoholic fatty liver disease [1–3]. Almost one in four outpatients with decompensated cirrhosis patients develop ACLF [4]. There are different definitions for ACLF but the two most widely accepted and validated are the one proposed by the Asian Pacific Association for the Study of Liver (APASL) [1–3] and the second by the European Association for the Study of Liver (EASL) Chronic Liver Failure (EASL-CLIF) consortium [5]. Following this, the world gastroenterology organization had combined the two definitions stratifying ACLF patients into three types [6] based on the underlying severity of chronic liver disease. It is challenging to have a unified definition of ACLF to develop treatment protocols, prognostic scores as well as stratifica-

tion for an emergency liver transplantation. Research exploring liver regenerative therapies, artificial liver support systems, strategies targeting systemic inflammation, and management of bacterial infections which are a key driver of extrahepatic organ failures is an unmet need [1]. Until, these therapies are able to conclusively improve transplant-free survival, liver transplant remains the only definitive treatment option for these patients [1–6].

43.2 Definitions of ACLF

The Asian pacific association for the study of liver (APASL) defines ACLF as an acute hepatic insult manifesting as jaundice (serum bilirubin ≥ 5 mg/dL) and coagulopathy (INR ≥ 1.5 or prothrombin activity $<40\%$) complicating within 4 weeks by clinical ascites and or encephalopathy in a patient with previously diagnosed or undiagnosed chronic liver disease and is associated with high 28-day mortality [1–3]. Conceptually, the APASL definition of ACLF specifies the syndrome wherein there is liver failure precipitated by an acute hepatic insult in a patient with compensated chronic liver disease. The acute insults include hepatitis B reactivation as the commonest cause in the Asia Pacific, followed by alcohol and drugs [1, 7–9]. Alcohol is the most common cause of acute insult in several Asian countries for instance in the Indian subcontinent. Superinfection with hepatitis E virus is also an important cause in the Indian subcontinent [1–3, 9]. Hepatotoxic drugs and complementary and alternative medicines (CAM) are other important contributing causes of acute insult causing the syndrome of ACLF. Drugs used for treatment of tuberculosis are next most important cause of drug induced acute liver failure especially reported from the Indian subcontinent [7]. The definition of ACLF excludes non-hepatic causes as acute insult for instance acute variceal bleed and particularly sepsis. According to APASL, sepsis is a consequence and not a cause for liver failure. The common causes of underlying chronic liver disease include alcohol, NASH, and hepatitis B and C [1–3].

The second most popular definition of ACLF is that proposed by the Chronic Liver Failure (CLIF) acute-on-Chronic Liver Failure in Cirrhosis (CANONIC) definition of ACLF [5, 10, 11]. According to this definition, ACLF is defined as "an acute deterioration of pre-existing chronic liver disease, usually related to a precipitating event and associated with increased mortality at 3 months due to multisystem organ failure." ACLF is defined and graded as ACLF grade 0 if patients had single non-kidney organ failure [5] or had no kidney dysfunction defined as serum creatinine level 1.5 mg/dL and absence of hepatic encephalopathy. Patients with ACLF grade 1 included patients with either single kidney failure (serum creatinine ≥ 2 mg/dL) or patients with single failure of either liver, coagulation, circulation, or respiration defined according to the CLIF-SOFA score. Patients with kidney dysfunction (serum creatinine between 1.5 and 1.9 mg/dL) and/or mild to moderate hepatic encephalopathy and patients with single cerebral failure (grade III or IV hepatic encephalopathy) and kidney dysfunction were classified as ACLF grade 1. ACLF grade 2 included patients with any two organ failures and ACLF grade 3 included patients with 3 organ failures. The 28-day and 90-day mortality rates increased with ACLF grades and were highest for ACLF grade 3, i.e., 76.7% and 79.1%, respectively. The 28-day and 90-day mortality rates of ACLF grade 1 were 22.1% and 40.7%, respectively and for ACLF grade 2 were 32.0% and 52.3%, respectively [5, 10, 11].

The North-American consortium has defined ACLF based on two or more organ failures. They define renal as requirement of dialysis, respiratory as requirement of mechanical ventilation, cerebral as grade III or IV hepatic encephalopathy and circulatory as requirement of vasopressors [12]. The way ACLF is defined based on these definitions is quite heterogenous and has generated confusion across the world. The context has become a bit more confused by inclusion of terms like hepatic and extrahepatic ACLF and infection related ACLF- iACLF. A unifying definition of ACLF is an unmet need to have a clarity for the syndrome and to differentiate it from patients with decompensated cirrhosis with organ failures. The APASL recommends for homogeneity by avoiding extrahepatic organ failures and sepsis in the definition of ACLF [1]. A comparison of the different definitions is given in Table 43.1 and a summary of existing studies on ACLF has been highlighted in Table 43.2.

Table 43.1 Comparison of different definitions of acute on chronic liver failure

	APASL	EASL-CLIF	NACSELD	WGO
Basis of definition	Consensus of international experts	CANONIC study	Prospective study	Consensus of international experts
Definition	Liver failure is defined as jaundice (a serum bilirubin level of ≥ 5 mg/dL) and coagulopathy (an INR of ≥ 1.5 or prothrombin activity of <40%). Liver failure is complicated within 4 weeks by clinical ascites and/or encephalopathy in patients with previously diagnosed or undiagnosed chronic liver disease (including cirrhosis)			ACLF is a syndrome characterized by acute hepatic decompensation resulting in liver failure (jaundice and prolongation of the INR) and one or more extrahepatic organ failures that is associated with increased mortality within a period of 28 days and up to 3 months from onset

(continued)

Table 43.1 (continued)

	APASL	EASL-CLIF	NACSELD	WGO
Study population		1343 patients in 12 European countries	507 patients in USA and Canada	
Included population	Decompensation on existing CLD (including cirrhosis) of any etiology	1. Decompensation in cirrhosis	1. Infection at admission or during hospital stay	Existing CLD (including cirrhosis)
		2. Prior episodes of decompensation of cirrhosis	2. Prior episodes of decompensation of cirrhosis	
Excluded population	1. Bacterial infections	1. HCC	1. HIV	
	2. Prior episodes of decompensation of cirrhosis	2. Chronic medical illnesses unrelated to hepatic disease	2. Organ transplant	
		3. HIV infection	3. Disseminated malignancies	
		4. Immunosuppression treatment		
Organ failure defined as:				
Liver	Total bilirubin ≥5 mg/dL and INR ≥1.5	Bilirubin level of >12 mg/dL		
Kidney	Acute kidney injury network criteria	Creatinine level of ≥2.0 mg/dL or renal replacement	Need for dialysis or other forms of renal replacement therapy	
Brain	West-haven hepatic encephalopathy grade 3–4	West-haven hepatic encephalopathy grade 3–4	West-haven hepatic encephalopathy grade 3–4	
Coagulation	INR ≥1.5	INR ≥2.5		
Shock		Use of vasopressors	MAP <60 mm hg or a SBP reduction of 40 mm hg from baseline, despite adequate fluid resuscitation and cardiac output	
Lungs		PaO2/FiO2 of ≤200 or SpO2/FiO2 of ≤214 or need for mechanical ventilation	Need for mechanical ventilation	

Table 43.2 Different types of artificial liver support systems available

System	Components	Source of albumin	Albumin recycling	Toxin removed	Outcomes	Shortcomings	Anticoagulation	Advantages
Molecular adsorbent recirculating system (MARS)	Blood circuit	Exogenous albumin	Through CRRT	Albumin bound	Improvement in HE, no survival benefit	More sophisticated	UFH	Most widely studied
	Albumin circuit			Water bound				
	Classic hemodialysis circuit			Cytokines				
Single-pass albumin dialysis (SPAD)	Standard CRRT, no additional adsorbent columns or circuits	Exogenous albumin	Not done	Albumin bound	Improvement in HE, no survival benefit	No studies on ACLF patients, all existing data is from ALF patients	Local anticoagulation with citrate	Simplest to use
				Water bound		More expensive as albumin is not reused		
						Difficulty in determining optimal albumin dialyzate concentration, dialyzate flow rate and treatment regimen		
Fractionated plasma separation and adsorption–FPSA (Prometheus)	First circuit: Albumin enters through AlbuFlow® filter and is returned to circulation using a neutral resin adsorber (Prometh®01) and an anion-exchange column (Prometh® 02)	Patient's albumin	Through CRRT	Albumin bound (more efficiently than MARS)	Improvement in HE, no survival benefit	Newest and yet to be fully studied		Increase in hepatic growth factor (HGF)
	Second circuit: Hemodialysis			Water bound				
				Cytokines				

CRRT continuous renal replacement therapy, *UFH* ultrafiltration hemodialysis

43.3 Pathogenetic Basis of ACLF (Fig. 43.1)

43.3.1 Systemic Inflammation

The presence of low-grade systemic inflammation in patients with stable or decompensated cirrhosis is considered to cause or augment relevant clinical signs and symptoms such as hyperdynamic circulation, fatigue, or minimal hepatic encephalopathy (MHE) [13, 14]. The etiology of cirrhosis could be chronic infections secondary to viruses, drugs, alcohol or autoimmune diseases. The progression of liver damage, fibro-

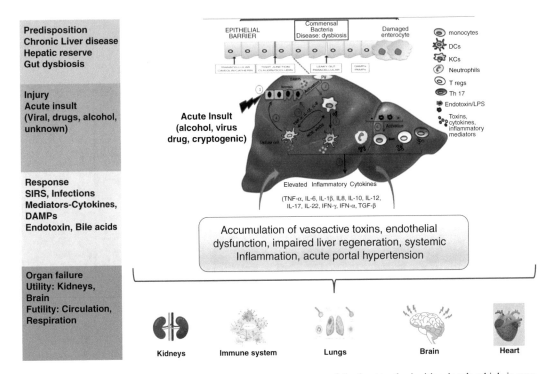

Fig. 43.1 The PIRO concept of ACLF. The PIRO concept i.e. (Predisposition, Injury, Response, Organ Failure) which has been used for stratifying patients of any acute illness can well be used for patients with ACLF. PIRO incorporates assessment of pre-morbid baseline susceptibility (predisposition) factors which includes the underlying hepatic reserve and gut dysbiosis which have an influence on the course of the disease. The injury includes the specific factor causing acute illness (insult) which includes viral, drugs, alcohol in patients with acute on chronic liver failure (ACLF). The acute insult in turn incites the host response. In patients with ACLF, the acute insult activates the Kupffer cells localized to the hepatic sinusoids, through toll-like receptor 4 (TLR4), complement receptors (C3R and C5R), and damage-associated-molecular-patterns (DAMPs) which results in increased release of proinflammatory and anti-inflammatory cytokines, endotoxin, prostaglandins, bile acids, lysosomal, and proteolytic enzymes. The activation of the hepatic stellate cells by the Kupffer cells produces vasoactive mediators like endothelin-1, thromboxane A2, nitric oxide, and prostaglandins which lead to a perturbed hepatic microcirculatory function, endothelial dysfunction, and an acute increase in the portal pressure. The

response of the host to the inciting insult which is measured as systemic inflammatory response syndrome which is commonly assessed by the physiological variables and can progress to a compensatory anti-inflammatory response syndrome (CARS) causes infections and secondary organ failures. The last component of the PIRO incorporates organ failures which includes organs of utility, i.e. the brain and kidneys and organs of futility that is circulation and respiration which contraindicate a liver transplant. The PIRO concept is especially useful in diseases like ACLF where the clinicians have limited therapeutic options in their armamentarium and therefore a stratification system enables identification of a possible clinical trajectory, to predict outcome much early, allowing allocation of the best treatment options to the patients before the development of organ failure what is called as the "golden window" of therapeutic intervention. *ACLF* acute-on-chronic liver failure, *SIRS* systemic inflammatory response syndrome, *DAMP* damage-associated molecular pattern, *DCs* dendritic cells, *KC* kupffer cells, *eNOS* endothelial nitric oxide synthase, *LPS* lipopolysaccharide, *MODS* multiorgan dysfunction syndrome, *PV* portal vein, *TGFβ* transforming growth factor beta, *TH17 cell* type 17T helper cell, *TREG cell* regulatory T cell genesis, and sinusoidal portal hypertension results in production of damage associated molecular patterns (DAMPS) which could be derived from the nucleus, i.e., high-mobility group protein B1 (HMGB1), histones, ATP, derived from cytoplasmic membrane, i.e. glypican and syndecan, from mitochondria or endoplasmic reticulum like calreticulin [15–17]. These DAMPs could initiate sterile inflammation and result in activation of the innate and adaptive immune system. At the same time, cirrhosis is characterized by gut dysbiosis, increase in gut permeability and enhancement of local intestinal inflammation with endogenous endotoxemia, and impairment of local intestinal defenses [15–17]. In animal models of liver cirrhosis, endotoxin-mediated tumor-necrosis-factor-alpha (TNF-α) is implicated in other organ dysfunction, worsening of systemic vasodilation with impairment of cardiac contractility. All these effects could be abrogated by fecal microbial transplantation [18, 19]. In a study from EASL-CLIF consortium it was demonstrated that higher grades of systemic inflammation in

ACLF were associated with higher incidence of organ failures which also differentiated them from patients with acute decompensation of cirrhosis [20]. Trebicka et al. evaluated baseline plasma levels of 15 cytokines, chemokines, and oxidized albumin) in 161 patients with ACLF which were compared to 40 healthy controls, 39 patients with stable compensated cirrhosis, and 342 patients with acute decompensation of cirrhosis. They observed that these markers were significantly elevated in patients with ACLF and in those patients with acute decompensation who finally succumbed at 28 days of systemic inflammation [21]. Considering systemic inflammation as the key driver of organ failures, the concept of "golden-window" has been proposed by the APASL (Fig. 43.2). In a study by Chowdhury and colleagues the relevance of SIRS was shown in patients with ACLF [22]. It was seen that presence, persistence, and development of new SIRS was associated with worse outcomes in patients with ACLF while resolution was associated with improved outcomes. Therefore, dynamicity of SIRS has an important prognostic

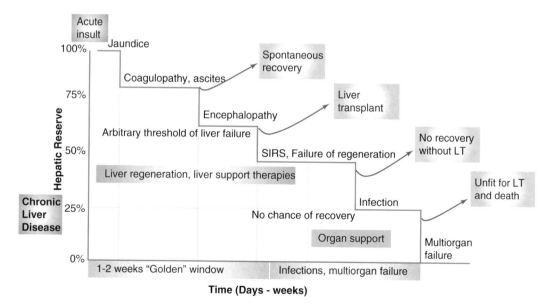

Fig. 43.2 The "Golden-Window" of therapeutic intervention in patients with ACLF. Systemic inflammation as the key driver of infection and multiorgan failure in patients with ACLF. The first 2 weeks provide the "golden-window" of targeted strategies for combating systemic inflammation using liver support therapies, immunomod-

ulation, and potentiation of liver regeneration using granulocyte colony stimulating factor (G-CSF) or modulation of gut dysbiosis using fecal microbial transplant for patients with ACLF as a possible bridge toward spontaneous recovery or liver transplant implication in patients with ACLF. Altogether, SIRS in patients with ACLF can lead to a state of immunodysfunction which is a harbinger of sepsis and multiorgan failure. SIRS and or infection in these patients results in cell-death by causing deprivation of oxygen and energy from the tissues [23].

43.3.2 Immunodysfunction in Patients with ACLF

Patients with ACLF not only have state of systemic inflammation but at the same time a state of prolonged and suppressed state of immune exhaustion has been well-described in these patients. These patients characteristically have increased concentrations of ant-inflammatory cytokines, i.e., interleukin-10 (IL-10) or IL-1 receptor antagonist (IL-1RA) [24]. The cells of the innate immune system, for instance, the monocytes are even though increased in frequency and display an activated phenotype but have failure to respond to stimulation with bacterial lipopolysaccharide (LPS). An increase in the number of peripheral blood monocytes expressing the tyrosine-protein kinase Mer (encoded by *MERTK*) which has anti-phagocytic functions has also been shown [25]. Changes in the adaptive immune system i.e. a lower frequency of naïve helper and suppressor T-cells while the number of activated T-cells is inappropriately noted in patients with ACLF. The state of cirrhosis-associated immune dysfunction is further exaggerated in patients with ACLF which is characterized by defects in phagocytosis, complement presentation, defects in innate and adaptive immunity, and defects in clearance of intestinal and bacterial pathogens [26]. Continuous exposure of bacterial derived pathogen-associated molecular patterns (PAMPs) and DAMPs amidst a state of sustained inflammation results concomitantly to state of immunosuppression in these patients [27].

43.3.3 Intestinal Inflammation and Gut Dysbiosis

Patients with cirrhosis have loss of gut barrier integrity secondary to an increase in the inflammatory mediators which downregulate the tight junctions causing leaky gut and associated bacterial translocation. Intestinal dysbiosis is a hallmark of patients with ACLF [28–32]. There is alteration of the gut microbial environment which is characterized by a shift to pathogenic bacterial species (e.g. *Enterococcus* spp.) and a decrease in the number of beneficial bacterial species (e.g. *Bifidobacterium* spp.) Concomitant to this, these patients have alteration in the gut motility, a reduction in the antimicrobial proteins, altered composition of bile salts and reduction in the gastric acid which gets exacerbated by the use of proton pump inhibitors. All this results in an increase in the translocation of gut-derived pathogens, i.e. LPS, flagellin, etc. which exacerbates systemic inflammatory response syndrome and leads to the development of bacterial infections. Amongst all etiologies, patients with alcohol have the highest gut associated dysbiosis and altered permeability because of the direct effects of alcohol itself in these changes [18, 19, 28–32].

43.3.4 Infections

Patients with ACLF develop an increased frequency of infections which are both community-acquired and nosocomial infections. Spontaneous bacterial peritonitis, gastrointestinal hemorrhage or hepatic encephalopathy are known risk factors for development of infections in patients with ACLF [1–6]. Patients of ACLF frequently develop both bacterial and fungal infections [33, 34]. Prophylactic antibiotics are therefore recommended in these situations to lower the risk of bacterial infections. The diagnosis of bacterial infection, however, remains a challenge. Currently, there are no rapid diagnostic methods for the diagnosis of occult infections and culture methods are the only definite proof of the presence of infections in these patients. Serum procalcitonin and C-reactive protein (CRP) in combination have a positive predictive value of more than 90% for the diagnosis of bacterial infection. A cut-off level of CRP of more than 24.7 ng/mL and serum procalcitonin of more than 0.47 μg/L is used for recommending prophylactic antibiotics [35]. The degree of systemic inflammation is could also be determined by the white cell counts and the use of neutrophil to lymphocyte ratio [5, 36]. A number of other pro-inflammatory markers, i.e. tumor necrosis factor alpha (TNF-α), interleukin-6 (IL-6), and IL-8 have been evaluated in these patients other markers, i.e., caspase-cleaved keratin18 (CK18) and keratin 18 (K18) are reflective of apoptotic and total cell death, respectively, and cK18: K18 ratio is known to increase with the severity of ACLF [37, 38]. However, currently none of the biomarkers can reliably differentiate sterile inflammation from infection. Infections are important triggers for the development of ACLF by causing organ failures which is associated with high mortality in the absence of liver transplantation. It is recommended to consider the site and acquisition of infection as well as the local microbiological profile to decide the choice of prophylactic antibiotics in patients with ACLF. In a large multicentric-multinational study global study performed to capture the data on bacterial infections across the globe regional differences were observed in the spectrum of infections in patients with cirrhosis. In the asian countries, particularly India a predominance of multidrug resistant infections was observed which was were associated with a higher incidence of organ failures, prolonged ICU stay, and higher mortality [39]. Choice of appropriate empirical antibiotics was associated with improved outcomes. As a protocol, the patients should be reassessed at 48–72 h for de-escalation of antibiotics after the culture report.

43.4 The Concept of Tolerance in ACLF

Sepsis is defined as the host response to a bacterial pathogen. Infections in patients with ACLF can directly impact or damage the tissues or cause stimulation of the immune system resulting in the release of pro-inflammatory cytokines which cause end-organ dysfunction or failure. The host response is related to the intrinsic tolerance. It has been well-documented that as compared to patients with decompensated cirrhosis, who are exposed to repeated prior episodes of bacterial infection and chronic endotoxemia, patients with ACLF respond poorly to containment of bacterial infections because of failure of protective mechanisms of tolerance [40].

43.4.1 Assessment of Liver and Extrahepatic Organs in Patients with ACLF

43.4.1.1 Liver Failure

According to the APASL definition the liver remains at the core of the entire syndrome of ACLF [1–3]. All patients therefore have liver failure which is manifested by jaundice, coagulopathy and/or ascites, and hepatic encephalopathy. Majority of patients with ACLF have ascites which is a consequence of underlying chronic liver disease, hemodynamic alterations secondary to systemic inflammation, and the development of acute portal hypertension. The severity of liver failure therefore is determined by the degree of jaundice, coagulation impairment, and the degree and severity of ascites [1–3]. Development of any grade of hepatic encephalopathy and its persistence is associated with worse clinical outcomes. Assessment of hepatic reserve would be worthwhile to determine the potential of spontaneous liver regeneration in patients with ACLF.

43.4.1.2 Coagulation Failure

Assessment of coagulation can be performed by standard tests, i.e., the international normalized ratio, platelet counts, and serum fibrinogen levels. In patients with decompensated cirrhosis, an intricate balance is noted between coagulation and fibrinolysis and is usually procoagulant [41]. The state of coagulation in patients with ACLF should be assessed by thromboelastography (TEG) or rotational thromboelastometry (ROTEM) [42, 43]. In a single-center prospective study consecutive patients of ACLF without sepsis were recruited and assessed by TEG and other specific assays (Factor VIII, von Willebrand factor, protein C and antithrombin III and followed for development of sepsis, bleeding events and overall outcomes [44]. A hypocoagulable TEG at baseline was an independent predictor of not only bleeding events but also mortality. The global coagulation index, lower levels of protein C, antithrombin III, and tissue plasminogen activator levels predicted 28-day mortality after adjusting for patient demographics and the MELD scores. Furthermore, during bleeding correction of coagulation using either ROTEM or TEG could also limit transfusion related adverse effects in patients with AC LF and may result in targeted coagulation correction.

43.4.1.3 Kidney Dysfunction or Failure

Kidneys are one of the most frequent extrahepatic organs that are affected in patients with ACLF. Acute kidney injury is reported in 22.8–34% of patients with ACLF [45]. Kidneys in patients with ACLF should be assessed using the relative changes in serum creatinine or by measuring urine output in hospitalized patients rather than relying on serum creatinine. This is because various factors influence the serum creatinine estimation which might result in underdiagnosis of renal dysfunction [45]. Use of biomarkers like serum cystatin C could be helpful in early detection of AKI in patients with ACLF. The AKI spectrum has also not been well-studied in patients with ACLF. These patients have predominance of structural AKI secondary to a higher prevalence of bacterial infections, systemic inflammation, high serum bilirubin, and predominance of circulatory dysfunction [46, 47].

43.4.1.4 Spectrum of AKI in ACLF

Patients with ACLF have acute portal hypertension, the main abnormality causing renal dysfunction in these patients is severe systemic and splanchnic vasodilatation which leads to decreased effective arterial blood volume and activation of the renin–angiotensin aldosterone (RAAS), the sympathetic nervous system and non-osmotic release of antidiuiretic hormone which causes salt and water retention. The pathogenetic basis of renal dysfunction in ACLF is quite different from that of patients with decompensated cirrhosis. Majority of patients have structural kidney damage as assessed by microscopic urinalysis and renal biomarkers. Severity of systemic inflammation, bacterial infections, cholemic nephropathy are most common reasons for structural kidney damage [1–3, 45–48].

43.4.1.5 Prediction of AKI in ACLF

In a large multicenter multinational prospective study of patients with ACLF from the Asia Pacific, a predictive score was developed for identification of the development or progression of AKI in patients with ACLF. The score was developed on the concept of PIRO, i.e. predisposition, injury, response and organ failure which was initially developed for patients with sepsis. Components of the predisposition component included high urea, serum creatinine, potassium, and serum bilirubin. In the injury component, the use of nephrotoxic drugs was identified as an important predictor, response component included presence of systemic inflammatory response syndrome, and organ failure included presence of low mean arterial pressure. Patients of ACLF could be risk stratified for AKI using the PIRO score for additional therapeutic interventions targeting the components of PIRO [48].

43.4.1.6 Diagnosis of AKI in Patients with ACLF

Considering the limitations of serum creatinine in patients with ACLF and especially in context of intensive care unit stay retention of urine output criteria may be relevant in the diagnosis of AKI in these patients [49]. However, this needs validation in patients with ACLF. The data from the AARC database suggested a lower value of serum creatinine is more relevant in patients with ACLF. Serum creatinine above 0.7 mg/dL (as derived from the AARC score) has a sensitivity of 78% and specificity of 36% for prediction of 30-day mortality in patients with ACLF. For the diagnosis of kidney failure, the conventional cut-off of 1.5 mg/dL even though had a low sensitivity of 48% but had a specificity of 99.8% for 30-day mortality [3]. The revised consensus criteria for AKI in patients with ACLF lead down by the international club of ascites suggest diagnosis of AKI using the AKIN criteria. In patients with stage 1 AKI or those with serum creatinine less than 1.5 mg/dL should be managed by removal of the precipitating cause and conservative measures. Patients who have stage 2 or 3 AKI and those with serum creatine above 1.5 mg/dL should undergo volume expansion with intravenous albumin. Kidney failure (serum creatinine $\geq$1.5 mg/dL) was seen in 22% of ACLF patients at baseline and developed in another 30% within a month [50]. The majority of patients of ACLF developed new episodes of AKI in the first 2 weeks (11%). Apart from the severity, the course of AKI was seen to be an important predictor of clinical outcomes. Patients with AKI resolution have improved outcomes while those with either AKI progression or persistence have worse outcomes [3].

43.5 Role of Biomarkers

43.5.1 Biomarkers of Glomerular Injury

43.5.1.1 Cystatin C

Cystatin C is a nonglycosylated protein with low molecular weight (13 kDa), has a constant rate of production and concentration of cystatin C is determined by glomerular filtration. It is, therefore, considered as an early marker of glomerular dysfunction. We have demonstrated the role of serum cystatin C in a large prospective cohort study in patients with cirrhosis, wherein it has been shown as a marker of renal reserve to predict development of new AKI episode and chronic kidney disease [47, 51]. In patients with hepatitis-B virus (HBV) related ACLF CysC was shown to accurately predict AKI even in patients with normal serum creatinine [52].

43.5.2 Biomarkers of Proximal Tubular Damage

43.5.2.1 Kidney Injury Molecule (KIM-1)

Kidney injury molecule-1 is a type 1 transmembrane glycoprotein which is comprised of an immunoglobulin and mucin domain. Under normal conditions, KIM-1 protein is only minimally expressed in kidney tissue or urine but is shed from the proximal tubules with tubular dysfunction wherein it can be detected in the urine by immunoassay. It is known to be upregulated in response to renal ischemia or nephrotoxic insult and is also believed to participate in the regeneration process after epithelial injury [53].

43.5.2.2 Liver Fatty Acid Binding Protein (L-FABP)

Fatty-acid protein bindings (FABPs) facilitate transfer of fatty acids between intra and extracellular membranes. They also have a role in the amelioration of cellular oxidative stress by inhibition of the toxic effects of oxidative intermediates on cellular membranes. In the normal healthy state, urinary L-FABP is undetectable; however, under states of renal ischemia there is decreased proximal tubular reabsorption of L-FABP which is detected as increased excretion in urine [53].

43.5.2.3 Interleukine-18

Interleukine-18 (IL-18) is a proinflammatory cytokine which is synthesized in renal proximal tubular epithelial cells as well as monocytes and macrophages. The concentrations of IL-18 have also been demonstrated to be increased in post-ischemic AKI following renal hypoxia. It can therefore be considered as an early biomarker of AKI in critically ill patients. It has also been shown to correlate with poor clinical outcomes (death or requirement of renal replacement therapy) in patients with sepsis [53].

43.5.3 Biomarkers of Distal Tubular Damage

43.5.3.1 Neutrophil Gelatinase-Associated Lipocalin

Neutrophil gelatinase-associated lipocalin (NGAL) NGAL belongs to the lipocalin superfamily (lipocalin 2, siderocalin). Both plasma and urine NGALs are increased after an episode of AKI. Elevated urine NGAL originates from both proximal and distal nephron after a nephrotoxic insult. Injury to proximal renal tubules precludes NGAL reabsorption and/or increase denovo NGAL synthesis secondary to upregulation of NGAL mRNA in the distal nephron segments (especially in the thick ascending limb of Henle's loop and the collecting ducts) [54].

43.5.4 Studies Assessing Markers of Tubular Injury in Patients with ACLF

The major challenge in patients with ACLF is to differentiate HRS associated with bacterial infections from ATN as it evolves through a continuous spectrum. In fact, HRS patients who are non-responders to vasoconstrictors are known to have tubular dysfunction requiring prolonged RRT [45]. In another prospective study in patients with cirrhosis and bacterial infections, measurement of urinary NGAL at infection diagnosis was reported to be useful in predicting clinical outcomes, persistent AKI and type of AKI [55]. Interestingly, N-GAL also accurately predicted development of a second infection and 3-month mortality. In this study significantly higher uNGAL was noted in patients who developed persistent AKI and amongst these patients was able to discriminate type-1 HRS from other causes of AKI with accuracy. In another study done in 55 patients with an acute decompensation of cirrhosis a panel of 12 biomarkers was studied to differentiate ATN from other causes of AKI. In this study also, NGAL was identified as the best biomarker, others being IL-18, albumin, trefoil-factor-3 (TFF-3) and glutathione-S-transferase-π (GST-π) [53]. In a large prospective study performed in 716 patients with ACLF, urine and plasma NGAL levels were analyzed. The authors noted that the levels of urine NGAL were markedly elevated in patients with ACLF (108(35–400) vs. 29 (12–73) µg/g creatinine; $p < 0.001$) and independently predicted 28-day mortality [54]. The authors proposed urine NGAL as a biomarker for patients with ACLF. In another study performed in patients with HBV-ACLF 280 patients were compared to 132 patients with HBV-related decompensated cirrhosis (DC). The authors studied the levels of five urinary tubular injury including neutrophil gelatinase-associated lipocalin (NGAL), interleukin-18 (IL-18), liver-type fatty acid binding protein (L-FABP), cystatin C (CysC), and kidney injury molecule-1 (KIM-1). This was correlated to patient demographics, development and progression of AKI, and response to terlipressin therapy were recorded. The levels of urinary biomarkers (NGAL, CysC, L-FABP, IL-18) were significantly elevated in patients with HBV-ACLF and AKI (ACLF-AKI), compared with that in patients with HBV-DC and AKI (DC-AKI) or those without AKI [56].

43.5.4.1 Management of AKI

According to the new consensus by the ICA for AKI, a new algorithm for the management of AKI based on the revised criteria has been proposed. Based on this algorithm it is recommended that patients with initial AKI stage 1 should be managed by removal of all precipitants (careful review of medications, diuretics, nephrotoxic drugs, vasodilators or non-steroidal anti-inflammatory drugs). Second step is to consider plasma volume expansion in patients with hypovolemia (the choice of fluid could either be a crystalloid or albumin or even blood as indicated) along with identification and early treatment of bacterial infections. Patients who respond with a decrease in serum creatinine value of 0.3 mg/dL of the baseline value should be subsequently followed up for any new episodes of AKI. Patients who have progression, should be managed as ICA-AKI stage 2 and 3. In this group of patients, along with the institution of all measures as recommended for patients with stage 1 AKI a work up for the differential diagnosis should be done on an immediate basis to identify whether it is HRS-AKI, intrinsic AKI or post-renal cause. It was further decided by the panel of experts that for patients with stage 1 AKI who do not improve but have no progression further management can be decided based on the absolute value of serum creatinine and if the serum creatinine is more than 1.5 mg/dL it was recommended to consider the same protocol as for management for stage 2 and 3 AKI. Patients with HRS-AKI are recommended to be managed with early use of vasoconstrictors based on the revised criteria for HRS-AKI (either with terlipressin or norepinephrine or midodrine plus octreotide). Management of non-responders to vasoconstrictors which constitute a large group of patients therefore still remains an ongoing challenge. There is paucity of data on dialysis in patients with cirrhosis therefore there are no specific recommendations regarding the dose, the intensity, duration and time of initiation of dialysis in these patients [45]. We propose different management algorithm with incorporation of antioxidants and anti-inflammatory strategies, early initiation of vasoconstrictors and extracorporeal support therapies considering a higher incidence of structural AKI and poor response to vasoconstrictors [45, 46, 48].

43.5.4.2 Cerebral Failure

Development and persistence of hepatic encephalopathy is associated with a grim prognosis in patients with ACLF. The pathophysiology of HE is multifactorial and complex important factors include hyperammonemia, systemic inflammation, gut dysbiosis, genetic factors, bacterial infection, and insulin resistance [1–3]. Alcohol use and hyponatremia are other factors implicated in brain dysfunction in patients with ACLF. Contrary to patients with acute liver failure, cerebral oedema is rare and is observed in 5% of the patients with hepatic encephalopathy as

reported in imaging studies [57]. Ammonia induces oxidative and cellular stress and in patients with ACLF. Whether higher levels of ammonia correlate with more severe grades of HE has not been studied in patients with ACLF [58]. Management involves identification and correction of precipitating factors should be identified and treated as required. Use of lactulose for bowel cleansing, non-absorbable antibiotics, novel ammonia lowering drugs, such as glycerol phenylbutyrate and ornithine phenylacetate, have shown some promise but are still experimental. Use of liver dialysis for refractory hepatic encephalopathy has shown some benefits. Abstinence of alcohol, strategies for systemic inflammation, use of antibiotics for infection, and treatment of diabetes may also improve hepatic encephalopathy by combating systemic inflammation [59].

43.5.4.3 Circulatory and Respiratory Failure

The revised consensus of APASL defined organs of utility and futility in patients with ACLF. Among the extrahepatic organ failures, brain and kidneys are considered as organs of utility because even though dysfunction or failure of these organs is associated with worse prognosis but these do contraindicate liver transplant. On the contrary, data from Europe and America has suggested that protocols of excluding patients with severe circulatory or respiratory failure. In patients wherein transplant is performed dysfunction or circulation or respiration is associated with worse outcomes as compared to patients who did not have these organ failures [60].

43.6 Management of Patients with ACLF (Fig. 43.3)

43.6.1 Albumin

Albumin has an important role in the treatment of ACLF. Normal liver synthesizes 11–15 g of albumin, however, this capacity is reduced by 60–80% in patients with ACLF. Albumin has colloid osmotic functions, is an important carrier of different substances, has anti-inflammatory and

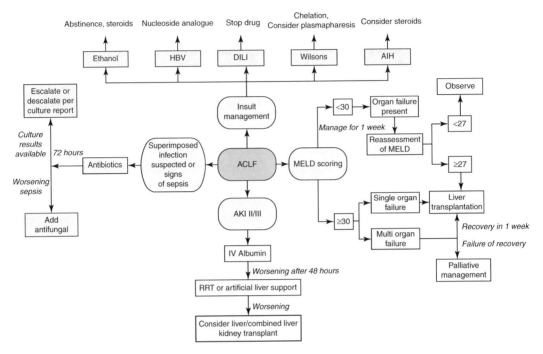

Fig. 43.3 Management algorithm for acute on chronic liver failure. *HBV* hepatitis B virus, *DILI* drug induced liver injury, *AIH* autoimmune hepatitis, *ACLF* acute on chronic liver failure, *AKI* acute kidney injury, *RRT* renal replacement therapy, *MELD* model of end-stage liver disease, *IV* intravenous

anti-oxidant property as well as maintenance of capillary permeability. Recent data has suggested utility of albumin in combating systemic inflammation and resolution of uncomplicated ascites [61–64]. Albumin is recommended for management for HRS-AKI, prevention of renal dysfunction in patients with spontaneous bacterial peritonitis (SBP), and prevention of paracentesis induced circulatory dysfunction (PICD). In a single-center randomized controlled trial in patients of ACLF who underwent modest-volume paracentesis the incidence of PICD and its associated complications was significantly reduced as compared to standard medical treatment [65].

43.6.2 Renal Replacement Therapy

The indications of renal replacement therapy are the same as those for other conditions, i.e. metabolic acidosis, volume overload, uremic complications, and electrolyte abnormalities. It should be considered in patients who are candidates for

orthotopic liver transplantation (OLT) or those with acute tubular necrosis (ATN), hypovolemia related renal failure or where renal functions are likely to be reversible. The leading indication identified in these patients has been volume overload. Continuous renal replacement therapy (CRRT) is better tolerated than intermittent hemodialysis because of improved cardiovascular stability, clear ammonia and pro-inflammatory cytokines, and improved cerebral oedema. Complications such as hypotension, bleeding secondary to coagulopathy, and catheter-related sepsis are commonly encountered with renal replacement therapy when used in patients with advanced liver disease. Hence, a multidisciplinary approach involving a hepatologist, a nephrologist, and an intensive care specialist is needed to decide the exact timing and modality of renal replacement therapy in patients with ACLF. Considering an extremely poor response to vasoconstrictors in only 35% of patients with HRS in patients with ACLF and higher prevalence of structural AKI in patients with ACLF, the utility of RRT remains to be explored [66, 67]. There is paucity of data on dialysis in patients with ACLF and decompensated cirrhosis therefore there are no specific recommendations regarding the dose, the intensity, and the duration of dialysis in these patients. In a recent multicentric prospective study from North American Consortium for the Study of End-Stage Liver Disease (NACSELD) database for cirrhotic patients hospitalized with an infection (I-ACLF) where RRT was not identified as an independent predictor of survival when it was done as a bridging therapy to liver transplantation [12]. There is emerging data to suggest that initiation of RRT early may attenuate both kidney-specific and non-kidney specific organ dysfunction as well as counteract systemic inflammation in critically ill patients. However, unfortunately complications such as hypotension, coagulopathy-related bleeding, and catheter-related sepsis are frequently encountered with RRT in patients with cirrhosis and therefore in the absence of absolute indications it is a daunting task for the clinicians to decide initiation of early RRT in such a severely sick group of patients. Randomized controlled trials are therefore needed to decide the timing of initiation of RRT (that is, "early" versus "late") in patients of ACLF who have structural kidney damage or have non-response to vasoconstrictors awaiting liver transplantation.

43.6.3 Extracorporeal Liver Support Systems

These can be non-cell based or cell-based systems. Non-cell based systems do not incorporate tissue and provide only detoxification functions using membranes and adsorbents which allow removal of both water-soluble and protein bound substances as against conventional hemodialysis which removes only water-soluble toxins. These newer developing therapies have demonstrated benefits in biochemical parameters, hemodynamic, hepatic encephalopathy and also renal functions but are expensive and still considered experimental in patients with ACLF [68, 69]. Currently, they are considered as an option in

patients as a bridge to liver transplantation or clinical recovery. The Molecular Adsorbent Recirculatory System (MARS), single-pass albumin dialysis (SPAD), and the Fractionated Plasma Separation and Adsorption (FPSA or Prometheus) have shown limited efficacy in improving transplant-free survival in patients with ACLF. In the HELIOS trial survival of patients with type 1 HRS when treated with FPSA was better compared to SMT (28-day survival 62% vs. 39%, 90-day survival probability, 42% vs. 6%, respectively; log-rank test, $P = 0.04$). Similarly in the RELIEF trial with MARS it was seen that the proportion of patients with a serum creatinine below 1.5 mg/dL at day 4 in patients with HRS at baseline tended to be higher in patients who were treated with MARS ($p = 0.07$). Considering a higher prevalence of structural AKI and cholemic nephropathy in patients with ACLF, the utility of MARS remains to be explored [45, 70, 71]. Larger randomized controlled trials are required for patients with ACLF as the patient populations enrolled in the large trials in Europe were performed using heterogenous definitions of ACLF [68–71]. Case reports and series have suggested beneficial effects of plasma-exchange in patients with ACLF [72–75]. In the large European multicentric trial performed in patients with ALF, plasma-exchange was shown to improve survival by dampening the immune response [76]. The results from the AARC database suggested a beneficial role of plasma-exchange in patients with ACLF in preventing multiorgan failure and ameliorating SIRS. Currently, a specific device (DIALIVE) with an aim to remove dysfunctional albumin and endotoxin and replacing it with functional albumin is being evaluated in ACLF patients [35]. Table 43.2 summarizes the studies on artificial liver support therapies in patients with ACLF.

43.6.4 Therapeutic Strategies Targeting Liver Regeneration in ACLF

Initial randomized controlled clinical trials from India suggested encouraging data for G-CSF. An impressive survival benefit was observed in these studies, however most of them were mono-centric [77–81]. Hence, the broad application of G-CSF in ACLF has not been routinely recommended outside clinical trials. The large multicentric trial performed in Europe, the. GRAFT-Study, did not Lreplicate the observed benefits observed in Asian trials. However, the differences in the definitions used to define ACLF may be a key factor explaining the observed differences [35].

43.6.5 Role of Anti-Oxidants in ACLF

Oxidative stress is hypothesized to play a crucial role in liver disease with the generation of advanced oxidative protein products (AOPP) playing a primary role in active inflammation. AOPP have been found to be in higher concentration in the serum in patients with viral hepatitis, diabetics, and advanced age. AOPP levels have also found to be higher in liver biopsies taken from severe ACLF secondary to alcohol compared to stable alcoholic cirrhosis, indicating role in ongoing damage [82].

Treatment with N-acetyl cysteine (NAC) in non-acetaminophen liver failure has been shown to improve survival in multiple studies. Nabi et al. showed that treatment of 40 patients with intravenous NAC for 72 h was associated with a decrease in mortality to 28% as compared to 53% in the control group [83]. These findings corroborated results of Mumtaz et al. study in 47 patients given oral NAC that showed a survival of 47% in treatment group and 27% in the non-treatment group [84]. Baniasadi et al. also showed benefit of NAC in antitubercular drug induced liver injury [85]. A meta-analysis of four prospective studies including 331 patients also showed that NAC was safe in non-acetaminophen liver disease and improved survival in both liver transplant and native liver patients [86]. However, studies are limited and NAC is not the standard of care for ACLF.

43.6.6 Liver Transplantation in ACLF

ACLF as a disease entity is characterized by dynamic course during hospital admission, with the course between day 3 and day 7 being the most integral in determining long-term management. An improvement in overall health opens the doors to other therapies such as bioartificial liver support (as summarized in Table 43.3), granulocyte colony stimulating factors, and stem cell transplant. These are in early phases of development and liver transplant is the only definite management option. Unlike acute liver failure (ALF), ACLF does not qualify for enlistment in the high urgency list. Furthermore, evaluation time is limited by the rapid evolution of disease with age, multiorgan failure, and recidivism forming key barriers to inclusion to the transplant list. Additionally, among those patients present on the waiting list, the incidence of mortality is high and exceeds that of ALF patients on the waiting list [87]. The key studies are summarized in Table 43.3.

Current data indicates that <50% ACLF patients are listed for transplant and < 20% ACLF patients actually successfully undergo transplantation. The 5-year survival in the patient that undergo successful transplantation is 74–90% [88]. This data highlights the necessity to validate prognostic tools to allow prioritization of patients with ACLF on the transplant list. Such patients should also be aggressively managed in the intensive care unit (ICU) with early management of known triggers of downward cascade such as infection and bleeding. The multiorgan failure seen as a defining feature of ACLF should be supported with vasopressors, mechanical ventilation, and continuous renal replacement as needed. It is notable that the highest quality of care can be provided with a well-balanced multidisciplinary team and early ICU admission [89].

The other options for these patients are living donor liver transplantation (LDLT) which has shown reasonable success, specifically with the

Table 43.3 Summary of studies on liver transplantation in patients with acute on chronic liver failure

Author, year	Sample size	Survival	Comments
Liu et al. (2003)	32	88% at 1 year	Hepatitis B patients
Wang et al. (2007)	42	83.3% at 1 year	Both DDLT and LDLT were done
Chan et al. (2009)	149	95.3% at 1 year 90% at 5 years	Both DDLT and LDLT were done
Bahirwani et al. (2011)	157	74.5% at 1 year	175 patients had no ACLF, post-transplant outcomes similar including eGFR
Ling et al. (2012)	126	73% at 1 year	Downgrading MELD improved survival, both DDLT and LDLT
Duan et al. (2013)	100	80% at 1 year 74% at 5 years	Both DDLT and LDLT
Xing et al. (2013)	133	78.1% at 1 year 72.8% at 5 years	Hepatorenal syndrome improved with LT, good outcome of combined liver kidney transplantation for patients with ESRD
Finkenstedt et al. (2013)	33	84.8% at 1 year 82% at 5 years	High wait list mortality in ACLF group, survival after LT comparable to non-ACLF
Gustot et al. (2014)	35	80.9% at 6 months	10% in those not transplanted for ACLF2–3
Levesque et al. (2017)	140	70% 1 year as compared to 92% in without ACLF	ACLF 3 poor than lower grades, 17/30 (56%) mortality at 1 year in this group
Artru et al. (2017)	73	83.9% at 1 year, baseline ACLF grade 3	7.9% survival in not LT, all patients had complications and longer hospital stay
Moon et al. (2017)	189 ACLF	76.8% at 1 year	ACLF longer stay in ICU as compared to without ACLF, survival worse than patients without ACLF (89.8% and 81.0%, respectively, at 1 and 5 years)
	136 (non-ACLF)	70.5% at 5 years	
Yadav et al. (2017)	52	88.5% at 90 days	Non-LT ($n = 68$) had 32.4% survival at 6 months
O'Leary et al. (2019)	768	93% each at 6 months	

use of right lobe liver grafts including the middle hepatic vein that ensures adequate venous drainage and speedy recovery. The 5-year survival rate with LDLT is also over 90% in patients with high MELD score at admission [90].

43.6.7 Assessing Futility in Patients with ACLF

In patients with deteriorating clinical course over the first week, a goals of care discussion should be undertaken. This patient population has shown to have the highest mortality in the second week of ICU admission. The CLIF-C ACLF score, designed to predict short-term mortality over 28 days in ACLF patients, has a 100% specificity in predicting mortality when the score is ≥ 70 has, despite all supportive treatment. The cumulative rate of survival in the ICU with MELD >28.2 is estimated to be 28.2% and SOFA greater than 10.5 is 10.5% [91]. Cirrhotic patients are prone to infection with higher risk of mortality as compared to non-cirrhotic, and the presence of septic shock is estimated to predict mortality independently (OR 50.3, 95% CI 8.99–281) [92].

Additionally, multiorgan failure involving >3 organs requiring support (i.e. ionotropic support, mechanical ventilation, and continuous renal replacement therapy) is independently associated with increased mortality [93].

43.6.8 Need of Dynamic Prognostic Models

Patients with ACLF rapidly develop infections, organ failures leading to high mortality in the absence of liver transplant. Currently, there is no universal prognostic model for deciding the liver transplant in patients with ACLF. The model for end stage liver disease score (MELD) is validated for patients with decompensated cirrhosis and King's College Hospital Criteria (KCH) for acute liver failure [94]. In patients with severe alcoholic hepatitis, the Lille's score has shown the need of an emergency liver transplant [95, 96]. In patients with autoimmune hepatitis, failure to improve the MELD scores at day 7 has been shown to be associated with worse outcomes and need for liver transplant [97, 98]. The AARC score has been developed from the large AARC database which is a composite of five variables [99]. The score includes bilirubin, creatinine, international normalized ratio (INR), arterial lactate, and hepatic encephalopathy. The score incorporates measures of liver failure (i.e., bilirubin, INR and lactate) and organs of utility, i.e., kidneys and brain. Kidneys are one of the most frequent extrahepatic organ failure in patients with ACLF and also have prognostic implication. Similarly, akin to ALF, brain involvement is an ominous sign and necessitates need of emergency liver transplantation. The AARC score additionally is dynamic and performed superior to other prognostic scores in predicting the outcome of ACLF patients. The score could therefore determine the need of emergency liver transplant in these patients, however, has not been validated in this context. Apart from these, the CLIF-C ACLF score developed by the EASL-CLIF consortium can be used in prognostication in ACLF patients admitted to the intensive care unit. A score above

70 has been shown to have a 100% specificity in predicting mortality in patients who are critically ill [100, 101]. However, considering the differences in the definitions, the score needs to be evaluated in ACLF patients defined according to the APASL.

43.7 Conclusion

ACLF is a distinct entity characterized by the development of liver failure on a background of chronic liver disease usually precipitated by an acute insult. Systemic inflammation is a key event in the pathogenesis of the syndrome. The management of the syndrome is a composite of identification and treatment of the etiological insult, systemic inflammation, and potentiation of liver regeneration. Development of infection and extrahepatic organ failure is a key event with a prognostic implication. The role of liver support therapies needs to be explored both as a bridge to transplant and to spontaneous recovery. Dynamic prognostic models for deciding transplant, reversibility, and futile ICU care are an unmet need in patients with ACLF.

Highlights
- Acute on Chronic Liver Failure (ACLF) is characterized by high 28-day mortality.
- Liver failure drives extrahepatic organ failures in patients with ACLF.
- ACLF occurs in the context of gut dysbiosis and systemic inflammation.
- The syndrome is characterized by a dynamic course and the rapidity of progression to organ failures providing the first 2 weeks as the "golden-window" for therapeutic interventions.
- Liver transplant is the ultimate savior in patients with ACLF.
- The syndrome of ACLF is a clinical challenge and an area of unwavering research for clinicians.

Financial Disclosures None.

Conflicts of Interest None to declare.

References

1. Sarin SK, Chandan K, Zaigham A, et al. Acute-on-chronic liver failure: consensus recommendations of the Asian Pacific Association for the study of the liver (APASL). Hepatol Int. 2014;8:453–71.
2. Sarin SK, Kumar A, et al. Acute-on-chronic liver failure: consensus recommendations of the Asian Pacific association for the study of the liver (APASL). Hepatol Int. 2009;3(269):282.
3. Sarin SK, Choudhury A, Sharma MK, et al. Acute-on-chronic liver failure: consensus recommendations of the Asian Pacific association for the study of the liver (APASL): an update. Hepatol Int. 2019;13(4):353–90. [published correction appears in Hepatol Int. 2019 Nov;13(6):826-828].
4. Piano S, Tonon M, Vettore E, et al. Incidence, predictors and outcomes of acute-on-chronic liver failure in outpatients with cirrhosis. J Hepatol. 2017;67(6):1177–84.
5. Moreau R, Jalan R, Gines P, et al. Acute-on-chronic liver failure is a distinct syndrome that develops in patients with acute decompensation of cirrhosis. Gastroenterology. 2013;144:1426–37.
6. Jalan R, Yurdaydin C, Bajaj JS, et al. Toward an improved definition of acute-on-chronic liver failure. Gastroenterology. 2014;147(1):4–10.
7. Devarbhavi H, Choudhury AK, Sharma MK, et al. Drug-induced acute-on-chronic liver failure in Asian patients. Am J Gastroenterol. 2019;114(6):929–37.
8. Chen T, Yang Z, Choudhury AK, et al. Complications constitute a major risk factor for mortality in hepatitis B virus-related acute-on-chronic liver failure patients: a multi-national study from the Asia-Pacific region. Hepatol Int. 2019;13(6):695–705.
9. Gawande A, Gupta GK, Gupta A, et al. Acute-on-chronic liver failure: etiology of chronic and acute precipitating factors and their effect on mortality. J Clin Exp Hepatol. 2019;9(6):699–703.
10. Arroyo V, Moreau R, Kamath PS, et al. Acute-on-chronic liver failure in cirrhosis. Nat Rev Dis Primers. 2016;2:16041. Published 2016 Jun 9. https://doi.org/10.1038/nrdp.2016.41.
11. Arroyo V, Jalan R. Acute-on-chronic liver failure: definition, diagnosis, and clinical characteristics. Semin Liver Dis. 2016;36(2):109–16.
12. Bajaj JS, O'Leary JG, Reddy KR, et al. Survival in infection-related acute-on-chronic liver failure is defined by extrahepatic organ failures. Hepatology. 2014;60(1):250–6.
13. Clària J, Stauber RE, Coenraad MJ, et al. Systemic inflammation in decompensated cirrhosis: characterization and role in acute-on-chronic liver failure. Hepatology. 2016;64(4):1249–64.
14. Bernardi M, Moreau R, Angeli P, Schnabl B, Arroyo V. Mechanisms of decompensation and organ failure in cirrhosis: from peripheral arterial vasodilation to systemic inflammation hypothesis. J Hepatol. 2015;63(5):1272–84.
15. Arroyo V, Moreau R, Jalan R, Ginès P, EASL-CLIF Consortium CANONIC Study. Acute-on-chronic liver failure: a new syndrome that will re-classify cirrhosis. J Hepatol. 2015;62(1 Suppl):S131–43.
16. Shi S, Verstegen MMA, Mezzanotte L, de Jonge J, Löwik CWGM, van der Laan LJW. Necroptotic cell death in liver transplantation and underlying diseases: mechanisms and clinical perspective. Liver Transpl. 2019;25(7):1091–104.
17. Zindel J, Kubes P. DAMPs, PAMPs, and LAMPs in immunity and sterile inflammation. Annu Rev Pathol. 2020;15:493–518.
18. Posteraro B, Paroni Sterbini F, Petito V, et al. Liver injury, endotoxemia, and their relationship to intestinal microbiota composition in alcohol-preferring rats. Alcohol Clin Exp Res. 2018;42(12):2313–25.
19. Mutlu E, Keshavarzian A, Engen P, Forsyth CB, Sikaroodi M, Gillevet P. Intestinal dysbiosis: a possible mechanism of alcohol-induced endotoxemia and alcoholic steatohepatitis in rats. Alcohol Clin Exp Res. 2009;33(10):1836–46.
20. Claria J, Stauber RE, Coenraad MJ, et al. Systemic inflammation in decompensated cirrhosis: characterization and role in acute-on-chronic liver failure. Hepatology. 2016;64:1249–64.
21. Trebicka J, Amoros A, Pitarch C, Titos E, Alcaraz-Quiles J, Schierwagen R, et al. Addressing profiles of systemic inflammation across the different clinical phenotypes of acutely decompensated cirrhosis. Front Immunol. 2019;10:476.
22. Choudhury A, Kumar M, Sharma BC, et al. Systemic inflammatory response syndrome in acute-on-chronic liver failure: relevance of 'golden window': a prospective study. J Gastroenterol Hepatol. 2017;32(12):1989–97.
23. Gustot T. Multiple organ failure in sepsis: prognosis and role of systemic inflammatory response. Curr Opin Crit Care. 2011;17:153–9.
24. Albillos A, Lario M, Alvarez-Mon M. Cirrhosis-associated immune dysfunction: distinctive features and clinical relevance. J Hepatol. 2014;61:1385–96.
25. Bernsmeier C, Pop OT, Singanayagam A, et al. Patients with acute-on-chronic liver failure have increased numbers of regulatory immune cells expressing the receptor tyrosine kinase MERTK. Gastroenterology. 2015;148(3):603–615.e14.
26. Hensley MK, Deng JC. Acute on chronic liver failure and immune dysfunction: a mimic of sepsis. Semin Respir Crit Care Med. 2018;39(5):588–97.

27. Jenne CN, Kubes P. Immune surveillance by the liver. Nat Immunol. 2013;14:996–1006.

28. Schnabl B, Brenner DA. Interactions between the intestinal microbiome and liver diseases. Gastroenterology. 2014;146:1513–24.

29. Wang L, Fouts DE, Starkel P, et al. Intestinal REG3 lectins protect against alcoholic steatohepatitis by reducing mucosa-associated microbiota and preventing bacterial translocation. Cell Host Microbe. 2016;19:227–39.

30. Qin N, Yang F, Li A, et al. Alterations of the human gut microbiome in liver cirrhosis. Nature. 2014;513:59–64.

31. Chen Y, Guo J, Qian G, et al. Gut dysbiosis in acuteon-chronic liver failure and its predictive value for mortality. J Gastroenterol Hepatol. 2015;30:1429–37.

32. Giannelli V, Di Gregorio V, Iebba V, et al. Microbiota and the gut-liver axis: bacterial translocation, inflammation and infection in cirrhosis. World J Gastroenterol. 2014;20:16795–810.

33. Fernández J, Acevedo J, Wiest R, et al. Bacterial and fungal infections in acute-on-chronic liver failure: prevalence, characteristics and impact on prognosis. Gut. 2018;67(10):1870–80.

34. Verma N, Singh S, Taneja S, et al. Invasive fungal infections amongst patients with acute-on-chronic liver failure at high risk for fungal infections. Liver Int. 2019;39(3):503–13.

35. Bechstein WO, Zeuzem S. Acute-on-chronic liver failure. Visc Med. 2018;34(4):243–4.

36. Moreau N, Wittebole X, Fleury Y, Forget P, Laterre PF, Castanares-Zapatero D. Neutrophil-to-lymphocyte ratio predicts death in acute-on-chronic liver failure patients admitted to the intensive care unit: a retrospective cohort study. Shock. 2018;49(4):385–92.

37. Kerbert AJC, Verspaget HW, Navarro ÀA, et al. Copeptin in acute decompensation of liver cirrhosis: relationship with acute-on-chronic liver failure and short-term survival. Crit Care. 2017;21(1):321.

38. Macdonald S, Andreola F, Bachtiger P, et al. Cell death markers in patients with cirrhosis and acute decompensation. Hepatology. 2018;67(3):989–1002.

39. Piano S, Singh V, Caraceni P, et al. Epidemiology and effects of bacterial infections in patients with cirrhosis worldwide. Gastroenterology. 2019;156(5):1368–1380.e10.

40. Moreau R. The pathogenesis of ACLF: the inflammatory response and immune function. Semin Liver Dis. 2016;36(2):133–40.

41. Stravitz RT. Algorithms for managing coagulation disorders in liver disease. Hepatol Int. 2018;12(5):390–401.

42. Goyal S, Jadaun S, Kedia S, et al. Thromboelastography parameters in patients with acute on chronic liver failure. Ann Hepatol. 2018;17(6):1042–51.

43. Blasi A, Calvo A, Prado V, et al. Coagulation failure in patients with acute-on-chronic liver failure and decompensated cirrhosis: beyond the international normalized ratio. Hepatology. 2018;68(6):2325–37.

44. Premkumar M, Saxena P, Rangegowda D, et al. Coagulation failure is associated with bleeding events and clinical outcome during systemic inflammatory response and sepsis in acute-on-chronic liver failure: an observational cohort study. Liver Int. 2019;39(4):694–704.

45. Maiwall R, Sarin SK, Moreau R. Acute kidney injury in acute on chronic liver failure. Hepatol Int. 2016;10(2):245–57.

46. Maiwall R, Kumar S, Chandel SS, et al. AKI in patients with acute on chronic liver failure is different from acute decompensation of cirrhosis. Hepatol Int. 2015;9(4):627–39.

47. Maiwall R, Pasupuleti SSR, Bihari C, et al. Incidence, risk factors, and outcomes of transition of acute kidney injury to chronic kidney disease in cirrhosis: a prospective cohort study. Hepatology. 2020;71(3):1009–22.

48. Maiwall R, Sarin SK, Kumar S, et al. Development of predisposition, injury, response, organ failure model for predicting acute kidney injury in acute on chronic liver failure. Liver Int. 2017;37(10):1497–507.

49. Amathieu R, Al-Khafaji A, Sileanu FE, et al. Significance of oliguria in critically ill patients with chronic liver disease. Hepatology. 2017;66(5):1592–600.

50. Angeli P, Garcia-Tsao G, Nadim MK, Parikh CR. News in pathophysiology, definition and classification of hepatorenal syndrome: a step beyond the International Club of Ascites (ICA) consensus document. J Hepatol. 2019;71(4):811–22.

51. Maiwall R, Kumar A, Bhardwaj A, Kumar G, Bhadoria AS, Sarin SK. Cystatin C predicts acute kidney injury and mortality in cirrhotics: a prospective cohort study. Liver Int. 2018;38(4):654–64.

52. Wan ZH, Wang JJ, You SL, et al. Cystatin C is a biomarker for predicting acute kidney injury in patients with acute-on-chronic liver failure. World J Gastroenterol. 2013;19(48):9432–8.

53. Ariza X, Solà E, Elia C, et al. Analysis of a urinary biomarker panel for clinical outcomes assessment in cirrhosis. PLoS One. 2015;10(6):e0128145.

54. Ariza X, Graupera I, Coll M, et al. Neutrophil gelatinase-associated lipocalin is a biomarker of acute-on-chronic liver failure and prognosis in cirrhosis. J Hepatol. 2016;65(1):57–65.

55. Fagundes C, Pépin MN, Guevara M, et al. Urinary neutrophil gelatinase-associated lipocalin as biomarker in the differential diagnosis of impairment of kidney function in cirrhosis. J Hepatol. 2012;57(2):267–73.

56. Jiang QQ, Han MF, Ma K, et al. Acute kidney injury in acute-on-chronic liver failure is different from in decompensated cirrhosis. World J Gastroenterol. 2018;24(21):2300–10.

57. Joshi D, O'Grady J, Patel A, et al. Cerebral oedema is rare in acute-on-chronic liver failure patients presenting with high-grade hepatic encephalopathy. Liver Int. 2014;34(3):362–6.

58. Sawhney R, Holland-Fischer P, Rosselli M, Mookerjee RP, Agarwal B, Jalan R. Role of ammonia, inflammation, and cerebral oxygenation in brain dysfunction of acute-on-chronic liver failure patients. Liver Transpl. 2016;22(6):732–42.

59. Romero-Gómez M, Montagnese S, Jalan R. Hepatic encephalopathy in patients with acute decompensation of cirrhosis and acute-on-chronic liver failure. J Hepatol. 2015;62(2):437–47.

60. Michard B, Artzner T, Lebas B, et al. Liver transplantation in critically ill patients: preoperative predictive factors of post-transplant mortality to avoid futility. Clin Transpl. 2017;31(12):10.

61. Fernández J, Clària J, Amorós A, et al. Effects of albumin treatment on systemic and portal hemodynamics and systemic inflammation in patients with decompensated cirrhosis. Gastroenterology. 2019;157(1):149–62.

62. Arroyo V, García-Martinez R, Salvatella X. Human serum albumin, systemic inflammation, and cirrhosis. J Hepatol. 2014;61(2):396–407.

63. Artigas A, Wernerman J, Arroyo V, Vincent JL, Levy M. Role of albumin in diseases associated with severe systemic inflammation: pathophysiologic and clinical evidence in sepsis and in decompensated cirrhosis. J Crit Care. 2016;33:62–70.

64. Caraceni P, Riggio O, Angeli P, et al. Long-term albumin administration in decompensated cirrhosis (ANSWER): an open-label randomised trial. Lancet. 2018;391(10138):2417–29. [published correction appears in Lancet. 2018 Aug 4;392(10145):386].

65. Arora V, Vijayaraghavan R, Maiwall R, et al. Paracentesis-induced circulatory dysfunction with modest-volume paracentesis is partly ameliorated by albumin infusion in acute-on-chronic liver failure. Hepatology. 2019;72(3):1043–55. [published online ahead of print, 2019 Dec 17]. https://doi.org/10.1002/hep.31071.

66. Jindal A, Bhadoria AS, Maiwall R, Sarin SK. Evaluation of acute kidney injury and its response to terlipressin in patients with acute-on-chronic liver failure. Liver Int. 2016;36(1):59–67.

67. Arora V, Maiwall R, Rajan V, et al. Terlipressin is superior to noradrenaline in the management of acute kidney Injury in acute on chronic liver failure. Hepatology. 2020;71(2):600–10.

68. Larsen FS. Artificial liver support in acute and acute-on-chronic liver failure. Curr Opin Crit Care. 2019;25(2):187–91.

69. Maiwall R, Maras JS, Nayak SL, Sarin SK. Liver dialysis in acute-on-chronic liver failure: current and future perspectives. Hepatol Int. 2014;8(Suppl 2):505–13.

70. Bañares R, Nevens F, Larsen FS, et al. Extracorporeal albumin dialysis with the molecular adsorbent recirculating system in acute-on-chronic liver failure: the RELIEF trial. Hepatology. 2013;57(3):1153–62.

71. Kribben A, Gerken G, Haag S, et al. Effects of fractionated plasma separation and adsorption on survival in patients with acute-on-chronic liver failure. Gastroenterology. 2012;142(4):782–789.e3.

72. Tan EX, Wang MX, Pang J, Lee GH. Plasma exchange in patients with acute and acute-on-chronic liver failure: a systematic review. World J Gastroenterol. 2020;26(2):219–45.

73. Ma Y, Chen F, Xu Y, et al. Safety and efficacy of regional citrate anticoagulation during plasma adsorption plus plasma exchange therapy for patients with acute-on-chronic liver failure: a pilot study. Blood Purif. 2019;48(3):223–32.

74. Stahl K, Busch M, Fuge J, et al. Therapeutic plasma exchange in acute on chronic liver failure. J Clin Apher. 2020;35(4):316–27.

75. Maiwall R, Moreau R. Plasma exchange for acute on chronic liver failure: is there a light at the end of the tunnel? Hepatol Int. 2016;10(3):387–9.

76. Larsen FS, Schmidt LE, Bernsmeier C, et al. High-volume plasma exchange in patients with acute liver failure: an open randomised controlled trial. J Hepatol. 2016;64(1):69–78.

77. Garg V, Garg H, Khan A, et al. Granulocyte colony-stimulating factor mobilizes CD34(+) cells and improves survival of patients with acute-on-chronic liver failure. Gastroenterology. 2012;142(3):505–512.e1.

78. Duan XZ, Liu FF, Tong JJ, et al. Granulocyte-colony stimulating factor therapy improves survival in patients with hepatitis B virus-associated acute-on-chronic liver failure. World J Gastroenterol. 2013;19(7):1104–10.

79. Singh V, Sharma AK, Narasimhan RL, Bhalla A, Sharma N, Sharma R. Granulocyte colony-stimulating factor in severe alcoholic hepatitis: a randomized pilot study. Am J Gastroenterol. 2014;109(9):1417–23.

80. Singh V, Keisham A, Bhalla A, et al. Efficacy of granulocyte colony-stimulating factor and N-acetylcysteine therapies in patients with severe alcoholic hepatitis. Clin Gastroenterol Hepatol. 2018;16(10):1650–1656.e2.

81. Shasthry SM, Sharma MK, Shasthry V, Pande A, Sarin SK. Efficacy of granulocyte colony-stimulating factor in the management of steroid-nonresponsive severe alcoholic hepatitis: a double-blind randomized controlled trial. Hepatology. 2019;70(3):802–11.

82. Cristani M, Speciale A, Saija A, Gangemi S, Minciullo PL, Cimino F. Circulating advanced oxidation protein products as oxidative stress biomarkers and progression mediators in pathological conditions related to inflammation and immune dysregulation. Curr Med Chem. 2016;23(34):3862–82. https://doi.org/10.2174/0929867323666160902154748.

83. Nabi T, Nabi S, Rafiq N, Shah A. Role of N-acetylcysteine treatment in non-acetaminophen-induced acute liver failure: a prospective study. Saudi J Gastroenterol. 2017;23(3):169–75. PMID: 28611340; PMCID: PMC5470376. https://doi.org/10.4103/1319-3767.207711.

84. Mumtaz K, Azam Z, Hamid S, Abid S, Memon S, Ali Shah H, Jafri W. Role of N-acetylcysteine in adults with non-acetaminophen-induced acute liver failure in a center without the facility of liver transplantation. Hepatol Int. 2009;3(4):563–70. Epub 2009 Aug 29. PMID: 19727985; PMCID: PMC2790590. https://doi.org/10.1007/s12072-009-9151-0.

85. Baniasadi S, Eftekhari P, Tabarsi P, Fahimi F, Raoufy MR, Masjedi MR, Velayati AA. Protective effect of N-acetylcysteine on antituberculosis drug-induced hepatotoxicity. Eur J Gastroenterol Hepatol. 2010;22(10):1235–8. PMID: 20461008. https://doi.org/10.1097/MEG.0b013e32833aa11b.

86. Hu J, Zhang Q, Ren X, Sun Z, Quan Q. Efficacy and safety of acetylcysteine in "non-acetaminophen" acute liver failure: a meta-analysis of prospective clinical trials. Clin Res Hepatol Gastroenterol. 2015;39(5):594–9. Epub 2015 Feb 26. https://doi.org/10.1016/j.clinre.2015.01.003.

87. Weiler N, Schlotmann A, Schnitzbauer AA, Zeuzem S, Welker MW. The epidemiology of acute liver failure. Dtsch Arztebl Int. 2020;117(4):43–50. PMID: 32036852; PMCID: PMC7036472. https://doi.org/10.3238/arztebl.2020.0043.

88. Artzner T, Michard B, Besch C, Levesque E, Faitot F. Liver transplantation for critically ill cirrhotic patients: overview and pragmatic proposals. World J Gastroenterol. 2018;24(46):5203–14. PMID: 30581269; PMCID: PMC6295835. https://doi.org/10.3748/wjg.v24.i46.5203.

89. Dong V, Karvellas CJ. Acute-on-chronic liver failure: objective admission and support criteria in the intensive care unit. JHEP Rep. 2019;1(1):44–52. PMID: 32039351; PMCID: PMC7001553. https://doi.org/10.1016/j.jhepr.2019.02.005.

90. Bhatti ABH, Dar FS, Butt MO, Sahaab E, Salih M, Shah NH, Khan NY, Zia HH, Khan EU, Khan NA. Living donor liver transplantation for acute on chronic liver failure based on EASL-CLIF diagnostic criteria. J Clin Exp Hepatol. 2018;8(2):136–43. Epub 2017 Nov 24. PMID: 29892176; PMCID: PMC5992305. https://doi.org/10.1016/j.jceh.2017.11.007.

91. Pan HC, Jenq CC, Lee WC, Tsai MH, Fan PC, Chang CH, Chang MY, Tian YC, Hung CC, Fang JT, Yang CW, Chen YC. Scoring systems for predicting mortality after liver transplantation. PLoS One. 2014;9(9):e107138. PMID: 25216239; PMCID: PMC4162558. https://doi.org/10.1371/journal.pone.0107138.

92. Wong F, Bernardi M, Balk R, Christman B, Moreau R, Garcia-Tsao G, Patch D, Soriano G, Hoefs J, Navasa M, International Ascites Club. Sepsis in cirrhosis: report on the 7th meeting of the international ascites Club. Gut. 2005;54(5):718–25. PMID: 15831923; PMCID: PMC1774473. https://doi.org/10.1136/gut.2004.038679.

93. Arroyo V. Acute-on-chronic liver failure in cirrhosis requires expedited decisions for liver transplantation. Gastroenterology. 2019;156(5):1248–9. Epub 2019 Mar 5. https://doi.org/10.1053/j.gastro.2019.03.004.

94. O'Grady JG. Acute liver failure. Postgrad Med J. 2005;81(953):148–54. PMID: 15749789; PMCID: PMC1743234. https://doi.org/10.1136/pgmj.2004.026005.

95. Mathurin P, O'Grady J, Carithers RL, Phillips M, Louvet A, Mendenhall CL, Ramond MJ, Naveau S, Maddrey WC, Morgan TR. Corticosteroids improve short-term survival in patients with severe alcoholic hepatitis: meta-analysis of individual patient data. Gut. 2011;60(2):255–60. Epub 2010 Oct 12. https://doi.org/10.1136/gut.2010.224097.

96. Mathurin P, Moreno C, Samuel D, Pruvot FR, Valle'e JC. Early liver transplantation for severe alcoholic hepatitis. N Engl J Med. 2011;365:1790–800.

97. Anand L, Choudhury A, Bihari C, et al. Flare of autoimmune hepatitis causing acute on chronic liver failure: diagnosis and response to corticosteroid therapy. Hepatology. 2019;70(2):587–96.

98. Yeoman AD, Westbrook RH, Portmann C, O'Grady OJ, Harrison PM, Heneghan MA. Early predictors of corticosteroid treatment failure in icteric presentations of autoimmune hepatitis. Hepatology. 2011;53:926–34.

99. Choudhury A, Jindal A, Maiwall R, et al. Liver failure determines the outcome in patients of acute-on-chronic liver failure (ACLF): comparison of APASL ACLF research consortium (AARC) and CLIF-SOFA models. Hepatol Int. 2017;11(5):461–71.

100. Engelmann C, Thomsen KL, Zakeri N, et al. Validation of CLIF-C ACLF score to define a threshold for futility of intensive care support for patients with acute-on-chronic liver failure. Crit Care. 2018;22(1):254.

101. Jalan R, Saliba F, Pavesi M, et al. Development and validation of a prognostic score to predict mortality in patients with acute-on-chronic liver failure. J Hepatol. 2014;61(5):1038–47.

Combined Liver and Kidney Transplant

44

Sonja Payne, Nelson Gonzalez, and Achal Dhir

44.1 Introduction

Single organ liver and kidney transplants are well established as standards of care for selected patients with severe liver and kidney disease, respectively [1]. Severe dysfunction in multiple organ systems, either due to a single pathological process or as a consequence of single system disease, creates a challenge for transplant medicine. Studies have demonstrated relatively poorer outcomes in patients with multiple organ dysfunction undergoing single organ transplant [2, 3]. This has led to an expansion of combined solid organ transplantation over recent years [4]. Renal insufficiency is very common among ESLD patients awaiting liver transplantation (LT) and affects clinical outcomes both before, and following LT [3]. Since renal function plays significant role in the outcome of patients awaiting LT, the model for end-stage liver disease (MELD) has almost universally replaced other wait list criteria which failed to incorporate a measure of renal function [5].

With implementation of the MELD allocation system, the proportion of combined liver–kidney transplantation (CLKT) has increased significantly. CLKT has become the procedure of choice for patients with severe primary disease of both organs [6]. Simultaneous replacement of two failing organs offers the advantage of single surgery, lower immunosuppression dose, and improved survival compared to single organ transplantation with significant disease remaining in the non-transplanted organ. However, the decision for CLKT can be difficult in the setting of the subtle differences in the natural history of kidney dysfunction associated with ESLD including hepatorenal syndrome (HRS), acute renal failure (ARF), and chronic kidney disease (CKD). The decision of single vs. combined transplant relies on multidisciplinary evaluation to discriminate patients with reversible and irreversible kidney failure.

Perioperative care of CLKT is challenging and requires thorough understanding of the disease specific physiology and implications as well as knowledge of the surgical procedure. Standardization of protocols for individual transplant centers may improve patient care and safety, ultimately leading to better outcomes.

44.1.1 Renal Function, Liver Disease, and Liver Transplantation

The kidney is a sensitive organ which may be negatively impacted by changes in renal hemodynamic derangements due to systemic disease as

S. Payne · N. Gonzalez · A. Dhir (✉)
Department of Anesthesia and Peri-Operative Medicine, London Health Sciences Centre, Western University, London, ON, Canada
e-mail: sonja.payne@lhsc.on.ca;
nelson.gonzalez@lhsc.on.ca; achal.dhir@lhsc.on.ca

well as direct damage due to local effects such as infection. Portal hypertension reduces effective circulating blood volume, increasing the risk of renal dysfunction and acute kidney injury (AKI) in patients with ESLD, especially in the setting of pre-existing renal disease. End-stage renal disease (ESRD) can cause hyperkalemia, platelet dysfunction, pulmonary edema, pericardial effusion, and coronary artery disease [1]. This physiological burden is compounded in combined kidney and liver disease leading to potentially significant metabolic acidosis, chronic anemia, and reduced drug metabolism with important perioperative implications [7, 8].

The perioperative period for LT exposes the patient to an acute kidney injury due to significant fluctuations in systemic and renal hemodynamics. The glomerular filtration rate (GFR) often decreases by about 10 mL/min immediately following LT with potential for further deterioration if the postoperative course is complicated [9, 10]. Unsuccessful recovery of kidney function after LT negatively impacts graft survival, patient survival, and quality of life [3, 11]. Prediction of renal recovery following liver transplantation in patients with preoperative renal dysfunction is challenging. Pre-existing comorbidities, presence of intrinsic renal disease, perioperative hemodynamic perturbations, and post-transplant immunosuppression are probably the most influential factors.

Pre-LT renal function has been found to be an independent predictor of post-LT patient and graft survival. Preoperative renal failure is associated with high perioperative morbidity and mortality during LT. There is higher incidence of primary nonfunction and 30-day mortality as well as lower long-term patient and graft survival in patients with pre-LT renal failure [3]. Studies have identified early liver allograft dysfunction, early development of stage 3 AKI following LT, and requirement for RRT at the time of liver transplantation as independent risk factors for the development of ESRD within first year of LT [11].

44.1.2 Why Is CKLT Important?

Patients with ESLD on dialysis undergoing liver transplantation have significantly better survival when CLKT is performed, compared to LT alone [12]. Five-year patient survival rates among patients selected to receive CLKT range from 64% to 76% [13]. Prior to introduction of the MELD score for allocation of LT in the USA, CLKT accounted for 1.7% and 2.5% in 1990 and 2001, respectively. It rose significantly to 8.2% in 2014 and 10% by 2017 after adoption of the MELD allocation system [14]. A 178% increase in the number of CLKT performed during the 9-year period post-MELD ($n = 2914$), when compared with the preceding 9-year period in the pre-MELD era ($n = 1049$) has also been reported [15]. At the authors' institute, the current rate of CLKT is also around 10% of all LTs. Data on renal outcomes after CLKT in the highest MELD recipients are scarce, as are accurate predictors of recovery of native kidney function. Well-designed clinical trials evaluating transplant futility in CLKT recipients are currently lacking. Controversy remains that MELD scoring system inappropriately prioritizes LT candidates with renal dysfunction [16].

44.1.3 Who Benefits from CKLT?

The decision to list a patient for CLKT carries important clinical implications. Ethical debates exist that discuss the inequity of organ distribution with transplantation of multiple organs in a single recipient [4]. Apart from having greater operative complexity, CLKT utilizes a precious resource from an already depleted kidney donor pool. CLKT is a clear treatment decision for patients with metabolic disease due to primary genetic defects of the liver, such as primary hyperoxaluria, or for patients with noncirrhotic diseases involving both liver and kidneys, such as polycystic organ disease where disease progression is certain. However, in many other clinical scenarios, decision-making is more complex for several reasons. Controversy is founded in the difficulty of predicting reversibility of renal function post-LT. CKD often deteriorates during and following LT due to the reasons described above. On the other hand, patients with hepatorenal syndrome (HRS) may have full renal recovery post-LT, even after in excess of 8 weeks of pre-transplant renal replacement therapy (RRT) [17, 18]. Though CLKT for patients with HRS is generally not recommended, improved outcome was observed with sequential kidney transplant if patients were RRT-dependent for over 8 weeks post-LT [19]. There is also uncertainty regarding the generalized survival benefit of combined kidney transplant in LT recipients. A large retrospective review of transplantation outcomes in the US demonstrated shorter kidney graft and patient survival in CLKT recipients compared to LT alone [20]. However, the same study found better patient and liver graft survival in CLKT recipients on long-term RRT prior to transplantation.

The mortality for LT candidates waiting for a kidney transplant is substantially higher than candidates on kidney alone wait list [21]. This may be explained by longer waiting times for two acceptable organs simultaneously, successful management of AKI or CKD with RRT, or the combined burden of disease.

In the universal setting of a finite donor pool, appropriate patient selection is critical to ensure best patient outcomes following CLKT. Heterogeneity in the criteria for CLKT allocation has resulted in significant variation across centers and regions. Currently in the USA, listing policy for CLKT is based on prior consensus recommendation, including factors such as duration of AKI, need for RRT, and evidence of CKD (Table 44.1) [22, 23]. However, other variables that may impact recovery of renal function after LT, such as age, comorbidities, etiology of AKI, and the fluctuation of renal function pre-LT, are not included in the CLKT selection criteria [24].

Common indications for CLKT are summarized in Table 44.2.

Table 44.1 CLKT summit consensus guidelines

Persistent AKI ≥ 4 weeks with one of the following	CKD for 3 months with one of the following
Stage 3 AKI as defined by modified RIFLE criteria: • Threefold increase in serum creatinine from baseline or • SCr ≥4 mg/dL with an acute increase of ≥0.5 mg/dL or • On renal replacement therapy eGFR ≤35 mL/min (MDRD-6) or GFR ≤25 mL/min (iothalamate clearance)	eGFR ≤40 mL/min (MDRD-6) or GFR ≤ 30 mL/min (iothalamate clearance) Proteinuria ≥2 g/day Kidney biopsy: >30% global glomerulosclerosis or > 30% interstitial fibrosis Metabolic disease

AKI acute kidney injury, *CKD* chronic kidney disease, *eGFR* estimated glomerular filtration rate, *RIFLE* risk, injury, failure, loss, end-stage renal disease, *SCr* serum creatinine

Table 44.2 Indications for CLKT

LT candidates with kidney disease	Kidney transplant candidates with liver disease
• ESLD with CKD • ESLD with AKI	• ESRD patients and liver cirrhosis • ESRD because of hyperoxaluria • polycystic kidney and liver disease with ESRD

ESLD end-stage liver disease, *CKD* chronic kidney disease, *AKI* acute kidney injury, *ESRD* end-stage renal disease

Transplant programs often follow locally adapted decision-making processes ensuring optimization of pre-transplant renal function while considering the appropriateness of CLKT.

Recent evidence demonstrates consistency in CLKT allocation criteria for patients with ESRD and cirrhosis and patients with cirrhosis and CKD [25]. However, allocation criteria in the setting of cirrhosis with AKI are quite variable, highlighting the clinical challenge in the diagnosis and predict reversibility of AKI in the setting of ESLD. Despite institutional guidelines, the final decision is best determined by a multidisciplinary discussion of individual patients. Ethical, social, and cultural context should also be considered in order to optimize the allocation process.

In line with many transplant centers in North America, the criteria for CLKT at the authors' institution have evolved over time. Criteria have been refined in the context of best evidence, growing clinical experience, and the contribution of Kidney Special Considerations Committee. In August 2017, the United Network for Organ Sharing (UNOS) /Organ Procurement and Organ Transplantation (OPTN) implemented a new CLKT allocation policy based on estimated GFR (eGFR) [26]. The primary reason for this change was driven by the fact that female patients were disadvantaged with the old MELD or NaMELD allocation system [27].

At the authors' institute, the current criteria to support CLKT include the following.

- Patients with ESLD and CKD who have been on dialysis for a period that is comparable to current wait times for kidney transplant alone.
- Patients with ESLD and CKD who are highly sensitized and would benefit from organs from the same donor. (Sequential transplant allows cross-match positive kidney transplants to proceed AFTER the liver transplant.)
- Patients with liver disease and CKD secondary to primary hyperoxalosis. One run of plasmapheresis should be performed prior to transplant.
- Patients with HRS who have required a minimum of 6 weeks RRT.
- Patients with metabolic disorders who have:
  - ESLD with eGFR less than 30.
  - ESLD and eGFR 30–40 may be considered for CLKT if the patient has either small sized kidneys or proteinuria (after discussion with Kidney Special Considerations Committee); kidney after liver transplant could be considered in these cases if there is a suitable living donor and kidney transplant can occur 1–3 months following LT.
- Patients with polycystic liver disease are assessed on a case by case basis considering the renal function to support the postoperative LT.

44.2 Anesthetic Considerations

Robust scientific evidence for combined liver-kidney transplant is limited by small case numbers. Practice guidelines often rely on extrapolation of best evidence from single organ transplant, results of cohort studies, and expert consensus.

44.2.1 Preoperative

Thorough preoperative assessment of potential transplant recipients is fundamental to achieving optimal patient outcomes. The overarching goals of preoperative evaluation are to facilitate appropriate patient selection for listing and to minimize post-transplant morbidity and mortality. A multidisciplinary approach facilitates identification, assessment, and potential optimization of multi-system involvement of end-organ failure, as well as relevant comorbidities. Particular emphasis is given to cardiorespiratory evaluation. Due to the unpredictable timing of transplant surgery, the optimal frequency to update pertinent investigations after listing to assess for interval change is not clear.

Cardiovascular disease is a leading cause of morbidity and mortality after single organ liver and kidney transplantation [28, 29]. The combined burden of dual-organ failure and significant physiological stress of transplant underpins the need for meticulous cardiovascular preoperative assessment. The American Heart Association issued a scientific statement of "Cardiac Disease Evaluation and Management Among Kidney and Liver Transplantation Candidates" [30]. Although this document provides guidance for single organ transplant surgery, the thorough review of best evidence remains useful in the context of combined solid organ transplantation. Relevant recommendations include the following.

- All stable patients on the waiting list should have resting ECG and echocardiogram repeated annually.
- Non-invasive cardiac stress testing (i.e., Dobutamine stress echocardiography) may be

considered even in the absence of active cardiac disease. The presence of multiple CAD risk factors represents an indication for non-invasive testing, regardless of functional status.

- A designated cardiology consultant may assist consideration of invasive cardiac evaluation, taking into account the risk of contrast-induced acute kidney injury.
- Patients deemed high risk for cardiovascular complications should be referred to a cardiologist for further evaluation and management.

In addition to preoperative assessment of features of end-stage liver disease, an evaluation of the impact of renal disease is essential. Local listing criteria may not necessitate the commencement of RRT. As such, a spectrum of functional volume and electrolyte status may exist. Abnormalities of sodium and potassium concentrations should be identified and optimized if time permits. In patients already initiated on RRT, an assessment of need for preoperative dialysis must be ascertained. Arteriovenous fistula and hemodialysis catheters may be present and must be protected in case of post-transplant renal graft failure. Intravenous access may be challenging in this patient population due to previous cannulation for dialysis resulting in vascular thrombosis/stenosis. Preoperative vascular mapping may be considered.

44.2.2 Intraoperative

There is sparsity of data in the literature concerning anesthetic and fluid management in CLKT. Hemodynamic goals vary during different stages of a combined liver-kidney transplant. Patients who have undergone hemodialysis with fluid removal prior to surgery may demonstrate increased cardiovascular instability during induction of general anesthesia and drainage of ascites. Substantial bleeding may occur during hepatic dissection in view of the fragile coagulation balance of end-stage liver disease, compounded by platelet dysfunction and anemia associated with chronic renal disease. In preparation for caval clamping prior to the anhepatic phase, judicious volume loading with potassium-deplete fluids can be guided by hemodynamic monitoring. Where possible, a piggyback caval clamping technique will assist in the preservation of preload. Avoidance of fluid overload during the neohepatic phase will minimize the risk of liver allograft congestion. Completion of vascular and bile duct anastomoses will provide time for stabilization of coagulation and volume status prior to commencement of renal transplantation.

Graft function is dependent on adequate oxygen delivery. Therefore, careful assessment of transfusion requirement, volume status, and maintenance of adequate perfusion pressure is essential at this stage [31]. Overzealous infusion for volume expansion may precipitate liver graft congestion, adversely affecting function. Although robust evidence is lacking to support the administration of mannitol to minimize ischemic-reperfusion and acute kidney injury in renal transplantation [32], mannitol is still widely used prior to renal reperfusion. However, the adverse effects of significant diuresis and potential hypovolemia due to diuretic administration must be considered in the setting of combined liver-kidney transplantation.

Due to significant hemodynamic changes observed during combined liver-kidney transplantation, invasive blood pressure monitoring is a standard of care. There is lack of clarity regarding the need for peripheral arterial monitoring (radial), central monitoring (femoral) or both. Some studies have demonstrated lack of correlation between invasive peripheral and central arterial pressure measurements, likely due to differences in vascular tone between measurement sites [33]. If invasive femoral artery pressure monitoring is to be considered, a discussion with the surgical team regarding the site of renal vascular anastomosis is required to avoid placement of an indwelling catheter in the operative field.

Pulmonary artery catheters (PAC) have long been a mainstay of hemodynamic monitoring during liver transplantation. The PAC allows direct measurement of pulmonary pressures, an estimate of left-heart filling volume and a means of intermittent measurement of cardiac output through thermodilution. The PAC may be used postoperatively for cardiac output monitoring in the intensive care unit. Limitations to use include the dependence on surrogate measurements for cardiac monitoring and the well-known risks of PAC placement and use. However, the use of PACs has decreased significantly worldwide.

Transesophageal echocardiography (TEE) is increasingly recognized as a useful method of real-time monitoring of cardiac function and volume status during non-cardiac surgery. Its use is supported by the American Society of Anesthesiology (ASA) when the nature of the surgery or the patient's underlying cardiovascular pathology may result in severe hemodynamic compromise. The greatest advantage of intraoperative TEE in liver transplantation is the continuous, direct assessment of the right and left sides of the heart in the setting of sudden changes in preload [33, 34]. There is growing consensus within the literature advocating for routine use of TEE during liver transplant surgery [35]. Given the complexities of hemodynamic goals during CLKT and the potential for hemodynamic instability, it seems sensible to extrapolate this standard of care to dual-organ transplant surgery. The use of TEE is likely to provide a more accurate assessment of intravascular volume status than the traditional CVP measurement [36]. There is a collective consensus in the current literature that TEE may be performed safely in patients with documented low-grade esophageal varices (Grade 1 and 2) without a recent acute upper gastrointestinal bleed [35].

Electrolyte abnormalities are common during combined liver-kidney transplantation. Pre-existing hyponatremia must be carefully considered as rapid correction may lead to central pontine myelinolysis. Commonly used therapies during liver transplantation, such as sodium bicarbonate and fresh frozen plasma, contain high concentrations of sodium. An alternative buffering agent THAM, devoid of sodium, has been discontinued by the manufacturer leaving little other options for management of severe aci-

dosis. Clotting factor concentrates contain significantly less sodium. Hyperkalemia occurs commonly during liver transplantation in patients with normal renal function. Intraoperative management is compounded by ESRD. "Washing" packed red cells prior to transfusion dramatically reduces potassium load [37]. The availability of intraoperative renal replacement therapy (IORRT) offers the advantage of relative electrolyte stability [38].

44.2.2.1 Renal Replacement Therapy

Intraoperative renal replacement therapy during LT has shown to be a feasible, safe, and effective approach to manage fluid shifts and electrolyte imbalance during surgery [38–40]. Although benefits of IORRT have been described in observational studies, namely prevention of significant electrolyte abnormalities and intravascular fluid removal, the evidence is not sufficiently robust to offer firm recommendations regarding its use. Institutional guidelines may aid decision-making and the successful implementation of this therapy. At the authors' institute, a multidisciplinary agreed trigger criterion has been developed to identify patients who may potentially benefit from IORRT (Table 44.3). Local logistics unique to each center, such as the availability of appropriately trained staff to operate the RRT machine, also play a significant role in this decision-making.

Any single major criteria or two and more minor criteria are generally sufficient to trigger a discussion on activation of CRRT in the operating room.

Table 44.3 Triggers for IORRT discussion

Major trigger (Recipient)	Minor trigger
• Acute liver failure • MELD >30 • CRRT/IHD pre-liver transplant • Two vasopressors • Redo-liver transplant	• DCD donor • Prolonged cold ischemic time • Severe metabolic derangement (Na+, K+) in recipientSS

44.2.3 Postoperative

CLKT patients tend to have higher incidence of bacterial infections and blood transfusion requirements with longer ICU and hospital stay compared to LT only patients. Though the incidence of renal dysfunction 6 months post-LT was similar, CLKT patients had quantitively worse renal function [41].

44.3 Conclusions

Combined liver and kidney transplantation can be a life-saving procedure for selected patients with combined liver and kidney failure. However, criteria for and timing to listing presents the liver and kidney transplant teams with challenges, as acute kidney injury may potentially be reversible. As well there is an issue of scarcity of organs and prioritization of allocation to combined organ failure patients over kidney failure patients on dialysis. As in all multi-organ failure, the additional presence of renal failure or the failure of recovery of renal function post-liver transplant is associated with increased mortality. The concerns raised in deciding the need for CLKT mainly rely on the benefit to the recipient in CLKT versus liver alone transplant and the fact that kidneys can potentially be diverted away from kidney alone patients on the waitlist who may derive greater benefit. In selected patients, CLKT is an appropriate use of a scarce resource, but better prognostic indicators for selection of patients are still needed. Further well-designed prospective studies as well as a reliable model to guide the decision-making in CLKT might help.

References

1. Stites E, Wiseman AC. Multiorgan transplantation. Transplant Rev (Orlando). 2016;30(4):253–60.
2. Gonwa TZ, McBride MA, Anderson K, Mai ML, Wadei H, Ahsan N. Continued influence of preoperative renal function on outcome of orthotopic liver transplant in the US: where will MELD lead US? Am J Transplant. 2006;2:2651–9.
3. Nair S, Verma S, Thuluvath PJ. Pretransplant renal function predicts survival in patients undergoing orthotopic liver transplantation. Hepatology. 2002;35:1179–85.
4. Organ Procurement and Transplantation Network. Ethical implications of multiorgan transplant. 2019. https://optn.transplant.hrsa.gov/media/2801/ethics_publiccomment_20190122.pdf. Accessed 26 Aug 2019.
5. Schilsky M, Moini M. Advances in liver transplantation allocation systems. World J Gastroenterol. 2016;22(10):2922–30.
6. Davis CL, Gonwa TA, Wilkinson AH. Identification of patients best suited for combined liver-kidney transplantation: part II. Liver Transpl. 2002;8:193–211.
7. Sampaio MS, Martin P, Bunnapradist S. Renal dysfunction in end-stage liver disease and post-liver transplant. Clin Liver Dis. 2014;18(3):543–60.
8. Chancharoenthana W, Leelahavanichkul A. Acute kidney injury spectrum in patients with chronic liver disease: where do we stand? World J Gastroenterol. 2019;25(28):3684–703.
9. Ojo AO, Held PJ, Port FK, Wolfe RA, Leichtman AB, Young EW, et al. Chronic renal failure after transplantation of a nonrenal organ. N Engl J Med. 2003;349(10):931–40.
10. Ruebner R, Goldberg D, Abt PL, et al. Risk of end-stage renal disease among liver transplant recipients with pre transplant renal dysfunction. Am J Transplant. 2012;12:2958–65.
11. Wadei HM, Lee DD, Croome KP, Mai ML, Golan E, Brotman R, et al. Early allograft dysfunction after liver transplantation is associated with short- and long-term kidney function impairment. Am J Transplant. 2016;16(3):850–9.
12. Hmoud B, Kuo YF, Wiesner RH, Singal AK. Outcomes of liver transplantation alone after listing for simultaneous kidney: comparison to simultaneous liver kidney transplantation. Transplantation. 2015;99(4):823–8.
13. Singal AK, Salameh H, Kuo YF, Wiesner RH. Evolving frequency and outcomes of simultaneous liver kidney transplants based on liver disease etiology. Transplantation. 2014;98(2):216–21.
14. Formica RN, Aeder M, Boyle G, Kucheryavaya A, Stewart D, Hirose R, et al. Simultaneous liver-kidney allocation policy: a proposal to optimize appropriate utilization of scarce resources. Am J Transplant. 2016;16(3):758–66.
15. Pham PT, Lunsford KE, Bunnapradist S, Danovitch GM. Simultaneous liver-kidney transplantation or liver transplantation alone for patients in need of liver transplantation with renal dysfunction. Curr Opin Organ Transplant. 2016;21(2):194–200.
16. Thompson JA, Lake JR. The impact of MELD allocation on simultaneous liver-kidney transplantation. Curr Gastroenterol Rep. 2009;11(1):76–82.

17. Wong F, Wl L, Al Beshir M, Marquez M, Renner E. Outcomes of patients with cirrhosis and hepatorenal syndrom type 1 treated with liver transplantation. Liver Transpl. 2015;21:300–7.

18. Ruiz R, et al. Long-term analysis of combined liver and kidney transplantation at a single center. Arch Surg. 2006;141(8):735–41.

19. Ruiz R, Barri YM, Jennings LW, Chinnakotla S, Goldstein RM, Levy MF, et al. Hepatorenal syndrome: a proposal for kidney after liver transplantation (KALT). Liver Transpl. 2007;13(6):838–43.

20. Locke JE, Warren DS, Singer AL, Segev DL, Simpkins CE, Maley WR, et al. Declining outcomes in simultaneous liver-kidney transplantation in the MELD era: ineffective usage of renal allografts. Transplantation. 2008;85(7):935–42.

21. Cassuto JR, Reese PP, Sonnad S, Bloom RD, Levine MH, Olthoff KM, et al. Wait list death and survival benefit of kidney transplantation among nonrenal transplant recipients. Am J Transplant. 2010;10(11):2502–11.

22. Eason JD, Gonwa TA, Davis CL, Sung RS, Gerber D, Bloom RD. Proceedings of consensus conference on simultaneous liver kidney transplantation (SLK). Am J Transplant. 2008;8(11):2243–51.

23. Davis CL, Feng S, Sung R, Wong F, Goodrich NP, Melton LB, et al. Simultaneous liver-kidney transplantation: evaluation to decision making. Am J Transplant. 2007;7(7):1702–9.

24. Cannon RM, Jones CM, Davis EG, Eckhoff DE. Effect of renal diagnosis on survival in simultaneous liver-kidney transplantation. J Am Coll Surg. 2019;228(4):536–44 e3.

25. Singal AK, Ong S, Satapathy SK, Kamath PS, Wiesner RH. Simultaneous liver kidney transplantation. Transpl Int. 2019;32(4):343–52.

26. Cullaro G, Hilrose R, Lai JC. Changes in simultaneous liver-kidney transplant allocation policy may impact postliver transplant outcomes. Transplantation. 2019;103:959–64.

27. Cholongitas E, Thomas M, Senzolo M, et al. Gender disparity and MELD in liver transplantation. J Hepatol. 2011;55:500–1.

28. Delville M, Sabbah L, Girard D, Elie C, Manceau S, Piketty M, et al. Prevalence and predictors of early cardiovascular events after kidney transplantation: evaluation of pre-transplant cardiovascular work-up. PLoS One. 2015;10(6):e0131237.

29. Nicolau-Raducu R, Gitman M, Ganier D, Loss GE, Cohen AJ, Patel H, et al. Adverse cardiac events after orthotopic liver transplantation: a cross-sectional study in 389 consecutive patients. Liver Transpl. 2015;21(1):13–21.

30. Lentine KL, Costa SP, Weir MR, Robb JF, Fleisher LA, Kasiske BL, et al. Cardiac disease evaluation and management among kidney and liver transplantation candidates: a scientific statement from the American Heart Association and the American College of Cardiology Foundation: endorsed by the American Society of Transplant Surgeons, American Society of Transplantation, and National Kidney Foundation. Circulation. 2012;126(5):617–63.

31. Calixto Fernandes MH, Schricker T, Magder S, Hatzakorzian R. Perioperative fluid management in kidney transplantation: a black box. Crit Care. 2018;22(1):14.

32. Lugo-Baruqui JA, Ayyathurai R, Sriram A, Pragatheeshwar KD. Use of mannitol for ischemia reperfusion injury in kidney transplant and partial nephrectomies—review of literature. Curr Urol Rep. 2019;20(1):6.

33. Rudnick MR, Marchi LD, Plotkin JS. Hemodynamic monitoring during liver transplantation: a state of the art review. World J Hepatol. 2015;7(10):1302–11.

34. Burtenshaw AJ, Isaac JL. The role of transoesophageal echocardiography for perioperative cardiovascular monitoring during orthotopic liver transplantation. Liver Transpl. 2006;12(11):1577–83.

35. Dalia AA, Flores A, Chitilian H, Fitzsimons MG. A comprehensive review of transesophageal echocardiography during orthotopic liver transplantation. J Cardiothorac Vasc Anesth. 2018;32(4):1815–24.

36. Aref A, Zayan T, Sharma A, Halawa A. Utility of central venous pressure measurement in renal transplantation: is it evidence based? World J Transplant. 2018;8(3):61–7.

37. Bansal I, Calhoun BW, Joseph C, Pothiawala M, Baron BW. A comparative study of reducing the extracellular potassium concentration in red blood cells by washing and by reduction of additive solution. Transfusion. 2007;47(2):248–50.

38. Nadim M, Annanthapanyasut W, Matsuoka L, Appachu K, Boyajian M, Ji L, Sedra A, Genyk Y. Intraoperative hemodialysis during liver transplantation: a decade of experience. Liver Transpl. 2014;20:756–64.

39. Baek SD, Jang M, Kim W, Yu H, Hwang S, Lee SG, et al. Benefits of intraoperative continuous renal replacement therapy during liver transplantation in patients with renal dysfunction. Transplant Proc. 2017;49(6):1344–50.

40. Zimmerman MA, Selim M, Kim J, Regner K, Saeian K, Zanowski S, et al. Outcome analysis of continuous intraoperative renal replacement therapy in the highest acuity liver transplant recipients: a single-center experience. Surgery. 2017;161(5):1279–86.

41. Baccaro M, et al. Combined liver–kidney transplantation in patients with cirrhosis and chronic kidney disease. Nephrol Dial Transplant. 2010;25:2356–63.

ABO-Incompatible Liver Transplantation

45

Vikram Raut

45.1 Introduction

"Organ demand versus supply" is the greatest obstacle to increase the frequency of liver transplantation, which has been one of the medical breakthroughs in recent times. Transplantation across the ABO blood groups is discouraged because of the risk of acute rejection, graft loss, and a poor outcome; thus, it is generally used only in emergency situations. In living-donor liver transplantation (LDLT), donor selection is restricted to family members, and ABO-incompatible (ABO-I) liver transplantation becomes inevitable as a means to breach this obstacle. This has compelled transplant surgeons to devise innovative strategies, such as local infusion therapy and rituximab, to prevent complications in ABO-I liver transplantation. However, with an increased risk of infection, antibody-mediated rejection, and consequent vascular and biliary complications, ABO-I liver transplantation continuous to be a formidable challenge in LDLT. In this review, we study the past and current immune strategies adopted by centers across the world for ABO-I LDLT, to provide insight for change or modification so as to improve outcomes and reduce ABO incompatibility-related complications in LDLT.

45.2 History of ABO-I Liver Transplantation

Since its inception by Thomas Starzl, ABO-I liver transplantation has evolved through an era of controversy and immunological violation to the current inevitable phase. The initial animal experiments conducted by Starzl demonstrated that the liver is "a privileged organ" with much greater resistance to acute rejection than the kidney or heart. With this understanding, Starzl breached ABO blood group barriers, particularly in the emergency situations when given no choice but to proceed with first available organ. In 1979, Starzl's group reported 11 human ABO-I liver transplantations without evidence of acute rejection. During this period, ABO incompatibility was not considered a contraindication to liver transplantation. In fact, ABO-I grafts were used children because of the difficulty of finding compatible small grafts, and in adults during emergencies. In 1986, Gordon et al. [1] reported 31 ABO-I liver transplants, carried out using cyclosporine and prednisolone for immunosuppression, and found that graft survival in the ABO-identical group was significantly better than that in the ABO-compatible and -incompatible groups. In children, he used ABO-I grafts in emergency as well as in elective conditions because of the shortage of small grafts. As the 1-year graft survival rate in adults was acceptable, he advocated the use of ABO-I grafts in

V. Raut (✉)
Apollo Hospital, Mumbai, India

adults only in emergency situations. Furthermore, Rego et al. [2] reported hyperacute rejection after ABO-I liver transplant, despite the "privileged" status of the liver. In 1989, Gugenhein et al. [3, 4] confirmed lower graft survival and hyper-acute rejection in ABO-I liver transplantation. In their series of 17 ABO-I liver transplants, Gugenhein et al. postulated immunological damage as the cause of low graft survival and reported antibody-mediated rejection as a cause of graft failure in six patients. They also acknowledged an increased incidence of arterial thrombosis and progressive cholangitis in ABO-I grafts. The debate continued about the increased incidence of complications of ABO-I liver transplants. In a control matched study including 15 ABO-I liver transplants, Sanchez-Urdazpal et al. [5] confirmed an increased incidence of cholangitis, bile leak, cellular rejection, and hepatic artery thrombosis in an ABO-I group. Because of the high incidence of complications, ABO-compatible liver transplantation became unpopular and was reserved for emergency transplant only.

45.3   Need of ABO-I Transplant in Setting of Living Donor

Since the donor of an LDLT is usually a first-degree relative, limiting choice, the use of grafts across the ABO blood groups is often inevitable. This has forced transplant surgeons to adopt various innovative methods to prevent the complications associated with ABO-I liver transplantation. In the early 1990s, various centers reported [6–8] improved the results of ABO-I liver transplantation in children by using pre- and postoperative plasma exchange and OKT-3. We have learned much from the experience of ABO-I kidney transplant surgeons who used peri-operative plasma exchange, splenectomy, and high-dose immunosuppressive drugs to ensure the success of ABO-I transplantation. Anti-donor antibody-induced complement fixation and endothelial damage leading to hemorrhagic necrosis by the formation of micro-thrombi in the graft vasculature is a major cause of early graft failure [9].

Diffuse intra-organ coagulation (DIC) can be confirmed by C4D immunofluorescent staining. To overcome this "single organ DIC," Tanabe's group from Keio University, Japan, endorsed portal vein infusion with prostaglandin E1, methylprednisolone, and gabexate mesilate [10]. Prostaglandin E1 improves microcirculation through vasodilatation and the prevention of platelet thrombi. Gabexate mesilate is a protease inhibitor that inhibits platelet aggregation and coagulation factors. Nakamura et al. [11] used a hepatic artery infusion of prostaglandin E1 to prevent biliary complications and improve the bile duct blood supply. In 2003, Monteiro et al. [12] gave rituximab (anti-CD20 monoclonal antibody) to a 15-year-old boy undergoing emergency ABO-I liver transplantation for resistant B cell lymphoma to reduce anti-donor antibody-producing B cells.

45.4   Current Strategies for ABO Incompatibility in LDLT Worldwide

ABO-I LDLT strategies are directed at eliminating or reducing the anti-ABO antibody. Apart from the routine immunosuppression given to all liver transplant patients, the following methods are also used in ABO-I LDLT.

45.4.1   Rituximab

Rituximab is the monoclonal chimeric human anti-CD20 antibody that revolutionized ABO-I LDLT. CD20 is expressed in most of stages of B cell development but not in plasma cells or stem cells. Rituximab was approved for resistant B cell lymphoma at a dose of 375 mg/m^2 weekly for 4 weeks. To deplete normal B cells in an ABO-I recipient, a single dose of rituximab is considered enough. In ABO-I liver transplantation, the timing of giving rituximab varies among centers from 7 to 15 days preoperatively. Today, most knowledge of the pharmacodynamics of rituximab comes from its use in B cell lymphoma. However,

Genberg et al. [13] recently studied the pharmacodynamics of rituximab in a renal transplant recipient. They found that a single dose of rituximab (375 mg/m2) was sufficient to completely eliminate B cells from the peripheral blood. Although reduced numbers of B cells were seen in the peripheral blood as early as 3 days after rituximab administration, complete elimination was seen only after 3 weeks. Nevertheless, a single dose of rituximab is not enough to completely eliminate B cells from the lymph node. These remnant cells became activated after antigen exposure from the graft and produced the anti-ABO antibody. The value of the complete elimination of B cells needs to be balanced against the need for 2–3 years of prolonged immunosuppression caused by 375 mg/m2 of rituximab. Conversely, the initial 4–6 weeks is critical for antibody-mediated rejection, and B cell suppression is required only for this period. Therefore, the ideal dose of rituximab remains unresolved.

45.4.2 Plasmapheresis

Anti-ABO antibodies are the trigger for antibody-mediated rejection after ABO-I LDLT. Thus, the anti-ABO antibody titers are reduced preoperatively by plasma exchange, plasma filtration, or immune adsorption in most centers across the world, aiming for immunoglobulin M and immunoglobulin G titers below 1:16 at the time of transplantation to prevent antibody-mediated rejection. These titers are maintained at these values because increasing antibody titers in the early postoperative period are associated with rejection. Plasmapheresis is the most effective way to control humoral antibody response to prevent rejection.

45.4.3 Mycophenolate Mofetil

Mycophenolate mofetil is a functionally selective drug that is cytotoxic to B and T lymphocytes. Since rituximab is ineffective against the plasma cells with active B cell-producing antibody, mycophenolate mofetil has been incorporated in a protocol used by groups from Chicago, Tohoku, Tokyo, Yokohama, and Italy. The preoperative administration of mycophenolate mofetil reduces plasma cells in the circulation.

45.4.4 Intravenous Immunoglobulin (IVIG)

Intravenous immunoglobulin causes FC-receptor-dependent B cell apoptosis and inhibits complement- and T cell-mediated allograft injury. A recent trial at Kyushu University, Japan, involving 30 patients showed the efficacy of IVIG given with rituximab and plasma exchange. Intravenous immunoglobulin is very promising in emergency ABO-I LDLT, when there is insufficient time for the action of rituximab. Cost is the major limiting factor in IVIG treatment.

Since the introduction of rituximab, the need for splenectomy in ABO-I LDLT is questionable. Raut et al. [14] showed no difference in anti-ABO-antibody response between a splenectomy group and a non-splenectomy group. In past local infusion of prostaglandin E, methylprednisolone, 1and gabexate mesilate, 1 through the portal vein or hepatic artery was used.

45.5 Outcomes and Long-Term Survival After ABO-I Liver Transplant

In meta-analysis by Lee et al. involving 8000 ABO-I liver transplant found, cases that used rituximab in ABO-I LT patients showed better 1-year graft survival after ABO-I LT than those that did not use rituximab. Furthermore, in patients with preoperative Rituximab 1-, 3-, and 5-year graft survivals of ABO-I LT were comparable to those of ABO-C LT. On the other hand, biliary stricture and ACR tended to be more prevalent after ABO-I LT when rituximab was not used. There were no differences in AMR and patient survival in accordance with the use of rituximab.

Key Points

- ABOI liver transplantation have become inevitable in this era of limited organ supply.
- Rituximab—The monochrome anti-CD20 antibody depletes the normal B cells in the ABOI recipients.
- Anti-ABO antibodies are removed by plasmapheresis.
- Mycophenolate reduces plasma cells in circulation.
- IVIG reduces compliment and T cells mediated allograft injury.
- Prostaglandin improves micro circulation and prevent platelet thrombus formation.

References

1. Gordon RD, Iwatsuki S, Esquivel CO, Tzakis A, Todo S, Starzl TE. Liver transplantation across ABO blood groups. Surgery. 1986;100(2):342–8.
2. Rego J, Prevost F, Rumeau JL, Modesto A, Fourtanier G, Durand D, et al. Hyperacute rejection after ABO-incompatible orthotopic liver transplantation. Transplant Proc. 1987;19(6):4589–90.
3. Gugenheim J, Samuel D, Fabiani B, Saliba F, Castaing D, Reynes M, et al. Rejection of ABO incompatible liver allografts in man. Transplant Proc. 1989;21(1 Pt 2):2223–4.
4. Gugenheim J, Samuel D, Reynes M, Bismuth H. Liver transplantation across ABO blood group barriers. Lancet. 1990;336(8714):519–23.
5. Sanchez-Urdazpal L, Sterioff S, Janes C, Schwerman L, Rosen C, Krom RA. Increased bile duct complications in ABO incompatible liver transplant recipients. Transplant Proc. 1991;23(1 Pt 2):1440–1.
6. Tokunaga Y, Tanaka K, Fujita S, Yamaguchi T, Sawada H, Kato H, et al. Living related liver transplantation across ABO blood groups with FK506 and OKT3. Transpl Int. 1993;6(6):313–8.
7. Renard TH, Andrews WS. An approach to ABO-incompatible liver transplantation in children. Transplantation. 1992;53(1):116–21.
8. Dunn SP, Halligan GE, Billmire DF, Vinocur CD, Lawrence J, Falkenstein K, et al. ABO-incompatible liver transplantation: a risk worth taking. Transplant Proc. 1993;25(6):3109.
9. Demetris AJ, Jaffe R, Tzakis A, Ramsey G, Todo S, Belle S, et al. Antibody-mediated rejection of human orthotopic liver allografts. A study of liver transplantation across ABO blood group barriers. Am J Pathol. 1988;132(3):489–502.
10. Tanabe M, Shimazu M, Wakabayashi G, Hoshino K, Kawachi S, Kadomura T, et al. Intraportal infusion therapy as a novel approach to adult ABO-incompatible liver transplantation. Transplantation. 2002;73(12):1959–61.
11. Nakamura Y, Matsuno N, Iwamoto H, Yokoyama T, Kuzuoka K, Kihara Y, et al. Successful case of adult ABO-incompatible liver transplantation: beneficial effects of intrahepatic artery infusion therapy—a case report. Transplant Proc. 2004;36(8):2269–73.
12. Monteiro I, McLoughlin LM, Fisher A, de la Torre AN, Koneru B. Rituximab with plasmapheresis and splenectomy in ABO-incompatible liver transplantation. Transplantation. 2003;76(11):1648–9.
13. Genberg H, Hansson A, Wernerson A, Wennberg L, Tyden G. Pharmacodynamics of rituximab in kidney allotransplantation. Am J Transplant. 2006;6(10):2418–28.
14. Raut V. Splenectomy does not offer immunological benefits in ABO-incompatible liver transplantation with a preoperative rituximab. Transplantation. 2012;93(1):99–105.

Non-Transplant Surgery for Post-Transplant Patient

Shweta A. Singh

46.1 Introduction

Liver transplantation (LT) has become a viable and acceptable modality of treatment for decompensated end stage liver disease (ESLD). Over the last decade, a large number of centres have started successful LT programmes and more than 1000 patients every year undergo LT surgery in our country [1]. However, most centres providing this facility are concentrated in certain metropolitan cities. Patients from different parts of the country return to their home towns after the procedure. With improved survival following transplant over the last two decades more and more of these patients would be requiring emergency or elective surgery in the future as they go about their daily lives. Often patients may not be able to return to the transplant centre for all procedures, so it is important for anaesthesiologists across the country, to be familiar with the peri-operative issues concerning this patient population.

46.2 Surgeries in Post-LT Recipients

Post-LT recipients may require a number of surgeries. These could be surgeries related to the transplant procedure itself, like repair of incisional hernia; or

incidental surgeries which could be required in any individual, e.g. appendectomy; or surgeries which are not directly related to the LT procedure but may be required more frequently in such patients, e.g. hip arthroplasty for an osteoporotic hip (due to long term steroid use) refer Table 46.1.

Table 46.1 Common surgical procedures after LT in the recipient

Interventions for complications post-transplant	• Postoperative haemorrhage • Vascular thrombosis (HAT/ PVT), Arterio-venous fistulas, Pseudoaneurysm • Colonic perforation, intestinal obstruction • Upper GI bleed, Variceal bleed • Incisional hernia repair • Anastomotic leaks, biliary tract interventions, Hepaticojejunostomy • Splenectomy • Diagnostic laparotomy
Diagnostic procedures to rule out rejection	• US/CT/MR guided biopsies • Endoscopy • Bronchoscopy
Patients at increased risk after transplant	• Pathologic fractures (long-term steroid use causing osteoporosis) • Lymph node biopsy • Bariatric surgery (full development of obesity)
Interventions unrelated to the transplantation	• Trauma • Neuro surgeries • Urological procedures • Obstetrics/gynaecology related surgeries • Emergency surgeries

S. A. Singh (✉)
Department of Anaesthesia and Critical care-CLBS, Max Super Speciality Hospital, Saket, New Delhi, India

Biliary tract interventions and repair of incisional hernia are some procedures often scheduled electively in this population. Although biliary strictures can present at any time after LT, the mean interval at the time of presentation is 5–8 months after transplant and the majority present within 1 year [2]. Biliary strictures and leaks are usually managed endoscopically but surgical management (hepaticojejunostomy) is sometimes necessary for strictures not amenable to endoscopic management [3].

Due to the large incision required for the LT procedure and placement of multiple indwelling peritoneal drainage catheters, the incidence of incisional hernias is not infrequent in this population. The reported incidence of incisional hernia ranges from 5 to 46% [4]. Incisional hernia repair is usually scheduled between 6 and 24 months post-transplant.

Other surgical procedures which are often required in this patient population is laparotomy for small bowel obstruction (secondary to adhesions), lymph node biopsy to rule out lymphoproliferative disease, abscess drainage, hip arthroplasty for a vascular necrosis from bone demineralization and management of fractures due to incidental falls or trauma [5]. These occur due to their predilection for infections, development of post-transplant lymphoproliferative disease, and side effects of prolonged steroid and other immunosuppressive medications.

Rarely bariatric surgery may be required in post-LT recipients for rapid weight gain secondary to tacrolimus induced metabolic syndrome. Such patients may have had the original surgery done for NASH related cirrhosis prior to LT [6].

46.3 Anaesthesia Concerns and Considerations

46.3.1 Preoperative Assessment of Transplant Recipients

The fundamental principles of evaluation and optimization during preoperative period and the anaesthetic management of post-LT patients posted for a non-transplant surgeries are similar to that of any other patient. However, the concerns unique to this population are increased susceptibility to infection as these patients are on immunosuppression, the adverse effects of immune-suppressive therapy, their interaction with anaesthetic drugs and the risk of allograft rejection in the absence of adequate immune-suppression. Besides this, usual evaluation for concomitant diseases, assessment of other organ function, and evaluation of functional status needs to be done.

46.3.2 Physiology of LT Recipient

46.3.2.1 Liver Functions

The liver synthetic functions as well as liver enzyme levels return to normal levels within a few days after transplantation. This recovery of functional capacity, drug metabolizing capacity, and synthesis of clotting factors is usually complete in the initial few weeks and much before the structural regeneration takes place [7].

46.3.2.2 Portal Hypertension

Patients with ESLD who undergo LT have long standing advanced portal hypertension (PHT) which leads to splenomegaly and varying degrees of pancytopenia, as part of hypersplenism. Recovery from this may be slow after LT and many patients will have clinically significant persistent thrombocytopenia. This has to be taken into consideration during the preoperative evaluation. Some patients may require splenectomy or splenic artery embolization post-LT if severe thrombocytopenia and splenomegaly persists early in the postoperative course. This reduces splenic vein flow to the transplanted liver and helps manage small for size syndrome.

46.3.2.3 Renal Functions in the Post-LT Recipient

Hepatorenal syndrome, by definition usually reverses gradually after LT, but many patients with pre-transplant renal dysfunction may not have a complete recovery of renal functions [8]. A significant proportion (5–50%) of post-LT patients may develop proteinuria and new onset AKI in the immediate postoperative period.

Although, renal recovery is common in liver recipients; 5 years cumulative incidence of chronic kidney disease is 18–22% [9].

Some patients may also undergo a sequential or combined liver–kidney transplant which may be responsible for an unpredictable recovery of renal functions.

Furthermore, calcineurin inhibitors which form the back bone of immunosuppressive regimens for LT patients can have significant nephrotoxicity and hence it is important to evaluate renal function using blood urea nitrogen and creatinine levels, urine analysis, and calculation of the glomerular filtration rate.

46.3.2.4 Cardiorespiratory System

Hepato-pulmonary syndrome (HPS) is a unique condition that develops in patients with ESLD and PHT, where in shunts form within the lungs leading to hypoxemia (platypnea and orthodeoxia). The hypoxemia related to ventilation/perfusion mismatch and intra-pulmonary shunts in these patients may take months to reverse [10].

Another unique condition which may persist post-LT is porto-pulmonary hypertension (PoPH) which may require pulmonary vasodilators for several months in the postoperative period. If a patient is on pulmonary vasodilators, such as sildenafil or epoprostenol, they need to be continued perioperatively to prevent aggaravation of pulmonary hypertension (PH) due to hypoxemia, hypercapnia, or acidosis. In this situation nitric oxide should be available to manage intraoperative PH.

The hyper-dynamic circulatory state of ESLD as well as cirrhotic cardiomyopathy regresses over the next few months after LT.

The overall risk of atherosclerotic heart disease is high in LT recipients [11]. For those with a functional capacity of less than four metabolic equivalents or development of metabolic syndrome post-LT, cardiac evaluation to rule out ischemic cardiac disease is recommended, especially for extensive surgeries.

Anaemia, which is multifactorial, is frequently present in the preoperative period in LT recipients. Up to 45–78% post-LT patients could have anaemia due to the antiproliferative effects of antimetabolite agents on the bone marrow [12]. Nutritional supplementation and erythrocyte-stimulating agents can be used to correct anaemia preoperatively, before an elective surgery.

46.4 Immunosuppression

All post-LT patients are on various regimens of immunosuppressive therapy.

The most commonly used immunosuppressive drugs in LT recipient are the calcineurin inhibitors (CNI), antimetabolites, like mycophenolate mofetil or azathioprine and steroids.

Newer drugs, such as tacrolimus, have largely replaced cyclosporine A, and mycophenolate mofetil has replaced azathioprine in most immunosuppression protocols [13].

These have a narrow therapeutic index and blood concentration shows significant variability. Immunosuppression needs to be maintained within therapeutic limits so as to avoid possibility of allograft rejection. On the other hand, immunosuppression can predispose to infection and/or drug-specific side effects. An abnormal LFT on basic testing may indicate rejection, infection or biliary stasis [14, 15]. It is also very important to continue immunosuppressive medications during peri-operative period.

46.4.1 Side Effects of Immunosuppressive Therapy

The immunosuppressive medications over long-term use can lead to several side effects that may have an impact on perioperative care of these patients Table 46.2.

These toxicities are many and varied, depending on the particular agent. Some of the side effects of chronic immunosuppression are development of metabolic syndrome which includes diabetes (DM), hypertension (HT), hyperlipidaemia, and weight gain as well renal dysfunction causing decreased glomerular filtration, proteinuria, hyperkalaemia, and hypomagnesaemia.

Table 46.2 Common side effects of some immunosuppressive drugs

	Tacrolimus	Cyclosporine	Mycophenolate mofetil	Steroids
Bone marrow suppression			+	
• Anaemia	−	−	−	−
• Leukopenia	−	−	+	−
• Thrombocytopenia	−	−	+	−
Metabolic syndrome	+	+	−	+
• Atherosclerosis	+	+	−	++
• Hypertension	+	++	−	+
• Dyslipidemia		+		+
Renal insufficiency	++	+	−	−
Cardiovascular hypertension	+	++	−	+
Endocrine • Diabetes	++	+	−	++
• Osteoporosis	−	−	−	++
• Adrenal suppression	−	−	−	++
• Obesity	−	−	−	++
Neurotoxicity				
• Seizures	+	+	−	−
• Headache	+	+	−	−
• Psychiatric disturbances	−	−	−	+
Hepatotoxicity	−	++	−	−
Gastrointestinal toxicity	+	++	++	+
Infections	−	−	−	+
Others				
• Anaphylactic reactions	++	−	−	−
• Cataract formation	−	−	−	+
• Electrolyte abnormalities	+	+	−	−

+ − causes, − not known to cause
TAC Tacrolimus, *CyA* Cyclosporine A, *MMF* mycophenolate mofetil, *DM* diabetes mellitus, *HTN* hypertension, + Present, − Absent

Azathioprine in particular was fraught with the complications of myelosuppression and an exogenous Cushing's syndrome. The side effect profile of cyclosporine included nephrotoxicity, premature atherosclerosis, hypertension, neurotoxicity, and hepatotoxicity [16–18].

The toxicity profile of tacrolimus is similar but less severe than cyclosporine; however, tacrolimus is associated with hyperglycaemia, and as many as 20% of tacrolimus recipients develop insulin-dependent diabetes [12]. LT recipients are known to develop new onset metabolic syndrome characterized by obesity, diabetes, HT, and dyslipidemia [19]. In a meta-analysis including 3043 transplant recipients, new-onset DM (NODM) was reported in 13.4% of patients after solid organ transplantation as early as within 3 months post-transplant [20, 21]. Calcineurin inhibitors are the most important drivers for the post-LT metabolic complications. NODM increases susceptibility to infectious and cardiovascular complications.

Among the complications encountered in post-LT population, nephrotoxicity is one of the most prevalent mandating a special mention [5]. Tacrolimus as well as cyclosporine induce production of thromboxane A_2 and endothelin, affecting renal microcirculation, causing a dose related decrease in renal blood flow and glomerular filtration rate even in therapeutic doses [22–24].

Co-administration of drugs such as amphotericin, NSAIDs, ranitidine, co-trimoxazole, tobramycin, gentamycin, and vancomycin with tacrolimus aggravates renal dysfunction and hence would require dose modification.

There is also lowering of seizure threshold, increased risk of infection and tumours, pancytopenia, osteoporosis, and poor wound healing.

Gastrointestinal ulcers may be caused by surgical stress, corticosteroids, and mycophenolate mofetil [25]. Hence, stress ulcer prophylaxis is necessary.

This state of induced immunosuppression predisposes patients to a number of bacterial, viral, fungal, and protozoal infections in addition to the community acquired ones adding significantly to morbidity and mortality [26]. It is important to remember that immunosuppressed patient may not mount fever and leucocytosis in response to infections, so absence of fever may not exclude infective complications. Certain viral infections may be more common due to the bone marrow suppressive effects of antimetabolites, for example, infection with cytomegalovirus. Pancytopenia may be present in some cases due to persistent splenomegaly and PHT. Treatment using colony stimulating factors many be warranted in such cases.

Besides identification and treatment of pre-existing infections before elective surgery, all aseptic measures for prevention of bacterial infections, e.g. close systems of intravenous fluids and invasive lines, must be taken along with surgical prophylaxis with broad spectrum antibiotics for ensuring a good outcome [27].

46.4.2 Drug Interactions of Immunosuppressive Therapy

Tacrolimus and cyclosporine are metabolized by cytochrome P-450 system of liver affecting bioavailability of many drugs. Doses of several antibiotics and antifungals may need to be tailored as mentioned in Table 46.3. Most drugs used for anaesthetic procedures do not require a dose mod-

Table 46.3 Interaction of immunosuppressive drugs with antibiotics. Overview of antibiotic dose modification

Antibiotic	CyA	TAC	MMF	Steroids		
				Prednisolone	Methyl-prednisolone	Dexa-methasone
Aminoglycocides	Nephrotoxicity					
Amikacine	D	D	C	C	C	C
Gentamycine	D	D	C	C	C	C
Tobramycine	D	D	D	C	C	C
Kanamycine	D	D	C	C	C	C
Macrolid						
Azithromycine	C	NA	C	D	C	D
Clarithromcine	D	D	C	D	D	D
Erythromycine	D	D	C	D	D	D
Roxithromycine	D	NA	C	D	D	D
Beta lactam						
Ampicillin	C	C	C	C	C	C
Amox clav	C	D	D	C	C	C
Aztreonam	C	C	D	C	C	C
Cefuroxime	C	C	C	C	C	C
Ceftriaxone	D	D	C	C	C	C
Ceftazidime	D	D	C	C	C	C
Imipenem	D	D	C	C	C	C
Quinolone						
Cipro	D	D	D	D	D	D
Levo	D	D	C	D	D	D
Antifungal						
Fluconazole	D	NA	NA	NA	NA	NA
Voriconazole	D	NA	NA	NA	NA	NA

D dose modification, *C* compatible, *NA* data unavailable

Table 46.4 Immunosuppressive drugs and anaesthetic agents

	Effect
Intravenous agents	
Propofol	Nil
Etomidate	Nil (caution for adrenal suppression)
Thiopentone	Nil
Benzodiazepines	Increased bioavailability
Opioids	CYA increases the analgesic effect of Fentanyl
Inhalational agents	
Isoflurane	CYA reduces the clearance
Muscle relaxants	Prolonged neuromuscular blockade
Local anaesthetic agents	Bupivacaine and Ropivacaine used safely

Table 46.5 Suggested preoperative investigations for evaluation

Investigations	
Blood	Haemoglobin, haematocrit
	Total leukocyte count
Coagulation	Platelets
	PT-INR
	APTT
LFT	SGOT, SGPT
	Bilirubin
	Albumin, protein
Renal function tests	BUN, creatinine, urea, sodium, potassium
Endocrine	FT_3, TSH
	FBS, PPBS, HbA1C
Cardiorespiratory	ECG, ECHO, CXR

ification especially in the absence of renal and hepatic dysfunction. However, cyclosporine and tacrolimus may alter blood levels of certain anaesthetic drugs as mentioned in Table 46.4 [28, 29].

46.5 Preoperative Evaluation

With a comprehensive understanding of the physiology of the post-LT patient, a thorough history and physical examination should be undertaken. Laboratory tests are needed to evaluate the functional status of the allograft and other organ systems as mentioned in Table 46.5.

The need for additional preoperative tests can be tailored on individual basis depending on the surgery required. A detailed cardiac evaluation may be required to rule out coronary heart disease in post LT patients as the incidence of cardiorespiratory problems within the first year of LT is high [30].

46.5.1 Premedication

Adequate fasting period is recommended as per ASA guidelines prior to surgery. In patients with associated comorbidities appropriate precautions to prevent aspiration should be taken. The usual anxiolytic premedication may be used, as in non-transplant patients. However, dose adjustment for

some drugs may be needed. The prophylaxis for stress ulcer and VTE is recommended.

In situations where steroids have been recently withdrawn prophylactic steroids may be considered prior to induction [31]. A glycaemic control plan is imperative for closely managing intraoperative and postoperative blood sugar levels in the diabetic.

Immunosuppressive drugs should be continued perioperatively in the same doses to maintain a steady concentration and reduce the risk of rejection. Cyclosporine can be given 4–6 h before surgery while other immunosuppressive drugs can be administered intravenously [32].

46.5.2 Considerations for General Anaesthesia

There is no ideal anaesthetic strategy. However, balanced anaesthesia with multimodal analgesia is usually the preferred approach. In the presence of normal hepatic and renal functions all standard anaesthetic medications and adjuncts may be used safely.

It is important to maintain adequate systemic blood pressure and volume intraoperatively. This is important as hypo perfusion and ischemia are both poorly tolerated by the liver allograft because the normal physiologic mechanisms that maintain and control blood flow in the liver are blunted in post-transplant patients [17].

In patients with renal dysfunction appropriate dosing of drugs metabolized by the kidney as well as hemodynamic management to optimize renal blood flow as autoregulation of renal blood flow is impaired.

Immunosuppressant medications may reduce seizure threshold hence hyperventilation during mechanical ventilation should be avoided [33, 34]. Hyperkalaemia and hypomagnesemia may be observed with cyclosporine or tacrolimus therapy [35–37]. Hence, electrolyte levels need to be monitored and managed.

46.5.3 Monitoring

Standard monitoring as per ASA guidelines are recommended. This includes continuous ECG, pulse oximetry, end tidal CO_2, and intermittent BP monitoring. Invasive monitoring might be indicated according to the nature of surgery and the clinical condition of the patient under strict asepsis and adequate antibiotic prophylaxis.

Invasive blood pressure monitoring using an arterial line may be indicated for haemodynamically unstable patients or those needing frequent blood gases, or for those requiring postoperative mechanical ventilation. Abdominal surgeries in LT recipients are likely to bleed so it is important to be prepared adequately with at large bore intravenous catheters, central venous access, arterial pressure monitoring, and blood cross match.

Urinary catheters can be avoided for short procedures to prevent catheter-associated urinary tract infection but would be required in prolonged surgeries or those with considerable fluid shifts.

46.5.4 Airway Management

The connective tissues in the joints are prone for glycosylation, especially in diabetic patients, resulting in reduction in range of movements. As a result the mouth opening maybe restricted, making intubation difficult. Lymphoproliferative overgrowth secondary to immunosuppressant drugs may compromise any part of the airway or mediastinum causing life threatening airway obstruction during sedation and anaesthesia [20].

Gingival hyperplasia secondary to cyclosporine may lead to bleeding during airway manipulation.

Oral endotracheal intubation is usually preferred over nasal intubation as it does not disrupt the nasal flora [38]. Use of second generation laryngeal mask devices may be prefered over endotracheal intubation, if not contra-indicated. In such cases, additional care must be taken to avoid gastric distention by air inffation [39, 40]. Overt hyperventilation may precipitate seizures by reducing the seizure threshold in patients taking cyclosporine and tacrolimus.

Early postoperative early extubation is preferred to prevent the development of nosocomial or ventilator associated pneumonia [41].

46.5.5 General Anaesthesia

All inhalational and intravenous anaesthetics have been used safely in transplant recipients. General principles are maintaining adequate depth of anaesthesia and avoiding hypoxia, hypercapnia, high airway pressures, and excessive PEEP to prevent a rise in splanchnic vascular resistance and decrease in hepatic blood flow as the normal physiologic mechanisms that maintain hepatic blood flow are blunted after LT.

46.5.6 Inhalation Agents

Although halothane is rarely used, it has potential hepatotoxicity and direct cardiac depressant effects. Prolonged use of N2O is best avoided due to the risk of bone marrow suppression and bowel distension [42].

Fluorinated inhalation agents such as sevoflurane, isoflurane, and desflurane can be safely used.

46.5.7 Intravenous Induction Agents like

Propofol, thiopentone, and etomidate do not require dose adjustments. Despite being metabolized by the liver and excreted by the kidney, there has been no need to modify propofol dosage in patients with hepatic or renal impairment [43]. Predetermined doses of propofol may further aggravate the adverse effects on heamodyamincs (hypotension) in patients with preoperative cardiovascular compromise. Care must be taken to titrate the doses of induction agents to the effect in such situation.

Etomidate provides cardiovascular stability in those at risk for decompensation during the induction. Similar to propofol, etomidate too does not require any dose modification. Single dose administration is shown to decrease serum cortisol levels for at least 24 h, but this has no clinical implication.

The clinical effects of ketamine are prolonged in the presence of hepatic insufficiency as it is metabolized by the hepatic cytochrome P-450 system. It can also aggravate neurotoxic effects of immunosuppressants.

46.5.8 Neuromuscular Blockers

Although most muscle relaxants can be used safely, atracurium and cisatracurium are preferred agents due to Hoffmann elimination. Patients on cyclosporine would require a smaller dose of nondepolarizing muscle relaxant, particularly vecuronium and pancuronium with prolonged recovery time [44–46].

Succinylcholine may be used in the need for rapid sequence intubation unless contraindicated [47].

46.5.9 Opioids

Multimodal analgesia is to be targeted during perioperative period. Fentanyl is safe for short-term use during surgery. However, the pharmacodynamic effects should be monitored due to accumulation effect. Morphine, codeine, oxycodone, and tramadol may be used with caution for postoperative analgesia [48]. Transdermal or on need based fentanyl boluses can be given.

Acetaminophen has been used without any adverse effects on the graft. NSAIDS may be contraindicated with concomitant tacrolimus use [49, 50].

46.5.10 Regional Anaesthesia

Liver recipient status is not an absolute contraindication of regional anaesthesia. The decision to administer central neuraxial blockade (CNB) and/or peripheral nerve blocks is based on the need of surgery and coagulation status of the patient. Some post-LT recipients maybe receiving low-dose heparin, dextran, or anti-platelet agents for graft thromboprophylaxis in the early post-transplant period which may need to be discontinued accordingly or anaesthetic plan modified as deemed appropriate after discussion with the transplant team.

An epidural or spinal can be planned if clotting studies (PT, INR, and APTT) and platelet count is normal under aseptic precautions. Bupivacaine and ropivacaine can be administered safely used through regional routes without any side effects.

The arguments in favour of regional anaesthesia are avoidance of systemic opioids, airway manipulation, and pulmonary complications due to mechanical ventilation [51].

However, the pre-existing autonomic neuropathy and cardiac denervation may cause hemodynamic collapse. Preloading with fluids before central neuraxial blockade may help to attenuate post-sympathetic blockade and hypotension. Direct and indirect-acting adrenergic agonists along with emergency airway management tools should be readily available for change of anaesthesia plan.

Peripheral nerve blocks are also a safe anaesthetic option, popular due to hemodynamic stability and better postoperative analgesia. Some studies show no difference in duration of peripheral nerve blocks in patients after transplantation compared to the general surgical population [52, 53].

46.5.11 Postoperative Management

ERAS protocol emphasises on early mobilsation and physical rehabilitation. This helps in early recovery and also reduces overall incidence of postopeative delirium.

Appropriate analgesia is an essential component of postoperative surgical care. Parenteral paracetamol is an effective analgesic agent and may spare narcotics. There is no evidence of an increased risk of hepatotoxicity [54].

Once extubated, patient-controlled analgesia (PCA) devices are effective and well received by patients and nurses.

Immunosuppressive therapy should be continued during the perioperative period and daily monitoring of steady-state cyclosporine or tacrolimus blood levels is recommended [55]. Adequate attention needs to be paid to the volume status, renal function, and prevention of infection.

The transplant patient population is considered as high-risk group for developing venous thromboembolism (VTE) [56]. However, the exact risk of developing VTEs in these patients is not clearly defined in literature, nor there are clear guidelines regarding the appropriate use of thromboprophylaxis in transplant recipients [57]. In our practice, VTE prophylaxis is tailored to the patient's specific needs in accordance with degree of ambulation and coagulation status as assessed by viscoelastic monitoring in combination with standard coagulation status [29, 58].

46.6 Conclusion

Perioperative anaesthetic management in majority of recipients is similar to the standard anaesthetic practice except for some essential considerations like the adverse effects of immunosuppression, its interaction with anaesthetic drugs, the risk of infection, and the potential for organ rejection. Preoperative assessment of any transplant recipient undergoing non-transplant surgery should also focus on postoperative course since transplant, comorbidities acquired by the patient, biochemical evaluation of function of liver allograft, and other organs.

As per literature and our own experience most LT recipients who undergo non-transplant surgery can do so safely under general anaesthesia without any drug interactions with anaesthetic drugs in the absence of liver and renal dysfunction. Depending on the type of surgery they could be transferred directly to the ward and discharged the next day after ensuring clinical and biochemical parameters to be normal. Immunosuppression needs to be continued perioperatively and drug levels can be tested prior to surgery.

Regional anesthesia including central neuraxial blocks and peripheral nerve blocks can safely be adminstered in post transplantation patients after confirming normal coagulation. The dose adjustement may not be necessary.

> **Key Points**
> - With improved survival more transplanted patients are coming for incidental surgeries.
> - The commonest surgery post-LT is repair of incisional hernia which is formed due to the large incision.
> - Biliary strictures and leaks may require surgical interventions.
> - Preoperative evaluation requires evaluation of the grafted organ.
> - Immunosuppressive medication should be modified, balancing risk of infection and the risk of rejection.
> - Transplant patient population is high risk developing VTE.

References

1. Narasimhan G. Living donor liver transplantation in India. Hepatobilary Surg Nutr. 2016;5(2):127–32.
2. Nemes B, Gaman G, Doros A. Biliary complications after liver transplantation. Expert Rev Gastroenterol Hepatol. 2015;9(4):447–66.
3. Testa G, Malago M, Valentin-Gamazo C, Lindell G, Broelsch CE. Biliary anastomosis in living related liver transplantation using the right liver lobe: tech-

niques and complications. Liver Transpl Surg. 2000;6(6):710–4.

4. de Goede B, Eker HH, Klitsie PJ, van Kempen BJ, Polak WG, Hop WC, et al. Incisional hernia after liver transplantation: risk factors and health-related quality of life. Clin Transpl. 2014;28(7):829–36.

5. Brusich KT, Acan I. Anesthetic considerations in transplant recipients for non transplant surgery. In: Organ donation and transplantation—current status and future challenges. London: IntechOpen; 2018.

6. Gentileschi P, Venza M, Benavoli D, Lirosi Francesca L, Camperchioli I, D'Eletto M. Intragastic balloon followed by biliopancreatic diversion in a liver transplant recipient: a case report. Obes Surg. 2009;19:1460–3.

7. Kang Y, Audu P. Coagulation and liver transplantation. Int Anesthesiol Clin. 2006;4:17–36.

8. Nguyen-Buckley C, Wong M. Anaesthesia for intestinal transplantation. Anesthesiol Clin. 2017;3:509–21.

9. Kida Y. Chronic renal failure after transplantation of a nonrenal organ. N Engl J Med. 2003;349(26):2563–5.

10. Eriksson JS, Soderman C, Ericzon B-G, Eleborg L, Wahren J, Hedenstierna G. Normalization of ventilation/perfusion relationships after liver transplantation in patients with decompensated cirrhosis: evidence for a hepatopulmonary syndrome. Hepatology. 1990;12:1350–7.

11. Pisano G, Fracanzani AL, Caccamo L, et al. Cardiovascular risk after orthotopic liver transplantation, a review of the literature and preliminary results of a prospective study. World J Gastroenterol. 2016;22(40):8869–82.

12. Tessier JM, Sirkin M, Wolfe LG, Duane TM. Trauma after transplant: hold the antibiotics please. Surg Infect (Larchmt). 2013;14(2):177–80.

13. Dias VC, Madsen KL, Mulder KE, Keelan M, Yatscoff RW, Thomson AB. Oral administration of rapamycin and cyclosporine differentially alter intestinal function in rabbits. Dig Dis Sci. 1998;43(10):2227–36.

14. Keegan MT, Plevak DJ. The transplant recipient for nontransplant surgery. Anesthesiol Clin North America. 2004;22(4):827–61.

15. Gelb AW, Freeman DJ, Robertson KM, Zhang C. Isoflurane alters the kinetics of oral cyclosporine. Anesth Analg. 1991;72(6):801–4.

16. Textor SC, Taler SJ, Canzanello VJ, Schwartz L, Augustine JE. Posttransplantation hypertension related to calcineurin inhibitors. Liver Transpl. 2000;6:521–30.

17. Neal DA, Alexander GJ. Can the potential benefits of statins in general medical practice be extrapolated to liver transplantation? Liver Transpl. 2001;7:1009–14.

18. Wijdicks EF. Neurotoxicity of immunosuppressive drugs. Liver Transpl. 2001;7:937–42.

19. Marchetti P. New-onset diabetes after transplantation. J Heart Lung Transplant. 2004;23(5 Suppl):S194–201.

20. Hammer GB, Cao S, Boltz MG, Messner A. Post-transplant lymphoproliferative disease may present with severe airway obstruction. Anesthesiology. 1998;89:263–5.

21. Xia Q. New onset diabetes after liver transplant. Enough attention required. J Diabetes. 2015;7:774–6.

22. Kopp JB, Klotman PE. Cellular and molecular mechanisms of cyclosporine nephrotoxicity. J Am Soc Nephrol. 1990;1:162.

23. McCauley J, Fung J, Jain A, Todo S, Starzl TE. The effects of FK506 on renal function after liver transplantation. Transplant Proc. 1990;22:17.

24. Khanna A. Tacrolimus and cyclosporine in vitro and in vivo induce osteopontin mRNA and protein expression in renal tissues. Nephron Exp Nephrol. 2005;101:119.

25. Courson AY, Lee JR, Aull MJ, Lee JH, Kapur S, McDermott JK. Routine prophylaxis with proton pump inhibitors and post-transplant complications in kidney transplant recipients undergoing early corticosteroid withdrawal. Clin Transpl. 2016;30(6):694–702.

26. Dunn DL. Problems related to immunosuppression. Infection and malignancy occurring after solid organ transplantation. Crit Care Clin. 1990;6(4):955–77.

27. Suzuki Y, Kenjo A, Togano T, Yamamoto N, Ohto H, Kume H. Infectious diseases in solid organ transplant recipients: analysis of autopsied cases in Japan. J Infect Chemother. 2017;23(8):531–7.

28. Campana C, Regazzi MB, Buggia I, Molinaro M. Clinically significant drug interactions with cyclosporin an update. Clin Pharmacokinet. 1996;30:141–79.

29. Rancic N, Vavic NN, Kovacevic AM, Mikov MM, Drgojevic-Simic VM. Drug-drug interactions of tacrolimus. Hosp Pharm. 2015;2:291–6.

30. Gill JS. Cardiovascular disease in transplant recipients: current and future treatment strategies. Clin J Am Soc Nephrol. 2008;3(2):S29–37.

31. Fussner LA, Heimbach JK, Fan C, Dierkhising R, Coss E, Leise MD, Watt KD. Cardiovascular disease after liver transplantation: when, what, and who is at risk. Liver Transpl. 2015;21(7):889–96.

32. Johnston TD, Katz SM. Special considerations in the transplant patient requiring other surgery. Surg Clin N Am. 1994;74:1211–21.

33. Csete M, Sopher MJ. Management of the transplant patient for nontransplant procedures. Adv Anesth. 1994;11:407–31.

34. Berden JH, Hoitsma AJ, Merx JL, et al. Severe central nervous system toxicity associated with cyclosporin. Lancet. 1985;1:219–20.

35. Adu D, Turney J, Michael J, et al. Hyperkalemia in cyclosporine-treated renal allograft recipients. Lancet. 1983;2:370–2.

36. June CH, Thomson CB, Kennedy MS, et al. Profound hypomagnesemia and renal magnesium wasting associated with the use of cyclosporine for marrow transplantation. Transplantation. 1985;39:620–4.

37. Mc Cauley J, Fung J, Jain A, et al. The effects of FK 506 on renal function after liver transplantation. Transplant Proc. 1990;22:17–20.

38. Bach A, Boehrer H, Schmidt H, Geiss HK. Nosocomial sinusitis in ventilated patients. Nasotracheal vs. orotracheal intubation. Anaesthesia. 1992;47(4):335–9.

39. Fuehner T, Wiesner O, DeWall C, Dierich M, Simon AR, Hadem J, Ivanyi P, Welte T, Gottlieb J. Self-expanding metallic stent placement with laryngeal mask in lung transplant recipients. Transplant Proc. 2010;42:4595–9.

40. Ejtehadi F, Carter S, Evans L, Zia M, Bradpiece H. General anaesthesia and emergency surgery in heart transplant recipient. Case Rep Surg. 2015;2015:256465.

41. Brusich KT, Can A, I, Filipčić NV. Ventilator-associated pneumonia: comparing cadaveric liver transplant and non-transplant surgical patients. Acta Clin Croat. 2016;55(3):360–9.

42. Ozbilgin M, Egeli T, Unek T, Ozkardesler S, Avkan-Oguz V, Sagol O, et al. Incidence of late acute rejection in living donor liver transplant patients, risk factors, and the role of immunosuppressive drugs. Transplant Proc. 2015;47(5):1474–7.

43. White P, Romero G. Nonopioid intravenous anaesthesia. In: Barash PG, Cullen BF, Stoelting RK, editors. Clinical anesthesiology. 5th ed. Philadelphia: Lippincott Williams& Wilkins; 2006. p. 334–52.

44. Crosby E, Robblee JA. Cyclosporine-pancuronium interaction in a patient with a renal allograft. Can J Anaesth. 1988;35(3 Pt 1):300–2.

45. Gramstad L. Atracurium, vecuronium, and pancuronium in end-stage renal failure. Br J Anaesth. 1987;59:995–1003.

46. Sidi A, Kaplan RF, Davis RF. Prolonged neuromuscular blockade and ventilatory failure after renal transplantation and cyclosporine. Can J Anaesth. 1990;37(5):543–8.

47. Barbara DW, Christensen JM, Mauermann WJ, Dearani JA, Hyder JA. The safety of neuromuscular blockade reversal in patients with cardiac transplantation. Transplantation. 2016;100(12):2723–8.

48. Carlos RV, Torres MLA, de Boer HD. Reversal of neuromuscular block with sugammadex in five heart transplant pediatric recipients. Braz J Anesthesiol. 2018;68:416–20.

49. Harris KP, Jenkins D, Walls J. Nonsteroidal anti-inflammatory drugs and cyclosporine: a poten-tially serious adverse interaction. Transplantation. 1988;46:598–9.

50. Mueller EA, Kovarik JM, Koelle EU, Merdjan H, Johnston A, Hitzenberger G. Pharmacokinetics of cyclosporine and multiple dose diclofenac during co-administration. J Clin Pharmacol. 1993;33:936–43.

51. Gupta PK, Hopkins PM. Regional anaesthesia for all? Br J Anaesth. 2012;109:7–9.

52. Brusich KT, Acan I, Vicic V, Filipcic NV. Supraclavicular nerve block: does kidney transplantation make a difference? In: Proceedings of 6th Croatian congress of regional anaesthesia and analgesia with international participation, at Zagreb, Croatia, vol. 117; 2015.

53. Freir NM, Murphy C, Mugawar M, LinnaneA Cunningham AJ. Transversus abdominis plane block for analgesia in renal transplantation: a randomized controlled trial. Anaesth Analg. 2012;115:953–7.

54. Ahlers SJ, Van Gulik L, Van Dongen EP, Bruins P, Tibboel D, Knibbe CA. Aminotransferase levels in relation to short-term use of acetaminophen four grams daily in postoperative cardiothoracic patients in the intensive care unit. Anaesth Intensive Care. 2011;39:1056–63.

55. Klintmalm GBG, Husberg BS, Starzl TE. The organ transplanted patient: immunological concepts and immunosuppression. In: Makowka L, editor. The handbook of transplantation management. Austin, TX: Landes; 1995. p. 72–108.

56. Abualhassan N, Aljiffry M, Thalib L, Coussa R, Metrakos P, Hassanain M. Post-transplant venous thromboembolic events and their effect on graft survival. Saudi J Kidney Dis Transpl. 2015;26(1):1–5.

57. Abdel-Razeq H. Venous thromboembolism prophylaxis for hospitalized medical patients, current status and strategies to improve. Ann Thorac Med. 2010;5:195–200.

58. Samama CM, Afshari A, ESA VTE Guidelines Task Force. European guidelines on perioperative venous thromboembolism prophylaxis. Eur J Anaesthesiol. 2018;35(2):73–6.